Cartilage Injury of the Knee

Aaron J. Krych
Leela C. Biant • Andreas H. Gomoll
João Espregueira-Mendes
Alberto Gobbi • Norimasa Nakamura
Editors

Cartilage Injury of the Knee

State-of-the-Art Treatment and Controversies

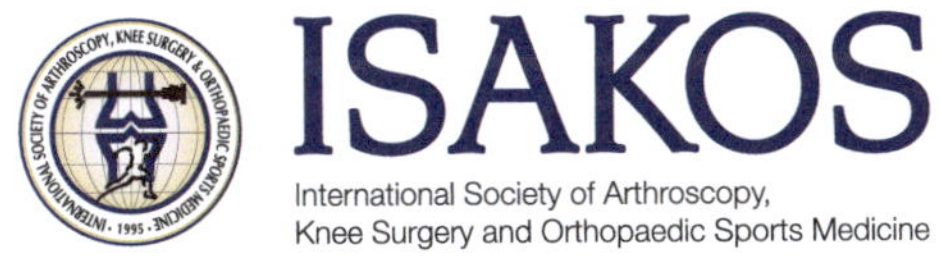

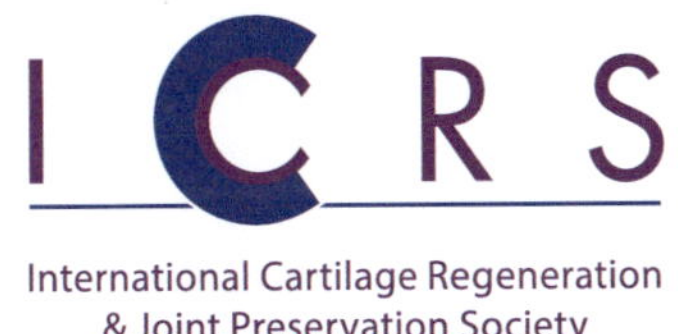

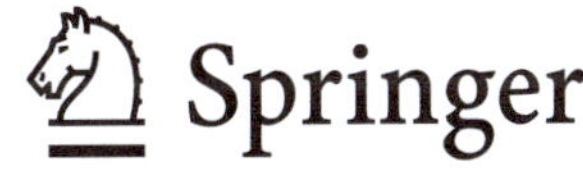

Editors
Aaron J. Krych
Orthopaedic Surgery and Sports
Medicine
Mayo Clinic
Rochester
MN
USA

Andreas H. Gomoll
Orthopedic Sugery
Hospital for Special Surgery
New York
USA

Alberto Gobbi
O.A.S.I. Bioresearch Foundation
Gobbi N.P.O.
Milan
Italy

Leela C. Biant
University of Manchester
Manchester
UK

João Espregueira-Mendes
Clínica Espregueira
FIFA Medical Centre of Excellence
Porto
Portugal

Norimasa Nakamura
Institute for Medical Science in Sports
Osaka Health Science University
Osaka
Japan

ISBN 978-3-030-78053-1   ISBN 978-3-030-78051-7   (eBook)
https://doi.org/10.1007/978-3-030-78051-7

This Springer imprint is published by the registered company Springer Nature Switzerland AG
The registered company address is: Gewerbestrasse 11, 6330 Cham, Switzerland

Preface

On behalf of the International Society of Arthroscopy, Knee Surgery and Orthopaedic Sports Medicine (ISAKOS) and International Cartilage Regeneration and Joint Preservation Society (ICRS), we are proud to introduce this multidisciplinary approach to patients with articular cartilage injuries. This book covers the entire spectrum of nonoperative and surgical management of articular cartilage injury—from diagnosis, imaging, and discussion of both gold standard treatment options and emerging therapies. Likewise, it covers the approach to common associated injuries, such as malalignment, meniscus injury and deficiency, as well as instability of the knee. In addition, comprehensive postoperative rehabilitation is also highlighted.

We are pleased to have an international panel of experts that are leaders in the field of articular cartilage treatment. This is a rapidly evolving field, and this book provides the latest and cutting-edge approaches to common presentations of articular cartilage injury of the knee. In our opinion, no knee cartilage surgeon should be without this important work. Our heartfelt gratitude goes out to the authors and the co-editors for their extraordinary commitment to achieve this comprehensive publication.

Rochester, MN, USA — Aaron J. Krych
Manchester, United Kingdom — Leela C. Biant
New York, NY, USA — Andreas H. Gomoll
Porto, Portugal — João Espregueira-Mendes
Milan, Italy — Alberto Gobbi
Osaka, Japan — Norimasa Nakamura

Contents

Articular Cartilage: Functional Biomechanics

Mário Ferretti, Lauro Augusto Veloso Costa,
and Noel Oizerovici Foni

1.1 Introduction

There are three different types of cartilage in the human body. The articular cartilage (focus of this chapter) is considered a hyaline cartilage, differing to the other types (elastic and fibrous) regarding function, biochemical composition, and biomechanical properties. The articular cartilage is found at the end of the bones and, in young and healthy patients, it has a white and translucent appearance. In the knee, the femoral cartilage has convex surfaces in both anteroposterior and medial-lateral directions, whereas tibial cartilage has concave surface in the medial compartment but it is convex for the anteroposterior direction in the lateral compartment [1–4]. In healthy knees, both the tibial and femoral cartilage appear to experience higher strain on the medial side under load conditions [5–7]. The thickness of the cartilage is variable across the different areas of the knee. The patella cartilage is the thickest, with an average of 4.1 mm, probably due to the high mechanical load to which it is subjected. In the absence of mechanical loading there is a reduction in the cartilage thickness [8]. Unlike other tissues in the body, articular cartilage does not have blood vessels or nerves. Therefore, its nutrition depends on diffusion and this limits the total number of cells. Probably, this further favors its biomechanical properties since there is an indirect relationship between the number of cells and cartilage thickness [9, 10]. Human knee cartilage also undergoes diurnal changes in strain that vary with the site in the joint. During the course of the day where the joint is undergoing the load, articular cartilage experiences significative compressive strain [11].

1.2 The Relationship Between Structure and Biomechanical Properties

The main components of the extracellular matrix (ECM) of the cartilage are collagen (75% of the dry weight), proteoglycans (20–30% of the dry weight), and water, which constitutes from 65% to 80% of the total weight of the cartilage. The mechanical properties of cartilage are conferred by interaction of the cartilage components of the ECM. Articular cartilage has a highly organized structure composed of zones, from the articulating surface to the subchondral bone: articulating surface (lamina splendens), superficial (tangential) zone, middle (transitional) zone, deep (radial) zone, and calcified zone. The proportion of the components varies through age, site in the joint, and depth from the surface (zones) [12, 13]. Because of this, mechanical properties also vary

M. Ferretti (✉) · L. A. V. Costa · N. O. Foni
Hospital Israelita Albert Einstein,
São Paulo, SP, Brazil
e-mail: mario.ferretti@einstein.br, ferretti@einstein.br;
lauro.veloso@einstein.br; noel.foni@einstein.br

© ISAKOS 2021
A. J. Krych et al. (eds.), *Cartilage Injury of the Knee*,
https://doi.org/10.1007/978-3-030-78051-7_1

through the depth [14]. The cellular type present in the cartilage is the chondrocyte. It responds to a mechanical and biochemical stimulus and it is responsible for the constant production of the components of the ECM, making from the cartilage a metabolically active tissue [2, 15]. On a microscope scale, the cartilage also exhibits an organizational structure oriented to distance from the chondrocyte membrane. Each cell is surrounded by a narrow pericellular matrix (PCM), forming units called chondrons. These units in turn are surrounded by the territorial and interterritorial matrices [16]. The composition and organizational structure of the articular cartilage are critical for the proper function of this tissue.

1.2.1 Collagens

Collagens are proteins with tissue-specific localizations. Type II collagen is the predominant collagen type in articular cartilage but cartilage also contains other types of collagens. They account for more than half of the dry weight of the tissue (50–90%) and form fibril fibers intertwined with proteoglycan [17]. The distribution of collagen fibrils in the cartilage is highly inhomogeneous. The fibrillar network is oriented parallel to the surface and gradually becomes essentially perpendicular with depth from the surface [2]. This arrangement provides the ability to resist shear and tension forces [1]. Because collagen fibers have a large ratio length/diameter, they offer little or no resistance to compression [18]. In the middle of the tissue, the organization is more random. The content of the collagen decreases with the depth from the articular surface [1].

Articular cartilage still contains other types of collagen other than collagen type II distributed differently depending on the region of the cartilage, such as type IX, X, XI, VI, XII, and XIV [19]. Although accounting for a small part of the ECM, these collagens not only play essential structural roles in the mechanical properties, organization, and shape of articular cartilage, but can also play an important role in the regulation of chondrocyte mechanotransduction mediated by the mechanical properties of the PCM [20].

1.2.2 Proteoglycans and Glycosaminoglycans

Proteoglycans are the second largest group of macromolecules in the tissue and account for 10–15% of the wet weight. They are comprised of a protein core with many attached glycosaminoglycans [14]. Glycosaminoglycans are unbranched polysaccharide chains composed of repeating disaccharides of amino sugars. Hyaluronic acid, chondroitin sulfate, keratan sulfate, and dermatan sulfate are common glycosaminoglycans present in articular cartilage [21]. The major and most abundant PG in articular cartilage is the aggrecan. These molecules are able to bind to hyaluronic acid and, through a link protein (glycoprotein), they can form large proteoglycan aggregates [22]. The biomechanical function of the hyaluronic acid is to aggregate the proteoglycans and immobilize them in the extracellular material [23]. From a mechanical point of view, the aggrecan molecules form a low-permeability structure when being compressed in the collagen network in order to retain fluid pressure, providing compressive stiffness for cartilage [24].

Glycosaminoglycans are negatively charged and extend out from the protein core, remaining separated from one another because of charge repulsion [25, 26]. Different of the collagen distribution, proteoglycan content is lowest at the superficial zone, increasing by as much as 50% into the middle and deep zones [26]. Together with collagens, proteoglycans are the dominant load-carrying structural components of the solid matrix [14]. As negatively charged, these structures are critical for the functionality of cartilage. They attract ions and water, helping in the maintenance of the mechanical properties and hydration of the ECM, providing resistance to compression.

1.2.3 Chondrocytes

Chondrocytes are specialized cells originated from the mesenchymal stem cells, responsible for synthesizing and maintaining the components of the EMC, accounting for less than 5% of the tissue volume in humans. Chondrocytes contribute little to the mechanical properties of the tissue [9]. The density of the cells is higher in the superficial zone than deeper zones. In addition, the shape and size of the cells also depend on the zone in which they are located, adjusting to the collagen fibril orientation [27]. In the superficial zone, chondrocytes are flatter and aligned parallel to the articular surface. In the middle zone, they are ovoid and randomly distributed inside the zone, and in the deep zone, they are round and aligned perpendicular to the tidemark [9, 18]. The complete process of stimulus of the cells and its interaction with the components of the ECM are not fully understood but it is known that chondrocytes respond to a variety of biochemical and mechanical stimuli that begin by stimulation of mechanoreceptors in the cellular membrane, including ion channels, integrin receptors, and primary cilia [28–30]. The response of chondrocytes depends on the applied load characteristics and the cartilage zone in which they are located [31].

1.2.4 Water

Water accounts for about 75% of the total wet weight of the articular cartilage. As well as the content of the collagen, the water content decreases with depth, from approximately 80% near the joint surface to 65% at the subchondral bone. Inorganic ions, such as sodium, calcium, chloride, and potassium, are dissolved in water [32]. In addition to its important function in the distribution of compressive forces, water acts in the lubrification of the joint and it plays a role in the transport of both nutrients and waste of products within the tissue [33, 34]. The movement of water within the tissue and the frictional resistance to water flow are the main mechanisms through which cartilage resists compressive forces [35]. The fluid flow is greater at the surface of the cartilage than in deep zones. The compaction of the superficial zone can result in compressive strains of up to 50%, while in the deep zones the compressive strain can be less than 5% due to

the impermeability of the subchondral bone and the bulk of the adjacent cartilage [1, 36, 37].

1.2.5 Zones

Articular cartilage is divided into zones, moving from the articulating surface to the subchondral bone. These zones are different with regard to cell morphology, collagen fiber orientation, and composition of water and proteoglycans, and such variation is closely related to the mechanical properties of each zone [38].

The most superficial zone, termed lamina splendens, has been primarily advocated by MacConaill in 1951 [39]. Posteriorly, the existence of this zone was confirmed by other studies [36, 40]. This zone lacks proteoglycan components and cells, and it contains collagen fibrils arranged in parallel [41]. The superficial zone is the largest zone, comprising up to 20% of the tissue. This layer contains flattened and horizontally arranged chondrocytes and the collagen fibrils run parallel to the articular surface. The proteoglycan content and the permeability in this layer are low. Thus, compressive forces redistribute radially across the cartilage [42–45]. On the other hand, the parallel organization of collagen in this zone provides resistance to tensile and shear forces [46]. The middle zone occupies 40–60% of the total tissue [1]. It contains spherical cells, and collagen fibers are oriented in a random way, allowing this zone to resist shear forces [47]. The proteoglycan content is higher than that in the superficial zone, and the water content is lower [44]. The deep zone occupies 20–50% of the tissue. The cells and the collagen fibrils are aligned in vertical columns perpendicular to the joint surface. The collagen fibrils in this zone are the largest in diameter and anchor the cartilage to the subchondral bone, making this zone effective in resisting compressive forces [44, 48]. Finally, the calcified zone is a thin zone between deep zone and subchondral bone that contains collagen type X. This type of collagen constitutes about 1% of total collagen in adult articular cartilage and it is found only in calcified zone. It functions anchoring the cartilage to the bone [19, 49].

1.3 Biomechanical Properties

1.3.1 General Concepts

The term biomechanics refers to the study of the mechanics in biological systems. Due to its eminent mechanical function of minimizing stress on the joint, articular cartilage has been widely studied from a biomechanical point of view.

The articular cartilage benefits from the moderate mechanical stimulation (tension, compression, and shear) for its development and homeostasis. Immobilization of the joint can cause loss of proteoglycans of the cartilage stimulating the degeneration of this tissue, while degeneration can also be caused by excessive joint loads [43, 50]. The proper biochemical composition and structure depend on the load to which articular cartilage is subjected [51]. Another feature that depends on the load is the thickness of the cartilage, with areas subjected to greater load exhibiting greater thickness [52]. Because of this, incongruent joints, such as knee, exhibit greater thickness of cartilage, whereas thin cartilage is found in congruent joints, such as ankle [52]. Besides that, there are differences in the biomechanical properties and load-bearing capabilities among articular surfaces inside the same joint. In the knee, patellar cartilage has a lower compressive aggregate modulus and higher permeability to fluid flow than that of the trochlea [53]. Regarding composition, the water content of the patella is higher by 5% and the proteoglycan content lower by 19% than that of the trochlea [53]. This variation helps to explain why the patellar cartilage has more degenerative changes than trochlea. The force exerted in the hip, knee, and ankle has been calculated in 3.3, 3.5, and 2.5 times body weight [54].

For the proper functioning of the tissue, the cartilage must be able to recover from any deformation induced by the load. The deformation, and the behavior after this deformation, of a material body subjected to mechanical force depends on its intrinsic properties, provided by composition, as well as its extrinsic geometric form [55]. The articular cartilage acts as a body that protects subchondral bone from mechanical

damage by reducing the static contact stress and the dynamic force transmitted to the bone, causing the reduction of the energy transmitted to the bone [56]. The mechanical behavior of cartilage is dependent on its osmotic swelling properties, anionic repulsion of the glycosaminoglycans, and steric and electrostatic interactions between the glycosaminoglycans and the collagen fibrils [57].

1.3.2 Mechanical Behavior of the Articular Cartilage

The cartilage can be described as a viscoelastic tissue since its load response exhibits both elastic and viscous behaviors [23, 57]. Viscosity is a behavior applied to fluids. It can be thought as the resistance of a fluid to the movement. Elasticity in turn is a concept applied for solid materials. It is the behavior of a material body to deform after the application of a load and the ability to return to its original shape when the stress is removed. This viscoelastic behavior of the cartilage can be still better explained by two mechanisms: movement of the fluid within the tissue (fluid phase) and deformation of the solid matrix (solid phase). This theory, which divides the biomechanical behavior of cartilage into two phases, is known as biphasic theory (a phase represents all of the chemical compositions with similar physical properties) [23, 58].

Water is the main component of the fluid phase. The movement of fluid within the tissue is crucial for shock absorption. The interstitial fluid may be transported through the ECM by application of a fluid pressure gradient or also the fluid transport can be achieved by deformation of the cartilage matrix [35]. Although the ECM is porous and permeable, the fluid transport does not occur freely, but it is resisted by frictional drag between the pore walls and the interstitial fluid and by the viscosity itself of the interstitial fluid [55]. The fluid phase also is composed of inorganic ions, such as sodium, calcium, chloride, and potassium. The relationship between proteoglycan aggregates and interstitial fluid provides compressive resilience to cartilage through negative electrostatic repulsion forces. The ion concentration of the tissue is higher than the concentration of the surrounding joint fluid, resulting in increased pressure within the tissue. This concentration difference results in fluid intake into the matrix and this resultant hydrostatic pressure results in cartilage swelling [32, 59]. In order to incorporate the effects of the negatively charged PG aggregates, Lai et al. [32] developed the triphasic theory in 1991. It provides a mathematical model that is capable to predict stress-strain fields in the solid matrix and interstitial fluid flow, along with the ion distribution and fluid pressure [32]. This theory includes both fluid and solid phases (biphasic theory), and an ion phase, which has many ionic species of dissolved electrolytes with positive and negative charges [47]. "Triphasic" models that incorporate the ionic phases of cartilage in addition to the solid and fluid phases suggest that an important role for the PCM and ECM may be to enhance and regulate the conversion of mechanical loading to physicochemical changes that can be sensed by the chondrocytes [16, 32]. By better quantifying the mechano-electrochemical parameters inside tissue, it will be easier to understand the biomechanical behavior of the normal and degenerative articular cartilage.

When subjected to a constant load, the cartilage exhibits a time-dependent and nonlinear behavior. When a stress is applied to the cartilage, the components of ECM move and the tissue deforms (strain). If this stress is removed quickly, the tissue returns to the original shape. However, if the stress continues to be applied through the tissue, water flows out the ECM, and the matrix reorganizes until it reaches a final equilibrium, at which the applied force is balanced by increased swelling pressure. Finally, when the stress is removed, interstitial fluid flows back into the cartilage and the original preloaded equilibrium is reestablished [56]. This recovery phase is slower than the creep deformation phase [60]. In this case of a constant load, the relation between stress and strain is not constant (dependent on the magnitude of strain) and the strain does not vanish instantaneously when the stress is removed (nonlinear behavior).

1.3.3 Behavior in Compression, Tension, and Shear

As a result of a load applied in the cartilage, a combination of compressive, tensile, and shear stresses is generated and distributed across the tissue. Due to the structure and composition of the cartilage, its response to these stresses is different [1, 61]. The response of the cartilage to the compression stress is mainly by the movement of the fluid within the tissue. Therefore, it is in response to the compression force that the viscoelastic property of cartilage becomes most important [23, 57]. The low permeability of the healthy tissue creates a high interstitial fluid pressure during compression, and this fact is responsible for the dissipation of this force [23]. As perceived, the content of the water within the cartilage is critical to the tissue biomechanics during compressive forces. Keeping the water into the tissue and therefore resisting the compressive forces is fundamentally a function of the interaction between proteoglycans and fibril collagen network. The large number of glycosaminoglycans negatively charged in the tissue attracts mobile cations generating an increase of the osmolarity. Thereby, a large amount of water is attracted to the tissue, causing it to swell [14, 62]. When a compressive force hits the cartilage, water flows in and out of the tissue, gradually transferring the importance of supporting the load to the solid matrix. Upon removal of the external load, the solid matrix recovers its initial dimension and water flows back into the cartilage, reestablishing the original equilibrium [56].

Fluid flow is essential for resisting the compressive stress and, on the other hand, the ECM is essential for resisting tensile and shear strains. The shear and tension force-resisting properties are fundamentally dependent on the amount, orientation, and molecular arrangement of the collagen fibers as well as its interaction with proteoglycans in the solid matrix [63, 64]. The tensile stiffness of the articular cartilage is higher than the compressive stiffness in equilibrium condition, and the tissue exhibits a tension-compression nonlinear mechanical behavior [65]. Shear stress is a force applied along the horizontal plane between the surfaces while the tension results in axial strain. For small deformations, collagen fibers realign in the direction of loading. With increasing deforming strength, collagen fibers will also be stretched [63, 66–68]. Under these conditions, the cartilage exhibits a flow-independent behavior. The tissue deforms with no significant fluid flow inside the matrix [1, 57, 69]. There is a relationship between the tensile stiffness and the depth of the cartilage. The tensile strength tends to decrease with depth below the surface. Collagen fibers in the superficial zone are oriented parallel to the surface, which makes this layer the most important to resist these forces [56].

Cartilage loading also occurs at a cellular level. Mechanical loading of articular cartilage, such as compressive loading, shear stress, and tension, stimulates the metabolism of chondrocytes and induces the synthesis of molecules in order to maintain the integrity of the tissue. This process by which physical forces are converted into biochemical signals is called mechanotransduction [8]. Mechanotransduction induces changes in gene expression, ECM remodeling, and proliferation [70]. Loading of articular cartilage involves force transmission through the interterritorial, territorial, and PCM before reaching the chondrocytes. These regions likely assist in modulating strains seen at the cellular level [71]. The PCM plays an important role in modulating the mechanical environment of the chondrocyte, serving as a transducer of both biomechanical and biochemical signals for the chondrocyte, and providing a uniform strain environment for the chondrocytes despite large zonal variations in ECM strain during loading [16, 71]. Thus, the PCM protects the chondrocyte in regions of high local strain such as the superficial zone, but amplifies lower magnitudes of local strain in the middle and deep zone [71]. Type VI collagen, which preferentially localizes to the PCM, is one of the structures that plays this role. It anchors the chondrocyte to the ECM, mediates cell-matrix interaction, and acts as a transducer for biomechanical signals [16, 19, 20]. Chondrocyte mechanoreceptors such as ion channels and integrins are also involved in the recognition of these signals and propagate them through cytoskeletal components that in turn extend from the cell surface to the PCM [28, 72–74]. The cytoskeletal structure not only acts in mechanotransduction but also plays a role in providing the chondrocyte with mechanical integrity to withstand compressive forces [75].

In summary, the integrity of the articular cartilage is dependent on the correct mechanical loading so that abnormal loads affect the matrix properties of the tissue at a cellular level [76]. It is known that underloading, static load, or excessive dynamic loading is associated with proteoglycan depletion and inhibition of matrix synthesis leading to joint degeneration [77, 78]. The chondrocytes from osteoarthritic cartilage differ in cellular responses to mechanical stimulation when compared with cells from normal joint cartilage [8]. The exact pattern of mechanical load to maintain tissue homeostasis is still unknown.

References

1. Athanasiou K, Darling E, Hu J, et al. Articular cartilage. 2nd ed. Boca Raton, FL: CRC Press/Taylor & Francis Group; 2016.
2. Muir H. The chondrocyte, architect of cartilage. Biomechanics, structure, function and molecular biology of cartilage matrix macromolecules. BioEssays. 1995;17:1039–48. https://doi.org/10.1002/bies.950171208.
3. Andriacchi TP, Mündermann A, Smith RL, et al. A framework for the in vivo pathomechanics of osteoarthritis at the knee. Ann Biomed Eng. 2004;32:447–57. https://doi.org/10.1023/B:ABME.0000017541.82498.37.
4. Koo S, Andriacchi TP. A comparison of the influence of global functional loads vs. local contact anatomy on articular cartilage thickness at the knee. J Biomech. 2007;40:2961–6. https://doi.org/10.1016/j.jbiomech.2007.02.005.
5. Liu F, Kozanek M, Hosseini A, et al. In vivo tibiofemoral cartilage deformation during the stance phase of gait. J Biomech. 2010;43:658–65. https://doi.org/10.1016/j.jbiomech.2009.10.028.
6. Bingham JT, Papannagari R, Van de Velde SK, et al. In vivo cartilage contact deformation in the healthy human tibiofemoral joint. Rheumatology. 2008;47:1622–7. https://doi.org/10.1093/rheumatology/ken345.

7. Sutter EG, Widmyer MR, Utturkar GM, et al. In vivo measurement of localized tibiofemoral cartilage strains in response to dynamic activity. Am J Sports Med. 2015;43:370–6. https://doi.org/10.1177/0363546514559821.

8. Ramage L, Nuki G, Salter DM. Signalling cascades in mechanotransduction: cell-matrix interactions and mechanical loading. Scand J Med Sci Sport. 2009;19:457–69. https://doi.org/10.1111/j.1600-0838.2009.00912.x.

9. Stockwell R. Biology of cartilage cells. Cambridge: Cambridge University Press; 1979.

10. Ulrich-Vinther M, Maloney MD, Schwarz EM, et al. Articular cartilage biology. J Am Acad Orthop Surg. 2003;11:421–30. https://doi.org/10.5435/00124635-200311000-00006.

11. Coleman JL, Widmyer MR, Leddy HA, et al. Diurnal variations in articular cartilage thickness and strain in the human knee. J Biomech. 2013;46:541–7. https://doi.org/10.1016/j.jbiomech.2012.09.013.

12. Lipshitz H, Etheridge R, Glimcher M. In vitro wear of articular cartilage. J Bone Jointt Surg. 1975;57A:527–37.

13. McDevitt C, Muir H. Biochemical changes in the cartilage of the knee in experimental and natural osteoarthritis in the dog. J Bone Jointt Surg. 1976;58B:94–101.

14. Mow VC, Guo XE. Mechano-electrochemical properties of articular cartilage: their inhomogeneities and anisotropies. Annu Rev Biomed Eng. 2002;4:175–209. https://doi.org/10.1146/annurev.bioeng.4.110701.120309.

15. Robin Poole A, Matsui Y, Hinek A, Lee ER. Cartilage macromolecules and the calcification of cartilage matrix. Anat Rec. 1989;224:167–79. https://doi.org/10.1002/ar.1092240207.

16. Wilusz RE, Sanchez-Adams J, Guilak F. The structure and function of the pericellular matrix of articular cartilage. Matrix Biol. 2014;39:25–32. https://doi.org/10.1016/j.matbio.2014.08.009.

17. Deshmukh K, Nimni ME. Isolation and characterization of cyanogen bromide peptides from the collagen of bovine articular cartilage. Biochem J. 1973;133:615–22. https://doi.org/10.1042/bj1330615.

18. Callaghan JJ. The adult knee. Philadelphia, PA: Lippincott Williams & Wilkins; 2003.

19. Luo Y, Sinkeviciute D, He Y, et al. The minor collagens in articular cartilage. Protein Cell. 2017;8:560–72. https://doi.org/10.1007/s13238-017-0377-7.

20. Zelenski NA, Leddy HA, Sanchez-Adams J, et al. Type VI collagen regulates pericellular matrix properties, chondrocyte swelling, and mechanotransduction in mouse articular cartilage. Arthritis Rheumatol. 2015;67:1286–94. https://doi.org/10.1002/art.39034.

21. Roughley P. The structure and function of cartilage proteoglycans. Eur Cells Mater. 2006;12:92–101. https://doi.org/10.22203/eCM.v012a11.

22. Hardingham TE, Fosang AJ, Dudhia J. The structure, function and turnover of aggrecan, the large aggregating proteoglycan from cartilage. Eur J Clin Chem Clin Biochem. 1994;32:249–57.

23. Mow VC, Lai WM. Recent developments in synovial joint biomechanics. SIAM Rev. 1980;22:275–317. https://doi.org/10.1137/1022056.

24. Klika V, Gaffney EA, Chen YC, Brown CP. An overview of multiphase cartilage mechanical modelling and its role in understanding function and pathology. J Mech Behav Biomed Mater. 2016;62:139–57. https://doi.org/10.1016/j.jmbbm.2016.04.032.

25. Sophia Fox AJ, Bedi A, Rodeo SA. The basic science of articular cartilage: structure, composition, and function. Sports Health. 2009;1:461–8. https://doi.org/10.1177/1941738109350438.

26. Carballo CB, Nakagawa Y, Sekiya I, Rodeo SA. Basic science of articular cartilage. Clin Sports Med. 2017;36:413–25. https://doi.org/10.1016/j.csm.2017.02.001.

27. Korhonen RK, Julkunen P, Wilson W, Herzog W. Importance of collagen orientation and depth-dependent fixed charge densities of cartilage on mechanical behavior of chondrocytes. J Biomech Eng. 2008;130 https://doi.org/10.1115/1.2898725.

28. Gilbert SJ, Blain EJ. Cartilage mechanobiology: how chondrocytes respond to mechanical load. In: Mechanobiology in health and disease. London: Elsevier; 2018. p. 99–126.

29. Lv M, Zhou Y, Chen X, et al. Calcium signaling of in situ chondrocytes in articular cartilage under compressive loading: roles of calcium sources and cell membrane ion channels. J Orthop Res. 2018;36:730–8. https://doi.org/10.1002/jor.23768.

30. Vaca-González JJ, Guevara JM, Moncayo MA, et al. Biophysical stimuli: a review of electrical and mechanical stimulation in hyaline cartilage. Cartilage. 2019;10:157–72. https://doi.org/10.1177/1947603517730637.

31. Liu H-Y, Duan H-T, Zhang C-Q, Wang W. Study of the mechanical environment of chondrocytes in articular cartilage defects repaired area under cyclic compressive loading. J Healthc Eng. 2017;2017:1–10. https://doi.org/10.1155/2017/1308945.

32. Lai WM, Hou JS, Mow VC. A triphasic theory for the swelling and deformation behaviors of articular cartilage. J Biomech Eng. 1991;113:245–58. https://doi.org/10.1115/1.2894880.

33. Mow VC, Ateshian GA, Spilker RL. Biomechanics of diarthrodial joints: a review of twenty years of progress. J Biomech Eng. 1993;115:460–7. https://doi.org/10.1115/1.2895525.

34. O'Hara BP, Urban JP, Maroudas A. Influence of cyclic loading on the nutrition of articular cartilage. Ann Rheum Dis. 1990;49:536–9. https://doi.org/10.1136/ard.49.7.536.

35. Torzilli PA, Mow VC. On the fundamental fluid transport mechanisms through normal and pathological articular cartilage during function—II. The analysis, solution and conclusions. J Biomech. 1976;9:587–606. https://doi.org/10.1016/0021-9290(76)90100-7.

36. Teeple E, Fleming BC, Mechrefe AP, et al. Frictional properties of Hartley guinea pig knees with and without proteolytic disruption of the articular surfaces.

Osteoarthr Cartil. 2007;15:309–15. https://doi.org/10.1016/j.joca.2006.08.011.

37. Eckstein F, Tieschky M, Faber S, et al. Functional analysis of articular cartilage deformation, recovery, and fluid flow following dynamic exercise in vivo. Anat Embryol (Berl). 1999;200:419–24. https://doi.org/10.1007/s004290050291.

38. Meng Q, An S, Damion RA, et al. The effect of collagen fibril orientation on the biphasic mechanics of articular cartilage. J Mech Behav Biomed Mater. 2017;65:439–53. https://doi.org/10.1016/j.jmbbm.2016.09.001.

39. MacConaill M. The movements of bones and joints; the mechanical structure of articulating cartilage. J Bone Joint Surg. 1951;33:251–7.

40. Aspden R, Hukins D. The lamina splendens of articular cartilage is an artefact of phase contrast microscopy. Proc R Soc London Ser B Biol Sci. 1979;206:109–13. https://doi.org/10.1098/rspb.1979.0094.

41. Fujioka R, Aoyama T, Takakuwa T. The layered structure of the articular surface. Osteoarthr Cartil. 2013;21:1092–8, https://doi.org/10.1016/j.joca.2013.04.021.

42. Setton LA, Zhu W, Mow VC. The biphasic poroviscoelastic behavior of articular cartilage: role of the surface zone in governing the compressive behavior. J Biomech. 1993;26:581–92. https://doi.org/10.1016/0021-9290(93)90019-B.

43. Buckwalter J, Anderson D, Brown T, et al. The roles of mechanical stresses in the pathogenesis of osteoarthritis: implications for treatment of joint injuries. Cartilage. 2013;4(4):286–94.

44. Wong M, Carter D. Articular cartilage functional histomorphology and mechanobiology: a research perspective. Bone. 2003;33:1–13. https://doi.org/10.1016/S8756-3282(03)00083-8.

45. Sakai N, Hashimoto C, Yarimitsu S, et al. A functional effect of the superficial mechanical properties of articular cartilage as a load bearing system in a sliding condition. Biosurface Biotribol. 2016;2:26–39. https://doi.org/10.1016/j.bsbt.2016.02.004.

46. Nugent GE, Aneloski NM, Schmidt TA, et al. Dynamic shear stimulation of bovine cartilage biosynthesis of proteoglycan 4. Arthritis Rheum. 2006;54:1888–96. https://doi.org/10.1002/art.21831.

47. Lu XL, Mow VC. Biomechanics of articular cartilage and determination of material properties. Med Sci Sports Exerc. 2008;40:193–9. https://doi.org/10.1249/mss.0b013e31815cb1fc.

48. Muir H, Bullough P, Maroudas A. The distribution of collagen in human articular cartilage with some of its physiological implications. J Bone Joint Surg Br. 1970;52-B:554–63. https://doi.org/10.1302/0301-620X.52B3.554.

49. Eyre D, Weis M, Wu J-J. Articular cartilage collagen: an irreplaceable framework? Eur Cells Mater. 2006;12:57–63. https://doi.org/10.22203/eCM.v012a07.

50. Haapala J, Arokoski J, Hyttinen M, et al. Remobilization does not fully restore immobilization induced articular cartilage atrophy. Clin Orthop Relat Res. 1999;362:218–29.

51. Brama PAJ, Tekoppele JMJ, Bank RA, et al. Functional adaptation of equine articular cartilage: the formation of regional biochemical characteristics up to age one year. Equine Vet J. 2010;32:217–21. https://doi.org/10.2746/042516400776563626.

52. Shepherd DET, Seedhom BB. Thickness of human articular cartilage in joints of the lower limb. Ann Rheum Dis. 1999;58:27–34. https://doi.org/10.1136/ard.58.1.27.

53. Froimson MI, Ratcliffe A, Gardner TR, Mow VC. Differences in patellofemoral joint cartilage material properties and their significance to the etiology of cartilage surface fibrillation. Osteoarthr Cartil. 1997;5:377–86. https://doi.org/10.1016/S1063-4584(97)80042-8.

54. Whitesides TE. Orthopaedic basic science. Biology and biomechanics of the musculoskeletal system. 2nd ed. J Bone Jointt Surg Am. 2001;83:482. https://doi.org/10.2106/00004623-200103000-00040.

55. Hall BK. Cartilage: structure, function, and biochemistry. New York: Academic Press, Inc.; 1983.

56. Kempson GE. The mechanical properties of articular cartilage. In: The joints and synovial fluid. New York: Elsevier; 1980. p. 177–238.

57. Hayes WC, Mockros LF. Viscoelastic properties of human articular cartilage. J Appl Physiol. 1971;31:562–8. https://doi.org/10.1152/jappl.1971.31.4.562.

58. Mow VC, Kuei SC, Lai WM, Armstrong CG. Biphasic creep and stress relaxation of articular cartilage in compression: theory and experiments. J Biomech Eng. 1980;102:73–84. https://doi.org/10.1115/1.3138202.

59. Urban J, Hall A, Gehl K. Regulation of matrix synthesis rates by the ionic and osmotic environment of articular chondrocytes. J Cell Physiol. 1993;154:262–70.

60. Hirsch C. The pathogenesis of chondromalacia of the patella. A physical, histologic and chemical study. Acta Chir Sand. 1944;83(1):1–06.

61. Salinas EY, Hu JC, Athanasiou K. A guide for using mechanical stimulation to enhance tissue-engineered articular cartilage properties. Tissue Eng Part B Rev. 2018;24:345–58. https://doi.org/10.1089/ten.teb.2018.0006.

62. Soltz MA, Ateshian GA. Experimental verification and theoretical prediction of cartilage interstitial fluid pressurization at an impermeable contact interface in confined compression. J Biomech. 1998;31:927–34. https://doi.org/10.1016/S0021-9290(98)00105-5.

63. Kempson GE, Muir H, Pollard C, Tuke M. The tensile properties of the cartilage of human femoral condyles related to the content of collagen and glycosaminoglycans. BBA Gen Subj. 1973;297:456–72. https://doi.org/10.1016/0304-4165(73)90093-7.

64. Akizuki S, Mow VC, Müller F, et al. Tensile properties of human knee joint cartilage: I. influence of ionic conditions, weight bearing, and fibrillation on the tensile modulus. J Orthop Res. 1986;4:379–92. https://doi.org/10.1002/jor.1100040401.

65. Huang C-Y, Soltz MA, Kopacz M, et al. Experimental verification of the roles of intrinsic matrix viscoelasticity and tension-compression nonlinearity in the biphasic response of cartilage. J Biomech Eng. 2003;125:84–93. https://doi.org/10.1115/1.1531656.

66. Woo SL-Y, Lubock P, Gomez MA, et al. Large deformation nonhomogeneous and directional properties of articular cartilage in uniaxial tension. J Biomech. 1979;12:437–46. https://doi.org/10.1016/0021-9290(79)90028-9.

67. Roth V, Mow VC. The intrinsic tensile behavior of the matrix of bovine articular cartilage and its variation with age. J Bone Joint Surg Am. 1980;62:1102–17.

68. Kempson GE, Freeman MAR, Swanson SAV. Tensile properties of articular cartilage. Nature. 1968;220:1127–8. https://doi.org/10.1038/2201127b0.

69. Hayes WC, Bodine AJ. Flow-independent viscoelastic properties of articular cartilage matrix. J Biomech. 1978;11:407–19. https://doi.org/10.1016/0021-9290(78)90075-1.

70. Jaalouk DE, Lammerding J. Mechanotransduction gone awry. Nat Rev Mol Cell Biol. 2009;10:63–73. https://doi.org/10.1038/nrm2597.

71. Choi JB, Youn I, Cao L, et al. Zonal changes in the three-dimensional morphology of the chondron under compression: the relationship among cellular, peri-cellular, and extracellular deformation in articular cartilage. J Biomech. 2007;40:2596–603. https://doi.org/10.1016/j.jbiomech.2007.01.009.

72. Martinac B. Mechanosensitive ion channels: molecules of mechanotransduction. J Cell Sci. 2004;117:2449–60. https://doi.org/10.1242/jcs.01232.

73. Ingber D. Integrins as mechanochemical transducers. Curr Opin Cell Biol. 1991;3:841–8. https://doi.org/10.1016/0955-0674(91)90058-7.

74. Driscoll TP, Cosgrove BD, Heo S-J, et al. Cytoskeletal to nuclear strain transfer regulates YAP signaling in mesenchymal stem cells. Biophys J. 2015;108:2783–93. https://doi.org/10.1016/j.bpj.2015.05.010.

75. Guilak F. Compression-induced changes in the shape and volume of the chondrocyte nucleus. J Biomech. 1995;28:1529–41. https://doi.org/10.1016/0021-9290(95)00100-X.

76. Buckwalter JA, Martin JA, Brown TD. Perspectives on chondrocyte mechanobiology and osteoarthritis. Biorheology. 2006;43:603–9.

77. Buckwalter JA, Mankin HJ. Articular cartilage: degeneration and osteoarthritis, repair, regeneration, and transplantation. Instr Course Lect. 1998;47:487–504.

78. Parkkinen JJ, Lammi MJ, Helminen HJ, Tammi M. Local stimulation of proteoglycan synthesis in articular cartilage explants by dynamic compression in vitro. J Orthop Res. 1992;10:610–20. https://doi.org/10.1002/jor.1100100503.

Laura Ann Lambert, James Convill,
Gwenllian Tawy, and Leela C. Biant

2.1 Introduction

Isolated chondral defects are associated with the onset and development of osteoarthritis (OA) [1]. The traumatic insult of the cartilage may initiate a cascade of events within the joint milieu, ultimately resulting in the degeneration of a joint [2].

Early diagnostic and discreet classification of chondral defects and OA are difficult due to the microscopic and macroscopic heterogeneity of both interrelated conditions. Diagnostic criteria must be sufficiently broad to incorporate all phenotypes, but accurate enough to discern an isolated injury from a healthy joint.

Biomarkers are 'characteristics that can be objectively measured and evaluated as indicators of normal biologic processes, pathogenic processes, or pharmacologic responses to a therapeutic intervention' [3]. We would also add, in this context, that effective biomarkers of chondral disruption and early osteoarthritis (eOA) should also be an indicator of response to surgical intervention. Current diagnoses of cartilage damage and eOA rely on radiological biomarkers. However, measurable molecular biomarkers present in human tissues could provide novel and objective methods for diagnosing and monitoring treatment effects. They may also pave the way for new therapeutic approaches in regenerative medicine.

Biomarkers in urine, blood and synovial fluid are the commonest targets for biomarker discovery, because of the ease of repeated sampling. Systemic biomarkers, such as blood and urine, effectively sample the whole body, making disease localisation difficult. Local biomarkers from synovial fluid have the advantage of being more specific and potentially higher in concentration, but the disadvantage of being more difficult to obtain in early disease.

In 2006, Bauer et al. classified biomarkers of OA to guide future research and clinical trials [4]. The BIPEDS method refers to six dimensions which each influences a biomarker's candidacy: B—burden of disease, I—investigative, P—prognostic, E—efficacy of intervention, D—diagnostic and S—safety. This method enables interpretation of the value a molecule may have as a clinical biomarker. The performance of a biomarker within each of the BIPEDS categories is commonly measured through sensitivity and specificity. Sensitivity is the capacity to detect a

L. A. Lambert · J. Convill · G. Tawy
University of Manchester, Manchester, UK
e-mail: lauraann.lambert@postgrad.manchester.ac.uk;
james.convill@student.manchester.ac.uk;
gwenllian.tawy@manchester.ac.uk

L. C. Biant (✉)
University of Manchester, Manchester, UK

Manchester University Foundation Trust,
Manchester, UK

Manchester Academic Health Science Centre,
Manchester, UK
e-mail: leela.biant@manchester.ac.uk

© ISAKOS 2021
A. J. Krych et al. (eds.), *Cartilage Injury of the Knee*,
https://doi.org/10.1007/978-3-030-78051-7_2

disease in individuals in whom the disease is truly present (true positive) and specificity is the capacity to rule out the disease in patients in whom the disease is truly absent (true negative). Positive predictive value (PPV) is a measure of a test's probability, when returning a positive result, to correctly identify, from a cohort where the condition may be present or absent, all those who do truly have a disease. Equally, negative predictive value (NPV) is the probability, when returning a negative result, to correctly identify, where the outcome may be binary, all of those who truly do not have a disease. It is important to note that PPV and NPV depend on the prevalence and the severity of the disease concerned [5]. Biomarker studies often evaluate their results using receiver operator characteristic (ROC) analysis. The goal is to demonstrate that there is a robust statistical association between the variable and the event when outcomes are binary. ROC analysis produces a curve of sensitivity against specificity at varying thresholds for the predicted risk. The area under the curve (AUC) indicates the probability that an individual with the event has a higher predicted probability than an individual without the event. An AUC of 0.5 is reflective of chance probability, whilst a statistic of 0.7 or above is accepted to be sufficiently discriminatory [6].

2.2 Biomarkers in Cartilage Damage

Recent research on chondral damage has focused on identifying and validating biomarkers that define general cartilage quality and cartilage injury or assess the efficacy of therapies in cartilage surgery. Although post-traumatic defects and osteochondritis dissecans are recognised causes, the exact aetiology of isolated cartilage defects in human articular cartilage is yet to be fully established [7]. This chondral damage is believed to impact the local metabolism within the joint, triggering a cascade of inflammatory mediators from adult chondrocytes and other sources. An imbalance in catabolic and anabolic activity may result in uncontrolled matrix degeneration in response to mechanical forces [8, 9].

2.3 Radiological Biomarkers in Cartilage Damage and Repair

Chondral defects are routinely diagnosed through a clinical history, physical examination and assessment of radiological features of the joint. Although weight-bearing plain radiographs are effective at demonstrating the reduction in joint space associated with established OA and other issues of bone and alignment, they cannot be used to detect earlier pathophysiological changes of a knee joint.

Cartilage imaging by magnetic resonance imaging (MRI) enables visualisation of the thickness and volume of the tissue and its subchondral borders [10]. The accuracy of cartilage imaging by MRI was once impeded by ill-defined margins with partially attached fragments and underestimation of deep fissures [11]. However, following the development of newer modalities and more powerful field strengths, only the smallest and most superficial defects are now not appreciable [7].

In 2003, the International Cartilage Repair Society (ICRS) published a standardised magnetic resonance imaging evaluation system for native and repaired articular cartilage [11]. The Magnetic Resonance Observation of Cartilage Repair Tissue (MOCART) Knee Score was published 1 year later [10, 12]. This scoring system utilises MRI biomarkers for a quantitative assessment of cartilage tissue following repair surgery for chondral defects [10, 12]. High-resolution images can be obtained from 1.0 T or 1.5 T MRI scanners by using a surface coil over the knee and employing fast-spin echo [12]. From these images, nine variables are used to grade cartilage quality (Table 2.1).

Improvements in MRI and cartilage surgery led to the score being updated (MOCART 2.0 Knee Score, 2019) [13]. The scoring system is now more sensitive, with subdivisions of the variables in 25% increments rather than 50% increments (Table 2.1) [13]. Currently MOCART scoring is operator dependent; however, with machine learning and evolving AI, automation in routine practice should be possible.

Table 2.1 The variables assessed by MOCART to grade cartilage quality [12]

Variable	Original MOCART	MOCART 2.0
1	Degree of defect repair and filling of the defect	Volume fill of cartilage defect
2	Integration of repair to border zone	Integration of repair into adjacent cartilage
3	Intactness of surface of the repair tissue	Intactness of surface of the repair tissue
4	Structure of the repair tissue	Structure of the repair tissue
5	Signal intensity of the repair tissue	Signal intensity of the repair tissue
6	Intactness of subchondral lamina	Bony defect or bony overgrowth
7	Intactness of subchondral bone	Subchondral changes
8	Presence of adhesions	–
9	Presence of synovitis	–

Certain MRI techniques can already be used in a semi-quantitative manner to measure the quality of cartilage. T2-weighted imaging produces the relaxation constant that provides information on the interaction of water and collagen molecules within cartilage. Compared to standard T2-weighted imaging, T2* techniques are able to yield 3D acquisitions with high spatial resolution of cartilage [14]. Mamisch examined knee cartilage with 3.0 T MRI after microfracture and found that global T2 and T2* values for cartilage repair tissue were significantly reduced compared to healthy cartilage sites in the patient group (T2: 47.1 ± 9.8 ms (29–73 ms); T2*: 19.1 ± 5.9 (9–31 ms)) [14]. Additionally, the relative decrease in T2* values (21% compared to 15% with T2) between healthy and repair tissue indicates its sensitivity to structural changes within the cartilage [14].

Quantifying the amount of glycosaminoglycan (GAG) within the articular cartilage using dGEMRIC (delayed gadolinium-enhanced MRI of cartilage) is another semi-quantitative method of evaluating articular cartilage. The dGEMRIC index gives a numeric value on a scale from around 300 to 700 ms [7]. This technique correlates well with arthroscopic evaluation of cartilage, and shows that beyond the lesion the adjacent cartilage

is normal [15, 16]. Vasiliadis demonstrated that the quality of cartilage repair with autologous chondrocyte implantation (ACI), 9–18 years after injury, was identical to normal adjacent cartilage using this evaluation technique [17].

A low dGEMRIC score is thought to correspond with a greater risk of developing OA [18]. However, longitudinal studies do not consistently support this. Engen did not detect a statistically significant difference in dGEMRIC indices for untreated focal cartilage defects between injured and uninjured knees at 12 years of follow-up [7]. dGEMRIC evaluation also does not consistently correlate with Kellgren and Lawrence (K-L) scoring or clinical outcomes [7, 17, 19].

Novel research is already indicating that 7 T MRI scanners may offer even greater improvements in obtaining radiological biomarkers of osteoarthritis [20, 21].

2.4 Systemic and Local Biomarkers of Cartilage Damage

Biomarkers reflecting cartilage turnover are found in human serum and urine [22, 23]. These could provide information about dynamic and quantitative changes in joint remodelling. Type II collagen is the most abundant protein of cartilage matrix; thus its synthesis and degradation can be monitored through the assessment of N and C propeptides and collagenous and non-collagenous proteins, respectively [24]. These markers have been evaluated mainly in known early or established OA [25, 26]. The assessment of biomarkers in vivo for those with a suspected acute or isolated cartilage injury is limited [27–30].

2.4.1 Collagen Biomarkers in Urine

C2C-HUSA (neoepitope of type II collagen human urine sandwich assay) is a cartilage-derived protein found to be elevated in early cartilage degradation, specifically pre-radiographic changes [28, 31, 32]. This is similar to cross-linked C-telopeptide of type II collagen (CTX-II), another biomarker of collagen turnover found in urine that reflects collagen degradation. It is found when there is increased turnover of cartilage secondary to increased mechanical loading [28, 33]. Boeth compared these biomarkers across an adult and adolescent cohort over a 2-year period. Regardless of the growth plate status, C2C-HUSA and CTX-II increased in the adolescent group overall.

2.4.2 Collagen Degradation Biomarkers in Serum

Serum cartilage oligomeric matrix protein (COMP) has been used as a biomarker in short-term studies of athletes. These studies show that COMP is increased following short-term high-impact activity [34, 35]. COMP is also increased following partial meniscectomy in young adults between 3 and 6 months post-operatively [27]. However, these observations are not seen with long-term follow-up [36]; COMP may only be transiently elevated in response to acute loading and to date has not yet clearly demonstrated an association with cartilage degradation [37].

Serum cartilage intermediate-layer protein 2 (CILP-2) may be reflective of long-term cartilage remodelling. In a comparison of an adult cohort over 40 years to a young healthy adolescent group, there was no increase from baseline to follow-up of CILP amongst adolescents. However, CILP is elevated over time in the adults, suggesting that the age of the cartilage influences the production of this biomarker. This is a linear increase with respect to cartilage volume as assessed by MRI [36, 38].

Serum type II collagen cleavage neoepitope (sC2C) is increased in OA [31]. Analysis of sC2C levels in those with an ACL injury compared to healthy controls shows a statistically significant difference in concentration over time [22]. In this cohort, baseline sC2C levels (average 22 months from injury) compared to follow-up (average time at 44 months from injury) serum concentrations significantly differed from the uninjured group. The temporal change in this molecular biomarker concentration indicates that the injury has disturbed the normal joint metabolism.

2.4.3 Collagen Synthesis Biomarkers in Serum

Procollagen molecule levels of type II collagen C-propeptide (PIICP) have been shown to be a valid index in the rate of type II collagen synthesis [39]. In patients with a recent history of meniscal injury, a significant decrease of PIICP was found between 3 and 6 months post-operatively in all patients compared to baseline levels [27]. Of all biomarkers used in this study, it had the highest diagnostic accuracy for *progressive* cartilage loss, AUC 0.75 (95% CI: 0.509–0.912).

However, singular serum biomarkers are unlikely to yield the most informative results and using the ratio of biomarkers in combination with each other may yield more accurate detection and degree of cartilage damage. In the aforementioned study of meniscal injury, multivariate logistic regression showed significant associations of *increased* COMP and type II collagen (COL II) and *decreased* PIICP with the presence of cartilage volume loss >10%, independent of age and duration after injury [27]. The combined impact of increased COMP and COL II and decreased PIICP exceeded the impact of each independent biomarker. However, none of the individual or combined biomarkers were a statistically significant predictor of future cartilage loss [27].

2.4.4 Local Biomarkers of Cartilage Damage

Local biomarkers produced in response to an acute insult are more likely to be elevated due to their proximity to the joint. Multiple studies have compared the elevation of sera and synovial biomarkers, and whilst often there is a positive correlation between the two, there is greater magnitude of increase in the latter group in response to an acute injury [29, 40].

Of all local biomarker sources, synovial fluid taken during arthroscopy or aspiration is less destructive than removal of local tissue such as synovium, bone or cartilage biopsy. In the early

1990s, Lohmander produced a series of papers on the presence of molecular markers such as aggrecan, proteoglycans and matrix metalloproteinases within synovial fluid in OA or joint injury [41–43]. More recently, Kumahashi demonstrated elevated levels of C2C in the synovial fluid of 235 patients 0–7 days after an acute knee injury, and a statistically significant positive correlation between synovial fluid and serum C2C concentrations, $r = 0.403$, $p < 0.001$. In accordance with the findings of Cibere [31], urinary concentrations of C2C did not show any relationship with MRI findings [29]. Yoshida also demonstrated that high levels of synovial C2C corresponded with an increased number of high-grade cartilage lesions at arthroscopy. They evaluated the samples for the presence of keratin sulphate (KS) and found that low-quartile KS levels in combination with high (upper quartile) C2C levels had the greatest impact on the number of high-grade cartilage lesions (odds ratio of 14.40 (95% CI = 1.35–153.0)) [30]. Again, reiterating a consistent theme throughout the literature, the right combination of biomarkers, may garner the most meaningful information on the extent of cartilage damage.

2.5 Biomarkers in Cartilage Repair

Biomarkers of cartilage repair therapies predominantly exist within the literature in the form of molecular markers, cell surface markers indicating the presence of chondrogenic cells, and chondrogenic gene markers.

2.5.1 Immunohistochemistry

Tissue biopsy enables microscopic and immunohistochemical evaluation of the section. It is regarded as the most objective and definitive method for the direct quality assessment of the repair tissue. As proof of concept in vitro or for assessment of cartilage explants seeded onto a scaffold, immunostaining for glycosaminoglycans, collagen and aggrecan is commonly undertaken. However, tissue biopsies cannot be obtained without harm to the cartilage itself, and therefore are not suitable as a biomarker for repeated sampling in clinical practice.

2.5.2 Cell Morphology

When cells are harvested for ACI they may lose differentiation capacity due to changes in shape and senescence [44]. One use of biomarkers is to monitor the potency of these cells during the ex vivo ACI process as a means of quality control prior to the later stage of the procedure. Diaz-Romero acquired cryopreserved human articular chondrocytes (HAC) from femoral heads and seeded them in culture media [45]. Following incubation, cell cohorts were either fixed, expanded or exposed to further chondrogenic stimuli. Analysis of gene expression profiles using a novel cellular enzyme-linked immuno-sorbent assay (CELISA) demonstrated a gradual decrease of calcium-binding proteins, S100A1 and S100B, accompanied with a decrease of COL I and an increase of COL II. Comparing this assay to cell pellet culture, which is the standard method of evaluating HAC dedifferentiation potential, it requires a lower cell number (10,000 cell/well vs. 2.5–5×10^5/pellet), a shorter incubation time (1 vs. 3 weeks) and more accurate quantitative results. The authors suggest that the S100B þ A1-CELISA could be used to evaluate the expression of alkaline phosphatase (AP), a marker of the undesirable hypertrophic phenotype [45].

2.5.3 Biochemical Analysis

There are many potential sources of stem cells for cartilage repair. Biomarkers may help select those that are most chondrogenic or other desirable attributes. For example, adipose-derived stem cells (hADSCs) are a type of mesenchymal stem cell that can be used as a source of pluripotent cells for cell therapy in articular cartilage repair. They have a high cell yield rate during in vitro expansion when obtained from liposuction of healthy females and seeded onto a 3-dimensional scaffold [46]. The production of s-GAG in both hyaluronic acid (HA) and hyaluronic acid/sodium alginate (HA/SA) scaffolds cultured with hADSCs was quantified. The released amount of s-GAG was higher in HA/SA scaffold compared to that in the HA scaffold on days 7 and 14, respectively ($p < 0.05$).

Gabusi treated 14 patients with a cell-free biomimetic osteochondral scaffold for knee osteochondral defects (size range of 1.5–4.0 cm^2) [47]. Baseline, 3-month and 12-month serum samples were assessed for biomarkers reflective of bone and cartilage turnover. CTXII and C2C (collagen type II cleavage), markers of collagen degradation, were not modulated during follow-up. However, CPII (procollagen II C-propeptide), a marker of cartilage synthesis, was found to significantly increase between 3 and 12 months ($p = 0.005$) and between baseline and 12 months ($p = 0.0005$). Tartrate-resistant acid phosphatase active isoform 5b (TRAP5b), a bone biomarker of degradation, did not show any modulation. In contrast, osteocalcin (OC), which is a marker of bone synthesis, showed a significant increase from baseline to 12 months ($p = 0.046$) [47].

2.5.4 Cell Surface Markers

Cell surface markers may facilitate the identification and sorting of multipotential progenitor cells located within articular cartilage and be a useful adjunct to evaluate the quality of cartilage biopsy utilised in ACI. Pretzel evaluated the markers and zonal location of mesenchymal progenitor cells (MPCs) from the cartilage of patients with end-stage OA and healthy donors with no evidence of OA [48]. Following enzymatic degradation of the cartilage donations, the remaining MPCs were passaged and cultured. After early expansion of the MPCs cell surface markers', CD105+ and CD166, concentrations were quantified. There was no difference between the quantity of multipotent stem cells using both immunohistochemistry and in situ immunodetection. 99% of the MPCs expressed both CD105+ and CD166, and on this basis CD166 may be a suitable biomarker for the identification of MPCs. These cells predominantly reside within the superficial and middle zones of the cartilage in both cohorts [48].

Neumann analysed cell surface antigens of cortico-spongiosis bone with the aim of identifying other potential cells within the subchondral bone with chondrogenic capacity [49]. The subchondral cortico-spongious bone-derived progenitor (CSP) cells exposed to transforming growth factor beta three (TGF-β3) and cultured in the presence of human serum demonstrated the antigens CD105, CD73, CD90 and CD166 and were homogeneously positive for the former three cell surface markers. These cell surface antigens are reflective of chondrogenic capacity [49].

2.5.5 Chondrogenic Gene Markers

Certain transcription factors manage stem cells towards the intended lineage, and the identification of these gene markers is frequently used in studies evaluating their own chondrogenic technique. Second- and third-generation ACI procedures preferentially use collagen sheets for cartilage defects or embed chondrocytes into resorbable scaffolds made of collagen, hyaluronan or polymers such as polylactic acid (PGLA) [50]. In a study, juvenile chondrocytes were obtained from paediatric patients with hip dysplasia and assembled onto PGLA scaffolds. Histological analysis was performed on mature graft explants. Gene expression analysis of typical chondrocyte marker genes showed the high expression of COL2A1 and type X collagen, moderate expression of COMP and low levels of aggrecan (ACAN) [51].

2.6 Biomarkers in Early Osteoarthritis

The role of molecular biomarkers in OA is vital to address current difficulties in eOA diagnosis and prognosis. A comprehensive review of biomarker research in OA was published in 2013 following a meeting of the European Society for Clinical and Economic Aspects of Osteoporosis and Osteoarthritis (ESCEO). The review highlighted biomarkers of interest related to collagen metabolism, ACAN metabolism, non-collagenous proteins as well as biomarkers related to other processes [52]. According to the BIPEDS method, type II collagen and ACAN were identified as being plausible targets for future research given their abundance in cartilaginous matrix. However, the authors concluded that no biomarker investigated had shown sufficient evidence to guide clinical trials or be used in a clinical environment [52]. One highlighted avenue for future research was the improved definition of eOA through the use of biomarkers [52].

In 2019, Kraus suggested that in order for an eOA marker to be truly effective, it must represent a state of preclinical OA [53]. Preclinical OA is the stage before OA is detectable by MRI or other sensitive imaging modalities. A biomarker that could reliably identify a patient in this state would allow early lifestyle changes and a better understanding of the efficacy of potential disease-modifying osteoarthritis drugs (DMOADs). However, not everyone who has radiographic OA progresses to severe forms of the disease, meaning it is reasonable to assume that not everyone with preclinical and pre-radiographic OA would progress to clinically significant OA.

Advanced discovery techniques such as Sequential Window Acquisition of All Theoretical Mass Spectra (SWATH-MS) to analyse the proteome and metabolomics of blood, urine and synovial fluid will undoubtedly become ever-more prominent in the search of valid biomarkers of preclinical and eOA.

Since Lotz's review on biomarkers in OA in 2013, further research on candidate molecular biomarkers for eOA of the knee has emerged, many of which have utilised these technologies. The types of biomarkers investigated can be subdivided into the following four categories: i) matrix-degrading enzymes, ii) matrix molecules, iii) regulatory molecules and iv) other molecules.

2.6.1 Matrix-Degrading Enzymes

Recent research has identified eight matrix-degrading enzymes that may represent potential candidate biomarkers of knee OA (Table 2.2) [54–57]. Matrix metalloproteinases are the most studied markers in this category. In 2018, Pengas investigated the effect of open total-knee meniscectomy on the development of OA later in life [58]. GAG and matrix metalloproteinase 3 (MMP-3) levels were quantified in synovial fluid and serum. Although GAG levels had reduced since meniscectomy, MMP-3 levels remained increased. This suggests that MMP-3 may be a potential biomarker of preclinical OA.

In another study, MMP-1 and MMP-3 were shown to be significantly elevated in OA patients compared to healthy subjects and eOA patients. MMP-3 also had an area under the curve (AUC) value of 0.690 when ROC analysis was carried out for its diagnostic ability. In this study eOA patients were defined as K-L grade ½ [54]. The study demonstrated that A disintegrin and metalloproteinase with thrombospondin motifs (ADAMTS)-4 and ADAMTS-5 were present in significantly different concentrations in eOA than in later stages of OA in serum [54]. Similar correlations were also reported for autotaxin in plasma and synovial fluid of individuals with knee OA [55]. According to the BIPEDS classification, these molecules have the potential to be used to diagnose eOA and identify the burden of disease of patients with the condition.

Promising research on MMP-13, tartrate-resistant acid phosphatase (TRAcP5b) and tissue transglutaminase 2 (TG2) in blood serum and OA tissue suggests that these molecules may also be considered as biomarkers of burden of disease [56, 57].

2.6.2 Matrix Molecules

Twenty-one potential biomarkers are categorised as matrix molecules (Table 2.2); 20 were investigated as burden of disease markers, 17 as diagnostic markers and 15 as prognostic markers. The Foundation for the National Institutes of Health

Table 2.2 Current candidate biomarkers in osteoarthritis

Type of biomarker			
Matrix-degrading enzymes	Matrix molecules	Regulatory molecules	Other molecules
A disintegrin and metalloproteinase with thrombospondin motifs: ADAMTS-4 ADAMTS-5 **Autotaxin** **Matrix metalloproteinases:** MMP-1 MMP-3 MMP-13 **Tartrate-resistant acid phosphatase** (TRAcP5b) **Tissue transglutaminase 2** (TG2)	**MMP-mediated degradation of type I collagen (C1M)** **Col2–3/4 C-terminal cleavage product of human type II collagen** (C2C) **MMP-mediated degradation of types 2 and 3 collagen:** C2M C3M **C-terminus of collagen X** (C-Col10) **Nitrated epitope of the α-helical region of type II collagen (Coll2-1NO2)** **Cartilage oligomeric matrix protein** (comp) **Matrix metalloproteinase-dependent degradation of C-reactive protein** (CRPM) **Chondroitin sulphate epitope 846** (CS846) **C-terminal cross-linked telopeptide types I and II collagen:** CTX-I CTX-Iα CTX-Iβ CTXII **Fibulin-3–1** **Hyaluronic acid** **High-sensitivity C-reactive protein** (hsCRP) **Cross-linked N-telopeptide of type I collagen** (NTX-1) **Osteocalcin** **N-terminal propeptide of collagens IIA and III:** PIIANP PIIINP **Uncarboxylated matrix Gla protein** (ucMGP)	**Adiponectin** **Adipsin** **Adropin** **Angiopoietin-2** **β-Catenin** **Bone morphogenetic protein** BMP2 BMP7 **Brain-derived neurotrophic protein** (BDNF) **Chemokine (C-C motif) ligand** (CCL2) **Calcitonin gene-related peptide** (CGRP) **C-X-C motif chemokine** (CXCL12) **Dickkopf-related protein** (DKK-1) **Fibroblast growth factor** (FGF-23) **Follistatin** **Fractalkine** **Granulocyte-colony-stimulating factor** (G-CSF) **Gremlin-1** **Hepatocyte growth factor** (HGF) **Hypoxia-inducible factor:** HIF-1α HIF-2α **Interleukin:** IL1Ra IL-6 IL-8 IL-10 IL-17 **Indian hedgehog** (IHh) **Leptin** **Prostaglandin E2** (PGE2) **Peroxiredoxin-6** (PRDX6) **Sclerostin** **Transforming growth factor** (TGF-β1) **Tumour necrosis factor** (TNF-α) **Transcription factor 4** **Tumour necrosis factor-inducible gene 6** (TSG-6) **Vascular endothelial growth factor** (VEGF) **Chitinase-3-like protein 1** (YKL-40)	**Hydroxyeicosatetraenoic acid** (15-HETE) **4-Hydroxy-L-proline** **Alanine** **Amyloid P** **Arginine** **Aggrecan** (ACAN) **Cluster of differentiation:** CD14 CD163 CD31/PECAM-1 CD40 **Fatty acid-binding protein 4** (FABP4) **Ghrelin** **Haptoglobin** **Lipopolysaccharide (LPS)-binding protein** (LBP) **Neuropeptide Y** (NPY)**Oxidised low-density lipoprotein** (ox-LDL) **Periostin** **Sialic acid** **Taurine** **Thymosin β4** **Vascular cell adhesion molecule** (VCAM-1) **von Willebrand factor** (vWF) **γ-Aminobutyric acid**

(FNIH) OA biomarker consortium evaluated the ability of 14 biomarkers in serum, urine or both to predict case status at 48 months and differentiate between 3 progressor types: pain progression, joint space loss progression and pain and joint space loss progression over 48 months. C-telopeptide of CTXII was shown to have the best predictive ability of case status and progression. This 12-month and 24-month time-integrated concentrations (TICs) of urinary Col2–3/4 C-terminal cleavage product of human type II collagen (C2C) predicted progression in all three progressor types [59]. Using K-L grade to define OA, *He* et al. reported a significant difference in C-Col10 between K-L grade 0 and K-L grade 2 ($P = 0.04$) [60]. Serum concentrations of hyaluronic acid (HA) were correlated with progression of joint space narrowing in patients classified as K-L grade 0/1 ($\beta = 0.15$, $P = 0.021$) [60].

2.6.3 Regulatory Molecules

Thirty-five regulatory markers are associated with OA (Table 2.2). With respect to the BIPEDS method, 33 were investigated as burden of disease markers, 21 as diagnostic markers and 6 as prognostic markers.

β-Catenin was significantly reduced in eOA compared to late/intermediate-stage OA ($P < 0.05$). The same study also demonstrated that serum concentrations of transcription factor 4 were significantly higher in eOA patients when compared to healthy controls ($P < 0.002$). Classification of the stage of OA was carried out for 32 patients using the Mankin scoring system following a total knee replacement [61].

Indian hedgehog (IHh) protein was elevated in the synovial fluid of eOA patients, classified as patients with Outerbridge scale 1/2 cartilage breakdown, compared to healthy controls ($P < 0.001$) [62]. If this relationship was further investigated and shown to be significant in other independent studies, then it would have positive implications for diagnosing eOA. Perhaps other biomarkers may follow the same pattern as IHh and are only dysregulated during eOA.

Using K-L grades 1/2 as a definition of eOA, serum concentrations of angiopoietin-2, interleukin 8 (IL-8), follistatin, granulocyte-colony stimulating factor (G-CSF), vascular endothelial growth factor and hepatocyte growth factor were shown to be significantly different in eOA than in healthy controls [63].

There is evidence that supports the use of regulatory markers as therapeutic targets in the development of disease-modifying osteoarthritis drugs (DMOADs). Clinical trials have used bone morphogenetic protein-7 (BMP7), fibroblast growth factor and β-nerve growth factor (β-NGF) as targets in an attempt to develop new OA drugs [64]. Tanezumab, a monoclonal antibody against β-NGF, reduced knee pain whilst walking by between 45% and 62% compared with 22% by placebo [65].

2.6.4 Other Molecules

A total of 25 markers did not fit into the other three categories (Table 2.2). 18 were investigated as burden of disease markers, 12 as diagnostic markers and 6 as prognostic markers as per the BIPEDS method. None of the markers in this category have been verified as potential biomarker candidates by more than one study. Two studies investigated amino acids. Chen investigated serum alanine and taurine and reported an AUC = 0.928 and AUC = 0.920 when used to diagnose OA in a study sample of 67 [66]. Arginine, investigated by Zhang, had an AUC = 0.984 [67].

2.6.5 Biomarker Panels

A total of 11 biomarker potential panels have been identified (Table 2.2). The source of all biomarkers for use in algorithms was either serum or urine and their use was demonstrated for predicting disease presence, severity and progression. Saberi presented an algorithm that consisted of patient demographics, biomarkers and radiology [68]. The algorithm was developed using 1335 patients' data from the Rotterdam Study and the algorithm had an excellent ability to predict disease progression over 2.5 years (AUC = 0.872).

Of the 12 algorithms described below, 2 specifically targeted the early diagnosis of OA [69, 70]. Both studies used the same methods of patient recruitment and sampling. To be deemed as having eOA, patients had to have new-onset knee pain, normal radiographs and Outerbridge grade I/II. The algorithm consisting of citrullinated proteins (CPs), hydroxyproline, anti-cyclic citrullinated peptide (anti-CCP) antibody, age and gender had the following statistics when distinguishing eOA from healthy controls and inflammatory arthritic diseases: AUC = 0.86, PPV = 0.733 and NPV = 0.885 [69]. The second algorithm for diagnosing eOA was intended for use after an individual had been excluded from the healthy control group. It combined anti-CCP antibody with biomarkers of protein oxidation, nitration and glycation to give an AUC of 0.98 [70]. Using patient demographics within the algorithm is an efficient method of increasing the algorithm's predictive ability.

IHh protein and IL-8 both performed well as single biomarkers so perhaps their combination along with patient demographics would create a highly sensitive and specific algorithm. Due to the heterogeneity and complexity of the disease, it is likely that an algorithm will be a more effective method for making a diagnosis.

2.7 Summary

Biomarker research of cartilage damage and eOA has continued to gain momentum due to the importance of the condition, diagnosis, assessment of prognosis and response to treatments. However, there is a lack of consensus on methods of diagnosis and classification of both interrelated conditions. Future research of prognostic value is likely to focus on biomarkers produced in serum and urine and locally within the joint. Whilst many of the aims set out by the ESCEO have made a clear difference in research direction, there are currently no single biomarkers that have been sufficiently validated for clinical use. Nevertheless, as observed in both cartilage injury

and early OA, biomarker panels, rather than singular biomarkers, may provide the most promising avenue for further evaluation.

References

1. Ondrésik M, Oliveira JM, Reis RL. Advances for treatment of knee OC defects. In: Oliveira JM, Pina S, Reis RL, San Roman J, editors. Osteochondral tissue engineering: challenges, current strategies, and technological advances. Cham: Springer International Publishing; 2018. p. 3–24.
2. Mobasheri A, Kalamegam G, Musumeci G, Batt ME. Chondrocyte and mesenchymal stem cell-based therapies for cartilage repair in osteoarthritis and related orthopaedic conditions. Maturitas. 2014;78(3):188–98.
3. Atkinson AJCW, DeGruttola VG, DeMets DL, Downing GJ, Hoth DF, Oates JA, Peck CC, Schooley RT, Spilker BA, Woodcock J, Zeger SL. Biomarkers and surrogate endpoints: preferred definitions and conceptual framework. Clin Pharmacol Ther. 2001;69(3):89–95.
4. Bauer DC, Hunter DJ, Abramson SB, Attur M, Corr M, Felson D, et al. Classification of osteoarthritis biomarkers: a proposed approach. Osteoarthr Cartil. 2006;14(8):723–7.
5. Trevethan R. Sensitivity, specificity, and predictive values: foundations, pliabilities, and pitfalls in research and practice. Front Public Health. 2017;5(307)
6. Ollier W, Muir KR, Lophatananon A, Verma A, Yuille M. Risk biomarkers enable precision in public health. Pers Med. 2018;15(4):329–42.
7. Engen CN, Løken S, Årøen A, Ho C, Engebretsen L. No degeneration found in focal cartilage defects evaluated with dGEMRIC at 12-year follow-up. Acta Orthop. 2017;88(1):82–9.
8. Pelletier JP, Martel-Pelletier J, Abramson SB. Osteoarthritis, an inflammatory disease: potential implication for the selection of new therapeutic targets. Arthritis Rheum. 2001;44(6):1237–47.
9. Attur MG, Dave M, Akamatsu M, Katoh M, Amin AR. Osteoarthritis or osteoarthrosis: the definition of inflammation becomes a semantic issue in the genomic era of molecular medicine. Osteoarthr Cartil. 2002;10(1):1–4.
10. Marlovits S, Singer P, Zeller P, Mandl I, Haller J, Trattnig S. Magnetic resonance observation of cartilage repair tissue (MOCART) for the evaluation of autologous chondrocyte transplantation: determination of interobserver variability and correlation to clinical outcome after 2 years. Eur J Radiol. 2006;57(1):16–23.
11. Brittberg M, Winalski CS. Evaluation of cartilage injuries and repair. J Bone Joint Surg Am. 2003;85-A(Suppl 2):58–69.

12. Marlovits S, Striessnig G, Resinger CT, Aldrian SM, Vecsei V, Imhof H, et al. Definition of pertinent parameters for the evaluation of articular cartilage repair tissue with high-resolution magnetic resonance imaging. Eur J Radiol. 2004;52(3):310–9.

13. Schreiner MM, Raudner M, Marlovits S, Bohndorf K, Weber M, Zalaudek M, et al. The MOCART (magnetic resonance observation of cartilage repair tissue) 2.0 knee score and atlas. Cartilage:2019, 1947603519865308.

14. Mamisch TC, Hughes T, Mosher TJ, Mueller C, Trattnig S, Boesch C, et al. T2 star relaxation times for assessment of articular cartilage at 3 T: a feasibility study. Skelet Radiol. 2012;41(3):287–92.

15. Årøen A, Brøgger H, Røtterud JH, Sivertsen EA, Engebretsen L, Risberg MA. Evaluation of focal cartilage lesions of the knee using MRI T2 mapping and delayed gadolinium enhanced MRI of cartilage (dGEMRIC). BMC Musculoskelet Disord. 2016;17:73.

16. Souza RB, Feeley BT, Zarins ZA, Link TM, Li X, Majumdar S. T1rho MRI relaxation in knee OA subjects with varying sizes of cartilage lesions. Knee. 2013;20(2):113–9.

17. Vasiliadis HS, Danielson B, Ljungberg M, McKeon B, Lindahl A, Peterson L. Autologous chondrocyte implantation in cartilage lesions of the knee: long-term evaluation with magnetic resonance imaging and delayed gadolinium-enhanced magnetic resonance imaging technique. Am J Sports Med. 2010;38(5):943–9.

18. Owman H, Tiderius CJ, Ericsson YB, Dahlberg LE. Long-term effect of removal of knee joint loading on cartilage quality evaluated by delayed gadolinium-enhanced magnetic resonance imaging of cartilage. Osteoarthr Cartil. 2014;22(7):928–32.

19. Neuman P, Owman H, Müller G, Englund M, Tiderius CJ, Dahlberg LE. Knee cartilage assessment with MRI (dGEMRIC) and subjective knee function in ACL injured copers: a cohort study with a 20 year follow-up. Osteoarthr Cartil. 2014;22(1):84–90.

20. Brinkhof S, Nizak R, Khlebnikov V, Prompers JJ, Klomp DWJ, Saris DBF. Detection of early cartilage damage: feasibility and potential of gagCEST imaging at 7T. Eur Radiol. 2018;28(7):2874–81.

21. Juras V, Mlynarik V, Szomolanyi P, Valkovič L, Trattnig S. Magnetic resonance imaging of the musculoskeletal system at 7T: morphological imaging and beyond. Top Magn Reson Imaging. 2019;28(3):125–35.

22. Svoboda SJ, Harvey TM, Owens BD, Brechue WF, Tarwater PM, Cameron KL. Changes in serum biomarkers of cartilage turnover after anterior cruciate ligament injury. Am J Sports Med. 2013;41(9):2108–16.

23. Bihlet AR, Byrjalsen I, Bay-Jensen A-C, Andersen JR, Christiansen C, Riis BJ, et al. Associations between biomarkers of bone and cartilage turnover, gender, pain categories and radiographic severity in knee osteoarthritis. Arthritis Res Ther. 2019;21(1):203.

24. Rousseau J, Garnero P. Biological markers in osteoarthritis. Bone. 2012;51(2):265–77.

25. Garnero P, Ayral X, Rousseau JC, Christgau S, Sandell LJ, Dougados M, et al. Uncoupling of type II collagen synthesis and degradation predicts progression of joint damage in patients with knee osteoarthritis. Arthritis Rheum. 2002;46(10):2613–24.

26. Cahue S, Sharma L, Dunlop D, Ionescu M, Song J, Lobanok T, et al. The ratio of type II collagen breakdown to synthesis and its relationship with the progression of knee osteoarthritis. Osteoarthr Cartil. 2007;15(7):819–23.

27. Koryem HK, Wanas MAAEQ, Rizk MMA, Kotb HT, Naguib AH, Shafei MMAHE, et al. Evaluation of early changes of cartilage biomarkers following arthroscopic meniscectomy in young Egyptian adults. Alex J Med. 2015;51(3):191–7.

28. Boeth H, MacMahon A, Poole AR, Buttgereit F, Önnerfjord P, Lorenzo P, et al. Differences in biomarkers of cartilage matrix turnover and their changes over 2 years in adolescent and adult volleyball athletes. J Exp Orthop. 2017;4(1):7.

29. Kumahashi N, Swärd P, Larsson S, Lohmander LS, Frobell R, Struglics A. Type II collagen C2C epitope in human synovial fluid and serum after knee injury – associations with molecular and structural markers of injury. Osteoarthr Cartil. 2015;23(9):1506–12.

30. Yoshida H, Kojima T, Kurokouchi K, Takahashi S, Hanamura H, Kojima M, et al. Relationship between pre-radiographic cartilage damage following anterior cruciate ligament injury and biomarkers of cartilage turnover in clinical practice: a cross-sectional observational study. Osteoarthr Cartil. 2013;21(6):831–8.

31. Cibere J, Zhang H, Garnero P, Poole AR, Lobanok T, Saxne T, et al. Association of biomarkers with pre-radiographically defined and radiographically defined knee osteoarthritis in a population-based study. Arthritis Rheum. 2009;60(5):1372–80.

32. Poole AR, Ha N, Bourdon S, Sayre EC, Guermazi A, Cibere J. Ability of a urine assay of type II collagen cleavage by collagenases to detect early onset and progression of articular cartilage degeneration: results from a population-based cohort study. J Rheumatol. 2016;43(10):1864–70.

33. O'Kane JW, Hutchinson E, Atley LM, Eyre DR. Sport-related differences in biomarkers of bone resorption and cartilage degradation in endurance athletes. Osteoarthr Cartil. 2006;14(1):71–6.

34. Kersting UG, Stubendorff JJ, Schmidt MC, Brüggemann G-P. Changes in knee cartilage volume and serum COMP concentration after running exercise. Osteoarthr Cartil. 2005;13(10):925–34.

35. Hoch JM, Mattacola CG, Bush HM, Medina McKeon JM, Hewett TE, Lattermann C. Longitudinal documentation of serum cartilage oligomeric matrix protein and patient-reported outcomes in collegiate soccer athletes over the course of an athletic season. Am J Sports Med. 2012;40(11):2583–9.

36. Boeth H, Raffalt PC, MacMahon A, Poole AR, Eckstein F, Wirth W, et al. Association between

changes in molecular biomarkers of cartilage matrix turnover and changes in knee articular cartilage: a longitudinal pilot study. J Exp Orthop. 2019;6(1):19.

37. Roberts HM, Law R-J, Thom JM. The time course and mechanisms of change in biomarkers of joint metabolism in response to acute exercise and chronic training in physiologic and pathological conditions. Eur J Appl Physiol. 2019;119(11):2401–20.

38. Boeth H, MacMahon A, Poole AR, Buttgereit F, Onnerfjord P, Lorenzo P, et al. Differences in biomarkers of cartilage matrix turnover and their changes over 2 years in adolescent and adult volleyball athletes. J Exp Orthop. 2017;4(1):7.

39. Nelson F, Dahlberg L, Laverty S, Reiner A, Pidoux I, Ionescu M, et al. Evidence for altered synthesis of type II collagen in patients with osteoarthritis. J Clin Invest. 1998;102(12):2115–25.

40. Catterall JB, Stabler TV, Flannery CR, Kraus VB. Changes in serum and synovial fluid biomarkers after acute injury (NCT00332254). Arthritis Res Ther. 2010;12(6):R229.

41. Lohmander LS, Ionescu M, Jugessur H, Poole AR. Changes in joint cartilage aggrecan after knee injury and in osteoarthritis. Arthritis Rheum. 1999;42(3):534–44.

42. Lark MW, Bayne EK, Lohmander LS. Aggrecan degradation in osteoarthritis and rheumatoid arthritis. Acta Orthop Scand Suppl. 1995;266:92–7.

43. Lohmander LS, Roos H, Dahlberg L, Lark MW. The role of molecular markers to monitor disease, intervention and cartilage breakdown in osteoarthritis. Acta Orthop Scand Suppl. 1995;266:84–7.

44. Diaz-Romero J, Gaillard JP, Grogan SP, Nesic D, Trub T, Mainil-Varlet P. Immunophenotypic analysis of human articular chondrocytes: changes in surface markers associated with cell expansion in monolayer culture. J Cell Physiol. 2005;202(3):731–42.

45. Diaz-Romero J, Kursener S, Kohl S, Nesic D. S100B + A1 CELISA: a novel potency assay and screening tool for Redifferentiation stimuli of human articular chondrocytes. J Cell Physiol. 2017;232(6):1559–70.

46. Son YJ, Yoon IS, Sung JH, Cho HJ, Chung SJ, Shim CK, et al. Porous hyaluronic acid/sodium alginate composite scaffolds for human adipose-derived stem cells delivery. Int J Biol Macromol. 2013;61:175–81.

47. Gabusi E, Paolella F, Manferdini C, Gambari L, Kon E, Filardo G, et al. Cartilage and bone serum biomarkers as novel tools for monitoring knee osteochondritis dissecans treated with osteochondral scaffold. Biomed Res Int. 2018;2018:9275102.

48. Pretzel D, Linss S, Rochler S, Endres M, Kaps C, Alsalameh S, et al. Relative percentage and zonal distribution of mesenchymal progenitor cells in human osteoarthritic and normal cartilage. Arthritis Res Ther. 2011;13(2):R64.

49. Neumann K, Dehne T, Endres M, Erggelet C, Kaps C, Ringe J, et al. Chondrogenic differentiation capacity of human mesenchymal progenitor cells derived from

subchondral cortico-spongious bone. J Orthop Res. 2008;26(11):1449–56.

50. Aurich M, Hofmann GO, Gras F, Rolauffs B. Human osteochondritis dissecans fragment-derived chondrocyte characteristics ex vivo, after monolayer expansion-induced de-differentiation, and after re-differentiation in alginate bead culture. BMC Musculoskelet Disord. 2018;19(1):168.

51. Kreuz PC, Gentili C, Samans B, Martinelli D, Kruger JP, Mittelmeier W, et al. Scaffold-assisted cartilage tissue engineering using infant chondrocytes from human hip cartilage. Osteoarthr Cartil. 2013;21(12):1997–2005.

52. Lotz M, Martel-Pelletier J, Christiansen C, Brandi ML, Bruyère O, Chapurlat R, et al. Value of biomarkers in osteoarthritis: current status and perspectives. Ann Rheum Dis. 2013;72(11):1756–63.

53. Kraus V. Preclinical osteoarthritis. Philadelphia, PA: Elsevier; 2019.

54. Li W, Du C, Wang H, Zhang C. Increased serum ADAMTS-4 in knee osteoarthritis: a potential indicator for the diagnosis of osteoarthritis in early stages. Genet Mol Res. 2014;13(4):9642–9.

55. Mabey T, Taleongpong P, Udomsinprasert W, Jirathanathornnukul N, Honsawek S. Plasma and synovial fluid autotaxin correlate with severity in knee osteoarthritis. Clin Chim Acta. 2015;444:72–7.

56. Nwosu LN, Allen M, Wyatt L, Huebner JL, Chapman V, Walsh DA, et al. Pain prediction by serum biomarkers of bone turnover in people with knee osteoarthritis: an observational study of TRAcP5b and cathepsin K in OA. Osteoarthr Cartil. 2017;25(6):858–65.

57. Tarquini C, Mattera R, Mastrangeli F, Agostinelli S, Ferlosio A, Bei R, et al. Comparison of tissue transglutaminase 2 and bone biological markers osteocalcin, osteopontin and sclerostin expression in human osteoporosis and osteoarthritis. Amino Acids. 2017;49(3):683–93.

58. Pengas I, Eldridge S, Assiotis A, McNicholas M, Mendes JE, Laver L. MMP-3 in the peripheral serum as a biomarker of knee osteoarthritis, 40 years after open total knee meniscectomy. J Exp Orthop. 2018;5(1):21.

59. Kraus VB, Collins JE, Hargrove D, Losina E, Nevitt M, Katz JN, et al. Predictive validity of biochemical biomarkers in knee osteoarthritis: data from the FNIH OA biomarkers consortium. Ann Rheum Dis. 2017;76(1):186–95.

60. He Y, Siebuhr AS, Brandt-Hansen NU, Wang J, Su D, Zheng Q, et al. Type X collagen levels are elevated in serum from human osteoarthritis patients and associated with biomarkers of cartilage degradation and inflammation. BMC Musculoskelet Disord. 2014;15:309.

61. Wu L, Guo H, Sun K, Zhao X, Ma T, Jin Q. Sclerostin expression in the subchondral bone of patients with knee osteoarthritis. Int J Mol Med. 2016;38(5):1395–402.

62. Zhang C, Wei X, Chen C, Cao K, Li Y, Jiao Q, et al. Indian hedgehog in synovial fluid is a novel marker for early cartilage lesions in human knee joint. Int J Mol Sci. 2014;15(5):7250–65.
63. Mabey T, Honsawek S, Saetan N, Poovorawan Y, Tanavalee A, Yuktanandana P. Angiogenic cytokine expression profiles in plasma and synovial fluid of primary knee osteoarthritis. Int Orthop. 2014;38(9):1885–92.
64. Zhang W, Ouyang H, Dass CR, Xu J. Current research on pharmacologic and regenerative therapies for osteoarthritis. Bone Res. 2016;4:15040.
65. Lane NE, Schnitzer TJ, Birbara CA, Mokhtarani M, Shelton DL, Smith MD, et al. Tanezumab for the treatment of pain from osteoarthritis of the knee. N Engl J Med. 2010;363(16):1521–31.
66. Chen R, Han S, Liu X, Wang K, Zhou Y, Yang C, et al. Perturbations in amino acids and metabolic pathways in osteoarthritis patients determined by targeted metabolomics analysis. J Chromatogr B Analyt Technol Biomed Life Sci. 2018;1085:54–62.
67. Zhang W, Sun G, Likhodii S, Liu M, Aref-Eshghi E, Harper PE, et al. Metabolomic analysis of human plasma reveals that arginine is depleted in knee osteoarthritis patients. Osteoarthr Cartil. 2016;24(5):827–34.
68. Saberi Hosnijeh F, Siebuhr AS, Uitterlinden AG, Oei EH, Hofman A, Karsdal MA, et al. Association between biomarkers of tissue inflammation and progression of osteoarthritis: evidence from the Rotterdam Study cohort. Arthritis Res Ther. 2016;18:81.
69. Ahmed U, Anwar A, Savage RS, Costa ML, Mackay N, Filer A, et al. Biomarkers of early stage osteoarthritis, rheumatoid arthritis and musculoskeletal health. Sci Rep. 2015;5:9259.
70. Ahmed U, Anwar A, Savage RS, Thornalley PJ, Rabbani N. Protein oxidation, nitration and glycation biomarkers for early-stage diagnosis of osteoarthritis of the knee and typing and progression of arthritic disease. Arthritis Res Ther. 2016;18(1):250.

How Do We Best Measure Outcomes Following Cartilage Repair Surgery?

Isabel Wolfe, Alissa Burge, Chisa Hidaka, and Stephen Lyman

3.1 Introduction

Early attempts at systematic assessment of patient outcomes focused on easily measurable, objective observations of clinical failure: surgical site infection, implant failure, revision surgery, or even death. These outcomes are still reported today as they remain objectively observable evidence of failure of surgical treatment. But how do we measure success? This is a particularly important question for cartilage repair where the evaluation of novel approaches, such as the implantation of stem cells, scaffolds, or other biologics against existing treatments, remains a significant hurdle for clinical development. The innovation of therapies for cartilage repair remains an active area of research because current treatments such as microfracture, tissue grafting, and chondrocyte transplantation do not lead to the formation of tissue with the normal, complex architecture of native articular cartilage within a treated lesion. Yet we have to understand whether and how tissue quality correlates with clinical treatment success, which considers such factors as return to full, pain-free activity and forestalling the progression to degenerative arthritis in the affected joint. Here, we review the most relevant outcome assessment tools for successful cartilage repair.

Over the decades of increasingly rigorous clinical investigation into outcomes after orthopedic therapies, our tools for measuring outcomes have evolved. The surgeon's experienced observations remain important, but with the development and use of methods for systematic assessment, researchers are more reliably able to compare outcomes across time and institutions. Gone are the days when a surgeon's careful, but ultimately biased, handwritten and thus error-prone clinical observations were the mainstay of medical documentation. New measurement tools make it possible to understand how one surgeon's "excellent" outcomes are compared to another's. Sophisticated research into the measurement instruments themselves has resulted in the development of surveys and assessment scales, which permit quantitative measurements of therapeutic outcomes with accuracy, repeatability, and clinical relevance.

A step forward in clinical measurement occurred with the introduction of the Hospital for Special Surgery (HSS) Hip Score, developed by famed hip surgeon, Philip D. Wilson, Jr. in 1972 [1]. The HSS Hip Score standardized the

I. Wolfe · A. Burge · C. Hidaka
Hospital for Special Surgery, New York, NY, USA

S. Lyman (✉)
Hospital for Special Surgery, New York, NY, USA

Weill Medical College of Cornell University, New York, NY, USA

Kyushu University School of Medicine, Fukuoka, Japan
e-mail: lymans@hss.edu

© ISAKOS 2021
A. J. Krych et al. (eds.), *Cartilage Injury of the Knee*,
https://doi.org/10.1007/978-3-030-78051-7_3

physician's assessment with regard to pain, motion, walking, and function on a numerical scale for the purpose of monitoring patient outcomes after total hip replacement. While these four domains were by no means a complete assessment of patient outcomes after hip surgery, this scoresheet permitted adequately systematic and quantifiable outcome measures to yield meaningful research until very recently [2].

Today, we have at our disposal several decades worth of experience in the development and testing of measurement instruments, such as that pioneered by Dr. Wilson. Scoring systems have been developed to permit the quantitative analysis of imaging modalities, such as magnetic resonance imaging (MRI) that could not have been imagined when Dr. Wilson began practice in 1948. In addition, as the entire field of healthcare has shifted towards patient-centered care, researchers have paid more attention to patients' perceptions of the treatment process, medical care, time of recovery, and return to prior level of activity [3]. As such, the use of psychometrically derived patient-reported outcome measures (PROMs), which directly assess patients' own perception of their state of health, without interpretation by a physician or other clinician has increased dramatically over the last 20 years [4]. The extent of improvement following cartilage or other surgery can now be documented on the tissue and patient level, as rigorously and quantitatively as the frequency of adverse outcomes or treatment failure.

Quantitative outcome measurement instruments have become essential in both clinical research and routine clinical practice, for different but complementary objectives. For many surgical procedures, including cartilage repair, outcome measures fall into the following main categories: imaging or radiographic analysis, survivorship analyses, surgeon-based outcome measures, performance-related assessments, and, of course, PROMs. What follows is a summary of the best assessment tools for measuring outcomes after cartilage repair surgery in the knee.

3.2 Objective vs. Subjective Measures

Outcome measures fall into two broad categories: "objective" measures such as knee range of motion and radiographic assessment, and "subjective" measures such as physician grading and patient self-reported outcomes. Both objective and subjective measures provide valuable information for clinical and research purposes. Whether objective or subjective, measurement instruments can be of greater or lesser quality depending on a number of considerations including the possibility of introducing physician or researcher bias, whether the measured outcomes are clinically relevant, and whether a scale or survey is adequately validated.

Clinical assessments are most useful if they are objective, as subjective assessment by a physician is prone to bias. Every physician wants their patient to do well. Knee range of motion is an objective clinical measure, but its relevance to patient satisfaction after cartilage repair is not known. Assessing the presence or absence of effusion and/or clicking or locking is somewhat subjective, but the binary nature of the observation helps the documentation be more reliable. A standardized scoring system, such as the one which Dr. Wilson used in his hip surgery patients, focusing on the most important clinical manifestations present with a cartilage lesion could be helpful, but has yet to be developed.

Cartilage grading is a widespread, reliable way to standardize the evaluation of treatment success after cartilage repair. New technological advancements have allowed for quantitative assessment of patients' joint cartilage pre- and postoperatively, at the radiographic, gross, and microscopic levels, providing quantitative assessments of the biochemical composition and morphologic characteristics of the cartilage before and after an intervention. Using these grading tools clinicians are able to detect and monitor longitudinal changes in cartilage tissue, especially the onset and progression of osteoarthritis [5]. Because a physician or researcher must interpret the radiographic, arthroscopic, or microscopic image, grading schemes are not impervious to bias and other inconsistencies. As detailed below, new technologies may be useful in overcoming this problem when radiographic images are considered.

While quantifiable and specific, objective measures may not reflect the patient's perception of outcome, as the correlation between radiographic changes and patients' symptoms may not be direct. In a recent systematic review of the relationship between quantitative magnetic resonance imaging (MRI) biomarkers and PROMs following cartilage repair surgery, a statistically significant correlation was detected in only about half of the included studies [6]. Overall, the authors concluded that the currently available body of literature does not offer sufficient information to draw strong conclusions regarding the role of advanced imaging for the postoperative assessment of cartilage surgery.

In contrast to objective measures, subjective measures more readily identify patient-related issues that are relevant to pain and functional limitations related to activities of daily life. Patient-reported outcome measures (PROMs) can assess a wide range of outcomes, and are generally divided into different domains (e.g., pain, function, satisfaction). When choosing a PROM, it is important to consider what domains or constructs are to be measured, which patients are to be included, and whether reliable, valid, and responsive outcome measures exist that assess parameters appropriate for your objective.

The general domains of pain, function, quality of life, and ability to perform daily activities that apply to all knee conditions are relevant following cartilage procedures. Activity-based outcomes are particularly important following cartilage surgery because of the young, active patient population. Chondral defects are especially common in active populations, and many patients include returning to activity as a primary reason for seeking treatment [7]. When the goal of treatment is to return to activity as quickly as possible, without pain and at a previous level of performance, PROMs that measure success in meeting these objectives must be used.

In Fig. 3.1 we organized various available outcome assessment tools based on their category (subjective or objective) as well as on their relative quality. Subjective measures, primarily PROMs, are valuable if they have been validated, and are relevant to cartilage repair. Objective measures, primarily advanced imaging analysis, are valued for providing detailed tissue-level information while minimizing physician or researcher bias. Subjective measures assessed by physicians are less valuable due to inherent bias. Even if they are from a patient's perspective, they

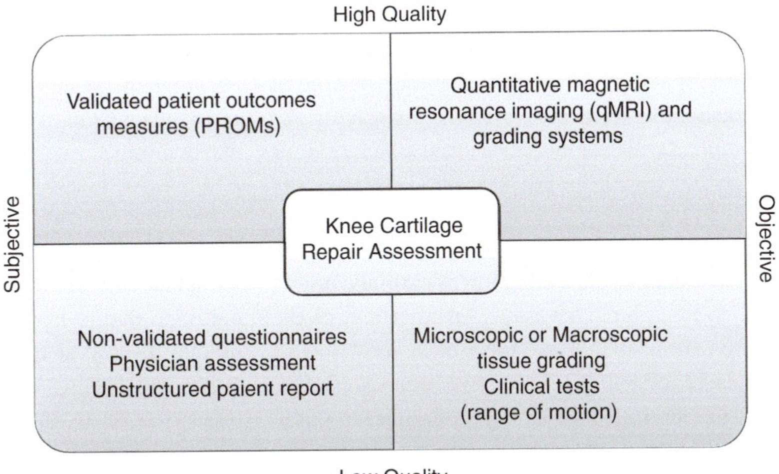

Fig. 3.1 Relative quality of subjective and objective measures of outcomes after cartilage surgery

are less valuable if they are not validated, are not systematic, or have been interpreted by the physician, researcher, or other person. Although quantitative, scoring systems for the microscopic or macroscopic cartilage tissue assessment are less valuable as reliance on grader interpretation can introduce bias or other inconsistencies.

3.3 Best Objective Measures

Assessment of structural outcome following cartilage repair can be performed using MRI or histology and macroscopic evaluation through (second-look) arthroscopy. Noninvasive and rigorously quantifiable MRI examination continues to be developed as an effective means for objective cartilage assessment, overcoming the limitations associated with micro- and macroscopic cartilage grading.

Histological scoring systems are used to assess biopsies, usually collected at second-look arthroscopy. Scoring systems used in cartilage repair include the comprehensive O'Driscoll, the simple Pineda scale, the Bern score, and the International Cartilage Repair Society (ICRS) Visual Histological Assessment Scale. Some of these have been validated and various modifications have been applied. These scales effectively standardize the assessment of microscopic images, but obtaining histologic samples has limitations. Biopsies are invasive, requiring a follow-up arthroscopic procedure. Sample selection can be affected by the location of the repair, as well as surgeon bias. Nonetheless, these measures are useful for studies where documenting the type of tissue in the repaired lesion is important. For example, with chondrocyte transplantation or other novel cell-based therapies, determining whether the repair tissue is fibrocartilage or articular cartilage may be germane.

For macroscopic evaluation of cartilage repair, the ICRS and Oswestry Arthroscopy Score (OAS) are available and have been shown to be valid and reliable [8]. These two scales were specifically designed to evaluate the macroscopic outcome of cartilage repair and to simplify and tailor the scoring system to clinical needs [8]. The recently developed ICRS II score has been identified as highly suitable to analyze in vivo-repaired cartilage [9], due to its validity, comprehensiveness, and usefulness for describing each cartilage characteristic individually. The ICRS II score contains several categories, which are divided into 13 subcategories, each scored on a 100 mm visual analogue scale (VAS). This enables evaluation of subtle differences and facilitates statistical comparisons of the individual cartilage characteristics [9]. A shortcoming of most of these cartilage repair scores is the absence of evaluation of integration of the repair tissue with its surroundings.

Other notable cartilage grading systems for macroscopic assessment include the Outerbridge and modified Noyes scoring systems. The Outerbridge classification system is based on direct visualization of the joint and was developed to be a simple, easy-to-use, and reproducible grading system of articular cartilage lesions [10]. The system assigns a grade of 0 (normal) through IV (most severe) to the chondral area of interest. While it remains the most widespread classification system for grading cartilage lesions, it has inconsistent reliability and validation studies with larger sample sizes are required to further evaluate the system [10]. Alternatively, the system may achieve the necessary reliability of a successful classification system by incorporation of advanced imaging (MRI) [10]. The Noyes scoring system is similar to earlier systems like Outerbridge. It was developed to correct deficiencies in these earlier systems in the description of the articular surface, depth of involvement, and size and location of the lesion [11].

Magnetic resonance imaging (MRI) provides direct visualization of articular cartilage and the surrounding tissues, permitting an effective and noninvasive means of assessing cartilage status. It has superior soft-tissue contrast in comparison to other radiographic modalities, and can be used to detect and monitor longitudinal changes in cartilage due to injury or progression of degenerative disease at the tissue and joint level [5]. Advanced grading systems for MRI offer advantages over those for microscopic or macroscopic tissue assessment: In contrast to the histologic grading of a biopsy specimen, MRI can be used to assess the tissue quality of the entire repair and the surrounding cartilage, including the interface. At the macroscopic level, MRI permits evaluation of not only the cartilage surface, but also the synovium and underlying bone in a systematic manner.

A variety of semiquantitative grading systems have been developed and validated for evaluation of cartilage repair on MRI. Two cartilage repair assessment scales, Magnetic Resonance Observation of Cartilage Repair Tissue (MOCART) and Osteochondral Allograft MRI Scoring System (OCAMRISS), as well as two scales for the assessment of joint cartilage degeneration, the Whole-Organ Magnetic Resonance Imaging Score (WORMS) and MRI Osteoarthritis Knee Score (MOAKS) are reviewed, below. Additionally, quantitative MRI (qMRI) has emerged as an objective metric to evaluate cartilage quality and can provide objective measures of the biochemical composition of cartilage and cartilage repair tissue. While conventional 2D sequences can provide information about overall cartilage status, qMRI allows for assessment of early ultrastructural changes that precede morphologic changes [5].

Magnetic resonance imaging evaluation following cartilage repair requires the use of MRI sequences tailored specifically for optimization of spatial resolution and tissue contrast in musculoskeletal structures. Normal hyaline articular cartilage is organized in layers, with each layer exhibiting predictable signal characteristics due to differences in collagen structure and distribution of matrix elements such as proteoglycan. Optimized MRI sequencing permits evaluation of changes in both chondral signal and morphology. The MRI protocols for postoperative evaluation following cartilage repair must also allow evaluation of all tissues within the joint, including fibrocartilaginous structures such as menisci and labrum, bone, and synovium. This is typically achieved through a combination of fat-suppressed fluid-sensitive sequences and high-resolution morphologic images such as proton density (PD)-weighted fast spin-echo (FSE) techniques.

Parametric, or quantitative, MRI techniques provide quantitative assessment of chondral tissue relaxation times on a pixel-by-pixel basis, allowing early detection of changes in chondral matrix elements and collagen organization. Such techniques include sequences such as T1rho, which has been established as a biomarker for changes in proteoglycan content, and T2 mapping, a biomarker for changes in mobile water content and collagen orientation. Following cartilage repair, regions of interest may be placed over areas of repair tissue in order to evaluate tissue relaxation times, with the patient's normal articular cartilage serving as an internal control for comparison.

For cartilage repair, two MRI assessment scales have been developed. Magnetic Resonance Observation of Cartilage Repair Tissue (MOCART) is a grading system for the assessment of repairs using allograft cartilage or autologous chondrocyte implantation. This system is based on the assessment of nine imaging features in the chondral repair tissue, subchondral bone, and synovium (Table 3.1, Fig. 3.2). The Osteochondral Allograft MRI Scoring System (OCAMRISS) is a similar scoring system for the assessment of osteochondral grafts. The OCAMRISS includes 13 imaging variables measuring cartilage and global joint health, as well as features relevant to incorporation of the osseous portion of the graft to the host bone (Table 3.1, Fig. 3.3). These systems do not mea-

Table 3.1 Examples of MR imaging features utilized in grading systems for evaluation of cartilage repair (reproduced with permission from Burge et al. [12])

MOCART	OCAMRISS
Degree of fill	Cartilage signal
Cartilage integration	Degree of fill
Surface integrity	Cartilage integration
Tissue structure	Surface congruity
Tissue intensity	Tidemark integrity
Subchondral plate	Subchondral congruity
Subchondral bone	Subchondral edema
Adhesions	Osseous integration
Synovitis	Cystic changes
	Opposing cartilage
	Meniscal tear
	Synovitis
	Fat pad scarring

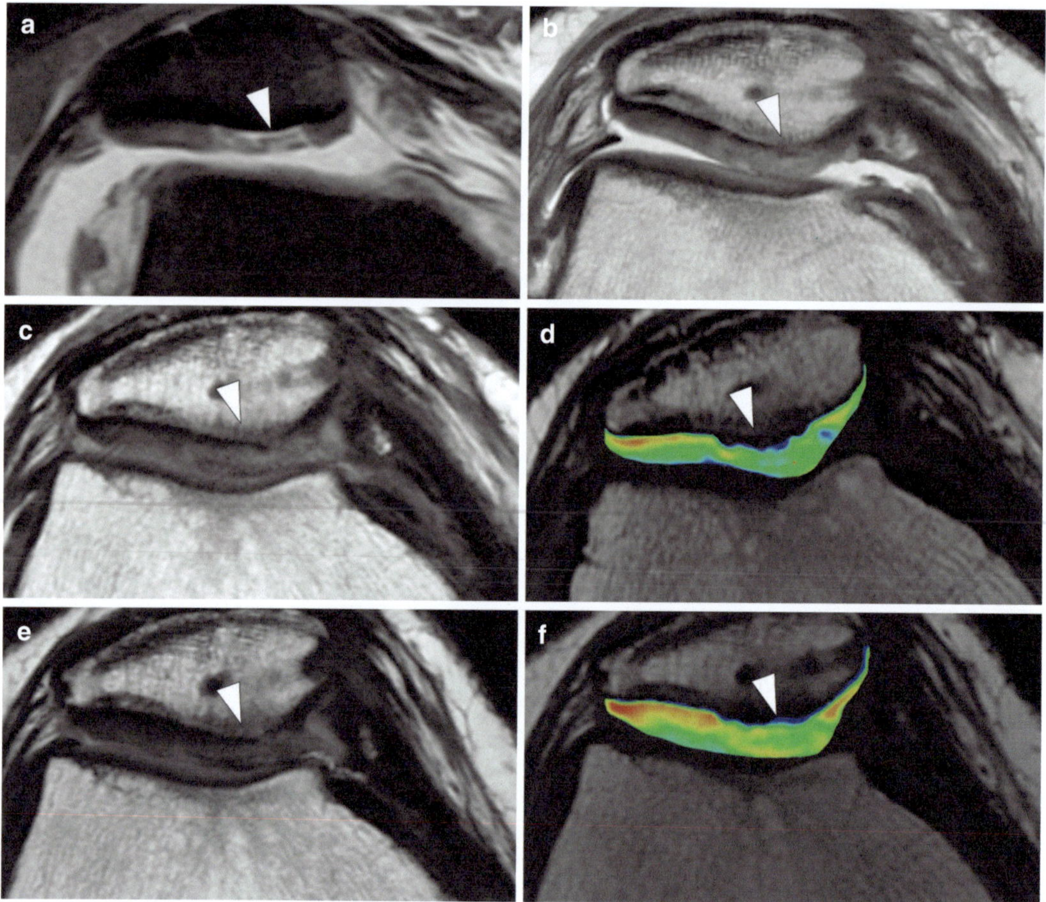

Fig. 3.2 Magnetic resonance imaging features following chondrocyte repair. (**a**) Axial T2 fat-saturated image in a 25-year-old woman following lateral patellar dislocation demonstrates chondral shear over the patellar apex (white arrowhead). (**b**) Axial PD FSE obtained 3 months following cartilage repair utilizing particulated juvenile allograft cartilage demonstrates fill of the previous defect by hyperintense repair tissue, which lacks the normal stratification of cartilage, but which is a normal appearance for the postoperative timeframe. Subsequent axial (**c**) PD FSE and (**d**) T2 map images obtained 6 months following cartilage repair demonstrate persistent graft hyperintensity with corresponding prolongation of relaxation times on mapping images (white arrowheads); however, graft signal appears relatively decreased compared to the prior study. Axial (**e**) PD FSE and (**f**) T2 map images obtained 1 year following repair demonstrate further decrease in graft signal intensity, with reduced prolongation of relaxation times since the prior study, and the suggestion of developing early chondral stratification (white arrowheads) on mapping images

Fig. 3.3 Magnetic resonance imaging features following osteochondral graft repair. Sagittal (**a**) IR and (**b**) PD FSE images in a 25-year-old man 2 years following osteochondral allograft repair of the lateral femoral condyle demonstrate overall good fill with restoration of the articular surface contour; however, there is pronounced edema with areas of cystic change along the osseous margins of the graft, and a focal linear hyperintense cleft along the subchondral plate at the posterior aspect of the graft (white arrowheads), suggesting developing subchondral delamination. Subsequent sagittal (**c**) IR and (**d**) PD FSE images obtained 1 year later demonstrate complete delamination yielding in situ osteochondral fragment (white arrowheads). Sagittal (**e**) IR and (**f**) PD FSE images obtained 6 months status post-interval revision allograft repair demonstrate excellent fill by repair tissue with restoration of the articular surface contour (white arrowheads). Subsequent sagittal (**g**) IR and (**h**) PD FSE images obtained 2 years following graft revision demonstrate persistent excellent fill (white arrowheads) with progressive osseous incorporation of the osseous portion of the graft

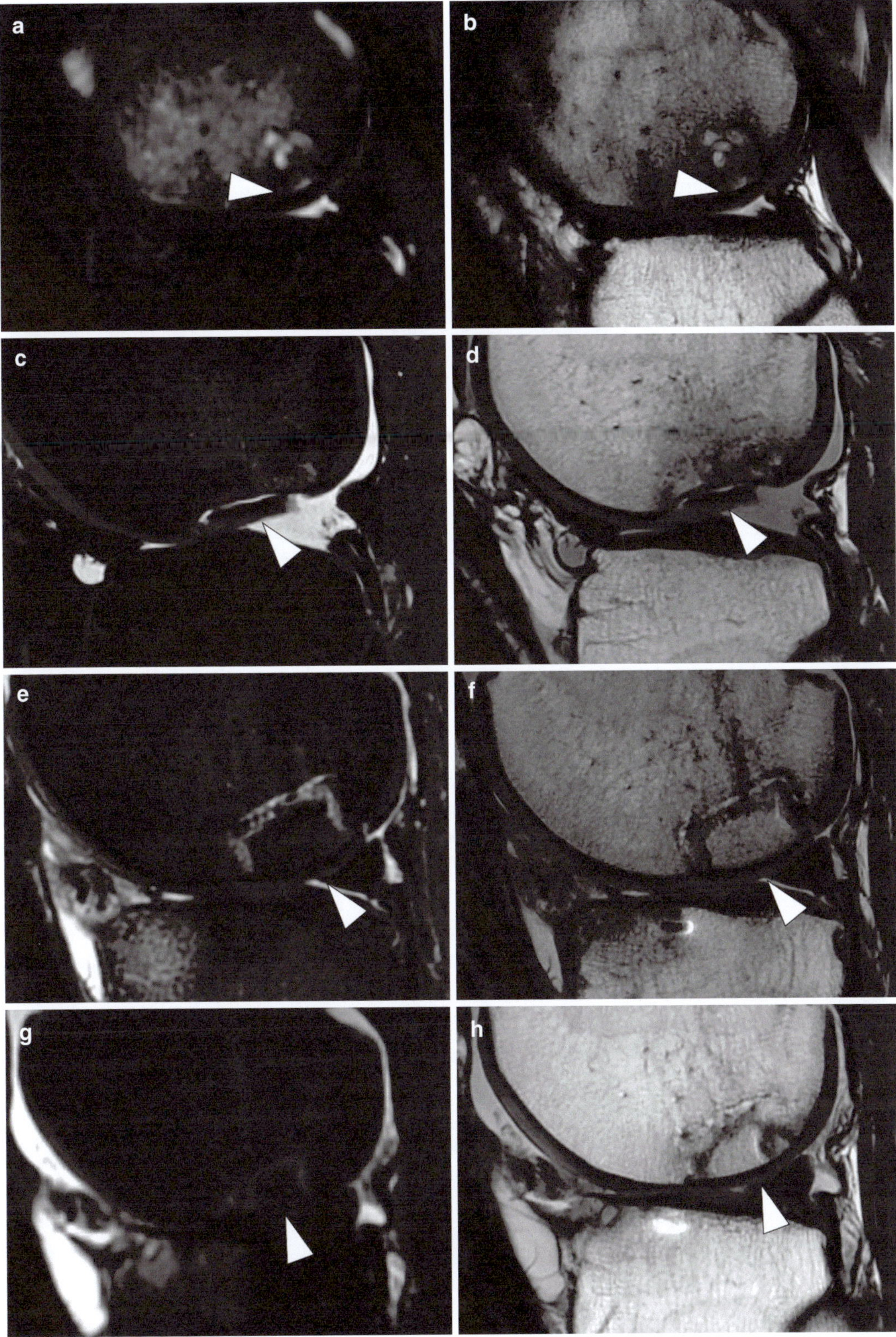

sure exactly the same parameters as microscopic grading schemes, but can provide detailed information about tissue quality and structure in a much more objective manner, as unlike small biopsies, the MRI image encompasses the entire repair. The ability to examine the interface between repair and surrounding tissue is also a strong advantage of MRI-based assessment.

Two additional MRI scales are useful for assessing global joint degeneration in the setting of cartilage repair. The Whole-Organ Magnetic Resonance Imaging Score (WORMS) is a method for semiquantitatively assessing knee MRIs for structural changes related to osteoarthritis, and has been widely used in clinical and epidemiological studies [13]. Articular surface features are scored in five subregions for WORMS. Morphological lesions of cartilage thinning or focal loss in each subregion are scored using a 7-point scale describing the areal extent of partial-thickness and full-thickness loss with one score [13]. Meniscal lesions are scored separately for the body and each horn of both menisci. For subchondral bone marrow lesions, the score assigned to each of the anatomic subregions reflects the volume of the subregion occupied by diffuse edema-like bone marrow lesion. The MRI Osteoarthritis Knee Score (MOAKS) is another semiquantitative cartilage measurement system on MRI. MOAKS uses a two-digit score for cartilage assessment that incorporates both area size per subregion and percentage of subregion affected by full-thickness cartilage loss [14].

Following cartilage repair, a grading system should ideally consider more than just the status of the repaired tissue. The most informative systems can model joint morphology quantitatively including measurements of cartilage thickness and volume. Thickness measurements, as well as other indicators of joint degeneration, are particularly helpful for longitudinal evaluation of the success of the repair in forestalling the onset and progression of osteoarthritis [5].

3.4 Best Subjective Measures

Subjective measures can be used to document the physicians' or patients' observations. Although physician grading may be useful for following individual patients, physicians' assessments are easily biased by their desire for good outcomes for their patients. In the context of knee arthroscopy, it has become clear that the relationship between impairment of the joint as traditionally measured by the clinician and patient-reported outcome is not direct [15]. Therefore, there is an emerging consensus that a patient's perspective regarding the outcome of a surgical intervention should serve as the primary outcome [15]. In knee arthroscopy and orthopedic sports medicine, generally, where many patients are young and/or active, measures of return to activity have risen to particular significance [15]. Validated PROMs are an excellent means to capture patients' perspectives in a quantitative manner without interpretation by a physician, researcher, or anyone else. These surveys have been validated not only for relevant knee-related outcomes, but also for their electronic administration [16], allowing for the assessment of large cohorts.

A recent systematic review of patient-reported outcome measures for the knee recommended the use of the International Knee Documentation Committee (IKDC) subjective knee score, the Knee Injury and Osteoarthritis Outcome Score (KOOS), and Lysholm Knee score for focal chondral defects based on psychometric data [17]. These are reviewed below. The Tegner and Marx surveys, which assess activity level, are particularly useful because of the young, active cartilage repair patient population, and are also included in our review. These PROMs are summarized in Table 3.2.

The purpose of the IKDC subjective knee score is to detect improvement or deterioration in symptoms, function, and sports activities due to knee impairment. It includes 18 items: 7 items on symptoms, 1 on sports, 9 on daily activities, and

Table 3.2 Knee-related patient-reported outcome measures (PROMs) for assessment of cartilage injury and repair

PROM	Number of questions	Domains/subscales	Scoring range
Knee-specific surveys			
International Knee Documentation Committee (IKDC) Subjective Knee Score	18	1. Symptoms 2. Sports 3. Daily activities 4. Current knee function (not included in total score)	0–100 with 100 representing highest level of function (subscales summed for aggregate score)
Knee Injury and Osteoarthritis Outcome Score (KOOS)	42	1. Pain 2. Symptoms 3. Function in daily living (ADL) 4. Function in sport and recreation (sport/rec) 5. Knee-related quality of life (QoL)	0–100 with 0 representing extreme knee problems and 100 representing no knee problems (five subscales scored separately)
Western Ontario and McMaster Universities Osteoarthritis Index (WOMAC)	24	1. Pain 2. Stiffness 3. Physical function	0–96 with 96 representing a higher level of pain, stiffness, and functional limitations (subscales summed for aggregate score)
Lysholm Knee Score	8	1. Limp 2. Support 3. Locking 4. Instability 5. Pain 6. Swelling 7. Stair climbing 8. Squatting	0–100 with 100 indicating highest function without knee symptoms or disability (scores for each domain summed for aggregate score)
Activity surveys			
Tegner Activity Score	1	Activity based on work and sports activities	0–10 with 0 representing disability due to knee symptoms and 10 representing participation in national or international elite-level soccer/football/rugby
Marx Activity Scale	4	1. Running 2. Deceleration 3. Cutting 4. Pivoting	0–16 with a higher score representing more frequent participation in the four knee functions (scores for each function summed for aggregate score)

1 on current knee function (not included in the total score). The scores for each item are summed to give a total score, with the maximum score of 100 indicating no limitation with daily or sporting activities and absence of symptoms. For patients who have had surgical intervention for cartilage injury, the IKDC shows moderate effect sizes at 6 months and large effect sizes at 1 year [7]. The minimal clinically important difference (MCID) is reported to be 6.3 points at 6 months and 16.7 points at 12 months following cartilage repair [18]. The IKDC's responsiveness to change following surgical interventions is one of its major strengths, along with the relevance of its domains to patients. However, the use of one aggregate score may mask deficits in one domain, and for highly active patients, return to sport may not be adequately assessed.

The KOOS is used to measure patients' opinions about their knee and associated problems over short- and long-term follow-up (1 week to decades). It includes five domains: pain frequency and severity during functional activities, symptoms (e.g., swelling, stiffness, catching), difficulty experienced during activities of daily living, difficulty experienced with sport and recreational activities, and knee-related quality of life. The five dimensions are scored separately, enhancing clinical interpretation. This also ensures content validity in groups of different ages and functional activity levels [7]. Other strengths of the KOOS include its reliability and validity across multiple languages and its high content validity, as patients with knee conditions were directly involved in its development. Additionally, the KOOS is particularly well suited following cartilage surgery because it contains all of the items of the Western Ontario and McMaster Universities Arthritis Scale (WOMAC), the most commonly used PROM for osteoarthritis. As such, it can provide insight into longitudinal studies regarding the development of secondary osteoarthritis [17].

Although the Lysholm Knee Scoring Scale is recommended in the setting of cartilage repair, based on its psychometric properties [17], it is surgeon derived and therefore may be the most useful for clinicians following their own patients, rather than for researchers assessing overall treatment success and patient satisfaction. The Lysholm Knee Scoring Scale has large effect sizes reported 1–6 years following microfracture [7]. It assesses eight items: limp, support, locking, instability, pain, swelling, stair climbing, and squatting.

Two more scales that have been widely reported following cartilage surgery, particularly in highly active populations, are the Tegner and Marx Activity Scales. Both scales can be used to describe general recreational activity before and after surgery as well as to assess the level of return to sport. The Marx scale may be preferred over the Tegner because it queries functional instead of sports-specific activity [17]. The Marx scale focuses on four activity points: running, deceleration, cutting, and pivoting. The recall period is over the past year and patients are asked to indicate approximately how many times they performed each of these activities at their healthiest and most active state. The scale has been extensively studied, validated, and internationally used [19].

3.5 Future Opportunities

While our modern objective and subjective measures would be almost unrecognizable to the early orthopedic surgeon carefully writing down his/her observations on his/her patients' conditions in his/her notebook by candle light, likewise these new methods may have seemed unnecessary or unbelievable to our forebears of just a couple generations before. As summarized above, the powerful combination of objective, MRI-based measurements and subjective PROMs provides clinicians and researchers with rigorous quantitative assessment tools to follow progress in single patients and to investigate therapeutic efficacy in large populations after cartilage repair. These tools will be particularly useful in assessing novel therapies such as the implantation of stem cells, scaffolds, or other biologics. Furthermore, continuing technological advances promise even more accurate and specific measurements in the near future, as we discuss below.

In a conversation with Dr. Wilson shortly before his passing, our senior author shared the details of a recent study using smartphones to evaluate patient mobility recovery after total-hip replacement [20]. Dr. Wilson listened patiently. He then smiled, shook his head, and said simply, "Who'd have thought it possible? Well, these are your problems to solve. I won't be here." And yet smartphone monitoring of patient activity is now common as wearable technologies have proven to be reliable measurement tools for monitoring patient movements [21]. These technologies, such as the Apple Watch, can measure heart rate [22] while others can even monitor sweat pH in real time [23]. The future of these wearable technologies seems bright as a tool for moving much of our previously subjectively measured patient outcomes into the objective digital domain.

Next-generation MRI and increasingly sophisticated MRI algorithms are also already being introduced. The 7 Tesla MRI should provide better resolution and faster scans to make MRI an even more useful clinical and research tool. Machine learning and other advanced computing methodologies may yield highly objective methodologies for analyzing these images with ever greater clinically relevant detail.

If you have ever had a study idea in which you said to yourself "If only we could measure X …" perhaps it is time to revisit that pipe dream. The technology may have arrived or may be on the horizon. Indeed, these are our problems to solve.

References

1. Wilson PD, Amstutz HC, Salvati EA, Mendes DG. Total hip replacement with fixation by acrylic cement: a preliminary study of 100 consecutive McKee-Farrar prosthetic replacements. J Bone Joint Surg. 1972;54A:207–36.
2. Wilson PD, Wong L, Lee Y, et al. Total hip arthroplasty performed for coxarthrosis preserves long-term physical function: a 40-year experience. HSS J. 2019;15:122–32.
3. Piedade SR, Filho MF, Ferreira DM, Slullitel DA, Patnaik S, Samitier G, Maffulli N. PROMs in sports medicine. In: Rocha Piedade S, Imhoff A, Clatworth M, Cohen M, Espregueira-Mendes J, editors. The sports medicine physician. Springer; 2019. p. 685–95.
4. Gagnier JJ. Patient reported outcomes in orthopaedics. J Orthop Res. 2017;35(10):2098–108.
5. Argentieri EC, Burge AJ, Potter HG. Magnetic resonance imaging of articular cartilage within the knee. J Knee Surg. 2018;31(2):155–65.
6. Lansdown DA, Wang K, Cotter E, Davey A, Cole BJ. Relationship between quantitative MRI biomarkers and patient-reported outcome measures after cartilage repair surgery: a systematic review. Orthop J Sports Med. 2018;6(4):2325967118765448.
7. Collins NJ, Misra D, Felson DT, Crossley KM, Roos EM. Measures of knee function: International Knee Documentation Committee (IKDC) Subjective Knee Evaluation Form, Knee Injury and Osteoarthritis Outcome Score (KOOS), Knee Injury and Osteoarthritis Outcome Score Physical Function Short Form (KOOS-PS), Knee Outcome Survey Activities of Daily Living Scale (KOS-ADL), Lysholm Knee Scoring Scale, Oxford Knee Score (OKS), Western Ontario and McMaster Universities Osteoarthritis Index (WOMAC), Activity Rating Scale (ARS), and Tegner Activity Score (TAS). Arthritis Care Res (Hoboken). 2011;63:S208–28.
8. Borne MP, Raijmakers N, Vanlauwe J, Victor J, Jong S, Bellemans J, Saris DBF. International cartilage repair society (ICRS) and Oswestry macroscopic cartilage evaluation scores validated for use in autologous chondrocyte implantation (ACI) and microfracture 1. Osteoarth Cartilage. 2008;15:1397–402.
9. Rutgers M, van Pelt MJ, Dhert WJ, Creemers LB, Saris DB. Evaluation of histological scoring systems for tissue-engineered, repaired and osteoarthritic cartilage. Osteoarthr Cartil. 2010;18(1):12–23.
10. Slattery C, Kweon CY. Classifications in brief: outerbridge classification of chondral lesions. Clin Orthop Relat Res. 2018;476(10):2101–4.
11. Noyes FR, Stabler CL. A system for grading articular cartilage lesions at arthroscopy. Am J Sports Med. 1989;17(4):505–13.
12. Burge AJ, Potter HGP. Imaging of failed cartilage repair. Operat Techn Sports Med. 2020;28(1):1–10.
13. Lynch JA, Roemer FW, Nevitt MC, et al. Comparison of BLOKS and WORMS scoring systems part I. cross sectional comparison of methods to assess cartilage morphology, meniscal damage and bone marrow lesions on knee MRI: data from the osteoarthritis initiative. Osteoarthr Cartil. 2010;18(11):1393–401.
14. Roemer FW, Guermazi A, Collins JE, et al. Semi-quantitative MRI biomarkers of knee osteoarthritis progression in the FNIH biomarkers consortium cohort-methodologic aspects and definition of change. BMC Musculoskelet Disord. 2016;17(1):466.
15. Irrgang JJ, Lubowitz JH. Measuring arthroscopic outcome. Arthroscopy. 2008;24(6):718–22.
16. Nguyen J, Marx R, Hidaka C, Wilson S, Lyman S. Validation of electronic administration of knee surveys among ACL-injured patients. Knee Surg Sports Traumatol Arthrosc. 2017 Oct 1;25(10):3116–22.
17. Wang D, Jones MH, Khair MM, et al. Patient reported outcome measures for the knee. J Knee Surg. 2010;23:137151.
18. Greco NJ, Anderson AF, Mann BJ, Cole BJ, Farr J, Nissen CW, et al. Responsiveness of the International Knee Documentation Committee subjective knee form in comparison to the Western Ontario and Mc-Master Universities Osteoarthritis Index, modified Cincinnati knee rating system, and short form 36 in patients with focal articular cartilage defects. Am J Sports Med. 2010;38:891–902.
19. Kanakamedala AC, Anderson AF, Irrgang JJ. IKDC subjective knee form and Marx activity rating scale are suitable to evaluate all orthopaedic sports medicine knee conditions: a systematic review. J ISAKOS. 2016;1:25–31.
20. Mehta N, Steiner C, Fields KG, Nawabi DH, Lyman SL. Using mobile tracking technology to visualize the trajectory of recovery after hip arthroscopy: a case report. HSS J. 2017;13(2):194–200.
21. Henriksen A, Haugen Mikalsen M, Woldaregay AZ, et al. Using fitness trackers and smartwatches to measure physical activity in research: analysis of consumer wrist-worn wearables. J Med Internet Res. 2018;20(3):e110.
22. Chow HW, Yang CC. Accuracy of optical heart rate sensing technology in wearable fitness trackers for young and older adults: validation and comparison study. JMIR Mhealth Uhealth. 2020;8(4):e14707.
23. Chung M, Fortunato G, Radacsi N. Wearable flexible sweat sensors for healthcare monitoring: a review. J R Soc Interface. 2019;16(159):20190217.

Quantitative Magnetic Resonance Imaging of Articular Cartilage Structure and Biology

4

Karyn E. Chappell, Ashley A. Williams, and Constance R. Chu

4.1 Introduction

Cartilage injury treatment remains a clinical challenge for which compositional magnetic resonance imaging (MRI) techniques can play an important role in the assessment of tissue damage and monitoring of treatment effects.

This chapter discusses semiquantitative joint scoring systems and quantitative compositional MRI techniques. In particular, the utility of compositional MRI in identifying how the tissue properties differ due to the structure and biology of articular cartilage is examined. The tissue properties of articular cartilage can be probed with different compositional MRI techniques including (i) semiquantitative cartilage morphology grading, (ii) T2 mapping, (iii) ultrashort echo times (UTE), (iv) dGEMRIC, and (v) T1rho (T1ρ). The magic angle effect—an inherent tissue property—that affects the majority of MRI techniques is also explained.

K. E. Chappell · A. A. Williams
Department of Orthopaedic Surgery, School of
Medicine, Stanford University, Stanford, CA, USA
e-mail: karynchappell@stanford.edu;
ashelyaw@stanford.edu

C. R. Chu (✉)
Department of Orthopaedic Surgery, School of
Medicine, Stanford University, Stanford, CA, USA

Department of Orthopaedic Surgery, Stanford
Medicine, Redwood City, CA, USA
e-mail: chucr@stanford.edu

4.2 Overview: Normal Cartilage Structure and Biology

Normal adult human articular cartilage is a complex composite material capable of withstanding and distributing compressive loads to subchondral bones. The articulating surfaces move on each other with minimal wear and friction. Articular cartilage also serves as a barrier separating bones from synovial fluid [1]. At the molecular level, cartilage consists of cells, a collagen fiber network, proteoglycans, and fluid containing mobile ions [2].

By weight, cartilage is approximately 60–85% water enmeshed in a network of mainly type II collagen fibers containing non-collagenous macromolecules (proteoglycan and hyaluronic acid), smaller non-collagenous matrix proteins, and cells [3, 4]. The collagen fibers make up the extracellular matrix (ECM), entrapping macromolecules and cells, and then lending tensile strength to the tissue [5, 6]. Scanning electron microscopy reveals that the architecture of the ECM varies depth-wise with different arrangements of the collagen fibrils at different depths [4, 7]. In adult human cartilage, four prominent zones are apparent; see Fig. 4.1:

1. Superficial or tangential zone: a thin sheet of collagen fibrils primarily arranged parallel to the cartilage surface, typically only 100–200 μm thick.

© ISAKOS 2021
A. J. Krych et al. (eds.), *Cartilage Injury of the Knee*,
https://doi.org/10.1007/978-3-030-78051-7_4

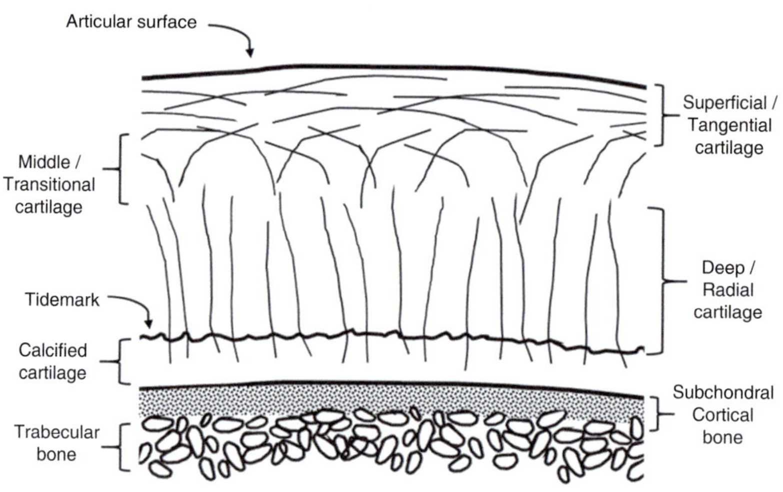

Fig. 4.1 Cartilage extracellular matrix architecture

2. Middle or transitional zone: collagen fibrils from the superficial layer bend or "arcade" into the cartilage midsubstance and demonstrate a more random orientation, typically accounting for 40–60% of the total tissue depth.
3. Deep or radial zone: collagen fiber bundle becomes radially arranged, perpendicular to the bone-cartilage interface and root in the calcified cartilage, where a distinct tidemark distinguishing the interface between calcified and noncalcified cartilage is apparent by histology. The deep zone typically accounts for 30–50% of the total tissue depth.
4. Calcified cartilage zone: a highly mineralized region acting as an interface between bone and cartilage. Accounts for around 3–8% of the total cartilage thickness and is separated from the overlying cartilage and the subchondral bone [8, 9].

Proteoglycans (PG) account for 4–10% of cartilage wet weight [3, 4]. PG also exhibits a strong depth-dependent distribution: the density of PG increases with depth plateauing in the deep zone [4]. Cartilage derives its compressive strength from water molecules attracted to glycosaminoglycan (GAG), a constituent of PG, in the ECM.

Numerous ionized and negatively charged side groups residing on GAG molecules cause the GAG side chains to repel each, while attracting water molecules [10]. Considerable osmotic pressures result from water in the ECM that are responsible for the remarkable compressive strength of articular cartilage [6].

Chondrocytes constitute only a small fraction of total cartilage tissue volume but are actively involved in maintaining tissue mechanical integrity. They regulate collagen and PG, sensing the mechanical environment to modify the PG in response to changing loads [3, 10]. Distribution and morphology of chondrocytes are depth dependent. Numerous small flat cells are present in the superficial cartilage. Moderately sized rounded cells occur in the middle zone, while fewer columns of larger elongated cells are present in the deep zone [11].

Interstitial water exists in two primary "pools" within the articular cartilage: the "free" water (approximately 70%) and the "bound" intrafibrillar water (approximately 30%) surrounding the collagen fibrils. The relative distribution and mobility of water in these pools have implications for MRI of articular cartilage primarily dedicated to proton imaging.

4.2.1 Trilaminar Appearance by Magnetic Resonance Imaging

Early MR appearance of articular cartilage was described as having a single layer of uniform intensity [12, 13]. As MR scanner strength increased, a bilaminar appearance of articular cartilage was reported [14, 15], consisting of a thin hyperintense outer layer and a thicker hypointense inner layer.

When field strengths increased to 1.5 T, Modl et al. [16] reported the first trilaminar appearance on both T1-W and T2-W images of patellar cartilage. Three distinct layers were now seen: a superficial low-intensity layer, a middle intermediate- to high-intensity layer, and a deep low-intensity layer at the bone cartilage interface. The variation in intensity was suggested to result from the collagen fibril orientation in the histological zones, drawing on the findings from Lehner et al. [17] bovine study. The collagen fibril anisotropy of the superficial and deep zone provided different intensities as the fibrils are oriented at ~90° to one another while the middle zone is randomly oriented.

Rubenstein et al. [18] confirmed that the signal intensity variations were dependent on the orientation of the collagen fibrils to the static magnetic field. A trilaminar appearance occurred when fibrils were aligned with the magnetic field. However the trilaminar appearance disappeared when collagen fibrils were rotated to 55°, the minimum dipolar coupling to the magnetic field. Now the cartilage had a uniform homogenous intensity because the superficial and deep zones behaved in the same way as the middle zone (Fig. 4.2). This experiment provided a direct observation of the "magic angle" effect in cartilage. The "magic angle" effect in cartilage manifests as an overall increase in the T2 relaxation time in the superficial and deep zones. The trilaminar MR appearance in cartilage was strongly influenced by the anisotropic organization of the collagen fibrils and their orientation relative to the magnetic field.

Henkelman et al. [19] identified that there was a strong orientation dependence of the T2 in bovine cartilage at different angles to the main field. Different T2 relaxation rates were noted at different angles for different layers of tissue. Xia [20] μMRI studies provided greater understanding of the T2 relaxation of cartilage showing it to be both depth dependent and orientation dependent. This raises the possibility of using T2 to determine the structural characteristics of carti-

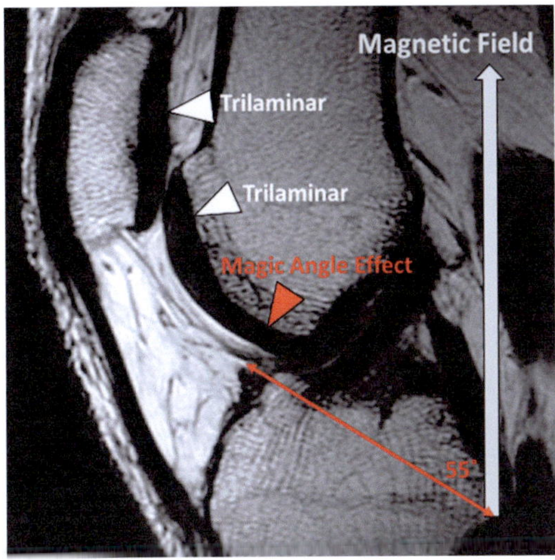

Fig. 4.2 A PD FSE sagittal knee image. The patellar cartilage and part of the femoral cartilage have a trilaminar appearance (white arrows) where collagen fibrils are aligned or perpendicular to the magnetic field. When the collagen fibrils are aligned around 55° they have a homogenous appearance (red arrow) due to the magic angle effect

lage such as in T2 mapping and UTE-T2* which will be described in more detail below.

It must be noted that the trilaminar appearance only occurs in healthy unloaded articular cartilage. The anisotropic organization of the superficial and deep zones changes in degenerative and compressed articular cartilage [21, 22].

4.3 Quantitative Magnetic Resonance Imaging Strategies to Noninvasively Assess and Monitor Cartilage Structure and Biology

MRI can visualize and measure articular cartilage changes before the gross changes to bone and joint space observed with radiography occur. Moreover, MRI is noninvasive and nondestructive and uses nonionizing radiation capable of visualizing tissues deep to the body surface. *Quantitative* MRI is a subspecialty of MR concerned with deriving quantitative measurements. Quantitative MRI techniques evaluate cartilage surface disruption, subsurface lesions, cartilage thickness loss, and compositional changes to the extracellular matrix.

4.3.1 Semiquantitative Assessments of Cartilage Morphology

Semiquantitative morphologic cartilage grading translates subjective image assessments into numbers for comparison across regions, subjects, cohorts, or longitudinally over time. Morphologic features of cartilage injury observed on MRI can be semi-quantitated using scoring systems specifically designed for cartilage, for example:

1. Modified versions of the Outerbridge for which the description by Potter (Table 4.1) is particularly relevant to MRI [23], ICRS (International Cartilage Repair Society) [24], or Noyes [25] scoring systems, derived from arthroscopic grading schemes
2. Chondromalacia patellae score [12] to describe defects pre-surgery
3. CaLS (Cartilage Lesion Score) [26] for longitudinal tracking of cartilage lesions
4. AMADEUS (Area Measurement and Depth and Underlying Structure) for assessment of preoperative cartilage and subchondral bone defect severity [27]

    Morphologic features of cartilage injury can also be semi-quantitated from subscores specific to cartilage within whole-joint scoring systems such as:
5. WORMS (Whole-Organ MRI Score) [28] or MOAKS [29] for cartilage assessment in the knee
6. SHOMRI (Scoring Hip Osteoarthritis with MRI) [30] for cartilage assessment in the hip

    Several semiquantitative scoring systems specific for postoperative evaluation of cartilage repair tissues have been developed:
7. MOCART (the Magnetic Resonance Observation of Cartilage Repair Tissue) [31] to assess repaired cartilage, Table 4.2
8. CROAKS (Cartilage Repair Osteoarthritis Knee Score) [32] for integrative assessment of

Table 4.1 Modified Outerbridge cartilage scoring system

Modified Outerbridge score[a]	Cartilage appearance on intermediate-weighted fast spin-echo MRI
0	Intact cartilage with normal signal
1	Increased signal intensity with no loss of cartilage thickness
2	Loss of cartilage thickness affecting less than 50% of the cartilage thickness
3	Loss of greater than 50% of the cartilage thickness without exposed bone
4	Full-thickness cartilage loss with exposed bone

[a]Adapted from Potter et al., Cartilage injury after acute, isolated anterior cruciate ligament tear: immediate and longitudinal effect with clinical/MRI follow-up. Am J Sports Med. 2012 Feb;40(2):276–85

both cartilage repair site and whole-joint recovery

Accurate morphologic assessment requires appropriate pulse sequence selection. Cartilage surface disruptions, lesions, and thinning are best observed with fluid-sensitive, fat-saturated T2-weighted, intermediate-weighted or proton density-weighted sequences acquired in three orthogonal planes. Additionally, T1-weighted sequences in at least one plane are recommended to provide intrasubstance cartilage detail.

4.4 Cartilage Morphometry

Quantitative MRI assessment of cartilage thickness and volume is termed cartilage "morphometry." MRI detects morphometric cartilage changes with more sensitivity than the indirect clinical standard of radiographic joint space narrowing [33]. For cartilage morphometry, clear delineation of both bone-cartilage and bone-synovium interfaces is required. Good boundary contrast is provided by T1-weighted fat-suppressed gradient-echo sequences with thin slices and close to isotropic resolution such as spoiled gradient recalled acquisition (SPGR),

Table 4.2 MOCART—Cartilage repair tissue assessment: grading scale

Variables

1. Degree of defect repair and filling of the defect

Complete (on a level with adjacent cartilage)

Hypertrophy (over the level of the adjacent cartilage)

Incomplete (under the level of the adjacent cartilage; underfilling):

   >50% of the adjacent cartilage

   <50% of the adjacent cartilage

   Subchondral bone exposed (complete delamination or dislocation or loose body)

2. Integration to border zone

Complete (complete integration with adjacent cartilage)

Incomplete (incomplete integration with adjacent cartilage)

   Demarcating border visible (split-like)

   Defect visible:

      <50% of the length of the repair tissue

      >50% of the length of the repair tissue

3. Surface of the repair tissue

Surface intact (lamina splendens intact)

Surface damaged (fibrillations, fissures, and ulcerations):

   <50% of repair tissue depth

   >50% of repair tissue depth or total degeneration

4. Structure of the repair tissue

Homogenous

Inhomogeneous or cleft formation

5. Signal intensity of the repair tissue

Dual T2-FSE:

   Isointense

   Moderately hyperintense

   Markedly hyperintense

3D-GE-FS:

   Isointense

   Moderately hypointense

   Markedly hypointense

6. Subchondral lamina

Intact

Not intact

7. Subchondral bone

Intact

Edema

Granulation tissue, cysts, sclerosis

8. Adhesions

No

Yes

9. Effusion

No

Yes

fast low-angle shot water excitation (FLASH), and dual-echo steady state (DESS) [33]. To date, most morphometric studies of cartilage have relied on extremely time-consuming manual cartilage segmentation. However, advances in machine learning and artificial intelligence approaches to cartilage segmentation have the potential to vastly improve the efficiency of this procedure.

4.4.1 Quantitative Assessments of Cartilage: Compositional MRI

Early changes to the composition and properties of the cartilage ECM after trauma or post-traumatic osteoarthritis are visualized with compositional imaging strategies. These precede the gross morphologic changes detected by conventional MRI. Detecting early changes identifies individuals most likely to benefit from therapeutic interventions. The most prominent MRI techniques to spatially map cartilage composition include T2 for hydration and collagen ECM integrity and organization [34]; delayed gadolinium-enhanced MRI of cartilage (dGEMRIC) for relative PG distribution [35]; and T1ρ for PG content and collagen structure, although the specificity of this measure remains controversial at the low spin-lock frequencies used clinically [36, 37]. Newer but promising techniques to

further assess collagen organization of joint tissues with an abundance of short-T2 species like tendons, ligaments, menisci, and deep and calcified articular cartilage include ultrashort-echo time (UTE) imaging [9, 38] and UTE-T2* mapping [39].

4.4.1.1 T2

T2 relaxation, also known as transverse or spin-spin relaxation, is a native tissue property and measurable MRI time constant (Fig. 4.3).

T2 mapping relies on intrinsic cartilage water to probe the organization and integrity of the extracellular collagen matrix. T2 relaxation in cartilage is strongly dependent on the anisotropic organization of the collagen fibrils in the ECM, the orientation of the collagen fibrils with respect to the external magnetic field, and the tissue water content [34]. It is only weakly dependent on the magnitude of the magnetic field, with decreasing T2 times measured with increasing field strength [34]. With the cartilage surface perpendicular or parallel to the main magnet field (i.e., the long axis of clinical MRI scanners), high-resolution T2 maps of normal human cartilage demonstrate low (short) T2 values in the superficial and deep zones. This arises because highly aligned collagen fibrils facilitate efficient dipole interactions between water protons (Fig. 4.4).

Higher (longer) T2 values are observed in the middle zone where the collagen fibrils are more

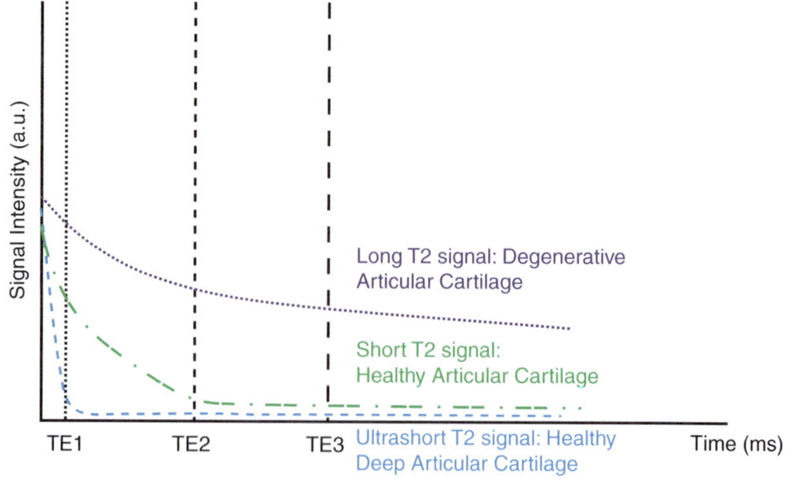

Fig. 4.3 A T2 decay graph comparing articular cartilage at 3 T. TE3 refers to long T2 signal (degenerative articular cartilage) while ultrashort T2 signal (deep articular cartilage) has TEs shorter than 1 ms. Healthy articular cartilage has short T2 signal with a range of TEs from approximately 10–80 ms

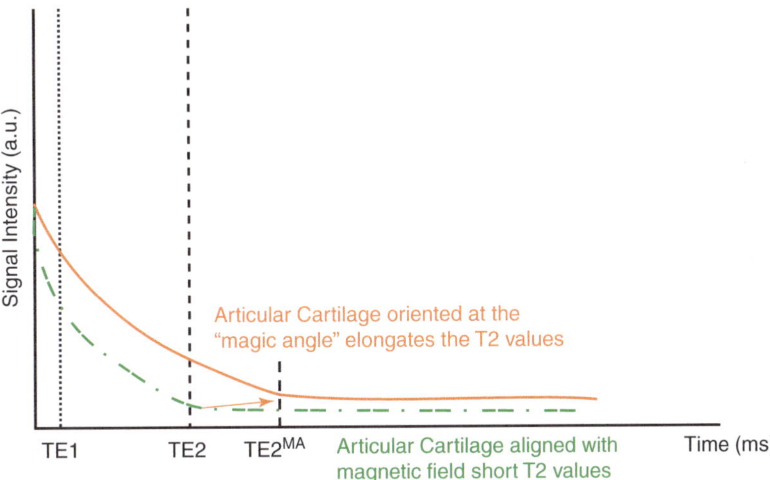

Fig. 4.4 T2 decay graph of articular cartilage aligned to the main magnetic field and at the "magic angle." The T2 is elongated at the "magic angle" (TE2^{MA})

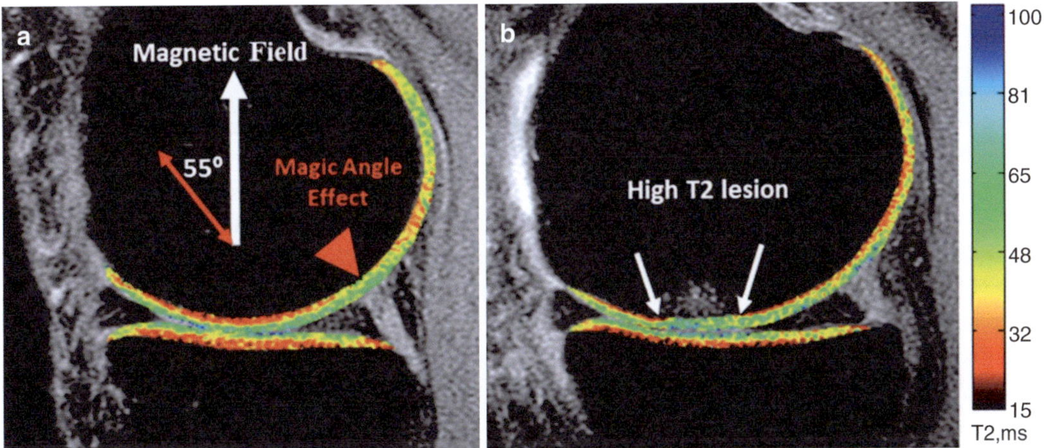

Fig. 4.5 Sample T2 maps acquired with a T2-weighted 2-D multi-echo FSE sequence (CartiGram, GE). (**a**) 53-Year-old healthy female with typical laminar T2 pattern in cartilage. Red arrowhead indicates T2 elongation due to magic angle effect. (**b**) 53-Year-old male with osteochondral dissecans and full-thickness high-T2 lesion in overlying cartilage

randomly organized and proton dipole interactions are less efficient. However, as the orientation of the cartilage fibrils with respect to the main magnetic field approaches the 55^0 "magic angle," as in anterior and posterior femoral knee cartilage observed in a sagittal view (Fig. 4.5), superficial and deep cartilage regions display elongated T2 values [34].

Departures from these expected T2 patterns indicate disruptions of collagen matrix architecture. In vivo, cartilage injury or disease resulting in disorganization of the extracellular collagen matrix typically causes an increase in measured T2 relaxation time that may manifest as a focal high-T2 lesion or global increase in T2 depending on the extent of the injury.

4.4.1.2 Ultrashort Echo Time (UTE)

UTE MRI captures T2 signals less than 1 ms. This improves the ability to visualize tissues with short-T2 components such as deepest layers of articular cartilage and menisci that are otherwise invisible by standard clinical T2 mapping and conventional musculoskeletal imaging sequences

[40]. In these tissues, long-T2 relaxation represents slow spin-spin interaction (e.g., interaction between free water molecules), while short T2 reflects fast spin-spin interaction (e.g., interaction between free and bound water molecules). UTE imaging picks up signals from both short- and long-T2 relaxations and produces hyperintensity for the deep radial zone of the knee cartilage, which usually has hypo-intensity in conventional gradient- or spin-echo images with long echo time (TE > 10 ms). Elevation of or interruption to this hypo-intense layer in deep cartilage on UTE-weighted images indicates disruption to the cartilage matrix organization at the osteochondral junction [41].

UTE-enhanced T2* (UTE-T2*) mapping, in which T2* values are calculated from a series of images with varying TEs including an UTE, is sensitive to changes in short-T2 signal (T2 < 10 ms) due to deep cartilage injury or disease [39]. 3-D in vivo UTE-T2* maps can be generated from a UTE Cones sequence (GE) [42] or an acquisition-weighted stack-of-spirals sequence (AWSOS, Siemens) [43]. Variable echo time (vTE) GRE imaging uses Cartesian k-space sampling with phase-encoding gradients to vary the effective echo time to achieve sub-millisecond

TEs for in vivo mapping of short-T2 tissues [44]. In ACL-reconstructed knees, elevated UTE-T2* values are frequently observed in deep weight-bearing cartilage as early as 2 years after ACL reconstruction surgery [45], Fig. 4.6, and are associated with known risk factors for osteoarthritis [46].

4.4.1.3 dGEMRIC

A reduction in cartilage GAG content due to injury or disease can be derived from cartilage T1 relaxation measurements in the presence of negatively charged gadolinium-based contrast agents [47–49]. Donnan theory of electrochemical neutrality dictates that negatively charged contrast distributes in cartilage in concentrations inversely proportional to the local fixed charge density (FCD) [2]. Thus, negatively charged contrast tends to be electrostatically repelled from regions of high GAG concentration while low-GAG regions admit more contrast. Measurement of the concentration of the contrast agent in cartilage (T1-Gd) allows for calculation of GAG content and visualization of the relative spatial distribution of GAG in the cartilage [49].

In clinical application of the delayed gadolinium-enhanced MRI of cartilage (dGEM-

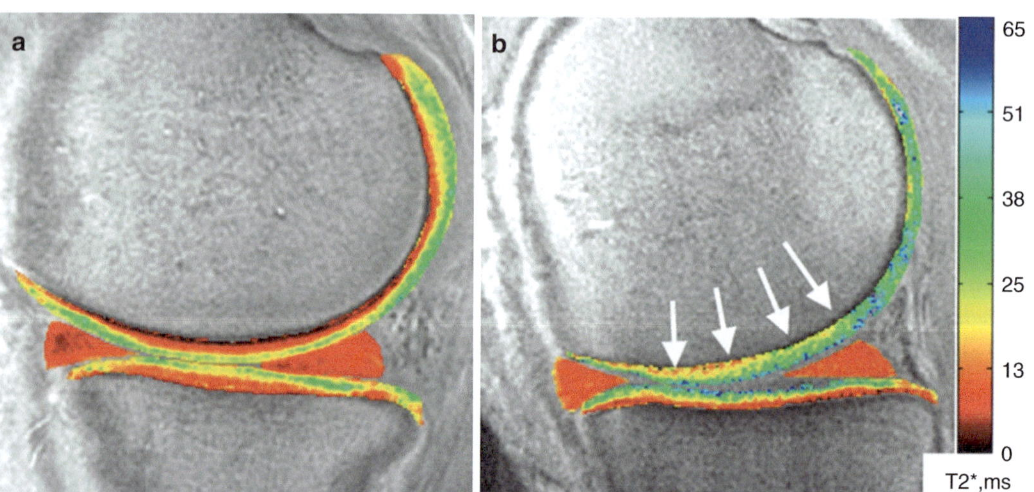

Fig. 4.6 Sample UTE-T2* maps acquired with 2 serial 4-echo Cones sequences (GE). (**a**) 20-Year-old healthy female with typical layer of low-UTE-T2* values in deep cartilage at the bone-cartilage interface. (**b**) 35-Year-old male 2 years after ACL reconstruction with no morpho-logical evidence of medial cartilage (Outerbridge grade 0) or meniscus pathology shows elevations to UTE-T2* values throughout medial femorotibial cartilage, particularly in deep medial femoral cartilage (white arrows)

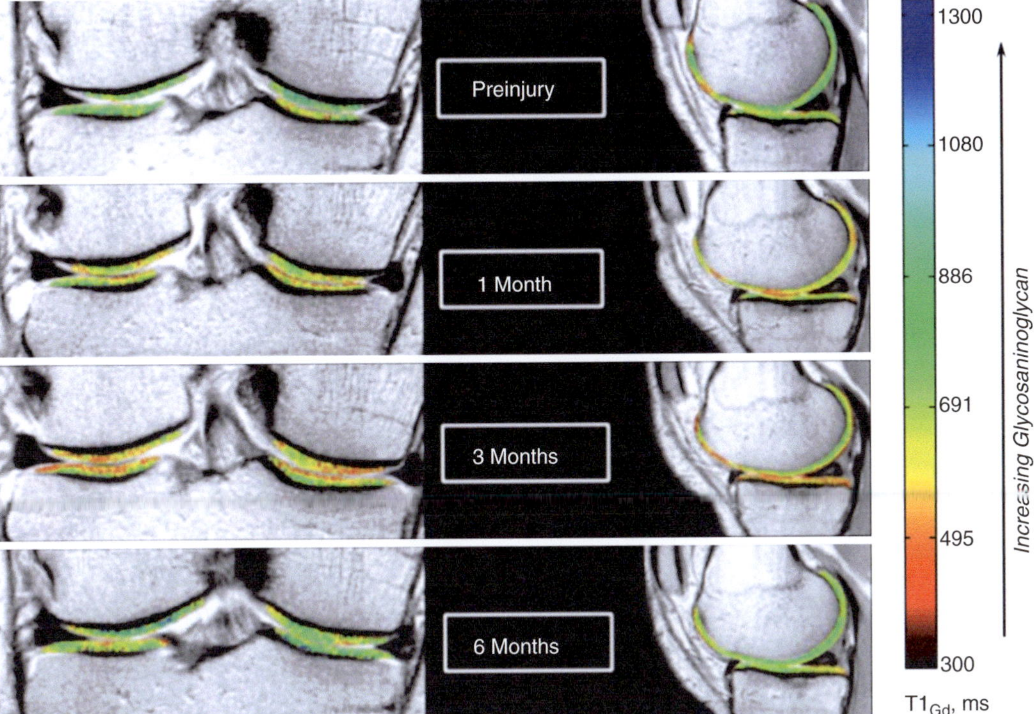

Fig. 4.7 Pre- and post-PCL-injury dGEMRIC images at 1, 3, and 6 months after the injury. dGEMRIC indices show a transient decrease, indicating a loss of cartilage GAG, which resolves to near-pre-injury levels by 6 months post-injury. Reprinted from Journal of Bone and Joint Surgery, Vol. 87, Is. 12, Young AA, et al. Glycosaminoglycan content of knee cartilage following posterior cruciate ligament rupture demonstrated by delayed gadolinium-enhanced magnetic resonance imaging of cartilage (dGEMRIC). A case report, pp. 2763–7, 2005, with permission from Wolters Kluwer Health Inc. www.ejbjs.org

RIC) technique, dGEMRIC maps show low-dGEMRIC indices (i.e., low-T1-Gd relaxation times) in regions of high contrast (low GAG), while showing high-dGEMRIC indices (i.e., high-T1-Gd relaxation times) in regions of low contrast (high GAG). Normal healthy cartilage exhibits a depth-wise increase of GAG concentration from relatively low levels in the superficial cartilage to higher levels in the deep cartilage. This corresponds with a similar depth-wise increase in dGEMRIC indices from lower values in superficial cartilage to higher values in deep cartilage. In a unique case study of an individual who suffered a posterior cruciate ligament tear in an automobile accident, a full-thickness but transient loss of GAG was observed over 6 months following the impact injury [50]; see Fig. 4.7.

dGEMRIC assessment poses challenges for implementation into routine clinical use where noncontrast MRI offers lower risk and greater acquisition efficiency. The protocol requires IV or IA administration of an anionic gadolinium-based contrast agent [35, 47, 48] followed by 10–15 min of exercise (e.g., walk or cycle on a stationary bike) to increase the delivery of the contrast to the joint [35], and then a joint-dependent delay before imaging (e.g., 90 min for knee, 60 min for hip) to facilitate contrast penetration into the cartilage [35]. Although dGEMRIC is most widely validated with the contrast agent Gd-DTPA (Magnevist) [51], Gd-BOPTA (MultiHance), an agent with lower risk for nephrogenic systemic fibrosis and nearly twofold higher relaxivity, may be preferred as it can be administered in half the dose of Gd-DTPA [47].

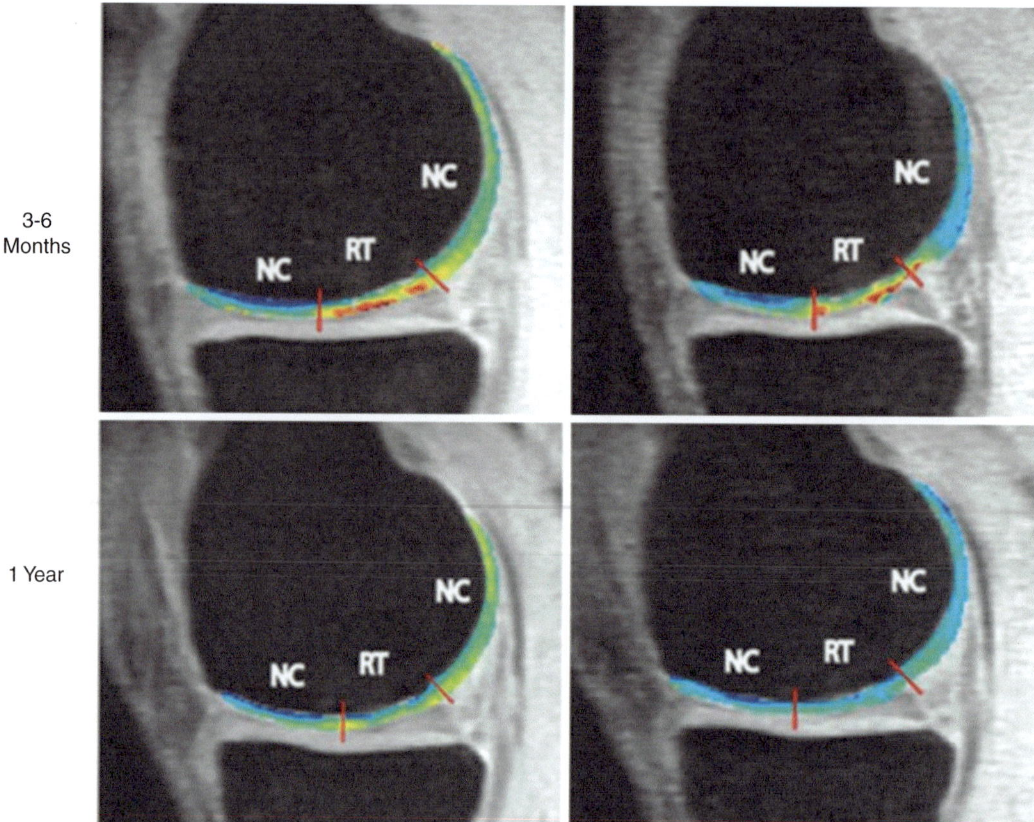

Fig. 4.8 T1ρ (left column) and T2 (right column) maps 3–6 months and 1 year after microfracture surgery. Repair tissue (RT) T1ρ and T2 appearance becomes similar to that of normal cartilage (NC) at 1 year after surgery. Reprinted from Holtzman et al. T(1ρ) and T(2) quantitative magnetic resonance imaging analysis of cartilage regeneration following microfracture and mosaicplasty cartilage resurfacing procedures. *J Magn Reson Imaging.* 2010;32(4):914–923, with permission of Wiley. © Wiley-Liss, Inc.

4.4.1.4 T1ρ

T1ρ measures longitudinal T1 relaxation (or spin-lattice relaxation) in the rotating frame, and thus is sensitive to slow-motion, low-frequency interactions between protons and local cartilage environment [52]. However the mechanism(s) governing T1ρ relaxation in cartilage are not fully understood [53]. In vitro, T1ρ has been correlated to fixed charge density in enzymatically degraded and human osteoarthritis specimens and is thought to have the potential to reflect cartilage PG content [54, 55]. But the specificity of T1ρ for cartilage PG measured in in vivo studies is much less clear [37, 56]. At 3 T and measured with spin-lock frequencies within RF power limitations and specific absorption rate (SAR) constraints, T1ρ appears to be more sensitive to tissue hydration, or a composite of cartilage matrix components of cartilage, than exclusively to PG content [37]. Despite that, T1ρ in vivo is a sensitive indicator of cartilage with established osteoarthritis as well as cartilage at risk of developing OA [56, 57], typically showing elevations in degenerate cartilage. Additionally, T1ρ has been used to monitor cartilage repair tissue recovery following mosaicplasty and microfracture [58, 59]; see Fig. 4.8.

To measure T1ρ relaxation, the net magnetization is tipped 90^0 into the transverse plane and then "spin-locked" by applying a low-energy long-duration radio-frequency (RF) pulse along the same direction. T1ρ relaxation can be assessed by a variety of commonly available sequences including 2-D or 3-D fast spin-echo (FSE) with multiple spin-lock times (i.e., typically at least four spin-lock images, with time to spin-lock (TSL) ranging from 0 to 80 ms). Similarly, 2-D or 3-D spoiled gradient echo (SPGR), 3-D gradient echo (GRE), fast low-angle shot (FLASH), balanced steady-state free precession (e.g., FISP), and 3-D magnetization-prepared angle-modulated partitioned k-space spoiled gradient echo snapshot (3-D MAPSS) [60] sequences with multiple TSL acquisitions can be used [61]. Although higher spin-lock frequency improves sensitivity to cartilage PG, spin-lock frequency is most commonly set to 500 Hertz due to RF power limitations and SAR constraints for in vivo studies.

4.4.2 Limitations of Morphologic and Compositional Cartilage MRI

Although there is generally excellent agreement between morphologic MRI assessments using fat-suppressed 3-D-SPGR or proton density-weighted FSE sequences compared to arthroscopic evaluations of cartilage damage as the gold standard [62], these techniques are relatively insensitive to subtle, subsurface changes to cartilage biochemical integrity. The primary advantage of compositional MRI is detection of changes to the composition and organization of cartilage's molecular constituents prior to gross morphologic damage. Consequently, compositional techniques are most useful in patients with subtle, mild, and early injury or disease who stand to benefit most from therapeutic interventions. By contrast, composition cartilage MRI may be less useful informing treatment decisions in patients with severe injury or advanced osteoarthritis.

Compositional MRI techniques in research settings have been found to be highly repeatable and reproducible in vivo [57]. In addition, T2 and T1ρ mapping each has good discriminatory abilities with respect to osteoarthritis detection; T2 and T1ρ are even able to differentiate subjects with only mild OA from healthy controls [57]. However, the test-retest reliability of composi-

tional cartilage imaging remains largely untested in multicenter settings potentially limiting their utility in routine clinical practice. Further, the value of using compositional cartilage information to improve diagnostic performance [63–65] and to follow acute traumatic injury [66] is only beginning to be reported.

4.4.3 Summary

The technological advances in compositional MRI over the last decade have evolved into a number of MRI techniques that can significantly improve the noninvasive evaluation of early cartilage damage and cartilage repair processes. While arthroscopy cannot be routinely used in the evaluation of asymptomatic patients, noninvasive MRI permits evaluation of patients and populations at risk for cartilage damage early along with longitudinal evaluation of patients after surgical or other therapeutic interventions. As our ability to speed up the scanning and processing times for compositional MRI techniques improves, they will likely become useful adjuvants to morphological MRI for evaluation of cartilage injury. Improving scan times would allow for validation with cross-site reproducibility and further our understanding of compositional MRI techniques as sensitive evaluation tools for individualized patient care.

References

1. Furey MJ. Joint Lubrication. In: Bronzino J, editor. Handbook of biomedical engineering. Boca Raton, FL: CRC Press, Inc.; 1995. p. 33–351.
2. Williams A. Regeneration of cartilage glycosaminoglycan after degradation by interleukin-1. Massachusetts Institute of Technology; 2001.
3. Handley C, Cheng K. Biological regulation of the chondrocytes. Boca Raton, FL: CRC Press, Inc.; 1992.
4. Mow VC, Ratcliffe A, Poole AR. Cartilage and diarthrodial joints as paradigms for hierarchical materials and structures. Biomaterials. 1992;13(2):67–97. https://doi.org/10.1016/0142-9612(92)90001-5.
5. Bank RA, Soudry M, Maroudas A, Mizrahi J, TeKoppele JM. The increased swelling and instantaneous deformation of osteoarthritic cartilage is highly

correlated with collagen degradation. Arthritis Rheum. 2000;43(10):2202–10. https://doi.org/10.1002/1529-0131(200010)43:10<2202::AID-ANR7>3.0.CO;2-E.

6. Bateman J, Lamande S, Ramshaw J. Molecular components and interactions; collagen superfamily. In: Comper WD, editor. Extracellular Matrix. Amsterdam: Harwood Academic Publishers; 1996.

7. Goodwin DW, Wadghiri YZ, Zhu H, Vinton CJ, Smith ED, Dunn JF. Macroscopic structure of articular cartilage of the tibial plateau: influence of a characteristic matrix architecture on MRI appearance. AJR Am J Roentgenol. 2004;182(2):311–8.

8. Bullough PG, Yawitz PS, Tafra L, Boskey AL. Topographical variations in the morphology and biochemistry of adult canine tibial plateau articular cartilage. J Orthop Res. 1985;3:1–16. https://doi.org/10.1002/jor.1100030101.

9. Du J, Carl M, Bae WC, Statum S, Chang EY, Bydder GM, et al. Dual inversion recovery ultrashort echo time (DIR-UTE) imaging and quantification of the zone of calcified cartilage (ZCC). Osteoarthr Cartil. 2013;21(1):77–85. https://doi.org/10.1016/j.joca.2012.09.009.

10. Temenoff JS, Mikos AG. Review: tissue engineering for regeneration of articular cartilage. Biomaterials. 2000;21(5):431–40. https://doi.org/10.1016/s0142-9612(99)00213-6.

11. Poole CA. Articular cartilage chondrons: form, function and failure. J Anat. 1997;191(Pt 1):1–13. https://doi.org/10.1046/j.1469-7580.1997.19110001.x.

12. Yulish BS, Montanez J, Goodfellow DB, Bryan PJ, Mulopulos GP, Modic MT. Chondromalacia patellae: assessment with MR imaging. Radiology. 1987;164(3):763–6. https://doi.org/10.1148/radiology.164.3.3615877.

13. König H, Sauter R, Deimling M, Vogt M. Cartilage disorders: comparison of spin-echo, CHESS, and FLASH sequence MR images. Radiology. 1987;164(3):753–8. https://doi.org/10.1148/radiology.164.3.3615875.

14. Tyrrell RL, Gluckert K, Pathria M, Modic MT. Fast three-dimensional MR imaging of the knee: comparison with arthroscopy. Radiology. 1988;166(3):865–72.

15. Hayes CW, Sawyer RW, Conway WF. Patellar cartilage lesions: in vitro detection and staging with MR imaging and pathologic correlation. Radiology. 1990;176(2):479–83.

16. Modl JM, Sether LA, Haughton VM, Kneeland JB. Articular cartilage: correlation of histologic zones with signal intensity at MR imaging. Radiology. 1991;181(3):853–5. https://doi.org/10.1148/radiology.181.3.1947110.

17. Lehner KB, Rechl HP, Gmeinwieser JK, Heuck AF, Lukas HP, Kohl HP. Structure, function, and degeneration of bovine hyaline cartilage: assessment with MR imaging in vitro. Radiology. 1989;170(2):495–9. https://doi.org/10.1148/radiology.170.2.2911674.

18. Rubenstein JD, Kim JK, Morova-Protzner I, Stanchev PL, Henkelman RM. Effects of collagen orientation on MR imaging characteristics of bovine articular cartilage. Radiology. 1993;188(1):219–26.

19. Henkelman RM, Stanisz GJ, Kim JK, Bronskill MJ. Anisotropy of NMR properties of tissues. Magn Reson Med. 1994;32(5):592–601.

20. Xia Y. Heterogeneity of cartilage laminae in MR imaging. J Magn Reson Imaging. 2000a;11(6):686–93. https://doi.org/10.1002/1522-2586(200006)11:6<686::AID-JMRI16>3.0.CO;2-#.

21. Alhadlaq HA, Xia Y. The structural adaptations in compressed articular cartilage by microscopic MRI (mu MRI) T-2 anisotropy. Osteoarthr Cartil. 2004;12(11):887–94. https://doi.org/10.1016/j.joca.2004.07.006.

22. Alhadlaq HA, Xia Y. Modifications of orientational dependence of microscopic magnetic resonance imaging T(2) anisotropy in compressed articular cartilage. J Magn Reson Imaging. 2005;22(5):665–73. https://doi.org/10.1002/jmri.20418.

23. Potter HG, Linklater JM, Allen AA, Hannafin JA, Haas SB. Magnetic resonance imaging of articular cartilage in the knee. An evaluation with use of fast-spin-echo imaging. J Bone Joint Surg Am. 1998;80(9):1276–84.

24. Roos EM, Engelhart L, Ranstam J, Anderson AF, Irrgang JJ, Marx RG, et al. ICRS recommendation document: patient-reported outcome instruments for use in patients with articular cartilage defects. Cartilage. 2011;2(2):122–36. https://doi.org/10.1177/1947603510391084.

25. Link T. Cartilage Imaging. New York: Springer Science and Business Media; 2011.

26. Alizai H, Virayavanich W, Joseph GB, Nardo L, Liu F, Liebl H, et al. Cartilage lesion score: comparison of a quantitative assessment score with established semiquantitative MR scoring systems. Radiology. 2014;271(2):479–87. https://doi.org/10.1148/radiol.13122056.

27. Jungmann PM, Welsch GH, Brittberg M, Trattnig S, Braun S, Imhoff AB, et al. Magnetic resonance imaging score and classification system (AMADEUS) for assessment of preoperative cartilage defect severity. Cartilage. 2017;8(3):272–82. https://doi.org/10.1177/1947603516665444.

28. Peterfy CG, Guermazi A, Zaim S, Tirman PF, Miaux Y, White D, et al. Whole-Organ Magnetic Resonance Imaging Score (WORMS) of the knee in osteoarthritis. Osteoarthr Cartil. 2004;12(3):177–90. https://doi.org/10.1016/j.joca.2003.11.003.

29. Hunter DJ, Guermazi A, Lo GH, Grainger AJ, Conaghan PG, Boudreau RM, et al. Evolution of semi-quantitative whole joint assessment of knee OA: MOAKS (MRI Osteoarthritis Knee Score). Osteoarthr Cartil. 2011;19(8):990–1002. https://doi.org/10.1016/j.joca.2011.05.004.

30. Lee S, Nardo L, Kumar D, Wyatt CR, Souza RB, Lynch J, et al. Scoring hip osteoarthritis with MRI (SHOMRI): a whole joint osteoarthritis evaluation system. J Magn Reson Imaging. 2015;41(6):1549–57. https://doi.org/10.1002/jmri.24722.

31. Marlovits S, Striessnig G, Resinger CT, Aldrian SM, Vecsei V, Imhof H, et al. Definition of pertinent parameters for the evaluation of articular cartilage

repair tissue with high-resolution magnetic resonance imaging. Eur J Radiol. 2004;52(3):310–9. https://doi.org/10.1016/j.ejrad.2004.03.014.

32. Roemer FW, Guermazi A, Trattnig S, Apprich S, Marlovits S, Niu J, et al. Whole joint MRI assessment of surgical cartilage repair of the knee: cartilage repair osteoarthritis knee score (CROAKS). Osteoarthr Cartil. 2014;22(6):779–99. https://doi.org/10.1016/j.joca.2014.03.014.

33. Eckstein F, Cicuttini F, Raynauld JP, Waterton JC, Peterfy C. Magnetic resonance imaging (MRI) of articular cartilage in knee osteoarthritis (OA): morphological assessment. Osteoarth Cartilage. 2006;14(Suppl A):A46–75. https://doi.org/10.1016/j.joca.2006.02.026.

34. Mosher TJ, Dardzinski BJ. Cartilage MRI T2 relaxation time mapping: overview and applications. Semin Musculoskelet Radiol. 2004;8(4):355–68. https://doi.org/10.1055/s-2004-861764.

35. Burstein D, Velyvis J, Scott KT, Stock KW, Kim YJ, Jaramillo D, et al. Protocol issues for delayed Gd(DTPA)(2-)-enhanced MRI (dGEMRIC) for clinical evaluation of articular cartilage. Magn Reson Med. 2001;45(1):36–41.

36. Regatte RR, Akella SV, Lonner JH, Kneeland JB, Reddy R. T1rho relaxation mapping in human osteoarthritis (OA) cartilage: comparison of T1rho with T2. J Magn Reson Imaging. 2006;23(4):547–53. https://doi.org/10.1002/jmri.20536.

37. van Tiel J, Kotek G, Reijman M, Bos PK, Bron EE, Klein S, et al. Is T1rho mapping an alternative to delayed gadolinium-enhanced MR imaging of cartilage in the assessment of Sulphated glycosaminoglycan content in human osteoarthritic knees? An in vivo validation study. Radiology. 2016;279(2):523–31. https://doi.org/10.1148/radiol.2015150693.

38. Du J, Takahashi AM, Bae WC, Chung CB, Bydder GM. Dual inversion recovery, ultrashort echo time (DIR UTE) imaging: creating high contrast for short-T(2) species. Magn Reson Med. 2010;63(2):447–55. https://doi.org/10.1002/mrm.22257.

39. Chu CR, Williams AA, West RV, Qian Y, Fu FH, Do BH, et al. Quantitative magnetic resonance imaging UTE-T2* mapping of cartilage and meniscus healing after anatomic anterior cruciate ligament reconstruction. Am J Sports Med. 2014;42(8):1847–56. https://doi.org/10.1177/0363546514532227.

40. Gatehouse PD, Bydder GM. Magnetic resonance imaging of short T2 components in tissue. Clin Radiol. 2003;58(1):1–19. https://doi.org/10.1053/crad.2003.1157.

41. Chang EY, Du J, Bae WC, Chung CB. Qualitative and quantitative ultrashort echo time imaging of musculoskeletal tissues. Semin Musculoskelet Radiol. 2015;19(4):375–86. https://doi.org/10.1055/s-0035-1563733.

42. Gurney PT, Hargreaves BA, Nishimura DG. Design and analysis of a practical 3D Cones trajectory. Magn Reson Med. 2006;55(3):575–82. https://doi.org/10.1002/mrm.20796.

43. Qian Y, Boada FE. Acquisition-weighted stack of spirals for fast high-resolution three-dimensional ultra-short echo time MR imaging. Magn Reson Med. 2008;60(1):135–45. https://doi.org/10.1002/mrm.21620.

44. Juras V, Apprich S, Zbyn S, Zak L, Deligianni X, Szomolanyi P, et al. Quantitative MRI analysis of menisci using biexponential T2* fitting with a variable echo time sequence. Magn Reson Med. 2014;71(3):1015–23. https://doi.org/10.1002/mrm.24760.

45. Williams AA, Titchenal MR, Do BH, Guha A, Chu CR. MRI UTE-T2* shows high incidence of cartilage subsurface matrix changes 2 years after ACL reconstruction. J Orthop Res. 2019;37(2):370–7. https://doi.org/10.1002/jor.24110.

46. Titchenal MR, Williams AA, Chehab EF, Asay JL, Dragoo JL, Gold GE, et al. Cartilage subsurface changes to magnetic resonance imaging UTE-T2* 2 years after anterior cruciate ligament reconstruction correlate with walking mechanics associated with knee osteoarthritis. Am J Sports Med. 2018;46(3):565–72. https://doi.org/10.1177/0363546517743969.

47. Rehnitz C, Do T, Klaan B, Burkholder I, Barie A, Wuennemann F, et al. Feasibility of using half-dose Gd-BOPTA for delayed gadolinium-enhanced MRI of cartilage (dGEMRIC) at the knee, compared with standard-dose Gd-DTPA. J Magn Reson Imaging. 2020;51(1):144–54. https://doi.org/10.1002/jmri.26816.

48. Rehnitz C, Klaan B, Do T, Barie A, Kauczor HU, Weber MA. Feasibility of gadoteric acid for delayed gadolinium-enhanced MRI of cartilage (dGEMRIC) at the wrist and knee and comparison with Gd-DTPA. J Magn Reson Imaging. 2017;46(5):1433–40. https://doi.org/10.1002/jmri.25688.

49. Bashir A, Gray ML, Hartke J, Burstein D. Nondestructive imaging of human cartilage glycosaminoglycan concentration by MRI. Magn Reson Med. 1999;41(5):857–65. https://doi.org/10.1002/(SICI)1522-2594(199905)41:5<857::AID-MRM1>3.0.CO;2-E.

50. Young AA, Stanwell P, Williams A, Rohrsheim JA, Parker DA, Giuffre B, et al. Glycosaminoglycan content of knee cartilage following posterior cruciate ligament rupture demonstrated by delayed gadolinium-enhanced magnetic resonance imaging of cartilage (dGEMRIC). A case report. J Bone Joint Surg Am. 2005;87(12):2763–7. https://doi.org/10.2106/JBJS.D.02923.

51. ACR Manual on Contrast Media, Version 10.3. By the ACR committee on drugs and contrast media. www.acr.org/-/media/ACR/Files/Clinical-Resources/Contrast_Media.pdf#page=83. Accessed 7 Feb 2020.

52. Sepponen RE, Pohjonen JA, Sipponen JT, Tanttu JI. A method for T1 rho imaging. J Comput Assist Tomogr. 1985;9(6):1007–11. https://doi.org/10.1097/00004728-198511000-00002.

53. Wang YX, Zhang Q, Li X, Chen W, Ahuja A, Yuan J. T1rho magnetic resonance: basic physics principles

and applications in knee and intervertebral disc imaging. Quant Imaging Med Surg. 2015;5(6):858–85. https://doi.org/10.3978/j.issn.2223-4292.2015.12.06.

54. Wheaton AJ, Casey FL, Gougoutas AJ, Dodge GR, Borthakur A, Lonner JH, et al. Correlation of T1rho with fixed charge density in cartilage. J Magn Reson Imaging. 2004;20(3):519–25. https://doi.org/10.1002/jmri.20148.

55. Keenan KE, Besier TF, Pauly JM, Han E, Rosenberg J, Smith RL, et al. Prediction of glycosaminoglycan content in human cartilage by age, T1rho and T2 MRI. Osteoarthr Cartil. 2011;19(2):171–9. https://doi.org/10.1016/j.joca.2010.11.009.

56. Taylor C, Carballido-Gamio J, Majumdar S, Li X. Comparison of quantitative imaging of cartilage for osteoarthritis: T2, T1rho, dGEMRIC and contrast-enhanced computed tomography. Magn Reson Imaging. 2009;27(6):779–84. https://doi.org/10.1016/j.mri.2009.01.016.

57. MacKay JW, Low SBL, Smith TO, Toms AP, McCaskie AW, Gilbert FJ. Systematic review and meta-analysis of the reliability and discriminative validity of cartilage compositional MRI in knee osteoarthritis. Osteoarthr Cartil. 2018;26(9):1140–52. https://doi.org/10.1016/j.joca.2017.11.018.

58. Holtzman DJ, Theologis AA, Carballido-Gamio J, Majumdar S, Li X, Benjamin C. T(1rho) and T(2) quantitative magnetic resonance imaging analysis of cartilage regeneration following microfracture and mosaicplasty cartilage resurfacing procedures. J Magn Reson Imaging. 2010;32(4):914–23. https://doi.org/10.1002/jmri.22300.

59. Theologis AA, Schairer WW, Carballido-Gamio J, Majumdar S, Li X, Ma CB. Longitudinal analysis of T1rho and T2 quantitative MRI of knee cartilage laminar organization following microfracture surgery. Knee. 2012;19(5):652–7. https://doi.org/10.1016/j.knee.2011.09.004.

60. Li X, Han ET, Busse RF, Majumdar S. In vivo T(1rho) mapping in cartilage using 3D magnetization-prepared angle-modulated partitioned k-space spoiled gradient echo snapshots (3D MAPSS). Magn Reson Med. 2008;59(2):298–307. https://doi.org/10.1002/mrm.21414.

61. Atkinson HF, Birmingham TB, Moyer RF, Yacoub D, Kanko LE, Bryant DM, et al. MRI T2 and T1rho relaxation in patients at risk for knee osteoarthritis: a systematic review and meta-analysis. BMC Musculoskelet Disord. 2019;20(1):182. https://doi.org/10.1186/s12891-019-2547-7.

62. Trattnig S, Winalski CS, Marlovits S, Jurvelin JS, Welsch GH, Potter HG. Magnetic resonance imaging of cartilage repair: a review. Cartilage. 2011;2(1):5–26. https://doi.org/10.1177/1947603509360209.

63. Kijowski R, Blankenbaker DG, Munoz Del Rio A, Baer GS, Graf BK. Evaluation of the articular cartilage of the knee joint: value of adding a T2 mapping sequence to a routine MR imaging protocol. Radiology. 2013;267(2):503–13. https://doi.org/10.1148/radiol.12121413.

64. Li Z, Wang H, Lu Y, Jiang M, Chen Z, Xi X, et al. Diagnostic value of T1rho and T2 mapping sequences of 3D fat-suppressed spoiled gradient (FS SPGR-3D) 3.0-T magnetic resonance imaging for osteoarthritis. Medicine (Baltimore). 2019;98(1):e13834. https://doi.org/10.1097/MD.0000000000013834.

65. van Eck CF, Kingston RS, Crues JV, Kharrazi FD. Magnetic resonance imaging for patellofemoral chondromalacia: is there a role for T2 mapping? Orthop J Sports Med. 2017;5(11):2325967117740554. https://doi.org/10.1177/2325967117740554.

66. Kijowski R, Roemer F, Englund M, Tiderius CJ, Sward P, Frobell RB. Imaging following acute knee trauma. Osteoarthr Cartil. 2014;22(10):1429–43. https://doi.org/10.1016/j.joca.2014.06.024.

MRI in Knee Cartilage Injury and Posttreatment MRI Assessment of Cartilage Repair

5

Marcus Raudner, Vladimir Juras, Markus Schreiner, Olgica Zaric, Benedikt Hager, Pavol Szomolanyi, and Siegfried Trattnig

5.1 Morphological MRI

Magnetic resonance imaging (MRI) has taken a central role in the diagnostic and longitudinal assessment of cartilage injuries [1]. This is especially important, as missed cartilage defects may put patients at risk for the early development of osteoarthritis (OA) [2]. Over the last few decades, multiple new treatment approaches for focal cartilage lesions have emerged, all with the unified goal of preventing OA and with a focus on athletes returning to sports activities at the preinjury level as early as possible [3].

Even though MRI has the highest sensitivity and specificity of all imaging modalities when it comes to assessing articular cartilage, a direct correlation with clinical outcome after surgical repair of cartilage defects is only described in a minority of studies [4, 5].

In order to improve structured morphological assessment after cartilage repair, the Magnetic Resonance Observation of Cartilage Repair Tissue (MOCART) was introduced by Marlovits et al. in 2006 and recently updated to the MOCART 2.0 in 2019 by Schreiner et al. [6, 7].

In order to reliably assess articular cartilage, an in-plane resolution of 0.3 x 0.3 mm or better is desirable with mainly fat-suppressed, fluid-sensitive, proton density-weighted (PDw) and T2-weighted (T2w) sequences used for the thorough assessment of potential signal alterations or evaluation of the cartilage surface [1, 8, 9].

The fact that PDw and T2w sequences offer optimal contrast between fluid, cartilage, and bone marrow makes them a stable choice for routine MRI protocols of the knee and other large joints, especially considering that gradient echo (GRE) sequences are much more prone to susceptibility artifacts [10, 11].

5.1.1 Microfracturing (MFX)

Directly after an MFX procedure, the repair tissue is typically hyperintense on T2w sequences, sometimes leading to the pitfall of fluidlike signal intensities [12]. With multiple longitudinal

M. Raudner
Department of Biomedical Imaging and Image-Guided Therapy, Medical University of Vienna, Vienna, Austria
e-mail: marcus.raudner@meduniwien.ac.at

V. Juras · O. Zaric · B. Hager · P. Szomolanyi
S. Trattnig (✉)
Department of Biomedical Imaging and Image-Guided Therapy, High Field MR Center, Medical University of Vienna, Vienna, Austria
e-mail: vladimir.juras@meduniwien.ac.at;
benedikt.hager@meduniwien.ac.at;
pavol.szomolanyi@meduniwien.ac.at;
siegfried.trattnig@meduniwien.ac.at

M. Schreiner
Department of Orthopaedics and Trauma-surgery, Medical University of Vienna, Vienna, Austria
e-mail: markus.schreiner@meduniwien.ac.at

© ISAKOS 2021
A. J. Krych et al. (eds.), *Cartilage Injury of the Knee*,
https://doi.org/10.1007/978-3-030-78051-7_5

controls, pluripotent stem cells migrate to the debrided defect and form fibrocartilaginous tissue. In an optimal scenario, the repair site shows the same signal intensity as the surrounding native cartilage. However, the repair site can often be depicted as hypointense on fluid-sensitive sequences [1, 13]. After an interval of 12–24 months, depending on the patient's age, size of defect, and perioperative incidents, the repair site should show a completely filled defect with a smooth surface and a seamless transition to the native cartilage, hinting at good integration (Fig. 5.1). Bone marrow edema is a common postoperative finding, but should not persist or enlarge over consecutive follow-ups as this can be associated with treatment failure [12, 13].

5.1.2 Osteochondral Auto- and Allograft (OAT and AOT)

The most important difference between auto- and allografts is that autografts have the inherent advantage of providing a thorough look at the donation site, which is naturally not present in allografts. Thus, allografts can, therefore, also be used in larger defects as donor-site limitations do not apply [14, 15].

Most importantly, filled defect volume, signal intensity, integration, and homogeneity of the repair tissue should be evaluated longitudinally. The integrity of the subchondral lamina and potential abnormalities in surrounding soft tissues or underlying bone marrow should also be examined. Bone marrow edema is a common finding in the majority of patients in the first months after cartilage repair, but should decline from there on, until, at the latest, 3 years after the surgery [16–18].

A major complication of OAT or AOT can be osteonecrosis, often showing demarcating borders alongside hypointense bone marrow lesions, with the worst case resulting in additional bone balding. Clinical implications of these MRI findings are to be thoroughly weighed, as the cartilage will still be passively nourished through the synovial membrane. Therefore, not every patient with osteonecrosis benefits from an arthroscopic intervention, and in some cases can be observed closely.

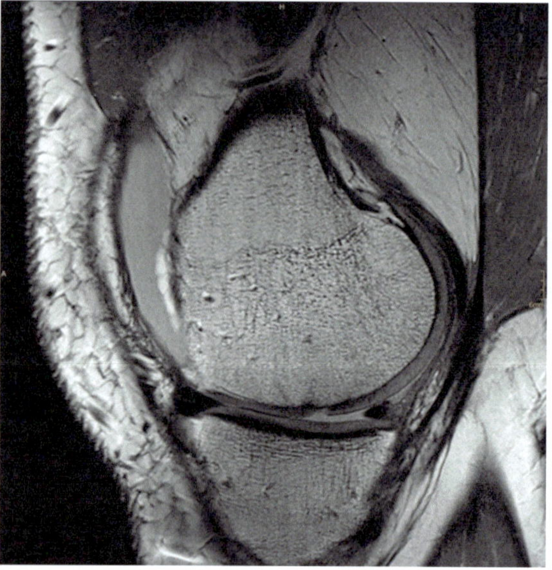
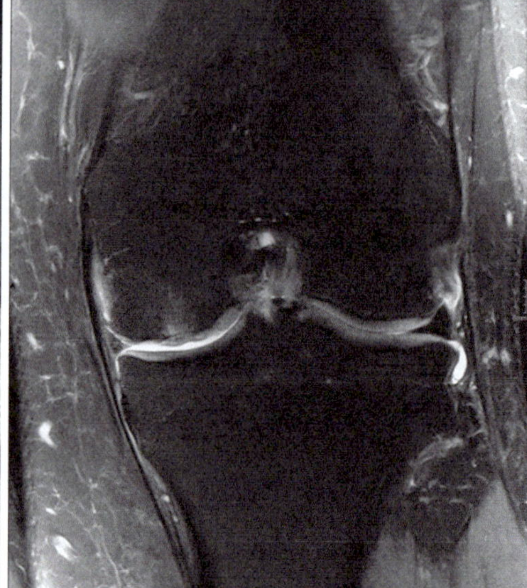
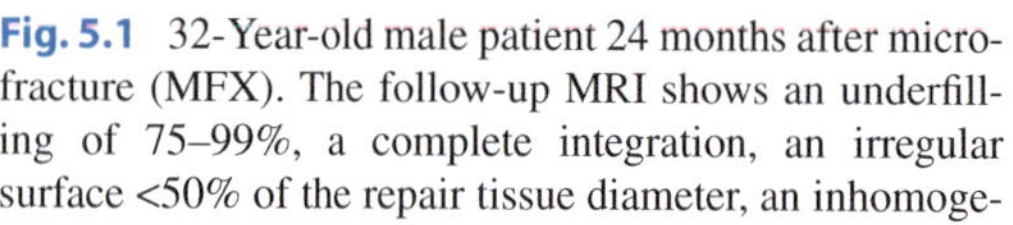

Fig. 5.1 32-Year-old male patient 24 months after microfracture (MFX). The follow-up MRI shows an underfilling of 75–99%, a complete integration, an irregular surface <50% of the repair tissue diameter, an inhomogeneous structure, minor hypointense signal, no bony overgrowth or defect, and a minor edema-like marrow signal with <50% maximum diameter of the repair tissue

5.1.3 Autologous Chondrocyte Implantation (ACI) and Matrix-Associated Chondrocyte Implantation (MACI)

These cell-based repairs go through a characteristic healing process. In the early postoperative follow-up, the repair tissue is typically hyperintense. These signal alterations decrease over time until the repair tissue is isointense (Fig. 5.2) to the surrounding cartilage [12, 19, 20]. Bone marrow edema is common with this repair procedure, but should not be seen in the follow-up examinations for more than 18 months after surgery [1]. An incomplete integration at the transitional border can manifest as streaky hyperintensity at the cartilage interfaces. It is a common finding in the early postoperative phase, but a sign of potential treatment failure at later examinations. Repairs via autologous periosteum are associated with a higher rate of hypertrophic filling and delamination than procedures using synthetic collagen or MACI with flaps [21]. A delamination is best depicted on a T2w sequence as a hyperintense signal aberration in the integrational border zone and underneath the repair tissue [12].

5.1.4 Successful Cartilage Repair

In 2006, Marlovits et al. published the first version of the "Magnetic Resonance Observation of Cartilage Repair Tissue" (MOCART) Score [6]. To date, it is the most often referenced score with which to systematically assess cartilage repair after MACI and has already been used in other repair procedures. In 2019, Schreiner et al. published the updated MOCART 2.0 for cartilage repair assessment [7].

The MOCART 2.0 consists of seven variables. The first is the volume of cartilage defect filling, as insufficient filling is a sign of insufficient repair [12]. The next variable is the integration into adjacent cartilage. This becomes more important with larger defects, as they are directly associated with a higher rate of integrational defects or delaminations [22]. The third

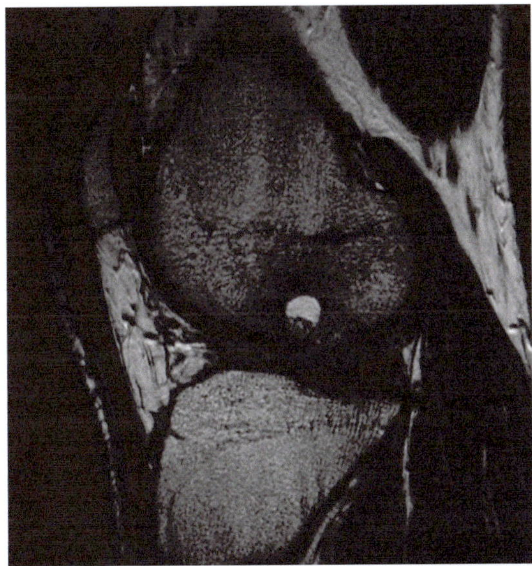
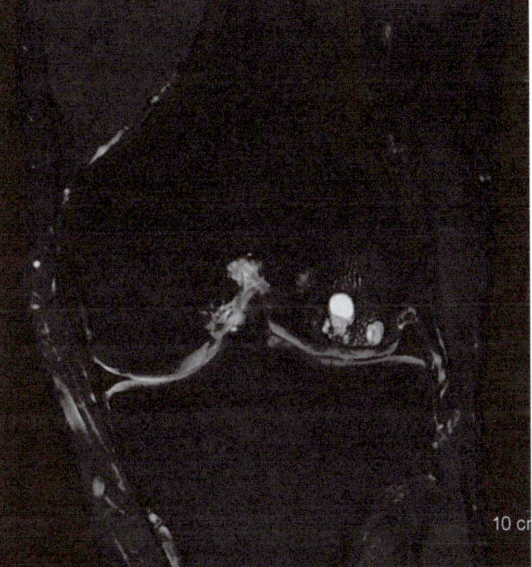
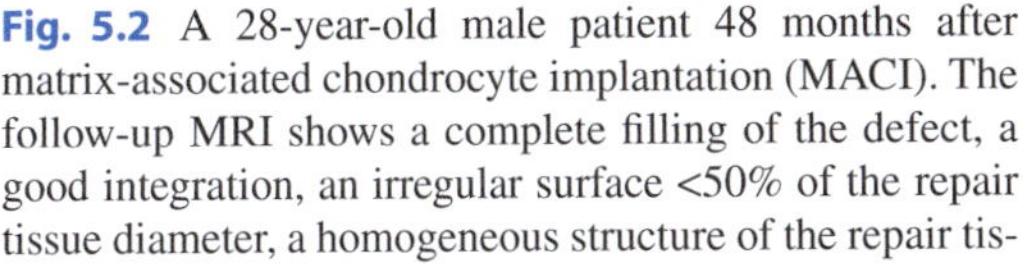

Fig. 5.2 A 28-year-old male patient 48 months after matrix-associated chondrocyte implantation (MACI). The follow-up MRI shows a complete filling of the defect, a good integration, an irregular surface <50% of the repair tissue diameter, a homogeneous structure of the repair tissue with isointense signal intensity, a bony overgrowth of less than 50% thickness of the adjacent cartilage, and a subchondral cyst exceeding 5 mm in the maximum diameter

variable is the surface of the repair tissue. As fissural surface defects facilitate inflammatory processes, they are associated with an unfavorable outcome [13]. Fourth is the structure of the repair tissue and the discrimination between homogeneous and heterogeneous cartilage repair tissue. The latter is a sign of defective cartilage integrity potential, which may also lead to treatment failure. Next is the signal intensity. This variable grades how the repair tissue compares to native cartilage on fluid-sensitive sequences. Favorably, the repair tissue is isointense to native cartilage. This should be the aim of every treatment procedure besides MFX, as bone marrow stimulation techniques, in general, are known to produce mainly fibro-cartilaginous tissue [13]. The next variable would be bony defects or bony overgrowth. Neither should be observed in a successful cartilage repair with the sole exception of OAT or AOT, which are transplanted with their subchondral interface.

5.1.5 Bony Defects

The subchondral lamina should have no defects and should heal in all dimensions to provide long-term stability and function of the joint. An exception is the implantation of an allograft, which comprises bony parts for reconstruction of osteochondral defects in the early stages. After 14 weeks, healing of the subchondral lamina should be visible [16]. Finally, the subchondral area should be assessed for changes, including bone marrow edema, subchondral cysts, or osteonecrosis-like signal.

Overall, the morphological postoperative assessment after cartilage repair and the MOCART 2.0 score are tasks that require the undivided attention of an experienced radiologist, but are important to improve long-term patient outcome.

5.2 T2/T2* Mapping in the Injured Knee

5.2.1 T2 and T2* Mapping

5.2.1.1 Technical Considerations

The transversal relaxation constant, T2, provides valuable information about the composition of healthy and degenerated connective tissues, such as cartilage, tendon, ligaments, and menisci. T2, as a quantitative biomarker, reflects the collagen content and organization and its interplay with water molecules. It also visualizes the zonal appearance of the cartilage, manifested by long-T2 values in the superficial zone, shorter in the transitional zone, and very short in the deep zone and subchondral bone. Goodwin et al. described, for the first time, the stratification of cartilage on T2 maps, attributing it to collagen fiber orientation, and described the magic angle effect as well [23]. In a further study, the same authors found a relationship between three-dimensional collagen organization and its influence on T2 values [24]. Dardzinski and colleagues demonstrated the in vivo feasibility of T2 mapping in human articular cartilage for the first time and found the most pronounced T2 stratification in patellar cartilage, with T2 increasing from the deep to the superficial zones from 45.3 ms to 67.0 ms, respectively [25]. These pivotal studies were followed by a number of works defining the influence of gender [26], age [27, 28], training and physical activity [27, 29], and loading [30, 31] on cartilage T2 values. The standardization of T2 is still a controversial point, which limits the widespread clinical application of this technique, although it was shown that the addition of a T2 mapping sequence to a routine MR protocol at 3 T can improve sensitivity in the detection of early cartilage degeneration [32]. Besides image acquisition, post-processing plays a crucial role in T2 mapping standardization in cartilage [33]. In addition to T2 mapping of articular cartilage, T2* relaxation time mapping is being discussed for the depiction of the collagen matrix [34]. As T2* is able to visualize fast-relaxing parts of the cartilage, especially the deep cartilage zone, with highly organized collagen fibers, it can provide additional information about cartilage status. As T2 and T2* maps provide the two-dimensional structural collagen dependence, recently, the evaluation of the maps was expanded using textural features and their correlation to cartilage status [35–37].

5.2.1.2 Cartilage Injury

Cartilage injury is characterized by collagen depletion and increased hydration. Recent technological advances in MRI, including field strength, coil design, and sequence development, allow for robust, reproducible T2 mapping with high in-plane resolution. High and ultrahigh fields provide the substantial benefit of a higher signal-to-noise ratio; however, there are physical limitations, such as lower B_1 homogeneity and power deposition, that limit the transfer of this technique to higher field strengths. A conventional multi-echo, multi-slice approach [38] is often alternated with advanced T2 mapping techniques, such as double-echo steady state (DESS) [39] and triple-echo steady state [40], which provide fair B_1 insensitivity and full joint coverage because of the three-dimensional capability.

A focal cartilage lesion may cause the onset of systematic disorders, such as osteoarthritis. It is, therefore, desirable to have available noninvasive diagnosis and patient monitoring imaging approaches. Low-grade cartilage lesions are difficult to diagnose since morphological changes are often subclinical and are accompanied by changes in hydration and disruption of collagen fibers. T2 mapping seems to be a helpful diagnostic tool that provides enough sensitivity to detect low-grade focal cartilage lesions. Juras et al. showed the diagnostic robustness of T2 mapping using TESS, in a study that involved 21 patients with focal cartilage lesions [41]. Patients were scanned repeatedly at four time points and the significant, continuous decrease of T2 values in patients with lesions was observed between baseline and 6 months in the superficial layer of the lesions at 3 T, where the T2 values decreased

from 41. 9 ± 9 ms to 36.2 ± 7 ms, which was a difference of 5.6 ± 2 ms ($p = 0.03$); see Fig. 5.3. Increased cartilage T2 values are associated with findings of pain in patients with focal lesions, whereas among morphologic knee abnormalities, only knee cartilage lesions are significantly associated with knee pain status. This was validated by a study of 126 patients from the Osteoarthritis Initiative using T2 mapping and the Whole-Organ Magnetic Resonance Imaging Score (WOMAC) pain assessment [42]. Årøen et al. investigated quantitative MRI techniques in focal cartilage lesions using arthroscopically verified findings. Both proteoglycan-specific (delayed gadolinium-enhanced MRI of cartilage (dGEMRIC)) and collagen-sensitive (T2 mapping) techniques were able to depict the focal cartilage changes, through either the decrease in proteoglycan content or the collagen disruption and greater hydration [43]. Hannila et al. compared the feasibility of morphological MRI and T2 mapping for the detection of early cartilage lesions. They showed that cartilage lesions diagnosed by T2 mapping better matched in size and location the arthroscopically confirmed lesion appearance [44].

5.2.1.3 Cartilage Repair

Cartilage has very limited capability for spontaneous healing. If this occurs, type I collagen and fibrocartilaginous tissue, as opposed to normal hyaline cartilage, are produced. A large number of surgical techniques have been developed to repair focal cartilage defects, including chondroplasty, debridement, drilling, microfracture (MFX), autologous chondrocyte implantation (ACI), osteochondral autograft transfer (OAT), osteochondral allograft, and matrix-associated chondrocyte transplantation (MACT) [45]. As T2 mapping provides information about hydration and collagen matrix organization, it helps to differentiate between the native cartilage and the repair tissue, to differentiate between different cartilage repair types, and to assess the maturation of the repair tissue over time. The first attempts to differentiate between repair and native cartilage were performed using animal models, either equine [46] or caprine [47]. White

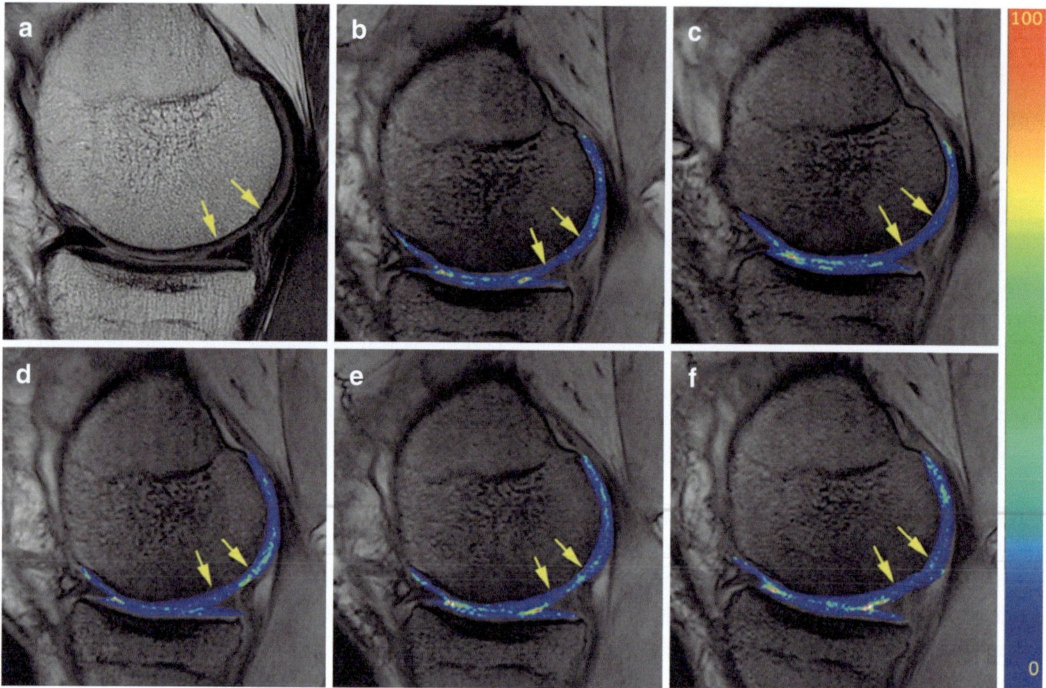

Fig. 5.3 A representative T2 map in a patient with low-grade cartilage lesion scanned at five time points: (**a**) morphological image; T2 map acquired at (**b**) baseline; (**c**) 8 days; (**d**) 3 months; (**e**) 6 months; and (**f**) 12 months. Reproduced with permission from [41]

et al. used ten equine subjects with OAT and MFX to show that zonal stratification depicted by T2 mapping is an indicator by which to distinguish fibrous tissue from hyaline cartilage [46]. Cartilage patterns in both tissue types were also confirmed with polarized light microscopy (PLM). Watanabe et al. investigated ten goats with MFX and they found T2 mapping useful for the differentiation of repair and native cartilage; however, they also pointed out the limitation of T2 to serve as a specific biochemical marker for collagen fibers [47]. The knowledge acquired from animal studies was subsequently transferred to in vivo human studies. Initial experience was published by Welsch et al., who compared cartilage repair with MFX and MACT (ten patients in each group) to healthy native cartilage [48]. Regarding the absolute values, a statistically nonsignificant T2 decrease was observed in MACT (56.4 ± 9.6 ms), and a statistically significant T2 decrease in MFX (47.3 ± 10.3 ms) when compared to healthy cartilage (57.8 ± 8.7 ms). However, zonal differentiation in cartilage repair using MACT was more like that in healthy cartilage than that in MFX. The example T2 map acquired with DESS in MFX and MACT patient is depicted in Fig. 5.4. T2 values also provide the information on cartilage function, as it is sensitive to loading-induced changes, and can be used as a functional quality marker. Mamisch et al. compared the influence of 45-min-long unloading to T2 values on MACT repair cartilage and healthy controls. The behavior of cartilage in terms of T2 was different in repair tissue (early unloading, 51.8 ± 11.7 ms; late unloading, 56.1 ± 14.4 ms) compared to healthy tissue (early unloading, 50.2 ± 8.4 ms; late unloading, 51.3 ± 8.5 ms), suggesting that T2 relaxation can be used to assess early and late unloading values of articular cartilage in a clinical setting and that the time point of the quantitative T2 measurement affects the differentiation between native and abnormal articular cartilage [49]. Similar behavior was

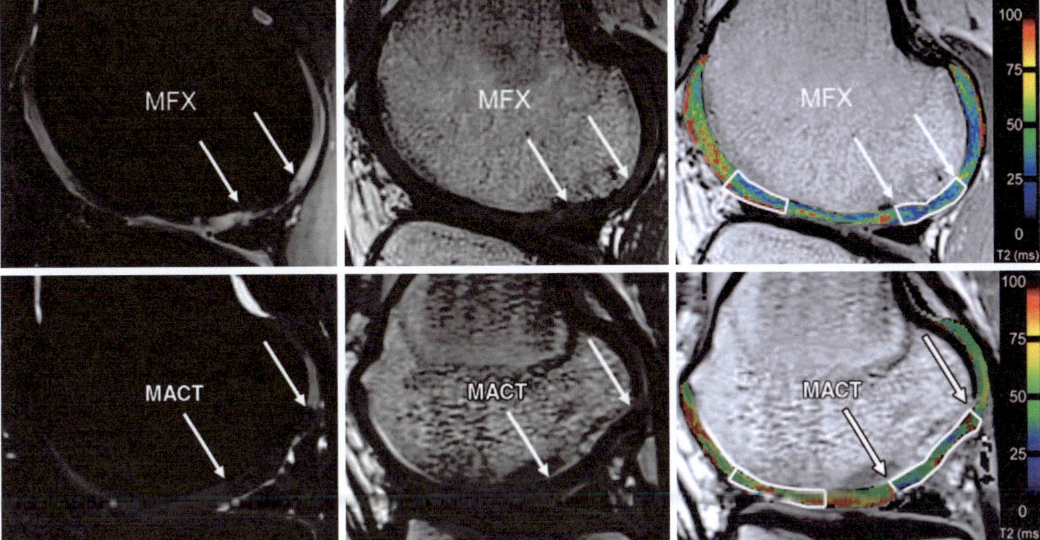

Fig. 5.4 Sagittal double-echo steady-state MR image (top-left), sagittal spin-echo raw T2 image (top-middle), and corresponding fused sagittal cartilage colored T2 map (top-right) in a patient after MFX. Sagittal double-echo steady-state MR image (bottom-left), sagittal spin-echo raw T2 image (bottom-middle), and corresponding fused sagittal cartilage colored T2 map (bottom-right) in age- and follow-up interval-matched patient after MACT. Cartilage repair area is located between the two arrows and control cartilage (outlined area on the left of each respective repair method) on colored T2 map. Reproduced with permission from [48]

observed in the patellar cartilage [31]. The effect of static loading on repair tissue (MACT) and healthy cartilage was studied by positioning the knee in the extended and the 40° flexed position [50]. Repair tissue showed different behavior in the loaded cartilage zone compared to healthy cartilage, suggesting that T2 may serve as a marker for the evaluation of repair-tissue quality after MACT and will allow for biomechanical assessment of cartilage transplants. Ultrahigh-field T2 applications allow for imaging at higher resolution [51, 52] or imaging joints with substantially thinner cartilage [53, 54]. T2 mapping can also be used to monitor patients after repair procedures to ensure the long-term success of cartilage repair surgeries in OCT [55, 56], MFX [57, 58], and ACI/MACI/MACT [59–61]. The clinical potential of T2 and T2* mapping is becoming more and more important in view of the number of studies published to date. The additional information about cartilage quality can potentially answer clinical questions related to cartilage repair tissue maturation, as well as differentiation after various repair techniques.

5.3 gagCEST

5.3.1 MRI of Cartilage Lesions and Repair: gagCEST

Glycosaminoglycan chemical-exchange saturation transfer (gagCEST) [62] is a promising biomarker for the noninvasive assessment and monitoring of articular cartilage defects and cartilage repair using magnetic resonance imaging [63]. In CEST imaging, selective saturation of exchangeable protons, which are subsequently transferred via chemical exchange and accumulated in the water pool, is used as contrast enhancement to indirectly detect specific endogenous metabolites, such as glycosaminoglycans [64]. Glycosaminoglycan (GAG) content is of particular interest in the assessment of cartilage lesions, as well as in the postoperative monitoring of cartilage repair, as it has been strongly correlated with cartilage biomechanics [65], particularly with compressive stiffness [66]. gagCEST offers distinct advantages over other GAG-specific imaging techniques, such as

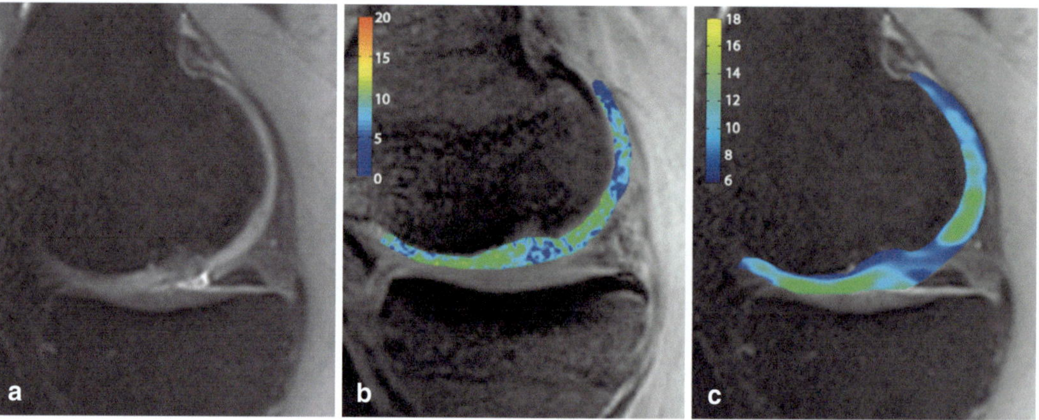

Fig. 5.5 Medial femoral condyle of a 30-year-old patient after microfracture displayed on (**a**) morphologic, (**b**) gagCEST map overlaid on a morphological image, and (**c**) 23 Na MR map overlaid on a morphological image. Color bars on b and c represent MTR_{asym} values summed over offsets from 0 to 1.3 ppm (gagCEST) and sodium SNRs, respectively. Reproduced with permission from [71]

dGEMRIC and sodium imaging. As opposed to dGEMRIC [67], it does not rely on the administration of contrast media. And, in contrast to sodium imaging, because it is a proton-based imaging technique, it does not need a multinuclear setup or dedicated radio-frequency coils. Furthermore, gagCEST offers an inherently better signal-to-noise ratio (SNR) than sodium imaging, which allows for a significantly higher spatial resolution, and thus less susceptibility to partial-volume effects [68].

The intricacy of the underlying technique and the challenging properties of articular cartilage, however, such as relatively short-T2 relaxation times and only small chemical shift differences between the exchangeable OH protons of GAGs and the water peak [69], give rise to distinct drawbacks as well. These include labeling efficiency, susceptibility to B_1 (RF field) and B_0 (static magnetic field) inhomogeneities, relatively long scan times, and thus susceptibility to motion artifacts [70]. Moving to higher field strengths (7 T) is helpful in two ways. First, the CEST effect depends on field strength, and second, the higher field strength provides increased spectral resolution, which helps to reduce direct saturation effects.

Schmitt et al. [71] examined 11 patients at a mean follow-up of 21 months after cartilage repair surgery (five patients after MFX and seven patients after MACT) using gagCEST and sodium imaging at 7 T (Fig. 5.5). In all patients, the MTR_{asym} (values summed for all offsets from 0 to 1.3 ppm) were significantly ($p = 0.003$) higher in healthy reference cartilage than in repair tissue. Furthermore, the authors observed a correlation between the MTR_{asym} and sodium SNR values, suggesting both a sensitivity of gagCEST to GAG content and lower GAG content in the repair tissue in these patients. Krusche-Mandel et al. [72] investigated nine patients at a follow-up of 8 years after autologous osteochondral transplantation using T2 mapping at 3 T and gagCEST, as well as sodium imaging at 7 T. Age at implantation was 49 years. Even though the clinical outcome was favorable, with a median Lysholm score of 90 points [IQR: 85.0–95.0, 95% CI: (85; 93)], statistically significant differences between the cartilage repair tissue and healthy reference cartilage in the same knee were observed with all three techniques. Corroborating the underlying theory, the strongest correlation was observed between gagCEST and sodium imaging. However, only for T2 mapping was a correlation found with clinical scores (i.e., the modified Lysholm score) [$\rho = -0.667$, 95% CI: (-0.922; -0.005)].

Subsequently, gagCEST was used at 3 T as well. Rehnitz et al. [73] employed T2 mapping, dGEMRIC, and gagCEST to quantitatively assess the knee cartilage of 10 healthy volunteers, 50 patients with suspected cartilage lesions, and 19 patients after microfracture. The authors observed significantly higher gagCEST values in cartilage defects grade 2 and 3 when compared to healthy reference cartilage (mean 4.8% vs. 1.4%, $p < 0.01$). In contrast to Schmitt et al., significantly higher gagCEST values were observed in cartilage repair tissue when compared to healthy reference cartilage (mean 7.3% vs. 0.7%, $p < 0.0001$). The results of this study, however, might have to be reappraised, since Singh et al. [74] have shown that proper correction of B_0 inhomogeneities leads to a negligible gagCEST effect at 3 T.

Brinkhof et al. [75] recently developed a 3D gagCEST sequence and applied it to healthy volunteers and patients with femoral cartilage lesions before cartilage repair surgery at 7 T in an acquisition time of 7 min. The authors observed good reproducibility and reported a significantly different gagCEST effect in cartilage lesions when compared to healthy cartilage, ranging from 1.3% to 5.1% versus 2.6% to 12.4%.

gagCEST is a promising, noninvasive, GAG-sensitive biomarker that does not require the application of contrast media. With currently available hardware and sequences, however, gagCEST seems to be restricted to 7 T systems. This, in turn, prevents widespread application for the assessment of cartilage lesions and repair, both in research and, even more so, in the clinic. Hence, continuous development and gradual improvement of hardware and sequences are pivotal for gagCEST to become a biomarker that can be applied in the clinical routine.

5.4 Sodium (^{23}Na) MRI

5.4.1 Biochemical Investigations of Cartilage Tissue Using Sodium MRI

Mechanical injury is a major cause of articular cartilage damage in young, active subjects. Within the last two decades, different surgical cartilage repair techniques have been proposed

for the treatment of cartilage defects, such as bone marrow stimulation techniques (BMS) (Pridie drilling, Microfracture (MFX)); first, second, and third generations of cell-based autologous chondrocyte implantation (ACI); autologous osteochondral transplantation (AOT); and cell-free implant techniques.

Proton (^{1}H) MR imaging allows for the morphological assessment of the cartilage or repair tissue, but it does not provide information about the sophisticated composition of the repair tissue. The complex repair structure, however, may affect the long-term outcome. MRI methods provide information about the morphology of the knee joint, but biochemical changes in the joint often occur before morphological changes are detectable. Therefore, there is an objective need for biochemical and quantitative MRI capable of providing early information about the biochemical changes of articular cartilage.

One of those techniques is sodium (^{23}Na) MR imaging, which can assess changes in Na ion content, linked to glycosaminoglycan (GAGs) molecules. The negatively charged GAGs are the essential molecules for cartilage molecular investigations, since GAGs provide strong electrostatic and osmotic forces, which have an important influence on cartilage function and homeostasis. Furthermore, the GAG content correlates with the biomechanical properties of cartilage [66]. In articular cartilage, the negatively charged GAGs are surrounded by positively charged sodium ions; thus, the sodium concentration can be used as an indirect measure of GAG content, which can be noninvasively assessed with sodium imaging [76, 77]. With the additional inclusion of quantification standards with known sodium concentrations, tissue sodium concentrations (TSC) can be calculated.

5.4.2 ^{23}Na-MRI for Different Cartilage Repair Technique Evaluations

Some of the initial studies that introduced ^{23}Na MR imaging of patients after cartilage repair were published by Trattnig et al. in 2010 [78]. In one study of 12 patients, examinations of femoral condyle cartilage were performed approximately 56 months after MACT. Sodium imaging results obtained at 7 T were compared with results generated at 3 T using the dGEMRIC technique. The sodium normalized signal intensity (NMSI) values were significantly lower in repair tissue than in reference cartilage ($p < 0.001$). dGEMRIC measurements also showed a significant difference in postcontrast T1 values between repair tissue and reference cartilage ($p = 0.005$). Moreover, a strong correlation was found between sodium imaging and dGEMRIC. These results indicated that [23]Na-MRI allows differentiation between MACT repair tissue and native cartilage of patients without the need for contrast agent application.

Zbyn et al. reported the results of [23]Na-MRI at 7 T, which were used to compare the quality of repair tissue of femoral condyle cartilage between two different repair procedures: MFX and MACT [79]. Every BMS patient was matched with one MACT patient according to age, postoperative interval, and defect location. NMSIs were significantly lower in BMS ($p = 0.004$) and MACT ($p = 0.006$) repair tissue than in corresponding reference cartilage (Fig. 5.6). The morphological appearance of the repair tissue, evaluated by the MOCART scoring system [6] and results, showed that differences in MOCART scores between

patients after BMS and after MACT were insignificant ($p = 0.915$). NMSI from repair tissue was significantly different between BMS and MACT ($p = 0.028$). The conclusion of the study was that the sophisticated, cell-based MACT technique produces a repair tissue with a more hyaline-like composition, while the result of the BMS technique is a fibrous repair tissue with very low GAG content. [23]Na-MRI is able to distinguish between repair tissues with different GAG content, and thus serves as a noninvasive evaluation of the performance of new cartilage repair techniques.

Cartilage repair procedures used in the knee joint are also performed in the ankle joint. However, there are biochemical and biomechanical differences between knee and ankle cartilage. Zbyn et al. investigated a feasibility of [23]Na-MRI for repair-tissue investigations in very thin ankle cartilage [80]. In the same study, Zbyn et al. scanned cadaver ankle samples and found a high correlation between GAG content and sodium signal ($r = 0.800$; $p < 0.001$; $R = 0.639$). These authors wanted to investigate the feasibility of quantitative sodium MRI in vivo for the evaluation of the thin cartilage of the ankle and subtalar joints at 7 T. Healthy volunteers—six MFX and six MACT patients with similar age, body mass index, and defect size—were measured and the results showed that both repair techniques

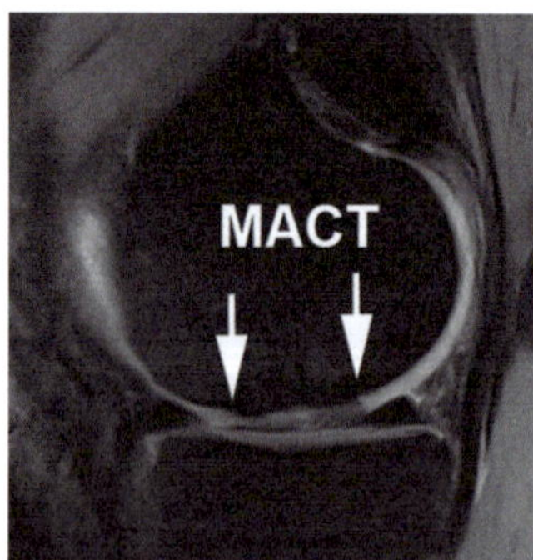

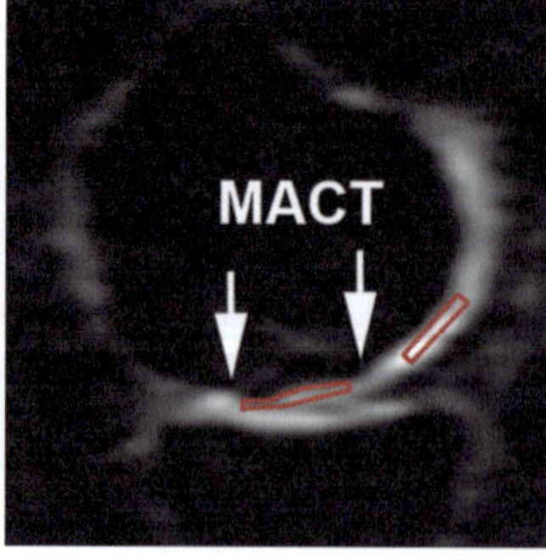

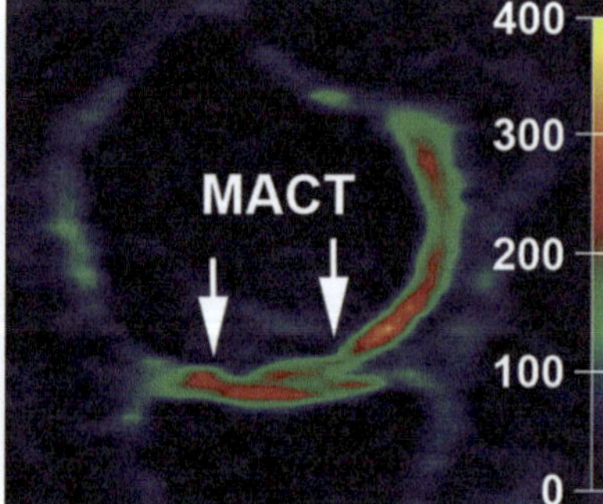

Fig. 5.6 Sagittal proton density-weighted 2D-TSE MR image with fat suppression (left); sagittal, sodium 3D-GRE image (middle); and color-coded sagittal sodium 3D-GRE image (right) in a 35-year-old woman obtained 50.6 months after MACT surgery. Cartilage repair tissue is situated between the two arrows. Red contours in the middle image represent the ROI analysis of repair tissue (left contour) and reference cartilage (right contour). Please note that repair tissue voxels situated closest to the repair tissue-native cartilage interface are not included into the ROI evaluations. Color scale represents the sodium signal intensity values (reproduced with permission from [79])

resulted in significantly lower mean sodium corrected signal intensities (cSI) in repair tissue than in reference cartilage (MFX, $p = 0.007$; MACT, $p = 0.008$). cSI and MOCART scores in repair tissue did not differ between MFX and MACT patients ($p = 0.185$). cSI from reference cartilage of the patients and cartilage of the volunteers did not reach the level of significant difference ($p = 0.355$).

In conclusion, both MFX and MACT produced repair tissue with lower ^{23}Na concentrations and, thus, of lower quality compared to native cartilage. Moreover, after MFX and MACT techniques, the generated repair tissue in the ankle joint has similar GAG content and similar morphological characteristics in patients with a comparable surgical outcome.

References

1. Guermazi A, et al. State of the art: MR imaging after knee cartilage repair surgery. Radiology. 2015;277(1):23–43.
2. Messner K, Maletius W. The long-term prognosis for severe damage to weight-bearing cartilage in the knee: a 14-year clinical and radiographic follow-up in 28 young athletes. Acta Orthop Scand. 1996;67(2):165–8.
3. Mithoefer K, et al. Return to sports participation after articular cartilage repair in the knee: scientific evidence. Am J Sports Med. 2009;37(Suppl 1):167S–76S.
4. de Windt TS, et al. Is magnetic resonance imaging reliable in predicting clinical outcome after articular cartilage repair of the knee? A systematic review and meta-analysis. Am J Sports Med. 2013;41(7):1695–702.
5. Blackman AJ, et al. Correlation between magnetic resonance imaging and clinical outcomes after cartilage repair surgery in the knee: a systematic review and meta-analysis. Am J Sports Med. 2013;41(6):1426–34.
6. Marlovits S, et al. Magnetic resonance observation of cartilage repair tissue (MOCART) for the evaluation of autologous chondrocyte transplantation: determination of interobserver variability and correlation to clinical outcome after 2 years. Eur J Radiol. 2006;57(1):16–23.
7. Schreiner MM, et al. The MOCART (magnetic resonance observation of cartilage repair tissue) 2.0 knee score and atlas. Cartilage. 2019:1947603519865308.
8. Rubenstein JD, et al. Image resolution and signal-to-noise ratio requirements for MR imaging of degenerative cartilage. AJR Am J Roentgenol. 1997;169(4):1089–96.
9. Disler DG, et al. Fat-suppressed three-dimensional spoiled gradient-echo MR imaging of hyaline cartilage defects in the knee: comparison with standard MR imaging and arthroscopy. AJR Am J Roentgenol. 1996;167(1):127–32.
10. Peterfy CG, et al. MR imaging of the arthritic knee: improved discrimination of cartilage, synovium, and effusion with pulsed saturation transfer and fat-suppressed T1-weighted sequences. Radiology. 1994;191(2):413–9.
11. Trattnig S, et al. Imaging articular cartilage defects with 3D fat-suppressed echo planar imaging: comparison with conventional 3D fat-suppressed gradient echo sequence and correlation with histology. J Comput Assist Tomogr. 1998;22(1):8–14.
12. Alparslan L, et al. Postoperative magnetic resonance imaging of articular cartilage repair. Semin Musculoskelet Radiol. 2001;5(4):345–63.
13. Choi YS, Potter HG, Chun TJ. MR imaging of cartilage repair in the knee and ankle. Radiographics. 2008;28(4):1043–59.
14. Farr J, et al. Clinical cartilage restoration: evolution and overview. Clin Orthop Relat Res. 2011;469(10):2696–705.
15. Hunziker EB, et al. An educational review of cartilage repair: precepts & practice--myths & misconceptions--progress & prospects. Osteoarthr Cartil. 2015;23(3):334–50.
16. Link TM, et al. Normal and pathological MR findings in osteochondral autografts with longitudinal follow-up. Eur Radiol. 2006;16(1):88–96.
17. Sanders TG, et al. Autogenous osteochondral "plug" transfer for the treatment of focal chondral defects: postoperative MR appearance with clinical correlation. Skelet Radiol. 2001;30(10):570–8.
18. Herber S, et al. Indirect MR-arthrography in the follow up of autologous osteochondral transplantation. Rofo. 2003;175(2):226–33.
19. Trattnig S, et al. Matrix-based autologous chondrocyte implantation for cartilage repair with HyalograftC: two-year follow-up by magnetic resonance imaging. Eur J Radiol. 2006;57(1):9–15.
20. Trattnig S, et al. Matrix-based autologous chondrocyte implantation for cartilage repair: noninvasive monitoring by high-resolution magnetic resonance imaging. Magn Reson Imaging. 2005;23(7):779–87.
21. Trattnig S, et al. MR imaging of osteochondral grafts and autologous chondrocyte implantation. Eur Radiol. 2007;17(1):103–18.
22. Vahdati A, Wagner DR. Implant size and mechanical properties influence the failure of the adhesive bond between cartilage implants and native tissue in a finite element analysis. J Biomech. 2013;46(9):1554–60.
23. Goodwin DW, Wadghiri YZ, Dunn JF. Micro-imaging of articular cartilage: T2, proton density, and the magic angle effect. Acad Radiol. 1998;5(11):790–8.
24. Goodwin DW, Zhu H, Dunn JF. In vitro MR imaging of hyaline cartilage: correlation with scan-

ning electron microscopy. AJR Am J Roentgenol. 2000;174(2):405–9.

25. Dardzinski BJ, et al. Spatial variation of T2 in human articular cartilage. Radiology. 1997;205(2):546–50.

26. Mosher TJ, et al. Effect of gender on in vivo cartilage magnetic resonance imaging T2 mapping. J Magn Reson Imaging. 2004;19(3):323–8.

27. Mosher TJ, Dardzinski BJ, Smith MB. Human articular cartilage: influence of aging and early symptomatic degeneration on the spatial variation of T2 - preliminary findings at 3 T. Radiology. 2000;214(1):259–66.

28. Nissi MJ, et al. T-2 relaxation time mapping reveals age- and species-related diversity of collagen network architecture in articular cartilage. Osteoarthr Cartil. 2006;14(12):1265–71.

29. Multanen J, et al. Effects of high-impact training on bone and articular cartilage: 12-month randomized controlled quantitative MRI study. J Bone Miner Res. 2014;29(1):192–201.

30. Shiomi T, et al. Loading and knee alignment have significant influence on cartilage MRI T2 in porcine knee joints. Osteoarthr Cartil. 2010;18(7):902–8.

31. Apprich S, et al. Quantitative T2 mapping of the patella at 3.0 T is sensitive to early cartilage degeneration, but also to loading of the knee. Eur J Radiol. 2012;81(4):E438–43.

32. Kijowski R, et al. Evaluation of the articular cartilage of the knee joint: value of adding a T2 mapping sequence to a routine MR imaging protocol. Radiology. 2013;267(2):503–13.

33. Raya JG, et al. T2 measurement in articular cartilage: impact of the fitting method on accuracy and precision at low SNR. Magn Reson Med. 2010;63(1):181–93.

34. Mamisch TC, et al. T2 star relaxation times for assessment of articular cartilage at 3 T: a feasibility study. Skelet Radiol. 2012;41(3):287–92.

35. Carballido-Gamio J, Link TM, Majumdar S. New techniques for cartilage magnetic resonance imaging relaxation time analysis: texture analysis of flattened cartilage and localized intra- and inter-subject comparisons. Magn Reson Med. 2008;59(6):1472–7.

36. Joseph GB, et al. Elevated cartilage T2 and increased severity of cartilage defects at baseline are associated with the development of knee pain over 7 years. Osteoarthr Cartil. 2013;21:S185–6.

37. Schooler J, et al. Longitudinal evaluation of T-1 rho and T-2 spatial distribution in osteoarthritic and healthy medial knee cartilage. Osteoarthr Cartil. 2014;22(1):51–62.

38. Pell GS, et al. Optimized clinical T2 relaxometry with a standard CPMG sequence. J Magn Reson Imaging. 2006;23(2):248–52.

39. Welsch GH, et al. Rapid estimation of cartilage T2 based on double echo at steady state (DESS) with 3 tesla. Magn Reson Med. 2009;62(2):544–9.

40. Juras V, et al. A comparison of multi-echo spin-echo and triple-echo steady-state T2 mapping for in vivo evaluation of articular cartilage. Eur Radiol. 2016;26(6):1905–12.

41. Juras V, et al. The comparison of the performance of 3 T and 7 T T-2 mapping for untreated low-grade cartilage lesions. Magn Reson Imaging. 2019;55:86–92.

42. Baum T, et al. Association of magnetic resonance imaging-based knee cartilage T2 measurements and focal knee lesions with knee pain: data from the osteoarthritis initiative. Arthritis Care Res. 2012;64(2):248–55.

43. Aroen A, et al. Evaluation of focal cartilage lesions of the knee using MRI T2 mapping and delayed gadolinium enhanced MRI of cartilage (dGEMRIC). BMC Musculoskelet Disord. 2016;17

44. Hannila I, et al. Patellar cartilage lesions: comparison of magnetic resonance imaging and T2 relaxation-time mapping. Acta Radiol. 2007;48(4):444–8.

45. Richter DL, et al. Knee articular cartilage repair and restoration techniques: a review of the literature. Sports Health. 2016;8(2):153–60.

46. White LM, et al. Cartilage T2 assessment: differentiation of normal hyaline cartilage and reparative tissue after arthroscopic cartilage repair in equine subjects. Radiology. 2006;241(2):407–14.

47. Watanabe A, et al. Ability of dGEMRIC and T2 mapping to evaluate cartilage repair after microfracture: a goat study. Osteoarthr Cartil. 2009;17(10):1341–9.

48. Welsch GH, et al. Cartilage T2 assessment at 3-T MR imaging: in vivo differentiation of normal hyaline cartilage from reparative tissue after two cartilage repair procedures - initial experience. Radiology. 2008;247(1):154–61.

49. Mamisch TC, et al. Quantitative T2 mapping of knee cartilage: differentiation of healthy control cartilage and cartilage repair tissue in the knee with unloading - initial results. Radiology. 2010;254(3):818–26.

50. Juras V, et al. Kinematic biomechanical assessment of human articular cartilage transplants in the knee using 3-T MRI: an in vivo reproducibility study. Eur Radiol. 2009;19(5):1246–52.

51. Chang G, et al. High resolution morphologic imaging and T2 mapping of cartilage at 7 tesla: comparison of cartilage repair patients and healthy controls. Magn Reson Mater Phys Biol Med. 2013;26(6):539–48.

52. Welsch GH, et al. In vivo biochemical 7.0 tesla magnetic resonance - preliminary results of dGEMRIC, zonal T2, and T2 * mapping of articular cartilage. Investig Radiol. 2008;43(9):619–26.

53. Brix M, et al. Cartilage repair of the ankle with microfracturing or autologous chondrocyte implantation/matrix associated autologous chondrocyte implantation: follow up from 1 to 14 years. Osteoarthr Cartil. 2012;20:S130–1.

54. Domayer SE, et al. Cartilage repair of the ankle: first results of T2 mapping at 7.0 T after microfracture and matrix associated autologous cartilage transplantation. Osteoarthr Cartil. 2012;20(8):829–36.

55. Holtzman DJ, et al. T-1 rho and T-2 quantitative magnetic resonance imaging analysis of cartilage regeneration following microfracture and mosaicplasty cartilage resurfacing procedures. J Magn Reson Imaging. 2010;32(4):914–23.

56. Krusche-Mandl I, et al. Long-term results 8 years after autologous osteochondral transplantation: 7 T gagCEST and sodium magnetic resonance imaging with morphological and clinical correlation. Osteoarthr Cartil. 2012;20(5):357–63.

57. Theologis AA, et al. Longitudinal analysis of T-1 rho and T-2 quantitative MRI of knee cartilage laminar organization following microfracture surgery. Knee. 2012;19(5):652–7.

58. Battaglia M, et al. Validity of T2 mapping in characterization of the regeneration tissue by bone marrow derived cell transplantation in osteochondral lesions of the ankle. Eur J Radiol. 2011;80(2):E132–9.

59. Kurkijarvi JE, et al. Evaluation of cartilage repair in the distal femur after autologous chondrocyte transplantation using T-2 relaxation time and dGEMRIC. Osteoarthr Cartil. 2007;15(4):372–8.

60. Trattnig S, et al. Quantitative T-2 mapping of matrix-associated autologous chondrocyte transplantation at 3 tesla - an in vivo cross-sectional study. Investig Radiol. 2007;42(6):442–8.

61. Giannini S, et al. Surgical treatment of osteochondral lesions of the talus by open-field autologous chondrocyte implantation a 10-year follow-up clinical and magnetic resonance imaging T2-mapping evaluation. Am J Sports Med. 2009;37:112s–8s.

62. Ling W, et al. Assessment of glycosaminoglycan concentration in vivo by chemical exchange-dependent saturation transfer (gagCEST). Proc Natl Acad Sci U S A. 2008;105(7):2266–70.

63. Link TM. Editorial comment: the future of compositional MRI for cartilage. Eur Radiol. 2018;28(7):2872–3.

64. Kogan F, Hariharan H, Reddy R. Chemical exchange saturation transfer (CEST) imaging: description of technique and potential clinical applications. Curr Radiol Rep. 2013;1(2):102–14.

65. Roughley PJ. The structure and function of cartilage proteoglycans. Eur Cell Mater. 2006;12:92–101.

66. Kempson GE, et al. Correlations between stiffness and the chemical constituents of cartilage on the human femoral head. Biochim Biophys Acta. 1970;215(1):70–7.

67. Watanabe A, et al. Delayed gadolinium-enhanced MR to determine glycosaminoglycan concentration in reparative cartilage after autologous chondrocyte implantation: preliminary results. Radiology. 2006;239(1):201–8.

68. Zbyn S, et al. Evaluation of cartilage repair and osteoarthritis with sodium MRI. NMR Biomed. 2015;

69. Zaiss M, Bachert P. Chemical exchange saturation transfer (CEST) and MR Z-spectroscopy in vivo: a review of theoretical approaches and methods. Phys Med Biol. 2013;58(22):R221–69.

70. Schreiner MM, et al. Reproducibility and regional variations of an improved gagCEST protocol for the in vivo evaluation of knee cartilage at 7 T. MAGMA. 2016;29(3):513–21.

71. Schmitt B, et al. Cartilage quality assessment by using glycosaminoglycan chemical exchange saturation transfer and (23)Na MR imaging at 7 T. Radiology. 2011;260(1):257–64.

72. Krusche-Mandl I, et al. Long-term results 8 years after autologous osteochondral transplantation: 7 T gagCEST and sodium magnetic resonance imaging with morphological and clinical correlation. Osteoarthr Cartil. 2012;20(5):357–63.

73. Rehnitz C, et al. Comparison of biochemical cartilage imaging techniques at 3 T MRI. Osteoarthr Cartil. 2014;22(10):1732–42.

74. Singh A, et al. Chemical exchange saturation transfer magnetic resonance imaging of human knee cartilage at 3 T and 7 T. Magn Reson Med. 2012;68(2):588–94.

75. Brinkhof S, et al. Detection of early cartilage damage: feasibility and potential of gagCEST imaging at 7T. Eur Radiol. 2018;28(7):2874–81.

76. Mankin HJ. Biochemical and metabolic aspects of osteoarthritis. Orthop Clin North Am. 1971;2(1):19–31.

77. Zbyn S, et al. Sodium magnetic resonance imaging of ankle joint in cadaver specimens, volunteers, and patients after different cartilage repair techniques at 7 T: initial results. Investig Radiol. 2015;50(4):246–54.

78. Trattnig S, et al. 23Na MR imaging at 7 T after knee matrix-associated autologous chondrocyte transplantation preliminary results. Radiology. 2010;257(1):175–84.

79. Zbyn S, et al. Evaluation of native hyaline cartilage and repair tissue after two cartilage repair surgery techniques with 23Na MR imaging at 7 T: initial experience. Osteoarthr Cartil. 2012;20(8):837–45.

80. Zbyn S, et al. Sodium magnetic resonance imaging of ankle joint in cadaver specimens, volunteers, and patients after different cartilage repair techniques at 7 T - initial results. NMR Biomed. 2014;50:246–54.

Assessment of Patient, Joint, Cartilage Injury Characteristics

Kevin R. Hayek and Jeffrey A. Macalena

6.1 Assessment of the Patient

6.1.1 Clinical History

A thorough history of prior injuries, treatments, and procedures should be conducted. It is important to acknowledge that not all cartilage injuries require intervention. Asymptomatic presentation is most common when considering all cartilage injuries. Many focal defects will be found on advanced imaging. It is the surgeon's role to determine which findings are significant.

The majority of symptomatic injuries of cartilage present with pain [1]. Associated findings include swelling and limited range of motion. The patient may report lack of confidence in the knee or inability to return to activities. The importance of a comprehensive understanding of knee symptomatology cannot be understated. Cartilage injuries often present in association with other injuries. Locking, catching, clicking, or popping are common complaints from the knee, and are suggestive of concomitant pathology.

The patient should be asked about a history of injury or instability. Mechanisms often predict injuries sustained. Acute injury, opposed to chronic, is a relatively better prognostic factor for

outcomes. Traumatic lesions have a higher rate of return to prior sport in athletes (87% vs. 33%) compared to degenerative lesions [2]. Patellar instability is essential to assess for when patellofemoral joint pain is present. Patellar dislocation can be associated with injury to the facets [3–7]. The presence of instability may necessitate stabilizing procedures. Age of onset, frequency, and severity are key history items.

Athletic, recreational, and work histories should be obtained. The sports history should consist of type of activity, level of competition, and anticipated patient goals for return to activity. Patients should be counseled that many individuals will be able to return to prior activities, but fewer will return to the same level, or presymptom performance [2]. Younger patients, <20 years of age, have a higher chance of returning to competition. Occupational history should be obtained including functional requirements. Assess specifically for ambulating, lifting, bending, squatting, and climbing. This information aids the surgeon in setting realistic goals and expectations for recovery. Many patients will sustain injuries at work. Workers' compensation injuries are associated with decreased patient-reported outcomes [8]. This should not discourage appropriate surgical intervention, but requires the surgeon to have a frank discussion about long-term expectations.

The patient should be asked about all prior treatments. This includes nonoperative treatments

K. R. Hayek · J. A. Macalena (✉)
Department of Orthopedic Surgery, University of Minnesota, Minneapolis, MN, USA
e-mail: maca0049@umn.edu

© ISAKOS 2021
A. J. Krych et al. (eds.), *Cartilage Injury of the Knee*,
https://doi.org/10.1007/978-3-030-78051-7_6

such as physical therapy, injections, and alternative therapies. Operative reports should be obtained for all prior procedures. Increasingly, medical records allow for the digital storage of intraoperative images. These are helpful as surgical reports may not be sufficiently detailed. It is important to know a history of prior cartilage procedures. Eventually most traumatized knees will show global degenerative sequela. Ekman *et al.* found that 50% of patients who underwent osteoarticular autograft transplant had progression of radiographic osteoarthritis at a median of 11.5 years [9]. Additionally, revision cartilage procedures have been noted to have higher rates of failure [10]. The cartilage surgeon needs to be mindful of the limits of restoration. Some knees with more diffuse and advanced changes and patients with lower demands may be better suited for arthroplasty.

Patient age is also an important consideration. The literature displays mixed results with the effect of age. In general, older age is correlated with poorer outcomes in cartilage surgery [8, 11–14]. Older age has a higher hazard ratio for graft failure in osteochondral allograft (OCA) for plateau lesions [8]. Patients over 40 years old with large lesions are more likely to have graft failure with OCA than younger patients [13]. Other data suggests that patients older than 40 with isolated medial or lateral femoral condylar lesions undergoing fresh osteochondral allografts had equivalent Knee injury and Osteoarthritis Outcome Scores (KOOS) [15]. Their work suggests the importance of choosing surgical patients who have a paucity of diffuse degenerative changes. Despite better graft incorporation, some studies have shown younger patients to have lower KOOS symptom scores. This may reflect their higher activity demands and overall expectations [16].

Patient body mass index is an importance consideration. Higher BMI is a risk factor for cartilage lesion progression [17] and is negatively correlated with patient-reported outcomes [13, 16] and graft survivorship [18]. Patients who are above their target weight should be encouraged to set goals for weight reduction. Consider referral to a dietician or discussion with the patient's primary care provider who may assist with management.

6.1.2 Special Populations

Female and pediatric patients are often considered unique populations. In cartilage surgery, they have been observed to do as well or better than male and skeletally mature counterparts, respectively. Female patients have been observed to have similar rates of clinical improvement, cartilage regeneration, and graft survival after cartilage surgery [16, 19]. For pediatric populations with cartilage injuries, surgery is a viable treatment for persistent traumatic defects or osteochondritis dissecans lesions. A systematic review of cartilage procedures in pediatric patients found beneficial evidence in support of several common surgical treatments including microfracture, osteochondral autograft (mosaicplasty), osteochondral allograft, and autologous chondrocyte implantation (ACI) [20]. The surgeon must take into account the specific pediatric considerations of remaining growth and the physis in their surgical plans.

6.1.3 Medical Comorbidities and Family History

It is important to determine and consider the patient's medical comorbidities. Personal or family history of venous thromboembolic event (VTE) including deep vein thrombosis (DVT) and pulmonary embolism (PE) should be noted. Appropriate prophylaxis or treatment should be addressed in the perioperative period. Diabetes carries increases risks of wound complications [21]. Smoking and nicotine consumption negatively affect the outcome of cartilage and ligament surgery [22]. Patients must be counselled to the risks and be encouraged to engage in cessation preoperatively. The patient should be referred to a cessation program or provider if they are agreeable.

Assess for personal or family history of rheumatoid arthritis, connective tissue disorders, or conditions associated with systemic laxity. Rheumatoid arthritis is a systemic disease, causing inflammatory destruction of the articular surface. Although the use of restoration techniques has been reported in limited numbers [23], caution is advised. Many providers consider rheumatoid arthritis a contraindication to cartilage surgery. Injury to the surrounding osteochondral unit during grafting may release pro-inflammatory mediators worsening the condition [24, 25]. Systemic laxity conditions including Ehlers-Danlos and Marfan syndromes affect joint stability and are heritable. Additionally, familial associations have been seen in osteochondritis dissecans (OCD) [26, 27].

6.2 Assessment of the Joint

6.2.1 Physical Examination

A thorough evaluation includes global lower extremity function assessment. Gait should be examined, and varus or valgus thrusts should be noted. The hip joints should be examined for pain or limited range of motion [28, 29]. Referred pain from the hip to the knee has an anatomic basis related to the branches of the femoral nerve [30]. While more commonly a cause of hip pain, consider the lumbar spine as a source of radicular pain when the patient has concomitant low-back symptoms [31, 32]. Examine the neurologic status of the limb for functional deficits which may contraindicate surgery.

6.2.2 Examination of the Knee Joint

The clinical history of cartilage injury may overlap with other intra-articular pathologies. The physical examination should be used to help confirm the diagnosis and identify alternative or coexisting pathologies. Both knees should be examined. In general, the less affected knee should be examined first. Examination should include inspection for prior surgical incisions which may affect procedures attempted or approaches used. Assess for effusion. Effusion indicates acute injury or ongoing irritation.

6.2.3 Tibiofemoral Articulation

Palpation should include the joint line, collateral ligaments, and subcutaneous bony landmarks. Examine the popliteal fossa for tenderness or masses. Baker's cysts are common. Range of motion should be assessed. Less than a 90-degree arc of motion preoperatively is concerning. Arthrofibrosis may limit any benefits of cartilage restoration. The collateral ligamentous exam consists of varus and valgus stress testing at 0° and 30° of flexion. The Lachman and pivot shift tests are used to assess for ACL injury. The posterior drawer and dial tests will assess for injury of the posterior cruciate ligament and posterolateral corner, respectively.

Provocative examination includes the Thessaly [33] and McMurray [34] tests. Typically, these tests are most helpful with large meniscal tears that become caught between the femur and tibia during motion. They may to a lesser degree be positive with cartilaginous injuries in overlapping anatomic areas.

6.2.4 Patellofemoral Articulation

The patellofemoral (PF) articulation comprises a complex anatomy balanced static and dynamic forces. Assessment of hyperlaxity by Beighton criteria [35] is a component of the instability exam. Tenderness over the medial patellofemoral ligament (MPFL) is known as the Bassett sign which may indicate injury or rupture [36]. Patellar crepitation is a poor prognostic sign for cartilage lesions in instability patients. Patients with preoperative crepitation are 3.6 times more likely to have a medial patellar facet lesion [37]. Crepitation is also indicative of larger and higher grade lesions.

The apprehension test assesses for incompetence of the MPFL ligament. This test described by Fairbanks [38] is performed in the supine position with a relaxed knee. The examiner directs a medial to lateral force on the patella attempting to gradually sublux the patella. If the patient stops the exam, or indicates that they feel their patella will dislocate, the result is positive. The exam has intermediate specificity for patellar instability of 70–92% [39, 40]. Dynamic variants of this test have been described [41, 42] and these have been reported to improve the sensitivities and specificities to the mid-90s and mid-80s, respectively.

Assessment of patellofemoral dynamic tracking includes observation for a pathologic J-sign. The J-sign occurs as the vector of patellar motion shifts medially when the patella overcomes the lateral ridge of the trochlea instead of entering the trochlea centrally when the knee moves from extension into flexion. The J-sign has relatively high intra-observer reliability and moderate concordance among observers for PF instability [43]. Extensor mechanism mal-tracking needs to be addressed to prevent recurrent PF cartilage injury. When J-tracking is apparent, it is helpful to observe the degree of flexion at which the patella relocates to facilitate surgical planning.

6.2.5 Radiographic Evaluation of Joint Alignment and Integrity

Knee joint alignment is a key consideration for the surgeon considering cartilage restoration or reconstruction. Alignment is best evaluated quantitatively. A regimented radiographic series should be obtained for every patient. Standard measurements are made on every series. Supplemental imaging techniques are described as well.

AP standing radiographs, as a component of full-length coronal hip-to-knee radiographs, should always be obtained. A PA weight-bearing flexion (Rosenberg) view allows for assessment of the functional portion of the condyles. The evaluator should assess for degenerative changes: subchondral cysts, joint space narrowing, osteophytes, and sclerosis. Focal cartilage lesions may not be evident unless there is an osteochondral lesion or significant degenerative changes. Assessment for osteochondritis dissecans lesions in pediatric patients is important, as these often present as lucent areas or irregular subchondral

bone along the lateral aspect of the medial femoral condyle.

On standing full-length AP coronal alignment radiographs, the mechanical axis of both lower extremities through the knee should be measured. To determine the alignment of the knee, two intersecting lines are drawn representing the intersection of the mechanical axes of the femur and tibia forming the hip-knee-ankle angle [44–46]. In young healthy males, the coronal alignment is near neutral, or 1–2° of varus at the knee [44]. Females have slightly more varus. The native joint line is set in 2–3° of varus compared to the mechanical axis [46]. Unsatisfactory alignment requires consideration of correction concomitantly, or prior to a cartilage restoration or reconstruction procedure.

Increased varus alignment of the knee has been noted in association with progression of osteoarthritis [47, 48]. Small amounts of varus deformity, as little at 3°, can cause significant increases in articular contact pressures [49]. Studies on the success of ACI and osteochondral grafting in the setting of osteotomy support correction of coronal knee malalignment. A meta-analysis of 389 high tibial osteotomies with adjunctive cartilage procedures showed a modest increase (97 vs. 92%) in HTO survival compared to HTO alone at 5 years post-procedure [50]. Retrospective analysis of 43 ACI procedures with varus alignment under 5° showed a higher proportion of survivorship for those that underwent concomitant high tibial osteotomy at 71 months postoperatively [51]. Leon et al. noted that a higher proportion of osteochondral allograft failures within 5 years had undercorrected alignment [52]. The available research for coronal plane deformities suggests that these should be addressed prior to or concurrently with cartilage restoration procedures.

The lateral knee view at 30° of flexion best evaluates the patellar height [53] and trochlear dysplasia [54], and provides a second view to localize lesions in the femoral condyles. The evaluator should examine the anterior femur for a crossover sign or prominence which is suggestive of dysplasia. Trochlear prominences, bumps, or supratrochlear spurs are pathologic when greater than 3 mm [54]. The evaluator should measure the Caton-Deschamps [54–56], Insall-Salvati [54, 56, 57], or Blackburne-Peel [53, 58] ratios to determine if the patellar height is in the normative range.

The axial 45-degree patellar (Merchant) view best evaluates the patellofemoral articulation in the zone of maximum engagement. Patellofemoral arthrosis, lateral tilt, and morphologic patellofemoral dysplasia can be assessed. The sulcus angle is measured between the two facets of the trochlea, and angles above 145° are considered dysplastic [54, 59, 60].

Anatomic abnormalities including patella alta, trochlear dysplasia, or excessive lateral patellar tilt are more prevalent in patients with patellofemoral cartilage lesions noted on MRI compared to controls without patellofemoral lesions [61]. There has been a long-standing association between aberrant patellofemoral anatomy and patellar dislocation [54]. Acute patella dislocations have been correlated with lesions of the inferomedial patella and lateral trochlea [3, 4]. For patellar or trochlear lesions, instability or overload should be addressed prior to or concomitantly with cartilage intervention. Recurrent instability has been noted to have a 4.5 times higher risk association with the development of osteoarthritis [62].

6.2.6 Supplemental Radiographs

When there is a concern for patellofemoral instability, the 20-degree axial patellar (Laurin) view is useful. In 20° of knee flexion the patella is at initial trochlear engagement [63]. Patients may have normal trochlear morphology and depth distally on the Merchant view, but Laurin's view may show abnormal patellar position more proximally due to abnormal patellar force vector, high trochlear dysplasia, or initial height mismatch.

Stress radiographs assist in the diagnosis of multi-ligamentous knee injuries, as well as collateral and posterior cruciate injuries [64–66].

There are many methods for stress application, with 16 different methods noted in a recent meta-analysis, making standardization challenging [65]. It is important for both the surgeon and technologist obtaining images to be knowledgeable regarding the techniques to maximize their validity. Higher volumes will improve reproducibility, suggesting that patients with complex ligamentous and cartilage injuries may benefit from being treated at referral centers.

6.2.7 Supplemental CT Scans

CT is valuable for the assessment of patellofemoral anatomy in cases of instability and rotational profile of the lower extremity. Many patients will present to clinic with an MRI scan ordered by another provider or clinic. The anatomic measurements discussed in this section can be made from MR images; however, their values may slightly differ from the CT.

Measure the tibial tubercle trochlear groove (TT-TG) distance on the axial CT. Values above 20 mm are abnormal, and values of 15–20 mm are borderline for contributing to patellar instability [54]. TT-TG can also be measured off MRI but may slightly underestimate the value [67]. Unloading of the lateral facet by anterior medialization of the tibial tubercle can correct forces causing lateral overload, but it is important to realize that overcorrection can worsen a damaged medial facet. Therefore, balance is preferred relative to overcorrection [61].

CT limited hip-knee-ankle for axial rotation assessment is the gold standard for assessing femoral torsion or anteversion and tibial torsion. This study should be considered in patients with patellofemoral cartilage injuries and concomitant instability when there are side-to-side abnormalities on physical exam or otherwise normal PF anatomy on CT. Intra-observer reliability is higher with CT than MRI making it preferred despite the downside of radiation exposure [68] (Table 6.1).

Table 6.1 Recommendations for standard knee cartilage injury radiographic series

Authors' recommendations for standard cartilage patient radiographic series:
1. 45° flexion PA weight-bearing radiographs (Rosenberg view)
2. AP full-length lower extremity standing coronal alignment views
3. 30° flexion lateral view
4. 45° flexion axial view (Merchant view)

6.3 Assessment of Cartilage Injury

Magnetic resonance imaging is the most valuable imaging study for assessing the articular surface (see Chap. 5 on MRI imaging). A high-quality MRI study with a minimum 3.0 Tesla magnet is preferred. Fast spin echo sequences (FSE), turbo spin echo sequences (TSE), fat suppression, and multichannel joint-specific coils improve the resolution and cartilage discrimination from surrounding tissues [69, 70]. Size and depth of lesions can be measured on MRI; however, it is important to recognize that MRI frequently underestimates size [71]. Assess for intact subchondral bone, edema, cysts, osteophytes, and resorption. Global degenerative changes are indicative of evolving osteoarthritis which has been associated with poorer outcomes and lower rates of graft integration [12]. MR-based cartilage scoring systems have been described. The MOCART and AMADEUS are meticulously crafted research tools, but can be cumbersome for clinical practice [72–74]. Focus the assessment on lesion location and area as these continue to be the major driving factors in treatment selection. Metallic implants from prior surgery can cause artifact limiting the MRI utility. CT arthrogram is of limited value. Proceeding with diagnostic arthroscopy for staging should be considered.

Diagnostic arthroscopy will definitively display the size, location, and character of the cartilage lesions. It can be performed immediately prior to interventions or as a separate procedure. Intra-articular structures, cartilage surfaces, and lesions should be photographed in regimented form. This provides consistency reviewing cases in follow-up, or when describing findings to other providers. Assess both the MR images and structures intraoperatively for associated ligament and meniscal cartilage injuries. Meniscal or ligamentous injuries or deficiencies should be addressed prior to or concurrently with a cartilage repair or restoration. It is important to document findings in the operative report in a systematic and specific manner. Location is a key factor. Patellar-trochlear lesions require assessment of instability or overload. Tibial lesions can be difficult to treat, due to the limited access. Isolated medial femoral condyle lesions typically have the best outcomes. When staged treatment is planned, consider a cartilage biopsy at the time of a diagnostic arthroscopy for autologous chondrocyte implantation.

Bipolar lesions can present treatment challenges (Fig. 6.1). Higher rates of failure are observed for the treatment of reciprocal femoral and tibial lesions with OCA [10, 75]. Importantly, bipolar lesions of the femur and tibia have shown clinical improvement with treatment of only femoral lesions [76]. Multifocal lesions, those requiring multiple adjacent grafts or plugs, show significant postoperative improvements in KOOS scores, but reoperation is common (>20%) [77]. Additionally, 33% of patients who had multiple directly adjacent plugs failed at 8 years postoperatively. As a caveat, despite the higher rates of failure with adjacent grafts, patients who have successful integration are significantly improved [10].

Description of the lesion should include size in mm in the medial-lateral and anteroposterior planes, depth, and base tissue (cartilage, subchondral bone, etc.). Using a ruler in the photograph or objects with known dimensions such as a shaver or probe can be valuable when revisiting photos. Direct visualization scoring systems for cartilage injury include the International Cartilage Repair Society (ICRS) [78] and Outerbridge classifications [79]. Lower grade lesions may be candidates for marrow stimulation techniques, though increasingly improved outcomes are being seen with osteochondral grafting and MACI (Table 6.2).

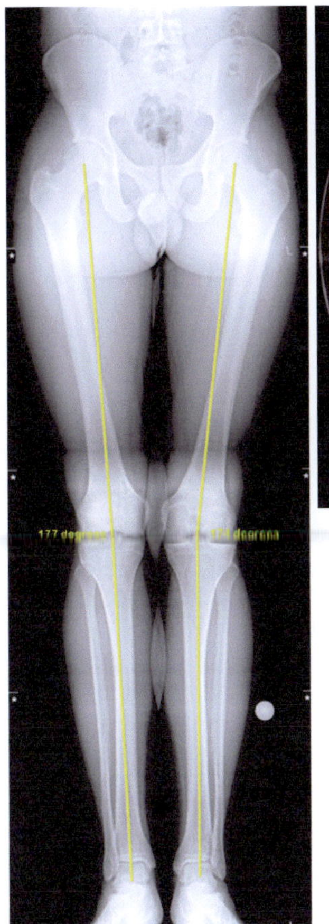

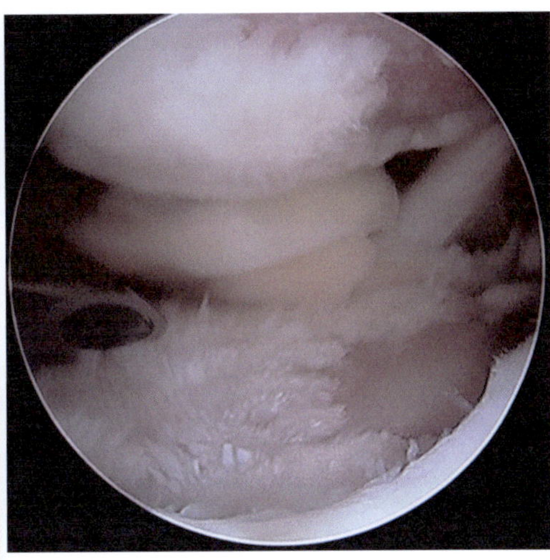

Fig. 6.1 Long leg alignment radiograph and arthroscopic images of grade 3 and 4 chondral changes in the lateral compartment of a 24-year-old male with a 6-degree valgus deformity in the setting of a radial meniscus tear

Table 6.2 International cartilage repair society classification for articular cartilage lesions [78]

ICRS cartilage injury grading system		
Grade 0	Normal cartilage	
Grade 1	Superficial lesions (fissures or cracks) without significant depth	
Grade 2	Lesions extending less than 50% of the cartilage depth	
Grade 3	Lesions extending greater than 50% of the cartilage depth	A. Above the calcified layer
		B. Down to the calcified layer
		C. Through the calcified layer but above subchondral bone
		D. Surface blisters with underlying >50% lesions
Grade 4	Severely abnormal lesions extending through the subchondral bone	

Square area of the lesion is important to determine during the evaluation as it will be a key factor in the treatments offered. There are two broad categories when considering the area of defects: <2 to 4 cm^2 and >2 to 4 cm^2. For defects <2 to 4 cm^2 squared both microfracture and osteochondral autografting (mosaicplasty) are reasonable treatment options. Mosaicplasty has been shown to have higher clinical scores than microfracture in long-term follow-up [80, 81]. Regarding larger defects, the SUMMIT trial showed that cartilage injuries 3 cm^2 or greater had improved KOOS pain and function scores at 2 and 5 years when comparing MACI to microfracture [82, 83]. Interestingly, a recent follow-up meta-analysis of all ACI trials versus

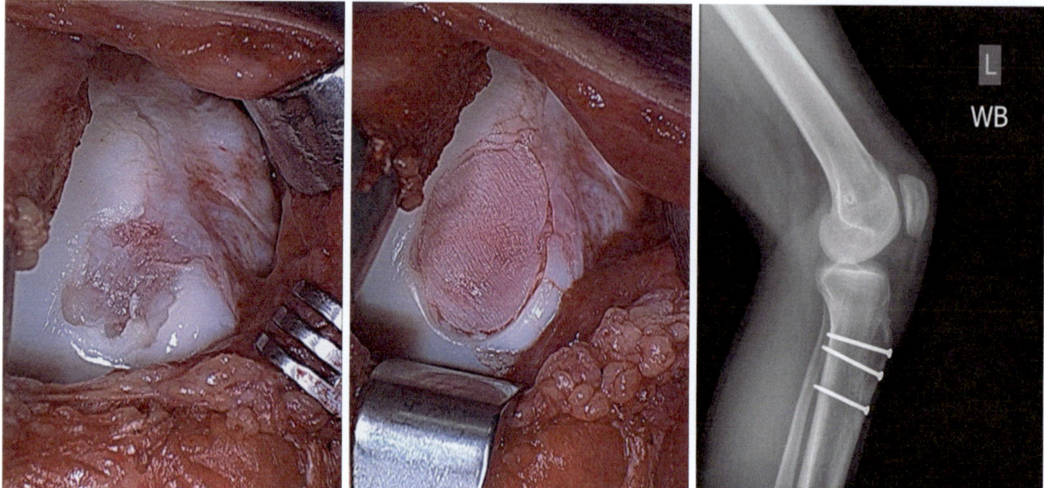

Fig. 6.2 16-Year-old male with an ICRS Grade 4.2 × 2.5 cm full-thickness chondral lesion of the lateral trochlea in the setting of recurrent patellar instability, with patella alta and increased TT-TT, who underwent a staging arthroscopy and later MACI to the trochlea with tibial tubercle osteotomy and MPFL reconstruction

microfracture found only partial sub-score improvements with MACI, which may have been affected by the heterogeneity of trial methodology and endpoints [84](Fig. 6.2).

Postoperatively, MRI can be used for the evaluation of cartilage graft integration. Patients undergoing MRI 12 years after MACI procedure showed good correlation between KOOS scores and MRI findings [85]. The surgeon should look for defect filling which is a beneficial finding. Graft hypertrophy, cartilage hyperintense signal, absence of cartilage signal, subchondral edema, or knee effusions are characteristics on MRI that would be consistent with poorer graft incorporation, and likely to be associated with residual symptoms.

6.4 Conclusions

Cartilage injuries of the knee are common. History, exam, and imaging should be used to determine which injuries are significant. Age, body mass index, and comorbidities are important patient factors. Concomitant ligamentous injuries, joint malalignment, and patellofemoral instability often require correction to improve cartilage surgery outcomes. High-quality MRI is essential for evaluation. Diagnostic arthroscopy provides definitive assessment of lesions. Location and area of lesions are key factors in treatment type. Excellent outcomes can be obtained with proper patient selection and optimization.

References

1. Pihlajamäki HK, Kuikka P-I, Leppänen V-V, Kiuru MJ, Mattila VM. The diagnosis of chondromalacia patellae reliability of clinical findings and magnetic resonance imaging for reliability of clinical findings and magnetic resonance imaging for the diagnosis of chondromalacia patellae. J Bone Joint Surg. 2010;92:927–34.
2. Zaffagnini S, Vannini F, Di Martino A, Andriolo L, Sessa A, Perdisa F, et al. Low rate of return to pre-injury sport level in athletes after cartilage surgery: a 10-year follow-up study. Knee Surg Sport Traumatol Arthrosc. 2019;27(8):2502–10.
3. Elias DA, White LM, Fithian DC. Acute lateral patellar dislocation at MR imaging: injury patterns of medial patellar soft-tissue restraints and osteochondral injuries of the Inferomedial Patella. Radiology. 2002;225(3):736–43.
4. Tompkins MA, Rohr SR, Agel J, Arendt EA. Anatomic patellar instability risk factors in primary lateral patellar dislocations do not predict injury patterns: an MRI-based study. Knee Surg Sport Traumatol Arthrosc. 2018;26(3):677–84.

5. Nomura E, Inoue M. Cartilage lesions of the patella in recurrent patellar dislocation. Am J Sports Med. 2004;32(2):498–502.

6. Nomura E, Kurimura M. Chondral and osteochondral injuries associated with acute patellar dislocation. Arthrosc J Arthrosc Relat Surg. 2003;19(7):717–21.

7. Luhmann SJ, Schoenecker PL, Dobbs MB, Gordon JE. Arthroscopic findings at the time of patellar realignment surgery in adolescents. J Pediatr Orthop. 2007;27(5):493–8.

8. Abolghasemian M, León S, Lee PTH, Safir O, Backstein D, Gross AE, et al. Long-term results of treating large posttraumatic Tibial plateau lesions with fresh osteochondral allograft transplantation. J Bone Joint Surg. 2019;101(12):1102–8.

9. Ekman E, Mäkelä K, Kohonen I, Hiltunen A, Itälä A. Favourable long-term functional and radiographical outcome after osteoautograft transplantation surgery of the knee: a minimum 10-year follow-up. Knee Surg Sport Traumatol Arthrosc. 2018;26(12):3560–5.

10. Familiari F, Cinque ME, Chahla J, Godin JA, Olesen ML, Moatshe G, et al. Clinical outcomes and failure rates of osteochondral allograft transplantation in the knee: A systematic review. Am J Sports Med. 2018;46(14):3541–9.

11. Knutsen G, Isaksen V, Johansen O, Engebretsen L, Ludvigsen TC, Drogset JO, et al. Autologous chondrocyte implantation compared with microfracture in the knee: a randomized trial. J Bone Joint Surg Ser A. 2004;86(3):455–64.

12. Wang D, Kalia V, Eliasberg CD, Wang T, Coxe FR, Pais MD, et al. Osteochondral allograft transplantation of the knee in patients aged 40 years and older. Am J Sports Med. 2018;46(3):581–9.

13. Lee S, Frank RM, Christian DR, Cole BJ. Analysis of defect size and ratio to condylar size with respect to outcomes after isolated osteochondral allograft transplantation. Am J Sports Med. 2019;47(7):1601–12.

14. de Windt TS, J Bekkers JE, Creemers LB, A Dhert WJ, F Saris DB. Patient profiling in cartilage regeneration prognostic factors determining success of treatment for cartilage defects. Am J Sports Med. 2009;37(S1):58S–62S.

15. Anderson DE, Robinson KS, Wiedrick J, Crawford DC. Efficacy of fresh osteochondral allograft transplantation in the knee for adults 40 years and older. Orthop J Sport Med. 2018;6(11):2325967118805441.

16. Frank RM, Cotter EJ, Lee S, Poland S, Cole BJ. Do outcomes of osteochondral allograft transplantation differ based on age and sex? A comparative matched group analysis. Am J Sports Med. 2018;46(1):181–91.

17. Carnes J, Stannus O, Cicuttini F, Ding Yz C, Jones G. Knee cartilage defects in a sample of older adults: natural history, clinical significance and factors influencing change over 2.9 years. Osteoarthr Cartil. 2012;20:1541–7.

18. Nuelle C, Nuelle J, Cook J, Stannard J. Patient factors, donor age, and graft storage duration affect osteochondral allograft outcomes in knees with or without comorbidities. J Knee Surg. 2016;30(02):179–84.

19. Kumagai K, Akamatsu Y, Kobayashi H, Kusayama Y, Koshino T, Tomoyuki S. Factors affecting cartilage repair after medial opening-wedge high tibial osteotomy. Knee Surg Sport Traumatol Arthrosc. 2017;25:779–84.

20. Valtanen RS, Arshi A, Kelley BV, Fabricant PD, Jones KJ. Articular cartilage repair of the pediatric and adolescent knee with regard to minimal clinically important difference: a systematic review. Cartilage. 2020;11(1):9–18.

21. Cianfarani F, Toietta G, Di Rocco G, Cesareo E, Zambruno G, Odorisio T. Diabetes impairs adipose tissue-derived stem cell function and efficiency in promoting wound healing. Wound Repair Regen. 2013;21(4):545–53.

22. Kanneganti P, Harris JD, Brophy RH, Carey JL, Lattermann C, Flanigan DC. The effect of smoking on ligament and cartilage surgery in the knee: a systematic review. Am J Sports Med. 2012;40(12):2872–8.

23. Kim S-J, Chang C-H, Suh D-S, Ha H-K, Suhl K-H. Case report autologous chondrocyte implantation for rheumatoid arthritis of the knee: a case report. J Med Case Rep. 2009;3:6619.

24. Hillen J, Geyer C, Heitzmann M, Beckmann D, Krause A, Winkler I, et al. Structural cartilage damage attracts circulating rheumatoid arthritis synovial fibroblasts into affected joints. Arthritis Res Ther. 2017;19(40)

25. Ringe J, Sittinger M. Tissue engineering in the rheumatic diseases. Arthritis Res Ther. 2009;11:211.

26. Paes RA. Familial osteochondritis dissecans. Clin Radiol. 1989;501:504.

27. Richie LB, Sytsma MJ. Matching osteochondritis dissecans lesions in identical twin brothers. Orthopedics. 2013;36(9):1213–6.

28. Lam S, Amies V. Hip arthritis presenting as knee pain. BMJ Case Reports. BMJ Publishing Group; 2015. https://doi.org/10.1136/bcr-2014-208625.

29. Khan AM, McLoughlin E, Giannakas K, Hutchinson C, Andrew JG. Hip osteoarthritis: where is the pain? Ann R Coll Surg Engl. 2004;86(2):119–21.

30. Sakamoto J, Manabe Y, Oyamada J, Kataoka H, Nakano J, Saiki K, et al. Anatomical study of the articular branches innervated the hip and knee joint with reference to mechanism of referral pain in hip joint disease patients. Clin Anat. 2018;31(5):705–9.

31. Sembrano JN, Polly DW. How often is low back pain not coming from the back? Spine (Phila Pa 1976). 34(1):27–32.

32. Defroda SF, Daniels AH, Deren ME. Differentiating radiculopathy from lower extremity arthropathy. Am J Med. 2016;129

33. Karachalios T, Hantes M, Zibis AH, Zachos V, Karantanas AH, Malizos KN. Diagnostic accuracy of a new clinical test (the Thessaly test) for early detection of meniscal tears. J Bone Joint Surg. 2005;87(5):955–62.

34. McMurray TP. Certain injuries of the knee joint. Br Med J. 1934;1(3824):709–13.

35. Beighton P, Solomon L, Soskolnet CL. Articular mobility in an African population. Ann Rheum Dis. 1973;32:413.
36. Davies GJ, Malone T, Bassett FH. Knee examination. Phys Ther. 1980;60(12):1565–74.
37. Luhmann SJ, Smith JC, Schootman M, Prasad N. Recurrent patellar instability. J Pediatr Orthop. 2019;39(1):33–7.
38. Fairbank H. Section of Orthopaedic internal derangement of the knee in children and adolescents. Proc R Soc Med. 1936;30:11.
39. Cook C, Mabry L, Reiman MP, Hegedus EJ. Systematic review best tests/clinical findings for screening and diagnosis of patellofemoral pain syndrome: a systematic review. Physiotherapy. 2012;98:93–100.
40. Haim A, Yaniv M, Dekel S, Amir H. Patellofemoral pain syndrome. Clin Orthop Relat Res. 2006;451:223–8.
41. Ahmad CS, McCarthy M, Gomez JA, Shubin Stein BE. The moving patellar apprehension test for lateral patellar instability. Am J Sports Med. 2009;37(4):791–6.
42. Zimmermann F, Liebensteiner MC, Peter B. The reversed dynamic patellar apprehension test mimics anatomical complexity in lateral patellar instability. Knee Surgery, Sport Traumatol Arthrosc. 2019;27:604–10.
43. Smith TO, Clark A, Neda S, Arendt EA, Post WR, Grelsamer RP, et al. The intra-and inter-observer reliability of the physical examination methods used to assess patients with patellofemoral joint instability. Knee. 2011;20:133–8.
44. Moreland JR, Bassett LW, Hanker GJ. Radiographic analysis of the axial alignment of the lower extremity. J Bone Joint Surg. 1987;69(5):745–9.
45. Paley D, Tetsworth K. Mechanical axis deviation of the lower limbs: preoperative planning of uniapical angular deformities of the tibia or femur. Clin Orthop Relat Res. 1992;280:48–64.
46. Cherian JJ, Kapadia BH, Banerjee S, Jauregui JJ, Issa K, Mont MA. Mechanical, anatomical, and kinematic axis in TKA: concepts and practical applications. Curr Rev Musculoskelet Med. 2014;7:89–95.
47. Bastick AN, Belo JN, Runhaar J, Bierma-Zeinstra SMA. What are the prognostic factors for radiographic progression of knee osteoarthritis? A Meta-analysis. Clin Orthop Relat Res. 1999;473:2969–89.
48. Sharma L, Chang AH, Jackson RD, Nevitt M, Moisio KC, Hochberg M, et al. Varus thrust and incident and progressive knee osteoarthritis. Arthritis Rehumatol. 2017;69(11):2136–43.
49. Guettler J, Glisson R, Stubbs A, Jurist K, Higgins L. The triad of varus malalignment, meniscectomy, and chondral damage: A biomechanical explanation for joint degeneration. Orthopedics. 2007;30(7):558–66.
50. Harris JD, Mcneilan R, Siston RA, Flanigan DC. Survival and clinical outcome of isolated high tibial osteotomy and combined biological knee reconstruction. Knee. 2013;20:154–61.
51. Bode G, Schmal H, Pestka JM, Ogon P, Südkamp NP, Niemeyer P. A non-randomized controlled clinical trial on autologous chondrocyte implantation (ACI) in cartilage defects of the medial femoral condyle with or without high tibial osteotomy in patients with varus deformity of less than 5°. Arch Orthop Trauma Surg. 2013;133:43–9.
52. León SA, Mei XY, Safir OA, Gross AE, Kuzyk PR. Long-term results of fresh osteochondral allografts and realignment osteotomy for cartilage repair in the knee. Bone Joint J. 2019;101-B(1_Supple_A):46–52.
53. Berg EE, Mason SL, Lucas MJ. Patellar height ratios A comparison of four measurement methods. Am J Sports Med. 1996;24(2):218–21.
54. Dejour H, Walch G, Nove-Josserand L, Guier C. Knee surgery sports traumatology I arthroscopy patellar problems factors of patellar instability: an anatomic radiographic study. Knee Surg, Sport Traumatol. 1994;2:19–26.
55. Caton J, Deschamps G, Chambat P, Lerat JL, Dejour H. Patella infera. Apropos of 128 cases. Rev Chir Orthop Reparatrice Appar Mot. 1982;68(5):317–25.
56. Koh JL, Stewart C. Patellar instability. Clin Sports Med. 2014;33:461–76.
57. Insall J, Salvati E. Patella position in the normal knee joint. Radiology. 1971;101(1):101–4.
58. Seil R, Müller B, Georg T, Kohn D, Rupp S, Müller B, et al. Reliability and interobserver variability in radiological patellar height ratios. Knee Surg Sport Traumatol Arthrosc. 2000;8:231–6.
59. Davies AP, Costa ML, Donnell ST, Glasgow MM, Shepstone L. The sulcus angle and malalignment of the extensor mechanism of the knee. J Bone Joint Surg Br. 2000;82-B(8):1162–6.
60. Tan SHS, Chng KSJ, Lim BY, Wong KL, Doshi C, Lim AKS, et al. The difference between cartilaginous and bony sulcus angles for patients with or without patellofemoral instability: a systematic review and meta-analysis. J Knee Surg. 2020;33(03):235–41.
61. Ambra LF, Hinckel BB, Arendt EA, Farr J, Gomoll AH. Anatomic risk factors for focal cartilage lesions in the patella and trochlea: a case-control study. Am J Sports Med. 2019;47(10):2444–53.
62. Sanders TL, Pareek A, Johnson NR, Stuart MJ, Dahm DL, Krych AJ. Patellofemoral arthritis after lateral patellar dislocation: a matched population-based analysis. Am J Sports Med. 2017;45(5):1012–7.
63. Laurin C, Dussaul R, Levesque H. The tangential X-ray investigation of the patellofemoral joint: X-ray technique; diagnostic criteria and their interpretation. Clin Orthop Relat Res. 1979;144:16–26.
64. Lafferty PM, Min W, Tejwani NC. Stress radiographs in orthopaedic surgery. J Am Acad Orthop Surg. 2009;17(8):528–39.
65. James EW, Williams BT, LaPrade RF. Stress radiography for the diagnosis of knee ligament injuries: a systematic review. Clin Orthop Relat Res. 2014;472(9):2644–57.

66. Laprade CM, Civitarese DM, Rasmussen MT, Laprade RF. Emerging updates on the posterior cruciate ligament. Am J Sports Med. 2015;43(12):3077–92.
67. Camp CL, Stuart MJ, Krych AJ, Levy BA, Bond JR, Collins MS, et al. CT and MRI measurements of tibial tubercle-trochlear groove distances are not equivalent in patients with patellar instability. Am J Sports Med. 2013;41(8):1835–40.
68. Botser IB, Ozoude GC, Martin DE, Siddiqi AJ, Kuppuswami S, Domb BG. Femoral anteversion in the hip: comparison of measurement by computed tomography, magnetic resonance imaging, and physical examination. Arthrosc J Arthrosc Relat Surg. 2012;28(5):619–27.
69. Hayashi D, Li X, Murakami AM, Roemer FW, Trattnig S, Guermazi A. Understanding magnetic resonance imaging of knee cartilage repair: A focus on clinical relevance. Cartilage. 2018;9(3):223–36.
70. Liu YW, Tran MD, Skalski MR, Patel DB, White EA, Tomasian A, et al. Musculoskeletal and emergency imaging MR imaging of cartilage repair surgery of the knee. Clin Imaging. 2019;58:129–39.
71. Campbell AB, Knopp MV, Kolovich GP, Wei W, Jia G, Siston RA, Flanigan DC. Preoperative MRI underestimates articular cartilage defect size compared with findings at arthroscopic knee surgery. PMID: 23324431. https://doi.org/10.1177/0363546512472044.
72. Jungmann PM, Welsch GH, Brittberg M, Trattnig S, Braun S, Imhoff AB, et al. Magnetic resonance imaging score and classification system (AMADEUS) for assessment of preoperative cartilage defect severity. Cartilage. 2017;8(3):272–82.
73. Marlovits S, Singer P, Zeller P, Mandl I, Haller J, Trattnig S. Magnetic resonance observation of cartilage repair tissue (MOCART) for the evaluation of autologous chondrocyte transplantation: determination of interobserver variability and correlation to clinical outcome after 2 years. Eur J Radiol. 2006;57:16–23.
74. Welsch GH, Zak L, Mamisch TC, Paul D, Lauer L, Mauerer A, et al. Advanced morphological 3D magnetic resonance observation of cartilage repair tissue (MOCART) scoring using a new isotropic 3D proton-density, turbo spin echo sequence with variable flip angle distribution (PD-SPACE) compared to an isotropic 3D steady-stat. J Magn Reson Imaging. 2011;33(1):180–8.
75. Meric G, Gracitelli GC, Gö Rtz S, De Young AJ, Mpa P-C, Bugbee WD. Fresh osteochondral allograft transplantation for bipolar reciprocal osteochondral lesions of the knee. Am J Sports Med. 2015;43(3):709–14.
76. Hannon CP, Weber AE, Gitelis M, Meyer MA, Yanke AB, Cole BJ. Does treatment of the tibia matter in bipolar chondral defects of the knee? Clinical outcomes with greater than 2 years follow-up. Arthrosc J Arthrosc Relat Surg. 2018;34(4):1044–51.
77. Cotter EJ, Hannon CP, Christian DR, Wang KC, Lansdown DA, Waterman BR, et al. Clinical outcomes of multifocal osteochondral allograft transplantation of the knee an analysis of overlapping grafts and multifocal lesions. Am J Sports Med. 2018;46(12):2884–93.
78. Brittberg M, Peterson L. Introduction to an articular cartilage classification. ICRS Newsl. 1998;1:5–8.
79. Slattery C, Kweon CY. In brief classifications in brief: Outerbridge classification of chondral lesions. Clin Orthop Relat Res. 2018;476:2101–4,
80. Solheim E, Hegna J, Strand T, Harlem T, Inderhaug E. Randomized study of long-term (15-17 years) outcome after microfracture versus mosaicplasty in knee articular cartilage defects. Am J Sports Med. 2018;46(4):826–31.
81. Zamborsky R, Danisovic L. Surgical techniques for knee cartilage repair: an updated large-scale systematic review and network meta-analysis of randomized controlled trials. Arthrosc J Arthrosc Relat Surg. 2020;36(3):845–58.
82. Saris D, Price A, Widuchowski W, Bertrand-Marchand M, Caron J, Drogset JO, et al. Matrix-applied characterized autologous cultured chondrocytes versus microfracture two-year follow-up of a prospective randomized trial. Am J Sports Med. 2014;42(6):1384–94.
83. Brittberg M, Recker D, Ilgenfritz J, Saris DBF. SUMMIT extension study group on behalf of the SES. Matrix-applied characterized autologous cultured chondrocytes versus microfracture: five-year follow-up of a prospective randomized trial. Am J Sports Med. 2018 May 22;46(6):1343–51.
84. Gou G-H, Tseng F-J, Wang S-H, Chen P-J, Shyu J-F, Weng C-F, et al. Systematic review autologous chondrocyte implantation versus microfracture in the knee: a meta-analysis and systematic review. Arthrosc J Arthrosc Relat Surg. 2020;36(1):289–303.
85. Kreuz PC, Kalkreuth RH, Niemeyer P, Uhl M, Erggelet C. Long-term clinical and MRI results of matrix-assisted autologous chondrocyte implantation for articular cartilage defects of the knee. Cartilage. 2019;10(3):305–13.

Nonoperative Management Options for Symptomatic Cartilage Lesions

Mathew J. Hamula, Abigail L. Campbell, and Bert R. Mandelbaum

7.1 Introduction

Articular cartilage is a vital component of an intricate system that constitutes the knee. The purpose of cartilage is to provide a low-friction surface for motion as well as a cushion on which to transmit forces efficiently and effectively. It lacks access to either abundant nutrients or progenitor cells rendering it vulnerable to injury and with little capacity to mount a regenerative response. Partial-thickness defects generally do not involve injury to the vasculature; however chondroprogenitor cells in marrow and blood cannot enter the damaged region. Therefore, these defects have a limited healing potential and typically progress. On the other hand, full-thickness lesions that penetrate the subchondral bone have a higher likelihood of intrinsic repair, though typically they will go on to heal with fibrocartilage with inferior mechanical properties to native articular cartilage [1]. Understanding and treating chondral lesions require a fundamental knowledge of physiology and pathophysiology.

The thickness and volume of articular cartilage follow a paradigm somewhat analogous to Wolff's law that form and mass follow function in bone remodeling. Cartilage demonstrates a directly proportional change in thickness that has a linear dose-response correlation with repetitive loading activities. There is also a critical threshold beyond which it can result in an alteration of cartilage homeostasis and lead to chondropenia. The chondropenic cascade leading to chondral lesions and joint degeneration can be exacerbated by the presence of additional pathology such as ligamentous instability, malalignment, and meniscal injury [2].

Cartilage injuries of the knee are ubiquitous and affect over one-third of athletes compared to less than one-fifth of the general population [3]. These injuries can cause significant morbidity and are frequently career ending. Acute chondral injuries occur in 9–60% of anterior cruciate ligament (ACL) ruptures and over 90% of patellar dislocations [3, 4]. Focal cartilage defects have been reported in 60–67% of individuals undergoing knee arthroscopy [5, 6]. Even when treated with state-of-the-art surgical modalities, it is often difficult to return to previous levels of performance. A 2018 ESSKA study of 31 high-level athletes undergoing matrix-associated cartilage transplantation reported that at 10-year follow-up, only 58% of patients returned to pre-injury level of sport [7]. Athletes in particular are at significant risk for symptomatic degenerative joint disease relatively early on in their lives [3, 8–11]. Long-term follow-up studies reveal that articular cartilage defects in athletes show a direct link

M. J. Hamula · A. L. Campbell · B. R. Mandelbaum (✉)
Kerlan-Jobe Institute, Los Angeles, CA, USA
e-mail: racquelm@smog-ortho.net

© ISAKOS 2021
A. J. Krych et al. (eds.), *Cartilage Injury of the Knee*,
https://doi.org/10.1007/978-3-030-78051-7_7

between chondral damage and development of osteoarthritis [10].

Cartilage injuries have the potential to limit patients' livelihood and athletes' future in their respective occupations, even when addressed operatively. It is therefore imperative for the managing physician to maximize their armamentarium of conservative treatments.

7.2 Clinical Evaluation and Classification

Clinical evaluation begins with a thorough history and physical examination. Care should be taken to elicit any history of trauma, recent or remote, swelling, instability, or mechanical symptoms. The physical examination should particularly include evaluation for the presence of swelling, effusion, pain to palpation, catching, locking, and special tests to evaluate for concomitant pathology. Range of motion is important and noting any pain with midrange, terminal flexion, or terminal extension.

Imaging is a crucial adjunct in assessing patients with chondral lesions. Plain radiographs are able to evaluate for osteochondral defects, loose bodies, joint space narrowing, alignment, and patellar tracking. Advanced imaging in the form of magnetic resonance imaging (MRI) is the current standard of diagnostic imaging affording great detail of chondral lesions and underlying bony involvement. Despite advances in MRI technology, chondral lesion may still remain undetected until arthroscopy. One potential application of in-office arthroscopy is to assist with diagnosis in cases where the MRI is not sensitive enough to pick up a lesion. Patient selection is important, however, since it can be difficult to tolerate in the office setting without sedation or pain medication.

The purpose of any classification system is threefold: distinguish subtle differences in pathology by capturing relevant factors, facilitate communication between clinicians, and guide management. There are several classification systems today including the Outerbridge, Bauer and Shariaree, and cartilage severity score (CSS).

Our preferred method is the CSS which provides a scoring system out of 100 including all of the articular surfaces of the knee as well as meniscal integrity. We have found that it is helpful in conveying to patients the severity of cartilage injury whether focal or global. There is also a comprehensive method developed by the International Cartilage Repair Society (ICRS). This score accounts for nine variables: etiology, defect thickness, lesion size, degree of containment, location, ligamentous integrity, meniscal integrity, alignment, and relevant factors in the patient history.

7.3 Indications for Nonoperative Management

With the recent advances in cartilage restoration it may seem trivial to discuss the nonoperative management of chondral lesions. However, there are substantial advances in treatment modalities that avoid invasive procedures and significant recovery time and rehabilitation. Additionally, with surgical management there is no guarantee of return to pre-injury levels of function. First, it is important to discuss the indications and contraindications for nonoperative management.

The indications for nonoperative management are essentially patients with no significant relative or absolute contraindications. Patients can consider nonoperative treatment of symptomatic cartilage lesions in the absence of any significant red flag symptoms such as mechanical symptoms of locking or catching secondary to a loose body or concurrent reparable meniscal tear. Those with partial-thickness or full-thickness cartilage lesions can consider an initial trial of nonoperative management as long as the risks and benefits are discussed thoroughly. Relative contraindications of nonoperative management include concomitant ligamentous or meniscal injury that may predispose the knee to more rapid degeneration. Any significant osteochondral or chondral loose body is an absolute contraindication to nonoperative management and should undergo arthroscopic loose body removal. Furthermore, there is a role for nonoperative treatments of patients who may at some point benefit from surgical intervention and for postoperative patients to optimize outcomes and prevent revision surgery.

7.4 Chondroprotection, Chondrofacilitation, and Resurfacing: A Framework for Management

When considering management of chondral lesions, it is helpful to have a framework that captures the nuances of pathophysiology and provides guidance for treatment options. Murray et al. [12] outlined in a previous paper three general categories to address chondral pathology:

1. Chondroprotection: strategies that aim to prevent loss of existing cartilage.
2. Chondrofacilitation: strategies that seek to facilitate intrinsic repair of damaged articular cartilage.
3. Chondrorestoration/resurfacing: improvements in chondral surface function are sought through replacement rather than intrinsic repair of cartilage defects with hyaline cartilage. These include autologous chondrocyte implantation (ACI) in all of its current permutations, autograft and allograft transplantation, and synthetics including scaffolds that fill the defect.

As this chapter focuses on nonoperative management of symptomatic cartilage lesions, we will focus on the first two categories. The caveat is that there is a significant cohort of patients that require either chondroprotection or chondrofacilitation postoperatively after a resurfacing procedure. Broadly speaking, we will discuss three groups of patients: nonoperative treatment entirely, patients that will go on to need cartilage repair, and postoperative patients from a cartilage repair or resurfacing that benefit from chondrofacilitation and chondroprotection in order to maximize outcomes and prevent the need for revision surgery.

7.5 Chondroprotection

The aim of chondroprotection is to promote cartilage homeostasis and prevent the chondropenic cascade that can ultimately lead to loss of structural integrity. As such there are numerous treatment recommendations with varying degrees of supporting evidence. These methods can be characterized as dynamic modifications or pharmacological interventions.

7.5.1 Weight Loss

Joint function is an interplay between motion and the forces that act on it. However, there are limits to modifications that we can recommend as clinicians that have overwhelming supporting evidence. For early osteoarthritis (OA), for example, there is evidence to support lower extremity muscle strengthening for pain and offloading effects [13–16]. Weight loss can reduce peak loads in the knee joint and abductor moment at the knee by a scale of 2.2 kg decrease in peak load for every 1 kg of weight loss [17]. However, the fact remains that the goal is to modify any modifiable risk factors with the best protocols to date. Injury prevention programs such as the FIFA 11+ are recommended to reduce the risk of intra-articular knee injury.

In addition to the weight loss benefits discussed previously, exercise is recommended for knee cartilage disease by the Osteoarthritis Research Society International and the American College of Rheumatology [18, 19]. A 2020 randomized trial published in the New England Journal of Medicine found physical therapy superior to glucocorticoid injection for knee osteoarthritis at 1 year, with those receiving therapy having less pain and functional disability (WOMAC) than those who received glucocorticoid injection [20]. Exercise programs in patients with exacerbations of knee osteoarthritis have been shown to improve symptoms with a relatively low rate of poor effects [21, 22]. Favorable inflammatory biomarker profiles were found with exercise programs in randomized studies [23]. Exercise may have an epigenetic effect as well.

MicroRNA-target interactions have been implicated in cartilage disease as well as muscle homeostasis related to exercise [24].

Blood flow restriction therapy is being utilized for various orthopedic applications, and there is some early evidence that it may improve pain while minimizing joint stress in knee osteoarthritis [25, 26]. Exercise is therefore recommended as a staple of first-line management for cartilage disease of the knee. Regarding the use of bracing, there is no level one evidence to support its effect and all available studies are equivocal [27].

7.5.2 Supplements

Glucosamine is a monosaccharide that in vitro has been shown to increase chondrocyte aggrecan production and decrease inflammatory and degradative mediators [28–30]. Chondroitin sulfate is a structural component of cartilage that adds compression strength to the cartilage matrix. Animal studies have demonstrated a chondroprotective effect by anti-inflammatory and anti-degradative effects, as well as stimulation of hyaluronic acid and proteoglycans [31–33].

There are dozens of studies assessing chondroitin sulfate and glucosamine supplementation for the use in cartilage disease of the knee. Examining oral supplementation in humans, a meta-analysis and systematic review of all randomized studies that were conducted in 2018 reported that the use of either glucosamine or chondroitin sulfate significantly improved visual analog scale (VAS) pain scores, but did not have this effect when combined and did not affect Western Ontario and McMaster Universities Osteoarthritis Index (WOMAC) score [34]. However, two randomized studies reported reduction on joint space narrowing with chondroitin sulfate [35, 36]. Based on the available evidence, chondroitin sulfate supplementation may improve symptoms and mitigate progression of cartilage degeneration in the knee.

Curcumin, a compound found in turmeric, has been studied for use in the knee for its potential anti-inflammatory effect. In animal studies, curcumin administration has a chondroprotective rather than chondrofacilitative action, leading to an increase in the number of chondrocytes and collagen content but not increasing cartilage thickness [37, 38]. However, despite its promising results in recent animal studies, there is little evidence in clinical outcomes with human use. It has been shown to be safe for use in humans for the indication of knee chondral disease [39].

7.5.3 Estrogen

Estrogen plays a well-understood role in the modulation of bone density. Its effect on cartilage has only been recently elucidated. Animal studies have demonstrated that estrogen inhibits degradation of cartilage's extracellular matrix, and that estrogen therapy can reduce the degree of cartilage degeneration [40, 41]. A large-cohort study in humans identified postmenopausal status as an independent risk factor for cartilage degeneration [42]. Certain estrogen receptors have been implicated in cartilage catabolism by upregulating matrix metalloproteinases [43, 44]. Due to this relationship, female patients in peri- or post-menopausal age groups experiencing knee pain due to cartilage disease should be referred to an endocrinologist or women's health specialist for hormonal evaluation. Developing a relationship with a local physician in this specialty is highly recommended to optimize patient care.

7.5.4 Steroid

Steroid injections are frequently performed in the knee. While the short-term improvement in pain has been established for use in the knee [45], there is evidence that extended use may have deleterious effects on articular cartilage [46, 47]. While there is concern for possible catabolic effect on cartilage, there is also evidence that intra-articular steroid injections in the knee may have an anabolic effect [48]. We recommend intra-articular steroid injection for use during the acute flare of knee pain, and one should not fear intermittent use as this treatment can be very effective for acute pain. However, the treating provider should keep in mind that a steroid injection is not a solution for a cartilage injury in the knee.

7.5.5 Future Directions in Chondroprotection

The positive effects of exercise continue to be elucidated as well as supplementation that may be related to diet. Whole-body health including diet and exercise will likely become a focus of both preventative and treatment approaches for cartilage injury and disease. As there are no simple and infallible invasive solutions to cartilage injury, prevention in the context of overall health and wellness is likely to become the focus of early management, thereby providing cartilage care before treatment becomes necessary.

7.6 Chondrofacilitation

Once structural damage has occurred, the goal is to facilitate intrinsic repair by creating a harmony between the innate biology and the local articular cartilage environment or milieu. The goals of nonoperative strategies are to deliver essential growth factors or temper inflammation in order to promote the regeneration or healing response of functional hyaline cartilage. These nonoperative techniques can often serve as adjuncts to surgical techniques. The focus of this chapter is to discuss them in the three groups of patients previously outlined.

7.6.1 Hyaluronic Acid

Hyaluronic acid (HA) is a major component of synovial fluid that has anti-inflammatory effects and may stimulate proteoglycan production. Initially developed as an avian-derived product, most HA is now produced by biological fermentation. HA has multiple functions in the native knee: lubrication, load absorption, fluid homeostasis, and analgesia [49]. Its mechanism of action in cartilage disease specifically comprises proteoglycan and glycosaminoglycan synthesis, anti-inflammatory effect, mechanical lubrication, and analgesia [50]. HA can be utilized as a multiple-injection series or one injection only, based on molecular weight and concentration.

There are myriad products available today including high molecular weight and extended release. Both molecular weight and HA concentration can influence HA's efficacy, which should be taken into consideration when reading literature on this subject. Animal studies show promising data in its chondrofacilitative effects [38, 51, 52]. Human studies examining intra-articular HA have been widely published, with positive clinical benefits in randomized trials [53, 54]. Of three randomized trials comparing HA and placebo that assessed structural changes on knee MRI, two trials reported no difference in joint space width loss between HA and placebo [55, 56], while one found significantly less joint space loss in both medial and lateral compartments [57]. Clinically, HA has been shown to delay total-knee arthroplasty [50, 58].

For these reasons, HA is a valuable asset to the provider managing knee pain due to cartilage injury or wear. In our clinic, we often administer HA with steroid in the first of a three-injection series. The addition of steroid to this first injection has anecdotally improved patients' pain faster and allowed earlier return to activities. HA can also be combined with PRP, though evidence behind combination therapy is currently limited. This combination will be discussed further in this chapter.

7.6.2 Platelet-Rich Plasma

Platelet-rich plasma (PRP) in its current iteration has been demonstrated to be safe and contains significant concentrations of autologous growth factors and proteins that may augment intrinsic repair [59]. The current definition includes quantitative criteria, specifically requiring PRP to contain more than 1 million platelets per milliliter (mL) of serum as this critical concentration shows the most promise in terms of stimulating a healing response [60, 61]. The other factor in

PRP formulations is the white blood cell concentration, with leukocyte-rich PRP (LR-PRP) and leukocyte-poor PRP (LP-PRP). While the use of PRP to treat cartilage injuries has rapidly expanded over the last decade, there remains a sparsity of evidence for use in isolated setting in the treatment of chondral lesions. Lui et al. [62] conducted a study showing superior cartilage healing with intra-articular injections of PRP compared to HA in a rabbit model with 5 mm focal chondral defects. Further animal studies on autologous conditioned plasma and platelet-enriched fibrin scaffolds have shown similar superior results [63, 64]. Additionally, combining PRP with HA has been shown to increase the release of growth factors [65].

There is limited clinical evidence to support the use of PRP in vivo for chondral lesions and OA. In some head-to-head comparisons, hyaluronic acid injections seem to outperform PRP alone in terms of pain relief [66–69]. Other studies, including recent meta-analyses and randomized controlled trials, have overall shown more consistent evidence for LP-PRP for intra-articular use in the treatment of chondral lesions and OA compared with placebo and hyaluronic acid [67, 70–73]. In general, LP-PRP likely produces less of an inflammatory response than LR-PRP within the intra-articular environment which may ultimately prove to be more therapeutically beneficial. Further studies on standardized formulations are needed to make definitive recommendations on isolated PRP for the nonoperative treatment of chondral lesions.

However, PRP has been reported to improve cartilage regeneration when used alongside microfracture and osteochondral allograft implantation. In a mouse model, leukocyte-rich PRP injection was compared to saline injection in femoral condylar focal cartilage defects, and increased cartilage regeneration and collagen II in the repair tissue in the PRP group were found. This suggests that there is a role for PRP at least as an adjunct, particularly in patients who may at some point benefit from a cartilage restoration procedure or following a surgery in order to enhance chondrofacilitation. A recent study by Everhart et al. [74] demonstrated an improved

healing rate in meniscal repairs with the use of PRP at the time of surgery although there was no difference when a concomitant anterior cruciate ligament (ACL) reconstruction was performed. For now, there is a growing body of evidence that PRP is helpful in conjunction with surgical procedures and can facilitate intrinsic repair of cartilage lesions. There is still not enough evidence to recommend its isolated use on focal chondral lesions. However, it may provide a useful temporizing measure for athletes mid-season as a nonsurgical treatment option prior to an arthroscopic debridement or cartilage restoration procedure.

7.6.3 Bone Marrow Aspirate Concentrate

Bone marrow aspirate concentrate (BMAC) has gained popularity and widespread use as it is relatively easy to harvest and one of the few treatment options acceptable under the US Food and Drug Administration (FDA) guidelines [75]. It can be used to give growth factors to the injury site, such as vascular endothelial growth factor, platelet-derived growth factor, transforming growth factor-beta, and bone morphogenic proteins. This is in addition to the mesenchymal stem cells (MSCs) present in the concentrate. BMAC shows a lot of potential, particularly in the treatment of osteochondral lesions of the tibial plateau where the use of osteochondral allograft is limited by size, shape, or location. There are several studies on the use of BMAC in chondral lesions [76–81], the vast majority with promising results. In general, there were more favorable results when BMAC was used with a scaffold. Given that some studies were inconclusive or showed negative results with BMAC alone, there is currently limited use for BMAC in isolation for the treatment of chondral lesions. However, in conjunction with a scaffold, including even HA, there is some promising data showing improvement in function. BMAC has been reported as a valuable augment to microfracture, matrix-associated chondrocyte implantation, and osteochondral allograft implantation. It has also improved cartilage repair compared with microfracture in an animal model [82]. At this time BMAC is a valuable addition to our armamentarium when combined with scaffolds. Its role in the nonoperative paradigm is confined to intra-articular injection combined with HA in patients who can tolerate the harvest in the clinic setting.

7.6.4 Cellular Based Therapies

Cellular based therapies are an attractive option in cartilage restoration. It is important to be cognizant of nomenclature when it comes to this heterogeneous group of therapeutic agents. Stem cells are defined as undifferentiated progenitor cells that are capable of proliferation, regeneration, self-maintenance, and replication [83]. Mesenchymal stem cells (MSCs) are of particular interest in the treatment of chondral lesion due to their accessibility and greater homogeneity in cell division [84]. The Mesenchymal and Tissue Stem Cell Committee of the International Society for Cellular Therapy in 2006 defined the minimal criteria for a human cell to be classified as an MSC: (1) the ability to adhere to plastic when maintained in standard culture conditions; (2) expression of CD105, CD73, and CD90; (3) the lack of expression of CD45, CD34, CD14, or CD11b, CD79alpha or CD19, and HLA-DR surface molecules; and (4) the ability to differentiate into osteoblasts, adipocytes, and chondroblasts in vitro [2]. Chang et al. [83] also postulated that MSCs also have an anti-inflammatory effect based on preclinical trials in small mammals. The two most popular options due to ease of collection are adipose-derived and bone marrow-derived MSCs.

Adipose-derived stem cells (ASCs) are relatively easy to harvest and result in a high yield of stem cells [85]. They have been shown to differentiate into chondrocytes in vitro and in vivo [86]. Intra-articular injections of ASCs have been reported to improve patient-reported outcomes for knee osteoarthritis but no studies have described its use for focal cartilage defects. Bone marrow-derived MSCs (BMSCs) are even more appealing due to their ease of collection. Sites of extraction include the iliac crest, tibia, or femur. One issue is that yield is typically low and the stem cells must be isolated and expanded in cell culture prior to utilization and this process can take up to 3 weeks. There are several animal models showing the positive effect of MSCs when combined with a matrix or scaffold [87, 88] as well as intra-articular injection of MSCs [89]. Although it seems highly promising, there is still a sparsity of literature showing clinical efficacy in humans. Chahla et al. [90] conducted a systematic review of studies evaluating the intra-articular injection of cell-based therapies in the knee. Only six studies were included, several of which were level III designs. While no major adverse events were reported, the improvement was modest and the quality of evidence was poor. Better studies are needed to definitively say that cellular based therapies are recommended for the nonoperative management of chondral lesions.

7.6.5 Osseous Involvement

Chondropenia results from a dose-response repetitive injury that leads to loss of articular cartilage volume. Once chondral lesions and osseous changes begin to occur the pathogenesis of osteoarthritis is well under way. Lesions can either extend through the full thickness of the cartilage and involve the bone or simply be accompanied by changes in the subchondral bone. Some of the structural changes that have been observed in the subchondral bone in severe osteoarthritis include bone marrow lesions, loss of mineralization, and progressive replacement of the marrow with fibroneurovascular mesenchymal tissue [91–93]. There is a growing interest in understanding and addressing both the osseous and chondral components of joint degeneration. Bone marrow lesions in osteoarthritis represent a late finding in degenerative joint disease and have been treated with various medications aimed at preventing bone resorption or promoting bone regeneration with varying degrees of success in clinical studies [94–99]. While no studies exist looking at the effect of bracing on bone marrow lesions in the tibiofemoral joint, a randomized controlled trial showed decrease in bone marrow lesion volume with 6 weeks of a pull-on patella sleeve in the patellofemoral joint [100].

There has been some recent investigation into combining intraosseous infiltration of injectable therapies combined with intra-articular to allow infiltration into the cartilage from both internal and external pathways, thereby treating the entire osteochondral unit. Early clinical results of combined intra-articular and intraosseous PRP therapy are promising [101, 102], but long-term data is not yet available. In the presence of subchondral bone edema this may provide an effective solution to address the inflammatory pathways related to pain and edema. The goal will be to intervene in this process early on and alter the natural history of joint degeneration before the onset of osteoarthritis.

7.6.6 Future Directions in Chondrofacilitation

The goal of facilitating intrinsic cartilage repair without surgical intervention is an ambitious one. As we continue to improve our understanding of the chondropenic cascade and catabolic process of joint degeneration, there will be more potential opportunities for therapeutic interventions. An example of this is Wnt signaling, which has been established as an important factor in the pathogenesis of osteoarthritis. It contributes to differentiation of osteoblasts and chondrocytes, as well as production of catabolic proteases. A relatively novel Wnt pathway inhibitor, small-molecule 04690 (SM04690), has been shown in a rodent model to induce the differentiation of functional chondrocytes and increase cartilage thickness and cartilage regeneration [103]. Additionally, Deshmukh et al. showed protection from cartilage catabolic activity. This novel therapeutic agent is currently undergoing phase 2B trials and has already demonstrated safety in human applications [104]. It is an exciting prospect to be able to stimulate chondral genesis, in addition to chondrofacilitation and chondroprotection.

There may not be a single therapy that provides effective treatment of cartilage lesions in the making. However, given the complexity of cartilage homeostasis, and by extension chondral pathology, it is more likely the answer will be some combination of therapies. The more immediate future may focus on combining the healing pro-inflammatory effects of PRP or mesenchymal stem cells of BMAC with a scaffold such as HA in a way that could target the chondral lesion effectively. As our understanding of the current modalities improves, we may be on the precipice of a transformation in our nonoperative approach to cartilage lesions. Additionally, chondroprotection of cartilage restoration or resurfacing procedures is of paramount importance.

7.7 Treatment Algorithm

We offer our current treatment algorithm focusing on nonoperative management of cartilage lesions involving the principles of chondroprotection and chondrofacilitation. Asymptomatic lesions, so long as there are no absolute indications for surgical management, should be monitored and treated with conditioning, minimizing high-impact joint loading when possible, and injury prevention protocols and "warm-ups." Diet and exercise can also play a pivotal role in maintaining functionality. The goal is to keep patients performing at their optimal level whether they are professional or recreational athletes, or simply have physically demanding occupations or hobbies. Once cartilage lesions become symptomatic, there are many ways to approach nonoperative treatment. First-line treatment should include a comprehensive analysis and discussion of dietary and exercise programs. This may include supplementation as discussed in the Chondroprotection section of this chapter. Second-line modalities can be broadly categorized as chondroprotective or chondrofacilitative. For either partial-thickness or full-thickness lesions, chondroprotective measures include conditioning, weight loss, medications, supplements, and endocrine evaluation. Chondroprotection also involves identifying concurrent pathology such as meniscal tears, instability, and malalignment. Finally, chondrofacilitation should be individualized to the patient and pathology. In cases where there is underlying osseous involvement, there may be a greater potential for PRP, BMAC, or other cell-based therapies to assist intrinsic repair. Hyaluronic acid may be better suited for those without concurrent osseous defects, although combined with an intraosseous PRP injection it may prove to be beneficial in cases where the subchondral bone is affected. Additionally, as nonoperative techniques are exhausted, the corresponding surgical options are highlighted in Fig. 7.1. Addressing osseous involvement is paramount, and orthobiologics such as PRP and BMAC serve as chondrofacilitators. Following operative intervention, the paradigm reverts to nonoperative management following chondroprotection and chondrofacilitation principles. The goal here is to prevent the need for revision surgery. As our understanding and therapeutic techniques continue to evolve, this algorithm will change or expand significantly.

7.8 Summary and Conclusion

A multitude of nonoperative modalities exist for the treatment of cartilage lesions. It is an exciting prospect as orthopedic surgeons and other practitioners become more critical of current surgical solutions for cartilage lesions or seek to help patients who previously would not have had any worthwhile treatment options. The goal is an ambitious one, to prevent chondropenia and protect chondral surfaces by stimulating regeneration of native functional hyaline cartilage using growth factors and anti-inflammatory therapies. Surgical techniques aimed at restoring chondral surfaces still play a crucial role, and the focus should be to facilitate and protect cartilage restoration or resurfacing procedures. Currently, there is no single satisfactory all-encompassing treatment for the broad spectrum of chondral lesions. Therefore, an individualized approach is required that fully involves the patient in the discussion. The aims are to maximize the potential for athletes and patients to return to their full sporting or working activities, prevent reinjury, and minimize the progression of joint degeneration.

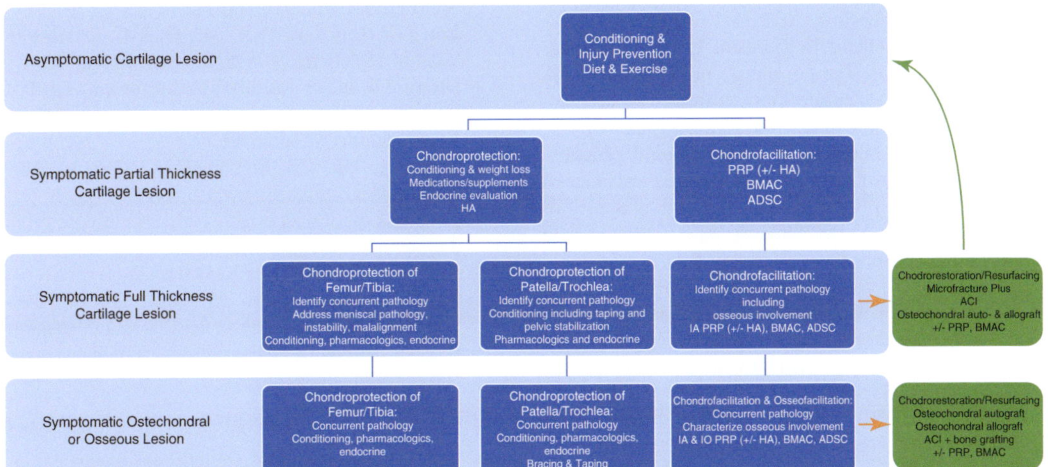

Fig. 7.1 A treatment algorithm for the nonoperative management of cartilage lesions based on chondroprotection, chondrofacilitation, and chondrorestoration/resurfacing surgical options in chondral, osteochondral, and osseous lesions. *HA* hyaluronic acid, *PRP* platelet-rich plasma, *BMAC* bone marrow aspirate concentrate, *ADSC* adipose-derived stem cells, *IA* intra-articular, *IO* intraosseous, *ACI* autologous chondrocyte implantation

References

1. Murray IR, Corselli M, Petrigliano FA, Soo C, Peault B. Recent insights into the identity of mesenchymal stem cells: Implications for orthopaedic applications. Bone Joint J. 2014;96-B(3):291–8.
2. Dominici M, Le Blanc K, Mueller I, Slaper-Cortenbach I, Marini F, Krause D, et al. Minimal criteria for defining multipotent mesenchymal stromal cells. The International Society for Cellular Therapy position statement. Cytotherapy. 2006;8(4):315–7.
3. Flanigan DC, Harris JD, Trinh TQ, Siston RA, Brophy RH. Prevalence of chondral defects in athletes' knees: a systematic review. Med Sci Sport Exerc. 2010;42(10):1795–801.
4. Brophy RH, Zeltser D, Wright RW, Flanigan D. Anterior cruciate ligament reconstruction and concomitant articular cartilage injury: incidence and treatment. Arthroscopy. 2010;26(1):112–20.
5. Widuchowski W, Widuchowski J, Trzaska T. Articular cartilage defects: study of 25,124 knee arthroscopies. Knee. 2007;14(3):177–82.
6. Curl WW, Krome J, Gordon ES, Rushing J, Smith BP, Poehling GG. Cartilage injuries: a review of 31,516 knee arthroscopies. Arthroscopy. 1997;13(4):456–60.
7. Zaffagnini S, Vannini F, Di Martino A, Andriolo L, Sessa A, Perdisa F, et al. Low rate of return to pre-injury sport level in athletes after cartilage surgery: a 10-year follow-up study. Knee Surg Sport Traumatol Arthrosc. 2019;27(8):2502–10.
8. Walczak BE, McCulloch PC, Kang RW, Zelazny A, Tedeschi F, Cole BJ. Abnormal findings on knee magnetic resonance imaging in asymptomatic NBA players. J Knee Surg. 2008;21(1):27–33.
9. Roos H, Lindberg H, Gärdsell P, Lohmander LS, Wingstrand H. The prevalence of gonarthrosis and its relation to meniscectomy in former soccer players. Am J Sports Med. 1994;22(2):219–22.
10. Messner K, Maletius W. The long-term prognosis for severe damage to weight-bearing cartilage in the knee: a 14-year clinical and radiographic follow-up in 28 young athletes. Acta Orthop Scand. 1996;67(2):165–8.
11. Brophy RH, Rodeo SA, Barnes RP, Powell JW, Warren RF. Knee articular cartilage injuries in the National Football League: epidemiology and treatment approach by team physicians. J Knee Surg. 2009;22(4):331–8.
12. Murray IR, Benke MT, Mandelbaum BR. Management of knee articular cartilage injuries in athletes: chondroprotection, chondrofacilitation, and resurfacing. Knee Surg Sport Traumatol Arthrosc. 2016;24(5):1617–26.
13. Berger MJ, McKenzie CA, Chess DG, Goela A, Doherty TJ. Quadriceps neuromuscular function and self-reported functional ability in knee osteoarthritis. J Appl Physiol. 2012;113(2):255–62.
14. Chang A, Hayes K, Dunlop D, Song J, Hurwitz D, Cahue S, et al. Hip abduction moment and protection against medial tibiofemoral osteoarthritis progression. Arthritis Rheum. 2005;52(11):3515–9.
15. Fransen M, McConnell S. Land-based exercise for osteoarthritis of the knee: a metaanalysis of randomized controlled trials. J Rheumatol. 2009;36(6):1109–17.
16. Segal NA, Glass NA, Torner J, Yang M, Felson DT, Sharma L, et al. Quadriceps weakness predicts risk for knee joint space narrowing in women in the MOST cohort. Osteoarthr Cartil. 2010;18(6):769–75.
17. Aaboe J, Bliddal H, Messier SP, Alkjaer T, Henriksen M. Effects of an intensive weight loss program on knee joint loading in obese adults with knee osteoarthritis. Osteoarthr Cartil. 2011;19(7):822–8.
18. Kolasinski SL, Neogi T, Hochberg MC, Oatis C, Guyatt G, Block J, et al. 2019 American College of Rheumatology/Arthritis Foundation Guideline for the Management of Osteoarthritis of the Hand, Hip, and Knee. Arthritis Rheumatol 2020;72(2):220–233.
19. Bannuru RR, Osani MC, Vaysbrot EE, Arden NK, Bennell K, Bierma-Zeinstra SMA, et al. OARSI guidelines for the non-surgical management of knee, hip, and polyarticular osteoarthritis. Osteoarthr Cartil. 2019;27(11):1578–89.
20. Deyle GD, Allen CS, Allison SC, Gill NW, Hando BR, Petersen EJ, et al. Physical therapy versus glucocorticoid injection for osteoarthritis of the knee. N Engl J Med. 2020;382(15):1420–9.
21. Bartholdy C, Klokker L, Bandak E, Bliddal H, Henriksen M. A standardized "rescue" exercise program for symptomatic flare-up of knee osteoarthritis: description and safety considerations. J Orthop Sport Phys Ther. 2016;46(11):942–6.
22. Lee K-H, Lim J-W, Park Y-G, Ha Y-C. Erratum to: vitamin D deficiency is highly concomitant but not strong risk factor for mortality in patients aged 50 year and older with hip fracture. J Bone Metabol Korea (South). 2016;23:49.
23. Bricca A, Juhl CB, Steultjens M, Wirth W, Roos EM. Impact of exercise on articular cartilage in people at risk of, or with established, knee osteoarthritis: a systematic review of randomised controlled trials. Br J Sports Med. 2019;53(15):940–7.
24. Shorter E, Sannicandro AJ, Poulet B, Goljanek-Whysall K. Skeletal muscle wasting and its relationship with osteoarthritis: a mini-review of mechanisms and current interventions. Curr Rheumatol Rep. 2019;21(8):40.
25. Ferraz RB, Gualano B, Rodrigues R, Kurimori CO, Fuller R, Lima FR, et al. Benefits of resistance training with blood flow restriction in knee osteoarthritis. Med Sci Sport Exerc. 2018;50(5):897–905.
26. Minniti MC, Statkevich AP, Kelly RL, Rigsby VP, Exline MM, Rhon DI, et al. The safety of blood flow restriction training as a therapeutic intervention for patients with musculoskeletal disorders: a systematic review. Am J Sport Med. 2019;363546519882652

27. Duivenvoorden T, Brouwer RW, van Raaij TM, Verhagen AP, Verhaar JA, Bierma-Zeinstra SM. Braces and orthoses for treating osteoarthritis of the knee. Cochrane Database Syst Rev. 2015;3:CD004020.

28. Azuma K, Osaki T, Tsuka T, Imagawa T, Okamoto Y, Takamori Y, et al. Effects of oral glucosamine hydrochloride administration on plasma free amino acid concentrations in dogs. Mar Drugs. 2011;9(5):712–8.

29. Imagawa K, de Andres MC, Hashimoto K, Pitt D, Itoi E, Goldring MB, et al. The epigenetic effect of glucosamine and a nuclear factor-kappa B (NF-kB) inhibitor on primary human chondrocytes--implications for osteoarthritis. Biochem Biophys Res Commun. 2011;405(3):362–7.

30. Dalirfardouei R, Karimi G, Jamialahmadi K. Molecular mechanisms and biomedical applications of glucosamine as a potential multifunctional therapeutic agent. Life Sci. 2016;152:21–9.

31. Hui JH, Chan SW, Li J, Goh JC, Li L, Ren XF, et al. Intra-articular delivery of chondroitin sulfate for the treatment of joint defects in rabbit model. J Mol Histol. 2007;38(5):483–9.

32. Monfort J, Pelletier JP, Garcia-Giralt N, Martel-Pelletier J. Biochemical basis of the effect of chondroitin sulphate on osteoarthritis articular tissues. Ann Rheum Dis. 2008;67(6):735–40.

33. Ronca F, Palmieri L, Panicucci P, Ronca G. Anti-inflammatory activity of chondroitin sulfate. Osteoarthr Cartil. 1998;6(Suppl A):14–21.

34. Simental-Mendia M, Sanchez-Garcia A, Vilchez-Cavazos F, Acosta-Olivo CA, Pena-Martinez VM, Simental-Mendia LE. Effect of glucosamine and chondroitin sulfate in symptomatic knee osteoarthritis: a systematic review and meta-analysis of randomized placebo-controlled trials. Rheumatol Int. 2018;38(8):1413–28.

35. Kahan A, Uebelhart D, De Vathaire F, Delmas PD, Reginster JY. Long-term effects of chondroitins 4 and 6 sulfate on knee osteoarthritis: the study on osteoarthritis progression prevention, a two-year, randomized, double-blind, placebo-controlled trial. Arthritis Rheum. 2009;60(2):524–33.

36. Hochberg MC, Zhan M, Langenberg P. The rate of decline of joint space width in patients with osteoarthritis of the knee: a systematic review and meta-analysis of randomized placebo-controlled trials of chondroitin sulfate. Curr Med Res Opin. 2008;24(11):3029–35.

37. Nicoliche T, Maldonado DC, Faber J, Silva M. Evaluation of the articular cartilage in the knees of rats with induced arthritis treated with curcumin. PLoS One. 2020;15(3):e0230228.

38. Zhang Z, Leong DJ, Xu L, He Z, Wang A, Navati M, et al. Curcumin slows osteoarthritis progression and relieves osteoarthritis-associated pain symptoms in a post-traumatic osteoarthritis mouse model. Arthritis Res Ther. 2016;18(1):128.

39. Shep D, Khanwelkar C, Gade P, Karad S. Safety and efficacy of curcumin versus diclofenac in knee osteoarthritis: a randomized open-label parallel-arm study. Trials. 2019;20(1):214.

40. Xu X, Li X, Liang Y, Ou Y, Huang J, Xiong J, et al. Estrogen modulates cartilage and subchondral bone remodeling in an ovariectomized rat model of postmenopausal osteoarthritis. Med Sci Monit. 2019;25:3146–53.

41. Xu K, Sha Y, Wang S, Chi Q, Liu Y, Wang C, et al. Effects of Bakuchiol on chondrocyte proliferation via the PI3K-Akt and ERK1/2 pathways mediated by the estrogen receptor for promotion of the regeneration of knee articular cartilage defects. Cell Prolif. 2019;52(5):e12666.

42. Lou C, Xiang G, Weng Q, Chen Z, Chen D, Wang Q, et al. Menopause is associated with articular cartilage degeneration: a clinical study of knee joint in 860 women. Menopause. 2016;23(11):1239–46.

43. Son YO, Park S, Kwak JS, Won Y, Choi WS, Rhee J, et al. Estrogen-related receptor gamma causes osteoarthritis by upregulating extracellular matrix-degrading enzymes. Nat Commun. 2017;8(1):2133.

44. Liang Y, Duan L, Xiong J, Zhu W, Liu Q, Wang D, et al. E2 regulates MMP-13 via targeting miR-140 in IL-1beta-induced extracellular matrix degradation in human chondrocytes. Arthritis Res Ther. 2016;18(1):105.

45. Arroll B, Goodyear-Smith F. Corticosteroid injections for osteoarthritis of the knee: meta-analysis. BMJ. 2004;328(7444):869.

46. McAlindon TE, LaValley MP, Harvey WF, Price LL, Driban JB, Zhang M, et al. Effect of intra-articular triamcinolone vs saline on knee cartilage volume and pain in patients with knee osteoarthritis: a randomized clinical trial. JAMA. 2017;317(19):1967–75.

47. Raynauld J-P, Buckland-Wright C, Ward R, Choquette D, Haraoui B, Martel-Pelletier J, et al. Safety and efficacy of long-term intraarticular steroid injections in osteoarthritis of the knee: a randomized, double-blind, placebo-controlled trial. Arthritis Rheum. 2003;48(2):370–7.

48. Klocke R, Levasseur K, Kitas GD, Smith JP, Hirsch G. Cartilage turnover and intra-articular corticosteroid injections in knee osteoarthritis. Rheumatol Int. 2018;38(3):455–9.

49. Adams ME, Lussier AJ, Peyron JG. A risk-benefit assessment of injections of hyaluronan and its derivatives in the treatment of osteoarthritis of the knee. Drug Saf. 2000;23(2):115–30.

50. Altman R, Lim S, Steen RG, Dasa V. Hyaluronic acid injections are associated with delay of total knee replacement surgery in patients with knee osteoarthritis: evidence from a large U.S. Health Claims Database. PLoS One. 2015;10(12):e0145776.

51. Pashuck TD, Kuroki K, Cook CR, Stoker AM, Cook JL. Hyaluronic acid versus saline intra-articular injections for amelioration of chronic knee osteoarthritis: a canine model. J Orthop Res. 2016;34(10):1772–9.

52. Barreto RB, Sadigursky D, de Rezende MU, Hernandez AJ. Effect of hyaluronic acid on chondrocyte apoptosis. Acta Ortop Bras. 2015;23(2):90–3.

53. Petterson SC, Plancher KD. Single intra-articular injection of lightly cross-linked hyaluronic acid reduces knee pain in symptomatic knee osteoarthritis: a multicenter, double-blind, randomized, placebo-controlled trial. Knee Surg Sport Traumatol Arthrosc. 2019;27(6):1992–2002.

54. Petrella RJ, Petrella M. A prospective, randomized, double-blind, placebo controlled study to evaluate the efficacy of intraarticular hyaluronic acid for osteoarthritis of the knee. J Rheumatol. 2006;33(5):951–6.

55. Pham T, Le Henanff A, Ravaud P, Dieppe P, Paolozzi L, Dougados M. Evaluation of the symptomatic and structural efficacy of a new hyaluronic acid compound, NRD101, in comparison with diacerein and placebo in a 1 year randomised controlled study in symptomatic knee osteoarthritis. Ann Rheum Dis. 2004;63(12):1611–7.

56. Listrat V, Ayral X, Patarnello F, Bonvarlet JP, Simonnet J, Amor B, et al. Arthroscopic evaluation of potential structure modifying activity of hyaluronan (Hyalgan) in osteoarthritis of the knee. Osteoarthr Cartil. 1997;5(3):153–60.

57. Wang Y, Hall S, Hanna F, Wluka AE, Grant G, Marks P, et al. Effects of Hylan G-F 20 supplementation on cartilage preservation detected by magnetic resonance imaging in osteoarthritis of the knee: a two-year single-blind clinical trial. BMC Musculoskelet Disord. 2011;12:195.

58. Dasa V, Lim S, Heeckt P. Real-world evidence for safety and effectiveness of repeated courses of hyaluronic acid injections on the time to knee replacement surgery. Am J Orthop (Belle Mead NJ). 2018:47(7).

59. Foster TE, Puskas BL, Mandelbaum BR, Gerhardt MB, Rodeo SA. Platelet-rich plasma: from basic science to clinical applications. Am J Sports Med. 2009;37(11):2259–72.

60. Dhillon RS, Schwarz EM, Maloney MD. Platelet-rich plasma therapy - future or trend? Arthritis Res Ther. 2012;14(4):219.

61. Rughetti A, Giusti I, D'Ascenzo S, Leocata P, Carta G, Pavan A, et al. Platelet gel-released supernatant modulates the angiogenic capability of human endothelial cells. Blood Transfus. 2008;6(1):12–7.

62. Liu J, Song W, Yuan T, Xu Z, Jia W, Zhang C. A comparison between platelet-rich plasma (PRP) and hyaluronate acid on the healing of cartilage defects. PLoS One. 2014;9(5):e97293.

63. Milano G, Deriu L, Sanna Passino E, Masala G, Saccomanno MF, Postacchini R, et al. The effect of autologous conditioned plasma on the treatment of focal chondral defects of the knee. An experimental study. Int J Immunopathol Pharmacol. 2011;24(1 Suppl 2):117–24.

64. Goodrich LR, Chen AC, Werpy NM, Williams AA, Kisiday JD, Su AW, et al. Addition of mesenchymal stem cells to autologous platelet-enhanced fibrin scaffolds in chondral defects: does it enhance repair? J Bone Joint Surg Am. 2016;98(1):23–34.

65. Iio K, Furukawa K-I, Tsuda E, Yamamoto Y, Maeda S, Naraoka T, et al. Hyaluronic acid induces the release of growth factors from platelet-rich plasma. Asia-Pacific J Sport Med Arthrosc Rehabil Technol. 2016;4:27–32.

66. Kon E, Mandelbaum B, Buda R, Filardo G, Delcogliano M, Timoncini A, et al. Platelet-rich plasma intra-articular injection versus hyaluronic acid viscosupplementation as treatments for cartilage pathology: from early degeneration to osteoarthritis. Arthrosc J Arthrosc Relat Surg Off Publ Arthrosc Assoc North Am Int Arthrosc Assoc. 2011;27(11):1490–501.

67. Sanchez M, Fiz N, Azofra J, Usabiaga J, Aduriz Recalde E, Garcia Gutierrez A, et al. A randomized clinical trial evaluating plasma rich in growth factors (PRGF-Endoret) versus hyaluronic acid in the short-term treatment of symptomatic knee osteoarthritis. Arthroscopy. 2012;28(8):1070–8.

68. Filardo G, Kon E, Di Martino A, Di Matteo B, Merli ML, Cenacchi A, et al. Platelet-rich plasma vs hyaluronic acid to treat knee degenerative pathology: study design and preliminary results of a randomized controlled trial. BMC Musculoskelet Disord. 2012;13:229.

69. Filardo G, Di Matteo B, Di Martino A, Merli ML, Cenacchi A, Fornasari P, et al. Platelet-rich plasma intra-articular knee injections show no superiority versus viscosupplementation: a randomized controlled trial. Am J Sports Med. 2015;43(7):1575–82.

70. Riboh JC, Saltzman BM, Yanke AB, Fortier L, Cole BJ. Effect of leukocyte concentration on the efficacy of platelet-rich plasma in the treatment of knee osteoarthritis. Am J Sports Med. 2016;44(3):792–800.

71. Patel S, Dhillon MS, Aggarwal S, Marwaha N, Jain A. Treatment with platelet-rich plasma is more effective than placebo for knee osteoarthritis: a prospective, double-blind, randomized trial. Am J Sports Med. 2013;41(2):356–64.

72. Cerza F, Carni S, Carcangiu A, Di Vavo I, Schiavilla V, Pecora A, et al. Comparison between hyaluronic acid and platelet-rich plasma, intra-articular infiltration in the treatment of gonarthrosis. Am J Sports Med. 2012;40(12):2822–7.

73. Cole BJ, Karas V, Hussey K, Pilz K, Fortier LA. Hyaluronic acid versus platelet-rich plasma. Am J Sports Med. 2017;45(2):339–46.

74. Everhart JS, Cavendish PA, Eikenberry A, Magnussen RA, Kaeding CC, Flanigan DC. Platelet-rich plasma reduces failure risk for isolated meniscal repairs but provides no benefit for meniscal repairs with anterior cruciate ligament reconstruction. Am J Sports Med. 2019;47(8):1789–96.

75. Gobbi A, Chaurasia S, Karnatzikos G, Nakamura N. Matrix-induced autologous chondrocyte implantation versus multipotent stem cells for the treatment of large patellofemoral chondral lesions: a nonrandomized prospective trial. Cartilage. 2015;6(2):82–97.

76. Gobbi A, Whyte GP. One-stage cartilage repair using a hyaluronic acid-based scaffold with activated bone marrow-derived mesenchymal stem cells compared with microfracture: five-year follow-up. Am J Sports Med. 2016;44(11):2846–54.

77. Enea D, Cecconi S, Calcagno S, Busilacchi A, Manzotti S, Gigante A. One-step cartilage repair in the knee: collagen-covered microfracture and autologous bone marrow concentrate. A pilot study. Knee. 2015;22(1):30–5.

78. Krych AJ, Nawabi DH, Farshad-Amacker NA, Jones KJ, Maak TG, Potter HG, et al. Bone marrow concentrate improves early cartilage phase maturation of a scaffold plug in the knee: a comparative magnetic resonance imaging analysis to platelet-rich plasma and control. Am J Sports Med. 2016;44(1):91–8.

79. Krych AJ, Pareek A, King AH, Johnson NR, Stuart MJ, Williams RJ 3rd. Return to sport after the surgical management of articular cartilage lesions in the knee: a meta-analysis. Knee Surg Sports Traumatol Arthrosc. 2017;25(10):3186–96.

80. Skowronski J, Skowronski R, Rutka M. Large cartilage lesions of the knee treated with bone marrow concentrate and collagen membrane--results. Ortop Traumatol Rehabil. 2013;15(1):69–76.

81. Skowronski J, Rutka M. Osteochondral lesions of the knee reconstructed with mesenchymal stem cells - results. Ortop Traumatol Rehabil. 2013;15(3):195–204.

82. Fortier LA, Potter HG, Rickey EJ, Schnabel LV, Foo LF, Chong LR, et al. Concentrated bone marrow aspirate improves full-thickness cartilage repair compared with microfracture in the equine model. J Bone Joint Surg Am. 2010;92(10):1927–37.

83. Potten CS, Loeffler M. Stem cells: attributes, cycles, spirals, pitfalls and uncertainties. Lessons for and from the crypt. Development. 1990;110(4):1001–20.

84. Chang Y-H, Liu H-W, Wu K-C, Ding D-C. Mesenchymal stem cells and their clinical applications in osteoarthritis. Cell Transplant. 2016;25(5):937–50.

85. Ruetze M, Richter W. Adipose-derived stromal cells for osteoarticular repair: trophic function versus stem cell activity. Expert Rev Mol Med. 2014;16:e9.

86. Wu L, Cai X, Zhang S, Karperien M, Lin Y. Regeneration of articular cartilage by adipose tissue derived mesenchymal stem cells: perspectives from stem cell biology and molecular medicine. J Cell Physiol. 2013;228(5):938–44.

87. Jang K-M, Lee J-H, Park CM, Song H-R, Wang JH. Xenotransplantation of human mesenchymal stem cells for repair of osteochondral defects in rabbits using osteochondral biphasic composite constructs. Knee Surg Sports Traumatol Arthrosc. 2014;22(6):1434–44.

88. Jung M, Kaszap B, Redöhl A, Steck E, Breusch S, Richter W, et al. Enhanced early tissue regeneration after matrix-assisted autologous mesenchymal stem cell transplantation in full thickness chondral defects in a minipig model. Cell Transplant. 2009;18(8):923–32.

89. Nam HY, Karunanithi P, Loo WC, Naveen S, Chen H, Hussin P, et al. The effects of staged intra-articular injection of cultured autologous mesenchymal stromal cells on the repair of damaged cartilage: a pilot study in caprine model. Arthritis Res Ther. 2013;15(5):R129.

90. Chahla J, Piuzzi NS, Mitchell JJ, Dean CS, Pascual-Garrido C, LaPrade RF, et al. Intra-articular cellular therapy for osteoarthritis and focal cartilage defects of the knee: a systematic review of the literature and study quality analysis. J Bone Joint Surg Am. 2016;98(18):1511–21.

91. Campbell TM, Churchman SM, Gomez A, McGonagle D, Conaghan PG, Ponchel F, et al. Mesenchymal stem cell alterations in bone marrow lesions in patients with hip osteoarthritis. Arthritis Rheumatol (Hoboken, NJ). 2016;68(7):1648–59.

92. Cox LGE, van Donkelaar CC, van Rietbergen B, Emans PJ, Ito K. Alterations to the subchondral bone architecture during osteoarthritis: bone adaptation vs endochondral bone formation. Osteoarthr Cartil. 2013;21(2):331–8.

93. Suri S, Walsh DA. Osteochondral alterations in osteoarthritis. Bone. 2012;51(2):204–11.

94. Klement MR, Sharkey PF. The significance of osteoarthritis-associated bone marrow lesions in the knee. J Am Acad Orthop Surg. 2019;27(20):752–9.

95. Pelletier J-P, Roubille C, Raynauld J-P, Abram F, Dorais M, Delorme P, et al. Disease-modifying effect of strontium ranelate in a subset of patients from the phase III knee osteoarthritis study SEKOIA using quantitative MRI: reduction in bone marrow lesions protects against cartilage loss. Ann Rheum Dis. 2015;74(2):422–9.

96. Varenna M, Zucchi F, Failoni S, Becciolini A, Berruto M. Intravenous neridronate in the treatment of acute painful knee osteoarthritis: a randomized controlled study. Rheumatology (Oxford). 2015;54(10):1826–32.

97. Laslett LL, Doré DA, Quinn SJ, Boon P, Ryan E, Winzenberg TM, et al. Zoledronic acid reduces knee pain and bone marrow lesions over 1 year: a randomised controlled trial. Ann Rheum Dis. 2012;71(8):1322–8.

98. Jäger M, Tillmann FP, Thornhill TS, Mahmoudi M, Blondin D, Hetzel GR, et al. Rationale for prostaglandin I2 in bone marrow oedema--from theory to application. Arthritis Res Ther. 2008;10(5):R120.

99. Mayerhoefer ME, Kramer J, Breitenseher MJ, Norden C, Vakil-Adli A, Hofmann S, et al. Short-term outcome of painful bone marrow oedema of the knee following oral treatment with iloprost or tramadol: results of an exploratory phase II study of 41 patients. Rheumatology (Oxford). 2007;46(9):1460–5.

100. Callaghan MJ, Parkes MJ, Hutchinson CE, Gait AD, Forsythe LM, Marjanovic EJ, et al. A randomised trial of a brace for patellofemoral osteoarthritis

targeting knee pain and bone marrow lesions. Ann Rheum Dis. 2015;74(6):1164–70.

101. Su K, Bai Y, Wang J, Zhang H, Liu H, Ma S. Comparison of hyaluronic acid and PRP intra-articular injection with combined intra-articular and intraosseous PRP injections to treat patients with knee osteoarthritis. Clin Rheumatol. 2018;37(5):1341–50.

102. Sánchez M, Delgado D, Pompei O, Pérez JC, Sánchez P, Garate A, et al. Treating severe knee osteoarthritis with combination of intra-osseous and intra-articular infiltrations of platelet-rich plasma: an observational study. Cartilage. 2019;10(2):245–53.

103. Deshmukh V, Hu H, Barroga C, Bossard C, Kc S, Dellamary L, et al. A small-molecule inhibitor of the Wnt pathway (SM04690) as a potential disease modifying agent for the treatment of osteoarthritis of the knee. Osteoarthr Cartil. 2018;26(1):18–27.

104. Yazici Y, McAlindon TE, Fleischmann R, Gibofsky A, Lane NE, Kivitz AJ, et al. A novel Wnt pathway inhibitor, SM04690, for the treatment of moderate to severe osteoarthritis of the knee: results of a 24-week, randomized, controlled, phase 1 study. Osteoarthr Cartil. 2017;25(10):1598–606.

The Role of Osteotomy in the Patellofemoral Joint with Cartilage Surgery

8

Lachlan M. Batty, Michelle E. Arakgi, and Alan M. J. Getgood

8.1 Introduction

Alignment and load distribution are critical factors to consider in the management of any chondral lesion of the knee. Joint-preserving surgical approaches to chondral lesions can broadly be grouped as palliative (debridement), reparative (marrow stimulation), restorative (autologous chondrocyte implantation (ACI)) or particulated juvenile allograft cartilage (PJAC) transplant or reconstructive procedures (osteochondral grafting) [1, 2]. Each of these treatment strategies can be performed in isolation or conjunction with a realignment procedure to optimise contact forces and load distribution. Realignment and load redistribution procedures are attractive in the context of restorative and reconstructive chondral procedures which are typically indicated for small, isolated, unipolar lesions. Because of this, the remainder of the knee is typically healthy allowing for a calculated and balanced load redistribution.

In the tibiofemoral joint, realignment procedures typically consist of osteotomy of the proximal tibia or distal femur to optimise coronal plane alignment although, importantly, the sagittal plane is also affected and should be considered. Indications for osteotomy in the tibiofemoral joint are usually for pain, instability or a combination of both. It is well established that alignment correction is critical in tibiofemoral cartilage procedures addressing chondral related knee pain [3–6]. In a similar fashion, when the PFJ is considered, osteotomies again have a potential role in the treatment of both pain and instability. The tibial tubercle osteotomy (TTO) (Figs. 8.1, 8.2e, f, and 8.3c, d) is the most common osteotomy used in managing patellofemoral joint (PFJ) conditions and in the context of PFJ chondral surgery. TTO is referred to as a distal realignment of the extensor mechanism. A proximal realignment refers to more proximally based soft-tissue procedures including lateral release, retinacular lengthening, or medial sided soft-tissue procedures. For a distal realignment, the TT can be moved proximal/distal, medial/lateral or anterior/posterior or in any combination of these directions. The aims of TTO in the setting of PF chondral surgery are to reduce contact pressures in a global fashion and/or to redistribute load to a more favourable location within the PFJ, thereby offloading the cartilage repair. Antero-medialisation of the TT,

L. M. Batty
Fowler Kennedy Sports Medicine Clinic, University of Western Ontario, London, Canada

OrthoSport Victoria Research Unit, Melbourne, VIC, Australia

M. E. Arakgi · A. M. J. Getgood (✉)
Fowler Kennedy Sports Medicine Clinic, University of Western Ontario, London, Canada
e-mail: alan.getgood@uwo.ca

© ISAKOS 2021
A. J. Krych et al. (eds.), *Cartilage Injury of the Knee*,
https://doi.org/10.1007/978-3-030-78051-7_8

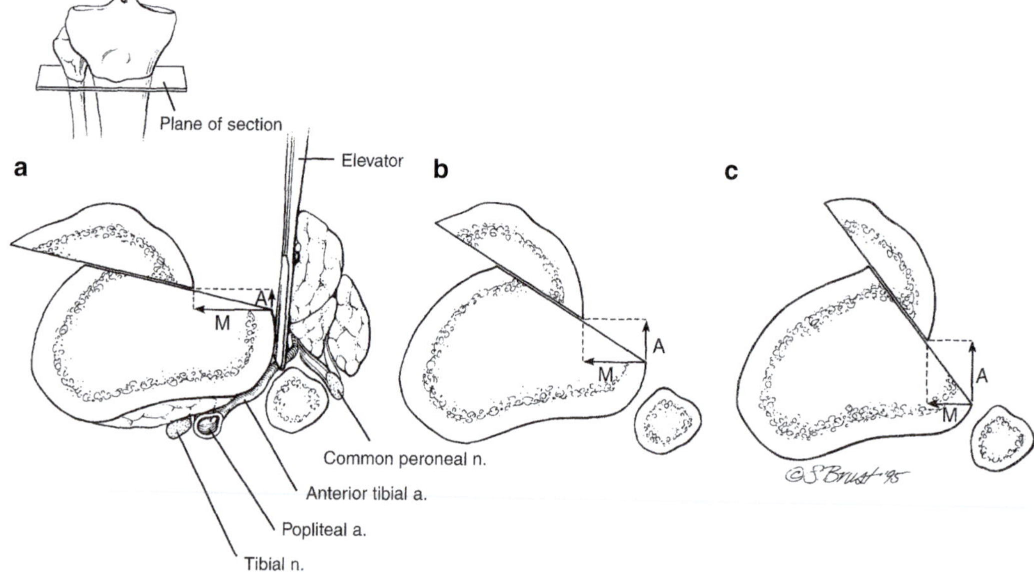

Fig. 8.1 Axial sections through the proximal tibia. A shallow (**a**), intermediate (**b**) and steep (**c**) antero-medialisation of the tibial tubercle. The relative amount of anteriorisation compared to medialisation is progressively increased from (**a**) to (**c**). This can be individually tailored to each patient. Reproduced with permission from: Buuck, DA, Fulkerson, JP. Anteromedialization of the tibial tubercle: A 4- to 12-year follow-up. Operative Techniques in Sports Medicine, Volume 8, Issue 2, 2000, Pages 131–137

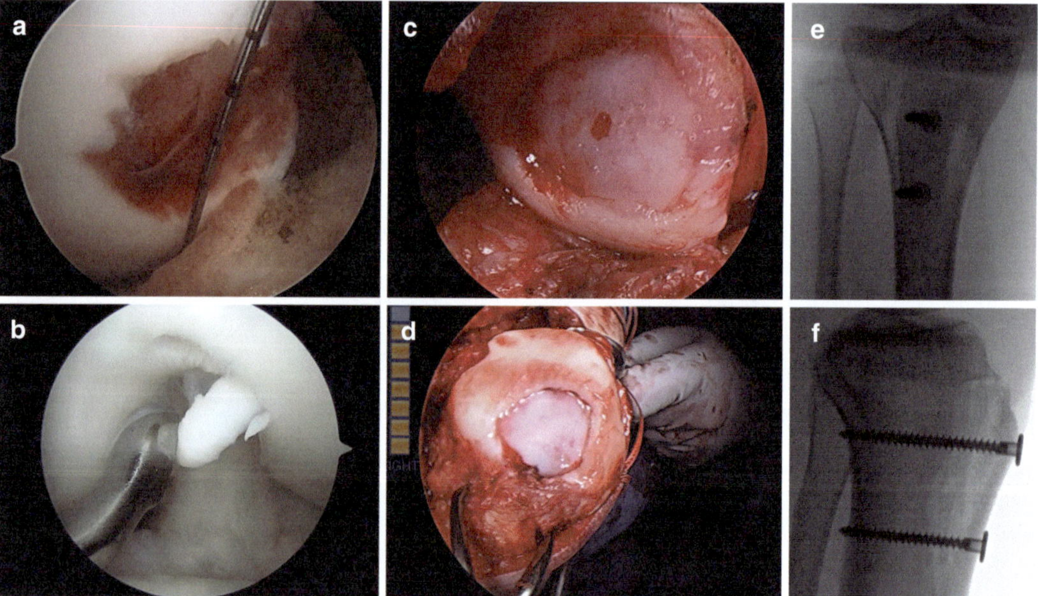

Fig. 8.2 Composite image of a central patella autologous chondrocyte implantation with a concomitant steep antero-medialisation of the tibial tubercle. (**a**) At initial arthroscopy, the location and size of the chondral defect are characterised. Patellofemoral tracking is also assessed under anaesthesia both clinically and arthroscopically. (**b**) A small portion of articular cartilage is removed with a curette from a non-articulating area of the distal trochlea to chondrocyte expansion. (**c** and **d**) At a second stage, the expanded chondrocytes are placed into the prepared chondral defect. The tibial tubercle osteotomy has been performed and aids in exposure for the ACI. (**e** and **f**) The steep tibial tubercle is secured with two low-profile screws using a lag technique. Note that the posterior cortex must be engaged. Images courtesy of Dr. Seth Sherman

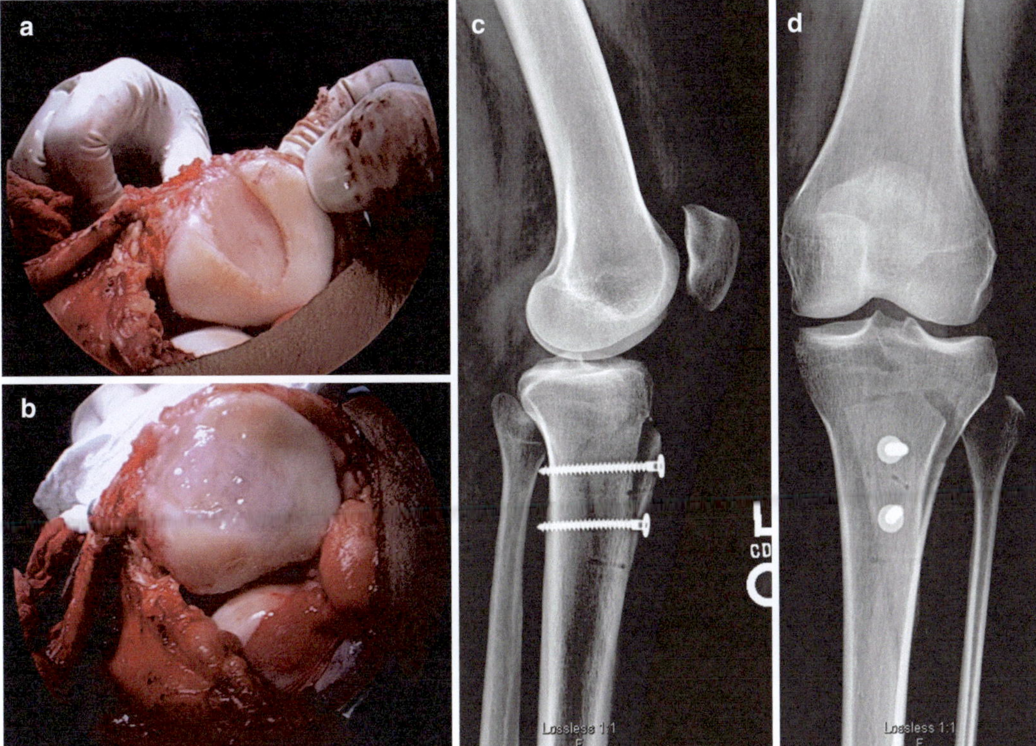

Fig. 8.3 A large patella chondral defect prepared to stable vertical margins (**a**). This has been treated with a particulated juvenile allograft cartilage transplantation (**b**) and a concomitant steep (anteriorisation > medialisation) tibial tubercle osteotomy (**c**, **d**). Images courtesy of Dr. Seth Sherman

as popularised by Fulkerson [7] (Fig. 8.1), is the most commonly used TTO in the context of PF chondral surgery and has been the most widely studied. Historically, direct anteriorisation of the TT, as popularised by Maquet [8, 9], fell out of favour for the treatment of chondral related anterior knee pain; however, there has been renewed interest as a concomitant procedure with advances in chondral restorative and reconstructive procedures [10]. A 2020 systematic review and meta-analysis identified that of 1937 PFJ cartilage procedures, a concomitant realignment procedure was performed in 575 cases (29.7%) [11]. TTO also has an important role in the management of PF instability; however, this is outside the scope of this chapter and the focus is on TTO as an adjunct to PF chondral surgery without PFJ instability.

8.2 Biomechanical Rationale

Numerous biomechanical studies have investigated PFJ kinematics. PF contact pressures and overall contact area increase and move proximally with progressive knee flexion [12–14]. Increasing the Q-angle, or a lateral vector of the extensor mechanism, increases lateral facet pressures and contact forces on the patella [12]. PFJ contact pressures can be modulated with displacement of the TT and change based on the direction and magnitude of displacement. Beck et al. [15] evaluated trochlea-sided contact pressures before and after antero-medialisation (7.5 mm medialisation, 13.5 mm anteriorisation) of the TT in ten cadaveric knees. PFJ pressures and the centre of force were measured using an electro-resistive pressure sensor on the trochlea at differing knee flexion angles.

After TTO, the mean total contact pressure was reduced in the order of 2–5 kg/cm^2, the centre of force was shifted medially 7.2–10.3 mm and there was a reduction in lateral trochlea contact pressures of 3–8 kg/cm^2 depending upon knee flexion angle and loading protocol. This was at the expense of increasing medial trochlea pressures by 2–8 kg/cm^2. Similar methodology was subsequently employed by Rue et al. [16] to investigate the effect of 10 mm of TT anteriorisation in ten cadaveric knees. Both mean and peak trochlear contact forces were reduced by 18–32% and 24%–32%, respectively, depending upon knee flexion angle. Unlike the antero-medialisation TTO by Beck et al., there was no medial shift in the centre of force. Stephen et al. [17] examined patellar contact pressures with isolated medialisation and lateralisation of the TT sequentially by 5, 10 and 15 mm. TT lateralisation significantly elevated lateral contact pressures with incremental displacement. However, medialisation reduced lateral contact pressures without significantly elevating peak medial pressures. Medial pressures appeared to plateau with progressive medial translation. The authors hypothesised that tension in lateral soft-tissue structures (ITB and lateral retinaculum) and lower stiffness of the medial structures (medial retinaculum and MPFL) could explain this phenomenon. Ramappa et al. [12] compared the efficacy of an isolated medialisation (10 mm) to a combined antero-medialisation (10 mm/10 mm) in addressing patellar maltracking due to a surgically increased Q-angle. Both were equally effective at normalising PF contact pressures and patellar tracking in this model in response to a more lateralised quadricep vector. Together, these studies highlight the efficacy of TTO as a means of altering PFJ contact pressures and kinematics. Of note, these biomechanical studies were performed on knees without known PF malalignment or pre-existing chondral disease, a common limitation in biomechanical work.

8.3 Clinical Outcomes

8.3.1 Tibial Tubercle Osteotomy with Palliative or Reparative Chondral Procedures

Traditionally, TTO was performed in isolation or with arthroscopic debridement only [7–9]. With the evolution in chondral procedures, this approach has somewhat fallen out of favour [18]. Many still advocate for an isolated TT antero-medialisation for the treatment of focal distal and lateral lesions of the patella [19]. This is largely based on an influential paper by Pidoriano et al. [20] that reviewed 36 patients undergoing arthroscopic patellar chondroplasty and TT antero-medialisation for patella chondral lesions. At a mean 46.8-month follow-up the authors highlighted that the geographical location of the chondral lesion significantly impacted the outcome. The 23 patients with distal and lateral facet lesions had 87% good-to-excellent subjective results and all would undergo the procedure again. Nine patients with medial facet lesions had 55% good-to-excellent results, and five patients with proximal or diffuse lesions had 20% good-to-excellent results. Interestingly, the severity of the chondral lesion as assessed by Outterbridge grade did not influence results. A later series of isolated antero-medialisation for chondral related PFJ pain in a military population demonstrated a mean improvement in patient-reported visual analogue scores (VAS) for pain of only 1.5 at 3.4-year follow-up. Although statistically significant, the clinical significance of this improvement was questioned by the authors [21]. Microfracture as an intervention for PFJ chondral lesions has seen a significant reduction in use and data on outcomes with and without TTO are lacking [18].

8.4 Tibial Tubercle Osteotomy with Restorative Chondral Procedures

8.4.1 Autologous Chondrocyte Implantation

In terms of PFJ restorative surgeries, TTO in combination with autologous chondrocyte implantation (ACI) has been the most extensively studied (Fig. 8.2). Early studies revealed suboptimal results of PFJ ACI as compared to tibiofemoral transplantation [22]. Only two of seven PF patients achieved good or excellent outcomes at 2 years in an initial ACI series by Brittberg et al. [22] The authors postulated that "the correction of underlying joint abnormalities concomitantly with the transplantation of chondrocytes may improve the success rate for patients with patellar defects." Although this concept was highlighted early in the experience with ACI, this statement likely applies to other chondral surgeries also. With further research, more favourable results do appear to be seen when PFJ ACI is performed in conjunction with TTO to correct any underlying malalignment or maltracking and offload the ACI graft [1, 23–27]. The challenge in interpreting these studies is understanding the decision-making process when a concomitant TTO was performed and identifying when an additional TTO is indicated at the individual patient level. Patient selection is critical as TTO is not without associated morbidity and risk. Documented rates of TTO performed in addition to PFJ ACI range from 0% [28] to 91% [29]. A 2020 systematic review and meta-analysis documented a 37.5% rate of realignment procedures being performed concomitantly with PFJ ACI [11]. A recent expert consensus statement found 96.43% agreement that significant patellar malalignment or maltracking should be addressed concomitantly

or prior to any PFJ cartilage restoration procedure. There was also 96.43% agreement that an unloading osteotomy should be strongly considered for a bipolar PFJ ACI procedure, regardless of patellar tracking and alignment [30].

Gomoll et al. [31] reported results of 110 patients undergoing patellar ACI in a multicentre series. Comparing the group mean pre- and post-operative PROM scores, the authors reported statistically significant and clinically important improvements (IKDC from 40 to 69; Cincinnati from 3.2 to 6.2; WOMAC from 50 to 29). Interestingly, there was variable use of concomitant TTO across the four centres ranging from 53% to 97%. Overall, antero-medialisation was performed for TTO in 75% of cases. There were no statistical differences in outcomes between the TTO group when compared to the no-TTO group; however, with non-random allocation to this treatment (based on maltracking or malalignment), this could be interpreted as supportive of selective TTO.

Gillogy and Arnold [32] followed 25 knees of patients who underwent a combined patellar ACI and TTO antero-medialisation. Preoperatively all patients showed persistent lateral patellar tracking clinically and failure to centralise in the trochlea by 45° of flexion. An increased Q-angle and arthroscopic visualisation of persistent lateral tracking with a large isolated full-thickness chondral defect on the patella were the essential indications for concomitant TTO antero-medialisation. At a mean follow-up of 7.6 years, there were significant improvements in all patient-reported outcome measures (PROM) and 83% rated their surgery as good or excellent. In a military population of 72 patients undergoing PFJ ACI, Zarkadis et al. [29] documented that 91% underwent a concomitant TTO. In this series, the indications for concomitant TTO included location of chondral disease (distal patella $n = 18$, lateral patella $n = 26$, lateral trochlear $n = 7$), combined patellar instability ($n = 4$) and/or TT-TG >15 mm ($n = 15$). At a mean 4-year follow-up, 78% had returned to their occupational specialties and mean VAS improved significantly. Three patients (4.1%) were classified as having surgical failures, requiring subsequent knee arthroplasty ($n = 2$) or revision chondral procedure ($n = 1$).

In a non-randomised trial, Pascal-Garrido et al. [25] followed 52 patients in 3 groups. These were isolated PFJ ACI ($n = 11$), PFJ ACI with TTO ($n = 12$) and PFJ ACI with TTO with a history of a failed microfracture ($n = 14$). Indications for TTO in this series were described as complex and based on multiple factors including the location of chondral disease, position of the patella relative to the trochlea and TT-TG offset. Distal and lateral patella lesions were treated with TT antero-medialisation. Central, proximal and medially located lesions were treated with modifications to avoid over-medialisation. Trochlea lesions were treated initially with ACI and TT antero-medialisation unless there was medial trochlea disease where a pure anteriorisation was performed. All three groups showed statistical improvement in most of the outcome scores at the time of follow-up of 4 years. Interestingly, patients treated with ACI with TT antero-medialisation with a history of microfracture showed significantly higher Knee Injury and Osteoarthritis Outcome Score (KOOS) for pain and KOOS ADL scores than those with ACI alone. In addition, 86% of these patients reported that they were mostly or completely satisfied with the procedure compared to 45% who received an ACI in isolation. The authors concluded that combined ACI with antero-medialisation improves outcomes more than ACI alone.

Henderson and Lavigne [24] also found superior outcomes for patients treated with combined ACI and extensor mechanism realignment for patella maltracking at 2-year follow up. In this series of 44 patients, the indication for concomitant TTO was failure of the patella to seat normally within the trochlea groove during the first 45° of flexion. Despite pre-existing maltracking and increased surgical morbidity from the TTO, this group had higher increases in all PROMs at 2-year follow-up. Vasiliadis et al. [27] reviewed 92 patients undergoing patellar or trochlea ACI at a mean 12.6 years of follow-up. In a similar fashion to the series from Henderson and Pascal-Garrido, patients with malalignment or instability who underwent a concomitant realignment procedure had comparable outcomes to ACI only. An increase in the serious complication rate (29% as compared to 13%) was seen with the addition of a TTO to ACI in this series including graft failures, arthrofibrosis, delamination and reoperation.

A 2014 systematic review published by Trinh et al. [26] compared clinical outcomes of patients undergoing PF ACI with or without a realignment procedure. Eleven studies (366 patients) were included in the review with a mean follow-up of 4.2 years. ACI was performed on the patella in 78% and on the trochlea in 22%. Twenty-three percent of subjects underwent concomitant osteotomy. Both groups demonstrated significant improvements following treatment. Three studies compared isolated ACI to combined ACI and TTO [24, 25, 27] with greater improvement in PROMs for patients undergoing combined osteotomy and ACI.

8.4.2 Particulate Juvenile Allograft Cartilage

Limited data are available for outcomes of PJAC in the PFJ (Fig. 8.3) [10, 33–37]. The indications for PJAC transplant are similar to ACI [38], and the indications for concomitant TTO are likely similar also. Of the published series, 43 concomitant TTOs were performed in the 126 reported patients (34.1%); however, indications were variable and included instability [10]. Buckwalter et al. [34] recommend an isolated antero-medialisation TTO for lateral patella lesions unless the TT-TG is <10 mm, in which case a direct anteriorisation is performed. For medial and central patella lesions, the authors recommend a combined TTO with the PJAC transplantation. The TT-TG distance was used to establish the relative amounts of anteriorisation and medialisation with a target correction of TT-TG less than 12 mm. Wang et al. [36] reviewed 27 patients at a mean of 3.84 years after

PFJ PJAC. They performed concomitant TTO to unload isolated lesions of the inferolateral patella (*n* = 6) and combined TTO with a medial patellofemoral ligament reconstruction in the setting of PFJ instability with TT-TG >20 mm (*n* = 4). There were significant improvements in pain and function outcome scores as measured by International Knee Documentation Committee (IKDC) and Knee Outcome Survey-Activities of Daily Living (KOS-ADL) PROMs but not for the Marx Activity Scale (MAS). The addition of TTO did not impact the outcome.

8.5 Tibial Tubercle Osteotomy with Reconstructive Chondral Procedures

Osteochondral autografting is technically demanding within the PFJ because of its complex 3-dimensional geometry. This makes restoring contour and achieving a uniform-level cartilage reconstruction extremely challenging (Fig. 8.4). This is compounded by differing chondral depths of the patella and trochlea that predisposes to a

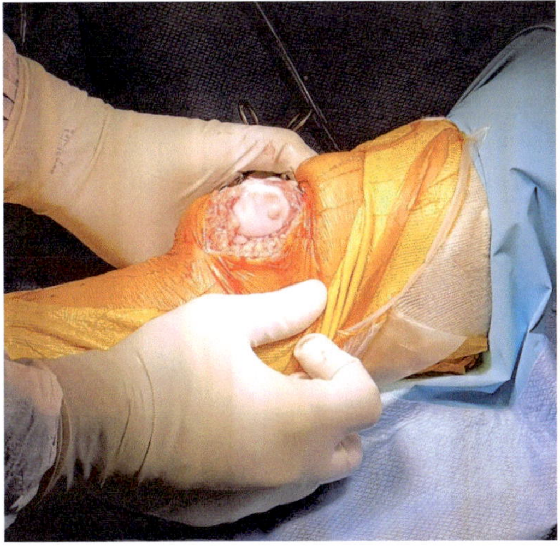

Fig. 8.4 A patellar autologous osteochondral transplantation to the superior pole of the patella for a focal chondral defect. The donor site was from the non-weight-bearing, non-articulating area of the medial femoral condyle. Note the challenging 3-dimensional contour of the patellar making achieving a uniform chondral surface level challenging

donor-graft chondral depth mismatch. Data are scarce for osteochondral autografting within the PFJ in general, and this is even more so for concomitant TTO with malalignment as this is an exclusion criterion in many series [39].

Gaweda et al. [40] reported on 19 patients undergoing a combined patella osteochondral autograft with a proximal (lateral release, medial plication) and distal (TT medialisation) realignment. Although the indication in this setting was instability, this is one of few papers reporting upon TTO with PFJ osteochondral autograft. A cohort of 30 patients undergoing an isolated proximal and distal realignment for instability but without patellar chondral wear was used as a control. Despite lower preoperative scores in the combined group, similar Marshall knee scores were achieved by 12 months and maintained to 24 months when comparing groups supporting the efficacy of a combined approach.

Nho et al. [41], however, demonstrated that patients with underlying PFJ maltracking performed worse after patellar osteochondral autograft transplantation. The authors reviewed 22 patients with isolated patellar lesions, 9 of whom underwent concomitant TTO for PFJ maltracking as per surgeon preference. Although the functional outcomes of patients who underwent a combined procedure increased at a mean 28.7-month follow-up, this was not statistically significant. In contrast, isolated patellar osteochondral autograft patients did have a significant improvement in IKDC scores although SF-36 and ADL improvements were not significant. It is unclear how the outcomes would have fared if the TTO had not been performed, but this highlights maltracking as a risk factor for a suboptimal result.

Osteochondral allograft transplantation can potentially minimise the issues associated with chondral depth mismatch and may be favourable for matching the contour of the complex PFJ anatomy as a site-specific donor plug can be used. Many of the published series, however, excluded patients with significant malalignment [42, 43], and other series had no indication for distal realignment [44]. Others report very high rates of distal realignment prior to PF osteochondral allograft transplantation [45], making it difficult to establish the indications for a combined TTO in this setting but these are presumably similar to osteochondral autografting.

8.6 Complications of Tibial Tubercle Osteotomy

Potential benefits of concomitant TTO need to be balanced against the associated risks and surgical morbidity. Risks associated with isolated chondral surgery are potentially increased with concomitant TTO. These include infection, wound-healing problems, venous thromboembolism, neurovascular compromise and anaesthesia-related complications. The addition of concomitant TTO adds osteotomy-specific complications to this list including non-union or delayed union, fracture, prominent hardware, compartment syndrome and skin necrosis. Payne et al. [1] conducted a systematic review on the complications following TTO. The authors included 19 studies including 787 TTOs. The overall complication risk was 4.6% (36 complications) with a major complication rate of 3.0%. The risk of osteotomy-site non-union was 0.8%, tibial fracture 1.0%, wound complication 0.8% and infection 1.0%. The risk of complications was higher when the TT was completely detached (10.7%) with a lower rate associated with antero-medialisation (3.7%). Hardware removal was performed in 36.7% of all osteotomies (49% for antero-medialisation).

8.7 Preoperative Planning: When to Add a Tibial Tubercle Osteotomy

If a cartilage-restorative procedure is to be performed within the PFJ and there is significant patellar maltracking, many advocate for a concomitant procedure to address this [24, 25, 27, 30, 41]. The assessment of maltracking and the threshold at which to intervene continue to be refined. Regardless, a comprehensive assessment of the entire limb and knee is mandatory for any patellofemoral chondral pathology or surgery.

Assessment for the underlying patellar instability is also critical. Here, we focus on the pertinent assessments in decision-making as to when an osteotomy should be combined with a chondral procedure in the absence of patellofemoral instability.

8.7.1 Clinical Assessment

Assessment of coronal and axial (rotational) alignment is critical when evaluating PF mechanics and kinematics. Femoral neck anteversion is assessed in the prone position by measuring hip internal rotation. External tibial torsion is assessed clinically with the foot-thigh angle. Anything greater than 50° or 20°, respectively, would necessitate a CT rotational profile. During gait we assess foot progression angle and for "squinting" patellae. We consider coronal and torsional alignment together as it is technically possible to correct both simultaneously with a femoral based osteotomy [46]; however, the indications for this are narrow and would be staged with a cartilage procedure if indicated.

Patellar tracking is assessed seated with a focus on J tracking. This refers to the "inverted J-path the patella takes in early flexion as the patella begins laterally subluxated and then suddenly shifts medially to engage with the femoral groove" [47]. The description of this motion can be classified as either "hard" or "soft," a subjective assessment based upon how sudden the patella jumps or glides into the groove. J tracking typically represents an underlying bony abnormality, most commonly trochlea dysplasia and/or patella alta. An initial assessment of patellar height can be made clinically in the seated position; the normal patella should sit in line with the long axis of the femur with the knee flexed 90°. Patella alta in conjunction with a distal patellar chondral lesion is one scenario where an isolated TT distalisation may be indicated; however, caution should be exercised as this can increase global PFJ pressures. The degree of knee flexion when the patellar is seated centrally within the trochlea is evaluated. Failure of the patella to engage centrally within the trochlear groove by 45° of knee flexion has been suggested to be clinically relevant patella maltracking [24, 32] and is a relative indication for a bony or soft-tissue extensor mechanism realignment in our practice. Assessment of medial patellar translation with the knee in extension and assessment of lateral patella tilt are our methods for evaluating lateral tightness. Where present, consideration is given to a lateral retinacular lengthening in addition to a TTO.

8.7.2   Radiographic Assessment

Weight-bearing knee X-rays including a true lateral are mandatory. Long leg alignment films are used to confirm clinical suspicion for coronal plane malalignment, in particular genu valgum. When clinically indicated (see above) we use a low-radiation-dose CT rotational profile to quantify torsional abnormalities. Assessment of the Q-angle has largely been replaced with assessment for lateralisation of the TT relative to the trochlea, as measured by the TT-TG distance on CT or MRI. The exact magnitude of the TT-TG distance where distal realignment is indicated in the setting of PFJ procedures is controversial. Some authors have suggested 15 mm [48, 49]; however, others have recommended numbers as low as 10 mm [34] or as high as 20 mm [36]. The TT-posterior cruciate ligament (PCL) distance has also been proposed as a method to quantify TT position on MRI [50]. Although described in the context of patellar instability, it is advantageous to have a tibial based reference (PCL) for TT position as this eliminates the impact of trochlear dysplasia as well as knee flexion and assesses lateralisation of the TT itself as opposed to the extensor mechanism [51]. Normal values have been reported as approximately 12 mm with over 20 mm considered pathological [50, 51]. Patella height is measured by the Caton-Deschamps (CD) ratio [52] and/or patellotrochlear index [53]. Patella alta with a CD ratio of over 1.4 and isolated distal patella wear is an indication for distalisation with or without a chondral procedure in our practice. MRI remains the best preoperative means to evaluate the size and location of a PFJ chondral defect.

8.7.3   Arthroscopic Assessment

Dynamic assessment of patellar tracking from an accessory superolateral viewing portal using dry arthroscopy can aid in evaluating PF kinematics and assessing or adjusting a realignment procedure. As previously discussed, arthroscopy also has a role in defining the exact location of the chondral lesion which is critical in determining if a TTO is indicated.

8.8   Senior Author's Current Practice

Non-operative management of anterior knee pain is the mainstay of treatment. The majority of patients may be treated with a combination of pain-relieving injections (corticosteroid/hyaluronic acid/platelet-rich plasma) and a thorough neuromuscular training rehabilitation programme. Particular attention is placed on core strength, gluteal, hip abductor and quadriceps muscle strength and hamstring flexibility. A summary of treatment algorithm is presented in Fig. 8.5.

In the event of failed non-operative management, careful patient selection, education and management of expectations are critical when embarking upon a PF cartilage-restorative procedure with or without TTO. A lateral based chondral lesion (lateral trochlea or distal/lateral patella) in the presence of patellar maltracking or malalignment is treated by antero-medialisation of the TT. This may be combined with a lateral retinacular lengthening in the setting of persistent lateral patellar tilt or reduced medial excursion. The relative amount of anteriorisation and medialisation is tailored to the individual patient. Radiologically, a TT-TG distance of >15 mm is an indication for medialisation of the TT with a general target of 10–15 mm. A secondary chondral procedure may be performed if the patient remains symptomatic; however, this is rarely required in our experience.

If the lesion is on the central/medial trochlea or central/medial patella, a TT anteriorisation may be performed along with a chondral resurfacing

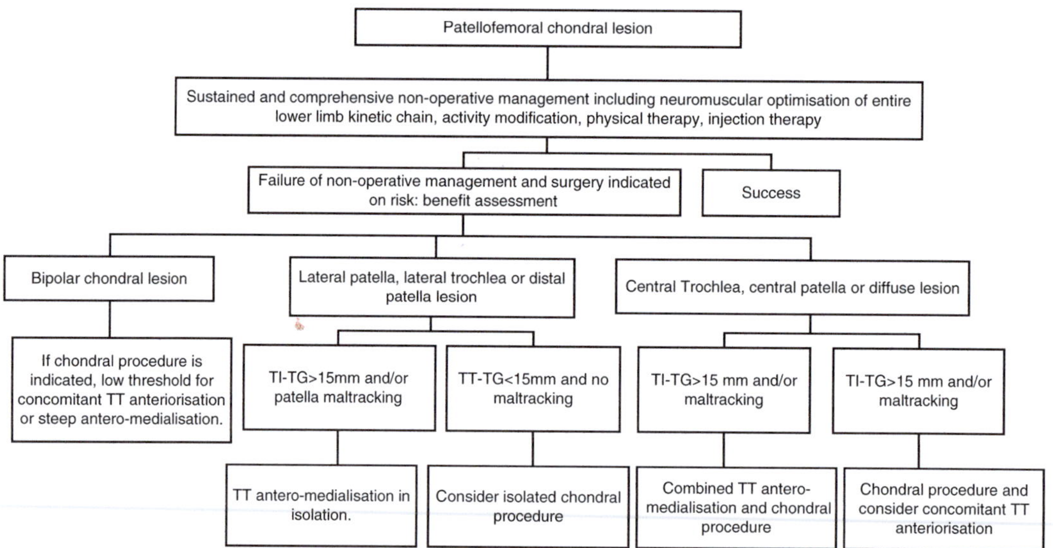

Fig. 8.5 Flow chart of the senior author's decision-making process regarding patellofemoral chondral surgery and role of concomitant tibial tubercle osteotomy. Importantly, an individualised approach is used and deviations are not uncommon. Chondral procedure selected based on patient and lesion characteristics. Relative amounts of TTO medialisation and anteriorisation are tailored to each patient targeting a TT-TG of approximately 10–12 mm and 10 mm of anteriorisation within limits of stability and contact area of the osteotomy

procedure. The choice of whether to perform an anteriorisation is based subjectively on maltracking and malalignment, which are assessed clinically, radiologically and arthroscopically. A decision is made as to whether to add in the TTO based upon the overall likelihood or abnormal kinematics causing the chondral lesion and balancing the risk profile of the patient by adding the TTO procedure. The choice of chondral procedure depends upon lesion size, location and patient characteristics. Osteochondral autograft or allograft transplantation and PJAC transplantation form the mainstay of treatment, partly due to the lack of availability of chondrocyte transplantation in Canada.

Bipolar reparative or reconstructive procedures are uncommon to perform in our practice; however, if performed, they are typically performed with an anteriorising osteotomy of 10 mm ± medialisation to obtain a TT-TG of 10 mm. In the presence of significant genu valgum and torsional malalignment, these are addressed simultaneously with a femoral osteotomy and a staged chondral procedure [46]. Smoking is a relative contraindication to any osteotomy in our practice and warrants a strong conversation with the patient regarding associated risks and need for smoking cessation.

Rehabilitation for chondral surgery is tailored to each patient and includes an assessment of the knee arc of motion when there is chondral articulation at the surgical site. Range of motion is restricted so as to reduce sheer forces upon the graft for 6 weeks. For ACI and PJAC, the patient is typically flatfoot feather-touch WB for 6 weeks. For osteochondral auto- and allograft transplantation, the patient is 50% weight bearing for 6 weeks. If a concomitant TTO is performed, active knee extension is avoided for 6 weeks. The patient is placed in a tracker brace with the range restriction from 0 to 90° for 2 weeks and then 0 to 120° from 2 to 6 weeks. Active flexion and passive knee extension exercises can be performed with range guided by the chondral surgery. During ambulation and sleeping, the patient's weight-bearing status is guided by the chondral surgery and the brace is locked in extension for 6 weeks.

8.9 Conclusions

Patellofemoral chondral lesions remain a challenging entity to treat; however, the TTO is a powerful tool that is likely synergistic with restorative and reconstructive chondral procedures. Ideally, larger comparative series will continue to inform the surgical decision-making process and allow a targeted approach at the individual patient level as to when this is indicated.

References

1. Cole BJ, Pascual-Garrido C, Grumet RC. Surgical management of articular cartilage defects in the knee. JBJS. 2009;91(7):1778–90.
2. Ackermann J, Cole BJ, Gomoll AH. Cartilage restoration in the patellofemoral joint: techniques and outcomes. Oper Techn Sports Med. 2019;27(4):150692.
3. Batty L, Dance S, Bajaj S, Cole BJ. Autologous chondrocyte implantation: an overview of technique and outcomes. ANZ J Surg. 2011;81(1–2):18–25.
4. Franceschi F, Longo UG, Ruzzini L, Marinozzi A, Maffulli N, Denaro V. Simultaneous arthroscopic implantation of autologous chondrocytes and high tibial osteotomy for tibial chondral defects in the varus knee. Knee. 2008;15(4):309–13.
5. Sterett WI, Steadman JR. Chondral resurfacing and high tibial osteotomy in the varus knee. Am J Sports Med. 2004;32(5):1243–9.
6. Sterett WI, Steadman JR, Huang MJ, Matheny LM, Briggs KK. Chondral resurfacing and high tibial osteotomy in the varus knee: survivorship analysis. Am J Sports Med. 2010;38(7):1420–4.
7. Fulkerson JP, Becker GJ, Meaney JA, Miranda M, Folcik MA. Anteromedial tibial tubercle transfer without bone graft. Am J Sports Med. 1990;18(5):490–7.
8. Maquet P. A biomechanical treatment of femoropatellar arthrosis: advancement of the patellar tendon. Rev Rhum Mal Osteoartic. 1963;30:779.
9. Maquet P. Advancement of the tibial tuberosity. Clin Orthop Relat Res. 1976;115:225–30.
10. Tompkins M, Hamann JC, Diduch DR, Bonner KF, Hart JM, Gwathmey FW, et al. Preliminary results of a novel single-stage cartilage restoration technique: particulated juvenile articular cartilage allograft for chondral defects of the patella. Arthroscopy. 2013;29(10):1661–70.
11. Hinckel BB, Pratte EL, Baumann CA, Gowd AK, Farr J, Liu JN, et al. Patellofemoral cartilage restoration: a systematic review and meta-analysis of clinical outcomes. Am J Sports Med. 2020;48(7):1756–72.
12. Ramappa AJ, Apreleva M, Harrold FR, Fitzgibbons PG, Wilson DR, Gill TJ. The effects of medialization and anteromedialization of the tibial tubercle on patellofemoral mechanics and kinematics. Am J Sports Med. 2006;34(5):749–56.
13. Huberti H, Hayes W. Patellofemoral contact pressures. The influence of q-angle and tendofemoral contact. J Bone Joint Surg Am. 1984;66(5):715–24.
14. Singerman R, White C, Davy DT. Reduction of patellofemoral contact forces following anterior displacement of the tibial tubercle. J Orthop Res. 1995;13(2):279–85.
15. Beck PR, Thomas AL, Farr J, Lewis PB, Cole BJ. Trochlear contact pressures after anteromedialization of the tibial tubercle. Am J Sports Med. 2005;33(11):1710–5.
16. Rue J-PH, Colton A, Zare SM, Shewman E, Farr J, Bernard RB Jr, et al. Trochlear contact pressures after straight anteriorization of the tibial tuberosity. Am J Sports Med. 2008;36(10):1953–9.
17. Stephen JM, Lumpaopong P, Dodds AL, Williams A, Amis AA. The effect of tibial tuberosity medialization and lateralization on patellofemoral joint kinematics, contact mechanics, and stability. Am J Sports Med. 2015;43(1):186–94.
18. Shanmugaraj A, Coughlin RP, Kuper GN, Ekhtiari S, Simunovic N, Musahl V, et al. Changing trends in the use of cartilage restoration techniques for the patellofemoral joint: a systematic review. Knee Surg Sports Traumatol Arthrosc. 2019;27(3):854–67.
19. Shen W, Jordan S, Fu F. Anatomic double bundle anterior cruciate ligament reconstruction. J Orthop Surg. 2007;15(2):216–21.
20. Pidoriano AJ, Weinstein RN, Buuck DA, Fulkerson JP. Correlation of patellar articular lesions with results from anteromedial tibial tubercle transfer. Am J Sports Med. 1997;25(4):533–7.
21. Fisher TF, Waterman BR, Orr JD, Holland CA, Bader J, Belmont PJ Jr. Tibial tubercle osteotomy for patellar chondral pathology in an active United States military population. Arthroscopy. 2016;32(11):2342–9.
22. Brittberg M, Lindahl A, Nilsson A, Ohlsson C, Isaksson O, Peterson L. Treatment of deep cartilage defects in the knee with autologous chondrocyte transplantation. N Engl J Med. 1994;331(14):889–95.
23. Farr J. Autologous chondrocyte implantation improves patellofemoral cartilage treatment outcomes. Clin Orthop and Relat Res. 2007;463:187–94.
24. Henderson I, Lavigne P. Periosteal autologous chondrocyte implantation for patellar chondral defect in patients with normal and abnormal patellar tracking. Knee. 2006;13(4):274–9.
25. Pascual-Garrido C, Slabaugh MA, L'Heureux DR, Friel NA, Cole BJ. Recommendations and treatment outcomes for patellofemoral articular cartilage defects with autologous chondrocyte implantation: prospective evaluation at average 4-year follow-up. Am J Sports Med. 2009;37(1_suppl):33–41.
26. Trinh TQ, Harris JD, Siston RA, Flanigan DC. Improved outcomes with combined autologous chondrocyte implantation and patellofemoral osteotomy versus isolated autologous chondrocyte implantation. Arthroscopy. 2013;29(3):566–74.

27. Vasiliadis HS, Lindahl A, Georgoulis AD, Peterson L. Malalignment and cartilage lesions in the patellofemoral joint treated with autologous chondrocyte implantation. Knee Surg Sports Traumatol Arthrosc. 2011;19(3):452–7.

28. Gobbi A, Kon E, Berruto M, Francisco R, Filardo G, Marcacci M. Patellofemoral full-thickness chondral defects treated with Hyalograft-C: a clinical, arthroscopic, and histologic review. Am J Sports Med. 2006;34(11):1763–73.

29. Zarkadis NJ, Belmont PJ Jr, Zachilli MA, Holland CA, Kinsler AR, Todd MS, et al. Autologous chondrocyte implantation and tibial tubercle osteotomy for patellofemoral chondral defects: improved pain relief and occupational outcomes among US Army servicemembers. Am J Sports Med. 2018;46(13):3198–208.

30. Chahla J, Hinckel BB, Yanke AB, Farr J, Group MoOA, Bugbee WD, et al., editors. An expert consensus statement on the management of large chondral and osteochondral defects in the patellofemoral joint. Orthop J Sports Med. 2020;8(3):2325967120907343.

31. Gomoll AH, Gillogly SD, Cole BJ, Farr J, Arnold R, Hussey K, et al. Autologous chondrocyte implantation in the patella: a multicenter experience. Am J Sports Med. 2014;42(5):1074–81.

32. Gillogly SD, Arnold RM. Autologous chondrocyte implantation and anteromedialization for isolated patellar articular cartilage lesions: 5-to 11-year follow-up. Am J Sports Med. 2014;42(4):912–20.

33. Farr J, Tabet SK, Margerrison E, Cole BJ. Clinical, radiographic, and histological outcomes after cartilage repair with particulated juvenile articular cartilage: a 2-year prospective study. Am J Sports Med. 2014;42(6):1417–25.

34. Buckwalter J, Bowman G, Albright J, Wolf B, Bollier M. Clinical outcomes of patellar chondral lesions treated with juvenile particulated cartilage allografts. Iowa Orthop J. 2014;34:44.

35. Grawe B, Burge A, Nguyen J, Strickland S, Warren R, Rodeo S, et al. Cartilage regeneration in full-thickness patellar chondral defects treated with particulated juvenile articular allograft cartilage: an MRI analysis. Cartilage. 2017;8(4):374–83.

36. Wang T, Belkin NS, Burge AJ, Chang B, Pais M, Mahony G, et al. Patellofemoral cartilage lesions treated with particulated juvenile allograft cartilage: a prospective study with minimum 2-year clinical and magnetic resonance imaging outcomes. Arthroscopy. 2018;34(5):1498–505.

37. Bonner KF, Daner W, Yao JQ. 2-year postoperative evaluation of a patient with a symptomatic full-thickness patellar cartilage defect repaired with particulated juvenile cartilage tissue. J Knee Surg. 2010;23(02):109–14.

38. Mosier BA, Arendt EA, Dahm DL, Dejour D, Gomoll AH. Management of patellofemoral arthritis: from cartilage restoration to arthroplasty. J Am Acad Orthop Surg. 2016;24(11):e163–e73.

39. Emre T, Atbasi Z, Demircioglu D, Uzun M, Kose O. Autologous osteochondral transplantation (mosaicplasty) in articular cartilage defects of the patellofemoral joint: retrospective analysis of 33 cases. Musculoskelet Surg. 2017;101(2):133–8.

40. Gawęda K, Walawski J, Węgłowski R, Drelich M, Mazurkiewicz T. Early results of one-stage knee extensor realignment and autologous osteochondral grafting. Int Orthop. 2006;30(1):39–42.

41. Nho SJ, Foo LF, Green DM, Shindle MK, Warren RF, Wickiewicz TL, et al. Magnetic resonance imaging and clinical evaluation of patellar resurfacing with press-fit osteochondral autograft plugs. Am J Sports Med. 2008;36(6):1101–9.

42. Cameron JI, Pulido PA, McCauley JC, Bugbee WD. Osteochondral allograft transplantation of the femoral trochlea. Am J Sports Med. 2016;44(3): 633–8.

43. Astur DC, Arliani GG, Binz M, Astur N, Kaleka CC, Amaro JT, et al. Autologous osteochondral transplantation for treating patellar chondral injuries: evaluation, treatment, and outcomes of a two-year follow-up study. JBJS. 2014;96(10):816–23.

44. Jamali AA, Emmerson BC, Chung C, Convery FR, Bugbee WD. Fresh osteochondral allografts. Clin Orthop Relat Res. 2005;437:176–85.

45. Spak RT, Teitge RA. Fresh osteochondral allografts for patellofemoral arthritis: long-term followup. Clin Orthop Relat Res 2006;444:193–200.

46. Imhoff FB, Schnell J, Magaña A, Diermeier T, Scheiderer B, Braun S, et al. Single cut distal femoral osteotomy for correction of femoral torsion and valgus malformity in patellofemoral malalignment-proof of application of new trigonometrical calculations and 3D-printed cutting guides. BMC Musculoskelet Disord. 2018;19(1):215.

47. Sheehan FT, Derasari A, Fine KM, Brindle TJ, Alter KE. Q-angle and J-sign: indicative of maltracking subgroups in patellofemoral pain. Clin Orthop Relat Res. 2010;468(1):266–75.

48. Sherman SL, Humpherys J, Farr J. Optimizing patellofemoral cartilage restoration and instability with tibial tubercle osteotomy. Arthroscopy. 2019;35(8):2255–6.

49. Sherman SL, Erickson BJ, Cvetanovich GL, Chalmers PN, Farr J, Bach BR Jr, et al. Tibial tuberosity osteotomy: indications, techniques, and outcomes. Am J Sports Med. 2014;42(8):2006–17.

50. Seitlinger G, Scheurecker G, Högler R, Labey L, Innocenti B, Hofmann S. Tibial tubercle–posterior cruciate ligament distance: a new measurement to define the position of the tibial tubercle in patients with patellar dislocation. Am J Sports Med. 2012;40(5):1119–25.

51. Brady JM, Rosencrans AS, Stein BES. Use of TT-PCL versus TT-TG. Curr Rev Musculoskelet Med. 2018;11(2):261–5.

52. Caton J, Deschamps G, Chambat P, Lerat JL, Dejour H. Les rotules basses: a propos de 128 observations. Rev Chir Orthop. 1982;68:317–25.

53. Biedert RM, Albrecht S. The patellotrochlear index: a new index for assessing patellar height. Knee Surg Sports Traumatol Arthrosc. 2006;14(8):707–12.

Osteotomy for the Varus Knee in Cartilage Surgery

9

Patricia M. Lutz, Andreas B. Imhoff, and Matthias J. Feucht

9.1 Introduction

Integrity of articular cartilage is based on a complex interplay of mechanical and biochemical factors. A certain amount of load is essential to maintain cartilage homeostasis [1, 2]. Joint loading exceeding the physiological level leads to an induction of proinflammatory and catabolic pathways, resulting in impaired synthesis and degradation of the extracellular matrix. In addition, high mechanical stress can lead to apoptosis and necrosis of chondrocytes [1, 2]. Mechanical alignment of the leg has a significant impact on load distribution in the knee joint [3–5]. Varus malalignment leads to increased load on the cartilage and subchondral bone in the medial compartment. Biomechanical studies have shown that even with a mild varus malalignment of 3–5°, approximately 80–90% of the total contact stress is located in the medial compartment [3–5]. Based on the interaction of alignment, contact stress, and cartilage homeostasis, malalignment and its correction play a crucial role in the development and treatment of cartilage lesions [6–8]. Within this chapter, we focus on varus malalignment in patients with focal cartilage lesions in the medial compartment of the knee.

P. M. Lutz · A. B. Imhoff (✉) · M. J. Feucht
Department of Orthopaedic Sports Medicine, Klinikum rechts der Isar, Technical University of Munich, Munich, Germany
e-mail: imhoff@tum.de

9.2 Rationale for Unloading Osteotomies in Cartilage Surgery

9.2.1 Relevance of Varus Malalignment in the Development and Progression of Cartilage Defects

A certain amount of load is essential to maintain cartilage homeostasis. However, a load exceeding the physiological level leads to irreversible damage to the cartilage in the long term [2]. Mechanical varus malalignment of the leg has a significant impact on pressure distribution in the knee [3, 5]. Even a mild varus malalignment of 3–5° results in overload of the medial compartment, since 80–90% of the total contact stress is located in the medial compartment [3, 5].

In large-cohort studies, even a small amount of mechanical varus malalignment (varus $\geq 2°$) has been identified as an independent risk factor for the development and progression of cartilage lesions and osteoarthritis in the medial compartment of the knee [9–11]. Mechanical malalignment also appears to be connected to osteochondral lesions: *Brown* et al. were able to show that two-thirds of patients with symptomatic osteochondritis dissecans (OCD) lesions had associated mechanical axis deviation [12]. Since

© ISAKOS 2021
A. J. Krych et al. (eds.), *Cartilage Injury of the Knee*,
https://doi.org/10.1007/978-3-030-78051-7_9

untreated focal cartilage lesions may progress over time, cartilage lesions must be regarded as a preliminary stage of osteoarthritis. It is therefore reasonable to assume that varus malalignment also has a negative impact on the natural course of focal cartilage lesions [13–16].

Biomechanically, contact pressure in the medial compartment increases with increasing varus angles. In knees with focal cartilage defects at the medial femoral condyle, contact pressure is concentrated around the defect rim [5]. Thus, especially the intact rim zone around the cartilage defect, which is considered essential for successful cartilage repair procedures, appears to be subject to high mechanical load in varus-aligned knees.

Based on these biomechanical data and the abovementioned relationship between varus malalignment and development and progression of cartilage damage, varus malalignment must be considered a risk factor for failure of cartilage repair procedures [16–18]. This consideration is supported by clinical studies [19, 20]. For example, *Krych* et al. have shown that untreated malalignment was the most commonly recognized reason for failure of cartilage repair procedures. In 59 patients undergoing revision surgery, untreated malalignment was observed in 56% [19].

9.2.2 Relevance of Varus Malalignment and Corrective Osteotomies in Cartilage Surgery

Several studies could demonstrate that the failure rate of cartilage repair procedures in the medial compartment is higher in cases of uncorrected varus malalignment:

A study with 123 patients showed a failure rate of 43% after transplantation of osteochondral allografts in patients with coronal malalignment, which was significantly higher compared to 9% in patients with a neutral leg axis [21]. In another study of 124 patients undergoing microfracture in the medial compartment, the failure rate was significantly higher (41%) in patients with varus malalignment compared to patients with a neutral axis (22%) [17].

Valgus-producing high tibial osteotomy (HTO) or distal femoral osteotomy (DFO) corrects varus malalignment, thereby transferring the load to the less damaged lateral compartment [3, 5]. Second-look arthroscopy studies after HTO in patients with varus malalignment with osteoarthritis of the medial compartment showed partial regeneration of the worn cartilage in most patients even without additive cartilage surgery [22]. This shows that repair mechanisms in chondrocytes can be induced by reducing the mechanical overload [23–25]. The aim of corrective osteotomies in cartilage surgery is to create physiological biomechanical conditions for the maturation of the induced or transplanted tissue [17, 18, 26]. In clinical studies, corrective osteotomies have proven to be advantageous for clinical outcome and long-term survival: Compared to isolated ACI in patients without malalignment, patients with combined corrective osteotomies and ACI showed a significantly higher survival rate after 15 years [27]. *Von Keudell* et al. were able to show a correlation between coronal malalignment and poorer clinical outcome scores (KOOS, Lysholm) after microfracturing. Especially patients with malalignment >5° had a high risk of failure and increase in defect size [16].

It remains unclear, however, as to which degree of varus malalignment has to be corrected. For decades, the expert opinion was that varus malalignment ≥5° should be corrected. In our opinion, however, valgus-producing osteotomies should be considered even for smaller deformities (<5°). This assumption is also supported by clinical studies: *Bode* et al. examined the failure rates in patients with cartilage damage of the medial femoral condyle and varus malalignment between 1° and 5° [18]. Treatment was performed using isolated ACI or combined ACI and valgus HTO. After a mean follow-up of 6 years, the survival rate after ACI + HTO was significantly higher (90%) compared to isolated ACI (58%). This study allows the conclusion that the indication for additive valgus HTO can be beneficial even in case of a small varus malalignment (<5°).

In our opinion, a cartilage repair procedure in the medial compartment should be combined with an unloading osteotomy if the mechanical varus exceeds 3°. Furthermore, isolated cartilage repair procedures in the medial compartment should not be performed in patients with varus malalignment >5°.

With regard to the extent of correction, there is also no clear evidence. In contrast to patients with osteoarthritis, where an overcorrection is usually aimed for, most authors aim for a straight-leg axis in patients with focal cartilage lesions [26]. Overcorrection should be avoided due to the risk of progressive cartilage degeneration in the contralateral compartment in these relatively young patients. In our clinical practice the post-operative weight-bearing line is therefore aimed at 50–55% of the medial-to-lateral tibial plateau width.

9.2.3 Outcomes After Combined Valgus Osteotomy and Cartilage Repair Procedures

Clinical outcomes and survival rates after cartilage surgery combined with valgus osteotomy are promising. A meta-analysis showed that there is a significantly higher 5-year survival rate after combined cartilage repair procedures and HTO compared to patients after isolated HTO (98% versus 92%) [28]. However, clinical studies after combined cartilage repair procedures and valgus osteotomy must be critically reviewed with regard to the indication. It must be differentiated if the cartilage repair procedure was performed in addition to the osteotomy with the aim of improving cartilage regeneration in osteoarthritis [23, 29–34], or if the valgus osteotomy was performed in addition to cartilage repair procedures in patients with focal cartilage defects [35–39]. For example, *Ferruzzi* et al. retrospectively compared the results after isolated HTO and combined ACI + HTO. After a mean follow-up of 11 years, the authors found no difference in clinical outcome and the conclusion was that ACI had no additional benefit to valgus HTO [30]. However,

when closely reviewing the inclusion criteria of this study, all patients were treated for advanced osteoarthritis [30]. Furthermore, *Bauer* et al. reported low survival rates and poor cartilage regeneration after combined ACI and HTO [29]. It must be noted, however, that patients with osteoarthritis in more than one compartment were treated. In our opinion and according to the literature, ACI is not indicated in advanced osteoarthritis, which is why these studies are not representative for patients with isolated focal cartilage lesions.

In the following, only studies in which a valgus osteotomy was performed combined with cartilage repair procedures in patients with isolated focal cartilage lesions without relevant osteoarthritis are summarized.

Minzlaff et al. reported the long-term results of 74 patients treated with combined valgus HTO and autologous osteochondral transplantation due to an osteochondral lesion at the medial femoral condyle and mechanical varus malalignment ≥2°. After an average follow-up of 7.5 years, pain VAS decreased by 4.8 points, and the Lysholm score increased by 33 points. The survival rate (defined as no conversion to partial- or total-knee arthroplasty) was 95% after 5 years, 93% after 7 years, and 90% after 9 years [39]. The return-to-sport rate in the same patient cohort was 77%, and there was no significant reduction of the previous activity level [38]. *Franceschi* et al. found a significant increase in the Lysholm score and Tegner scale in patients treated with arthroscopic ACI of the medial tibial plateau and valgus HTO. Additionally, the pain VAS decreased [37]. *Bode* et al. analyzed the clinical outcome and return to work of 40 patients after combined ACI and valgus HTO. After a follow-up of 5 years, a significantly improved pain VAS and Lysholm score were observed. Regarding return to work, the authors found an average incapacity of work after surgery of 94 days, with a correlation to workload. The average incapacity of work in patients who did not perform any physical activity was significantly lower (68 days) compared to patients with heavy physical work (155 days) [35].

9.3 Technical Approach

9.3.1 Preoperative Diagnostic and Patient Selection

A detailed preoperative workup and careful patient selection are crucial for the success of combined unloading osteotomies and cartilage repair procedures. The ideal patient has a focal cartilage lesion at the medial femoral condyle, frontal plane mechanical varus alignment of more than 3°, intact menisci, intact ligaments, and a normal lateral and patellofemoral compartment.

Diagnostics include patient history and clinical examination, MRI, X-rays of the knee in three planes, and a weight-bearing full-leg radiograph. The clinical examination should also assess ligament stability of the knee.

Joint-preserving therapy is not contraindicated in the case of instability, as long as it is treated as a part of the surgical procedure. From the authors' point of view, a careful deformity analysis based on the weight-bearing full-leg radiograph is an important step of the preoperative planning [40]. The mechanical leg axis is utilized to measure the amount of varus angulation. Furthermore, the mechanical lateral distal femoral angle (mLDFA) and the medial proximal tibial angle (MPTA) are measured to identify the site of the bony deformity (tibial based vs. femoral based deformity). Based on these measurements, it must be decided whether to perform a tibial, femoral, or double-level osteotomy (Figs. 9.1 and 9.2). The goal should be to achieve physiological values of the LDFA and MPTA, and to avoid an oblique joint line. When considering a medial open-

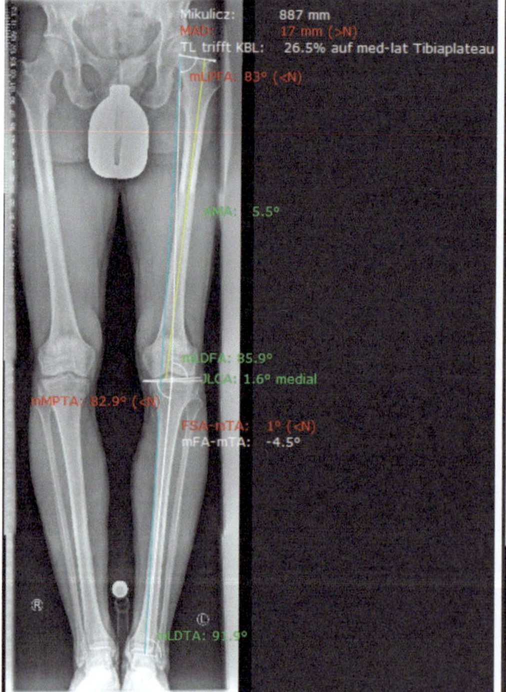

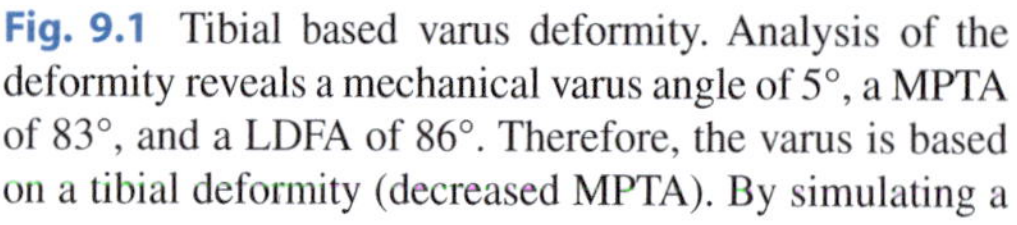

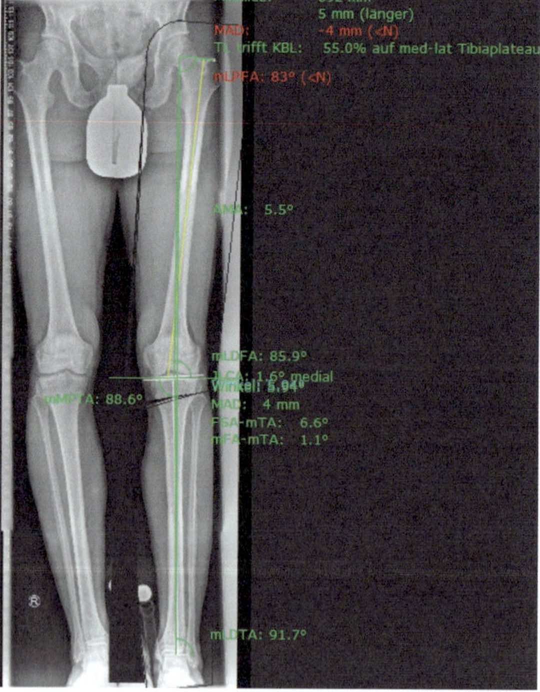

Fig. 9.1 Tibial based varus deformity. Analysis of the deformity reveals a mechanical varus angle of 5°, a MPTA of 83°, and a LDFA of 86°. Therefore, the varus is based on a tibial deformity (decreased MPTA). By simulating a medial open-wedge HTO to 55% of the medial-to-lateral tibial plateau width, the MPTA is normalized and the varus deformity is corrected to 1° of mechanical valgus

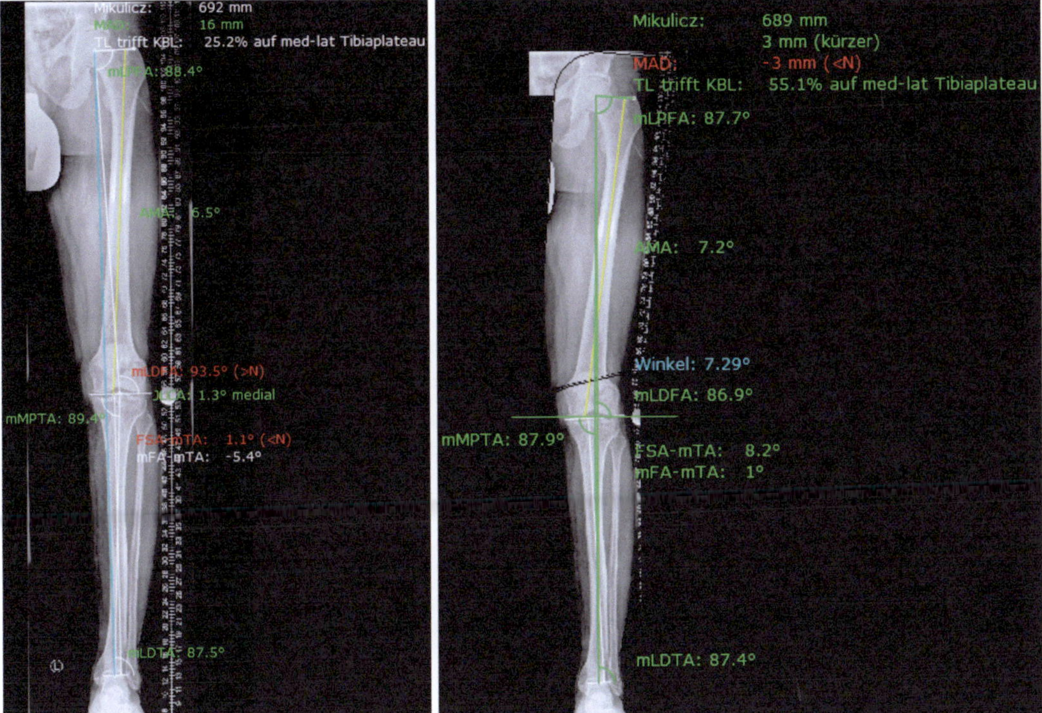

Fig. 9.2 Femoral based varus deformity. Analysis of the deformity reveals a mechanical varus angle of 5°, a MPTA of 89°, and a LDFA of 94°. Therefore, the varus is based on a femoral deformity (increased LDFA). By simulating a lateral closing-wedge DFO to 55% of the medial-to-lateral tibial plateau width, the LDFA is normalized and the varus deformity is corrected to 1° of mechanical valgus

wedge HTO, the tibial bone varus angle has also proven to be an important prognostic factor [41]. This angle allows for a differentiation between congenital metaphyseal varus (primary varus) and acquired varus (secondary varus). Patients with congenital metaphyseal varus are good candidates for realignment osteotomies, whereas patients with secondary varus may not be suitable for valgus osteotomies.

Preoperatively, the "brace test" has been shown to be helpful in patient selection [42]. If the patient benefits from a valgus brace in terms of a noticeable pain reduction, realignment osteotomy can be indicated. Finally, a diagnostic arthroscopy just before osteotomy is mandatory, since it allows qualitative assessment of the cartilage in the contralateral compartment, which will be more loaded after the osteotomy. If arthroscopy reveals a significant lesion or more advanced wear, we only correct to neutral (50%).

9.3.2 Principles of the Surgical Technique and Rehabilitation

In case of a planned ACI, we prefer a staged procedure in most patients. First, the osteotomy is performed and an arthroscopic cartilage biopsy at the intercondylar notch is gained for chondrocyte cultivation. ACI is then performed 3–6 weeks later. Nevertheless, it is also possible to combine osteotomy and ACI [35], depending on the surgeon's preference. Based on product availability, ACI can be performed either arthroscopically or in an open fashion. If another cartilage repair procedure is planned which does not require chondrocyte cultivation, such as microfracturing, matrix-assisted marrow stimulation, or autologous osteochondral transplantation, a single-stage procedure is usually performed.

Careful planning of the osteotomy is one of the most important steps towards success. We recommend to use specific computer software (e.g., mediCAD Hectec, Germany); however, also conventional planning using radiographs is possible. The surgeon must identify the level of deformity and decide whether to perform an HTO (in case of a pathologic MPTA) or DFO (in case of a pathologic LDFA). In occasional cases, a double-level osteotomy is necessary to avoid an oblique joint line. With regard to the desired amount of correction, we usually plan the postoperative axis at 50–55% of the width of the tibial plateau (medial border = 0%, lateral border = 100%) [26]. Aggressive overcorrection to more than 55% should be avoided since patients undergoing combined osteotomy and cartilage

repair procedures are usually younger than patients treated for osteoarthritis.

In our clinical practice, the vast majority of patients is treated with either a medial open-wedge HTO or a lateral closing-wedge DFO. For both osteotomy sites, we recommend a biplanar technique and angle-stable implants (e.g., PEEKPower HTO Plate, Arthrex, or TomoFix, Synthes).

The postoperative rehabilitation is usually dictated by the cartilage repair procedure, which requires non-weight bearing for 6 weeks. No brace is used and range of motion is not restricted. If a staged procedure is performed, full weight bearing is allowed at 2 weeks after the osteotomy.

9.3.3 Case Presentation (Figs. 9.3 and 9.4)

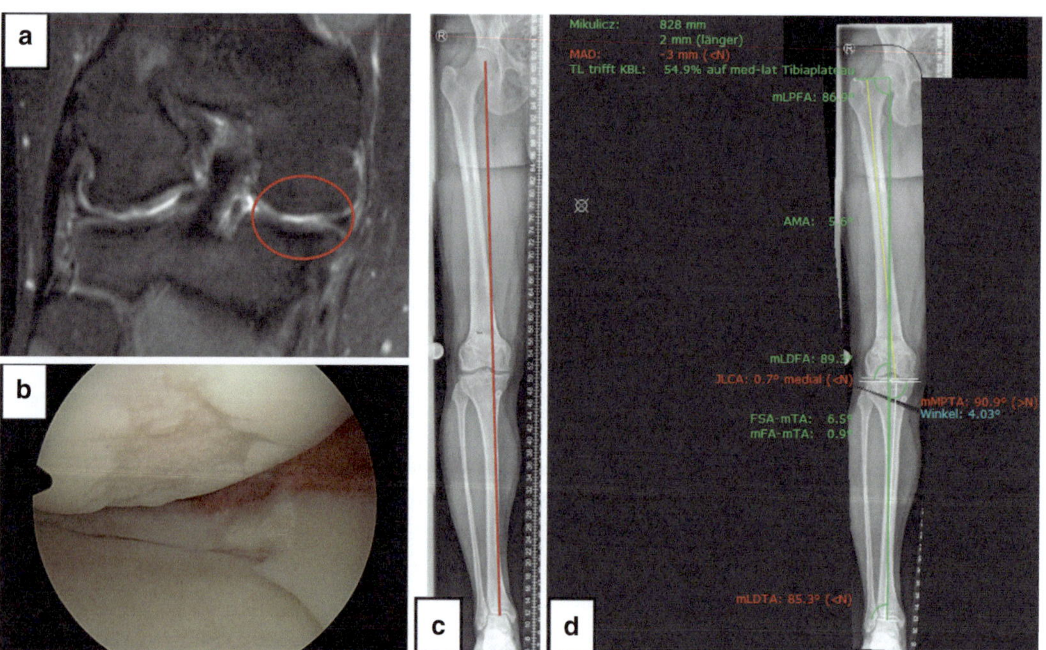

Fig. 9.3 A 32-year-old male presented with pain in the medial compartment after ACL reconstruction and partial medial meniscectomy. MRI (**a**) and arthroscopy (**b**) revealed a focal cartilage defect of the femoral condyle (3x2 cm, ICRS grade III). Weight-bearing full-leg radiographs showed a tibial based varus deformity of 4° (**c, d**)

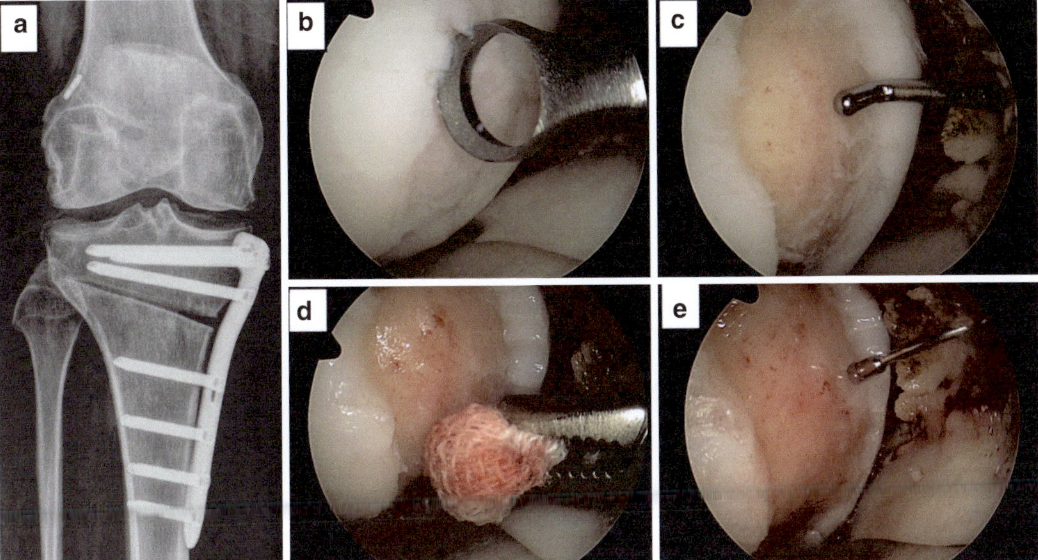

Fig. 9.4 The patient was treated with a staged procedure. First, a medial open-wedge HTO was performed to correct the varus deformity (**a**) and a cartilage biopsy was harvested from the intercondylar notch for chondrocyte cultivation. After 4 weeks, ACI was performed arthroscopically (Tetec Novocart Inject) (**b–e**)

9.4 Conclusions

Varus malalignment must be considered an important risk factor for failure of cartilage repair procedures in the medial compartment. Unloading osteotomies are therefore important to improve the biomechanical environment for the induced or transplanted repair tissue. Good clinical results have been reported after combined valgus osteotomies and cartilage repair procedures and there is growing evidence that even small deviations from a neutral axis (<5° of varus) should be corrected. In our opinion, a cartilage repair procedure in the medial compartment should be combined with an unloading osteotomy if the mechanical varus exceeds 3°. Furthermore, isolated cartilage repair procedures in the medial compartment should not be performed in patients with varus malalignment >5°.

References

1. Buckwalter JA, Martin JA, Brown TD. Perspectives on chondrocyte mechanobiology and osteoarthritis. Biorheology. 2006;43:603–9.

2. Heijink A, Gomoll AH, Madry H, et al. Biomechanical considerations in the pathogenesis of osteoarthritis of the knee. Knee Surg Sports Traumatol Arthrosc. 2012;20:423–35.

3. Agneskirchner JD, Hurschler C, Wrann CD, et al. The effects of valgus medial opening wedge high tibial osteotomy on articular cartilage pressure of the knee: a biomechanical study. Arthroscopy. 2007;23:852–61.

4. Bruns J, Volkmer M, Luessenhop S. Pressure distribution at the knee joint. Arch Orthop Trauma Surg. 1993;113:12–9.

5. Mina C, Garrett WE Jr, Pietrobon R, et al. High tibial osteotomy for unloading osteochondral defects in the medial compartment of the knee. Am J Sports Med. 2008;36:949–55.

6. Arnold MP, Hirschmann MT, Verdonk PC. See the whole picture: knee preserving therapy needs more than surface repair. Berlin: Springer; 2012.

7. Dye SF. The knee as a biologic transmission with an envelope of function: a theory. Clin Orthop Relat Res. 1996;325:10–8.

8. Waller C, Hayes D, Block JE, et al. Unload it: the key to the treatment of knee osteoarthritis. Knee Surg Sports Traumatol Arthrosc. 2011;19:1823–9.

9. Sharma L, Chmiel JS, Almagor O, et al. The role of varus and valgus alignment in the initial development of knee cartilage damage by MRI: the MOST study. Ann Rheum Dis. 2013;72:235–40.

10. Sharma L, Song J, Dunlop D, et al. Varus and valgus alignment and incident and progressive knee osteoarthritis. Ann Rheum Dis. 2010;69:1940–5.

11. Tanamas S, Hanna FS, Cicuttini FM, et al. Does knee malalignment increase the risk of development

and progression of knee osteoarthritis? A systematic review. Arthritis Care Res. 2009;61:459–67.

12. Brown ML, Mccauley JC, Gracitelli GC, et al. Osteochondritis dissecans lesion location is highly concordant with mechanical axis deviation. Am J Sports Med. 2020;48:871–5.

13. Cicuttini F, Ding C, Wluka A, et al. Association of cartilage defects with loss of knee cartilage in healthy, middle-age adults: a prospective study. Arthritis Rheum. 2005;52:2033–9.

14. Linden B. Osteochondritis dissecans of the femoral condyles: a long-term follow-up study. JBJS. 1977;59:769–76.

15. Messner K, Maletius W. The long-term prognosis for severe damage to weight-bearing cartilage in the knee: a 14-year clinical and radiographic follow-up in 28 young athletes. Acta Orthop Scand. 1996;67:165–8.

16. Von Keudell A, Atzwanger J, Forstner R, et al. Radiological evaluation of cartilage after microfracture treatment: a long-term follow-up study. Eur J Radiol. 2012;81:1618–24.

17. Bae DK, Song SJ, Yoon KH, et al. Survival analysis of microfracture in the osteoarthritic knee—minimum 10-year follow-up. Arthroscopy. 2013;29:244–50.

18. Bode G, Schmal H, Pestka JM, et al. A non-randomized controlled clinical trial on autologous chondrocyte implantation (ACI) in cartilage defects of the medial femoral condyle with or without high tibial osteotomy in patients with varus deformity of less than 5. Arch Orthop Trauma Surg. 2013;133:43–9.

19. Krych AJ, Hevesi M, Desai VS, et al. Learning from failure in cartilage repair surgery: an analysis of the mode of failure of primary procedures in consecutive cases at a tertiary referral center. Orthop J Sports Med. 2018;6:2325967118773041.

20. Robb CA, El-Sayed C, Matharu GS, et al. Survival of autologous osteochondral grafts in the knee and factors influencing outcome. Acta Orthop Belg. 2012;78:643.

21. Ghazavi M, Pritzker K, Davis A, et al. Fresh osteochondral allografts for post-traumatic osteochondral defects of the knee. J Bone Joint Surg. 1997;79:1008–13.

22. Jung W-H, Takeuchi R, Chun C-W, et al. Second-look arthroscopic assessment of cartilage regeneration after medial opening-wedge high tibial osteotomy. Arthroscopy. 2014;30:72–9.

23. Akizuki S, Yasukawa Y, Takizawa T. Does arthroscopic abrasion arthroplasty promote cartilage regeneration in osteoarthritic knees with eburnation? A prospective study of high tibial osteotomy with abrasion arthroplasty versus high tibial osteotomy alone. Arthroscopy. 1997;13:9–17.

24. Koshino T, Wada S, Ara Y, et al. Regeneration of degenerated articular cartilage after high tibial valgus osteotomy for medial compartmental osteoarthritis of the knee. Knee. 2003;10:229–36.

25. Odenbring S, Egund N, Lindstrand A, et al. Cartilage regeneration after proximal tibial osteotomy for medial gonarthrosis. An arthroscopic, roentgeno-graphic, and histologic study. Clin Orthop Relat Res. 1992;277:210–6.

26. Feucht MJ, Minzlaff P, Saier T, et al. Degree of axis correction in valgus high tibial osteotomy: proposal of an individualised approach. Int Orthop. 2014;38:2273–80.

27. Minas T, Von Keudell A, Bryant T, et al. The John Insall Award: a minimum 10-year outcome study of autologous chondrocyte implantation. Clin Orthopaedics Rel Res. 2014;472:41–51.

28. Harris JD, Mcneilan R, Siston RA, et al. Survival and clinical outcome of isolated high tibial osteotomy and combined biological knee reconstruction. Knee. 2013;20:154–61.

29. Bauer S, Khan R, Ebert J, et al. Knee joint preservation with combined neutralising high tibial osteotomy (HTO) and matrix-induced autologous chondrocyte implantation (MACI) in younger patients with medial knee osteoarthritis: a case series with prospective clinical and MRI follow-up over 5 years. Knee. 2012;19:431–9.

30. Ferruzzi A, Buda R, Cavallo M, et al. Cartilage repair procedures associated with high tibial osteotomy in varus knees: clinical results at 11 years' follow-up. Knee. 2014;21:445–50.

31. Jung W-H, Takeuchi R, Chun C-W, et al. Comparison of results of medial opening-wedge high tibial osteotomy with and without subchondral drilling. Arthroscopy. 2015;31:673–9.

32. Matsunaga D, Akizuki S, Takizawa T, et al. Repair of articular cartilage and clinical outcome after osteotomy with microfracture or abrasion arthroplasty for medial gonarthrosis. Knee. 2007;14:465–71.

33. Sterett WI, Steadman JR. Chondral resurfacing and high tibial osteotomy in the varus knee. Am J Sports Med. 2004;32:1243–9.

34. Sterett WI, Steadman JR, Huang MJ, et al. Chondral resurfacing and high tibial osteotomy in the varus knee: survivorship analysis. Am J Sports Med. 2010;38:1420–4.

35. Bode G, Ogon P, Pestka J, et al. Clinical outcome and return to work following single-stage combined autologous chondrocyte implantation and high tibial osteotomy. Int Orthop. 2015;39:689–96.

36. Cameron JI, Mccauley JC, Kermanshahi AY, et al. Lateral opening-wedge distal femoral osteotomy: pain relief, functional improvement, and survivorship at 5 years. Clin Orthop Relat Res. 2015;473:2009–15.

37. Franceschi F, Longo UG, Ruzzini L, et al. Simultaneous arthroscopic implantation of autologous chondrocytes and high tibial osteotomy for tibial chondral defects in the varus knee. Knee. 2008;15:309–13.

38. Minzlaff P, Feucht MJ, Saier T, et al. Can young and active patients participate in sports after osteochondral autologous transfer combined with valgus high tibial osteotomy? Knee Surg Sports Traumatol Arthrosc. 2016;24:1594–600.

39. Minzlaff P, Feucht MJ, Saier T, et al. Osteochondral autologous transfer combined with valgus high tibial

osteotomy: long-term results and survivorship analysis. Am J Sports Med. 2013;41:2325–32.

40. Paley D, Herzenberg JE, Tetsworth K, et al. Deformity planning for frontal and sagittal plane corrective osteotomies. Orthop Clin N Am. 1994;25:425–66.

41. Niemeyer P, Schmal H, Hauschild O, et al. Open-wedge osteotomy using an internal plate fixator in patients with medial-compartment gonarthritis and varus malalignment: 3-year results with regard to preoperative arthroscopic and radiographic findings. Arthroscopy. 2010;26:1607–16.

42. Minzlaff P, Saier T, Brucker PU, et al. Valgus bracing in symptomatic varus malalignment for testing the expectable "unloading effect" following valgus high tibial osteotomy. Knee Surg Sports Traumatol Arthrosc. 2015;23:1964–70.

D. Hansom and M. Clatworthy

10.1 Introduction

Alignment of the lower limb is an important contributing factor to the development of knee arthritis and is related to the wear pattern of articular cartilage [1]. The surgical treatment of unicompartmental knee arthritis was historically in the form of an osteotomy, aimed at overcorrecting the angular deformity at the knee, with the rationale being to transfer the weight-bearing load from the degenerate compartment to the more normal contralateral compartment to provide symptomatic relief. With the continued improvement of arthroplasty implants however, osteotomy enthusiasm has declined. Whilst arthroplasty remains an excellent option for many patients, the young active patient with knee osteoarthritis (OA), chondral pathology or mechanical malalignment continues to present a treatment dilemma [2]. Indeed, poor outcomes following arthroplasty have been reported in this age group [3–5], with some registries showing higher fail-

ure rates in the under-55 arthroplasty patient population [6]. In this patient subgroup, osteotomies around the knee are a recognised treatment option, aiming to preserve the native knee joint and delay knee arthroplasty [7, 8].

Varus deformity or genu varum is the most common mechanical malalignment seen [9], and can be successfully treated with either a medial opening-wedge or a lateral closing-wedge high tibial osteotomy (HTO) [10–12].

Valgus malalignment or genu valgum, however, is far less common. Excessive physiological valgus (5°–8°) leads to mechanical overload of the lateral compartment [13], progressive lateral meniscal and cartilage damage [9] and increases the risk of developing lateral knee OA. Whilst a valgus deformity may be idiopathic due to a hypoplastic lateral femoral condyle [7], it is most commonly due to an extensive tear of the lateral meniscus at a young age or other pathologies such as trauma, rheumatoid arthritis, metabolic disorders, rickets or poliomyelitis to name a few [14]. The convex anatomy of both the lateral femoral condyle and tibial plateau requires an intact lateral meniscus (LM) to provide congruency. Thus the absence of the LM, whether congenital [15], traumatic or as a result of previous surgery, causes increased contact stresses in the lateral compartment and will accelerate lateral knee OA. Additionally, damage to the lateral femoral condyle (LFC) can occur in conjunction with an acute ACL ± PCL injury or chronic instability,

D. Hansom (✉)
Department of Orthopaedics, Forth Valley Royal
Hospital, Larbert, Scotland, UK

Department of Orthopaedics, Middlemore Hospital,
Auckland, New Zealand

School of Medicine, University of Glasgow,
Glasgow, Scotland, UK

M. Clatworthy
Department of Orthopaedics, Middlemore Hospital,
Auckland, New Zealand

© ISAKOS 2021
A. J. Krych et al. (eds.), *Cartilage Injury of the Knee*,
https://doi.org/10.1007/978-3-030-78051-7_10

resulting in further lateral joint damage and ultimately degeneration [2]. In today's society, the association between a valgus deformity and obesity is becoming increasingly abundant. This causes rapid early degeneration of the meniscus and subsequent cartilage, resulting in early-onset OA of the lateral compartment [2]. Whilst these causative factors are generally universally accepted, the specific indications and contraindications are less so. This dubiety is succeeded only by the question of which osteotomy to perform and when. In general, surgical options can be divided into two anatomical groups: either the distal femoral osteotomy (DFO), either medial closing or lateral opening, or the high tibial osteotomy (HTO), either medial closing or lateral opening. This chapter outlines the current views on these topics, focusing on indications/contraindications, preoperative planning, osteotomy options and methods, post-operative management and complications in relation to the correction of the valgus knee.

10.2 Indications and Contraindications

It has been well documented that patient selection is vital in achieving good clinical outcomes after osteotomies for the valgus knee [2, 13]. Assuming that a valgus malalignment is recognised, as well as any associated pathological conditions as previously mentioned, patient age is the most commonly disputed indicator for osteotomy. Whilst some suggest that osteotomies should only be performed in patients under the age of 55 [16], others extend this to include those under 60 [17] and 65 [2]. It should be highlighted, however, that other factors should be considered such as activity level, lifestyle and general health. Once considered, the ideal osteotomy patient is an active patient, under the age of 55 [8]. In addition, any joint degeneration or osteoarthritic change should be isolated to the lateral compartment [13]. Whether patellofemoral involvement is a contraindication or not is a debatable topic. Some authors believe that an opening-wedge DFVO may reduce the Q-angle, and therefore

will unload the PFJ [8]. In addition, it has been demonstrated that patients with PFJ OA in conjunction with lateral compartment OA have comparable outcomes at final follow-up [18]. Whilst this study included patients with all grades of PFJ OA (Grade I—9%; Grade II—45.4%; Grade III—36.3%; and Grade IV—4.5%) only 26 knees were included and therefore its power has to be questioned. In comparison, many other authors consider PFJ OA an absolute [17] or relative [16, 19] contraindication. Perhaps therefore, taking into consideration potential mechanical advantages suggested by the work of Zarrouk et al., moderate PFJ OA may not be considered an absolute contraindication to DFO [13].

In addition, osteotomies should not be performed in patients with rheumatoid arthritis (RA), significant knee instability or a fixed valgus deformity of >20° [2, 13]. Puddu suggests that the valgus correction in such severe knees can result in ligament instability and, if associated with tibial subluxation of >1 cm, represents an absolute contraindication and osteotomy should not be performed. Additionally, it has been suggested that both nicotine use and osteoporosis are associated with poor outcomes following osteotomy [13, 20].

The patient with a valgus deformity and anterior cruciate ligament (ACL) insufficiency provides a unique and technically challenging situation. By combining an osteotomy with ACL reconstruction, the malalignment problem can be addressed as well as the resolution of instability. Whilst research on combined procedures for the valgus knee is scarce, several studies exist supporting a combined approach in the varus knee [21, 22]. Such studies produced good results, with resolution of normal daily activities and recreational sports, and did not find any increase in complications compared to an isolated HTO. This view is supported by a case series presented by Dejour et al., who also favour the simultaneous approach [23]. It should be stressed however that this view is far from universal, with some authors recommending alignment correction with HTO before considering ACL reconstruction [24, 25]. In a case series of eight patients undergoing combined procedures, Latterman et al. found a major complication rate of 75%, with a third being ACL re-rupture. These rates were found to be lower in the staged procedure groups [25].

Obesity and osteotomy for the valgus knee is another controversial topic. Whilst obesity is widely viewed as having a negative impact on the outcome of surgery, it is felt by some that being overweight may make a patient a better candidate for osteotomy rather than arthroplasty [2]. It should be recognised however that obesity does increase post-operative complications and more recent studies have shown that a BMI of greater than 30 kg/m^2 is associated with worse outcomes after DFVO [26, 27]. It is therefore recommended that weight should be reduced to as near to normal as possible before embarking on osteotomy correction.

10.3 Assessment

A full radiographic assessment is essential in the preoperative planning for any osteotomy. This should include weight-bearing anteroposterior and lateral views, skyline patella and Rosenberg views. The Rosenberg view is critical for the assessment of the valgus disease as this is predominantly a flexion disease. The standard weight-bearing AP X-ray will therefore not typically show the lateral compartment disease (Fig. 10.1) as there is minimal distal femoral wear. The 45° weight-bearing view will show the OA as there is posterior wear (Figs. 10.2 and 10.3). The use of computed tomography (CT) is not routinely recommended; however, magnetic resonance imaging (MRI) is required to determine the extent of disease in the lateral compartment and evaluate the integrity of the medial compartment and associated ligamentous/soft-tissue injury and may therefore aid preoperative planning in specific cases.

When planning, the first stage should be to determine where the weight passes through the knee joint. This can be achieved by drawing a line from the centre of the femoral head to the centre of the talar dome. The mechanical axis of

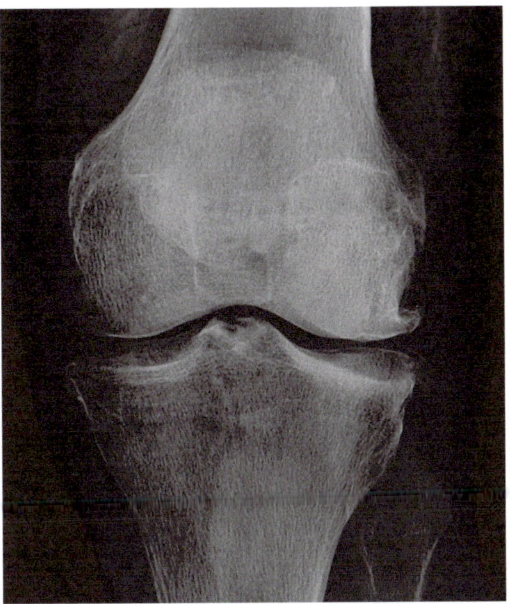

Fig. 10.1 Weight-bearing AP X-ray, demonstrating minimal lateral joint degeneration with preservation of the joint space

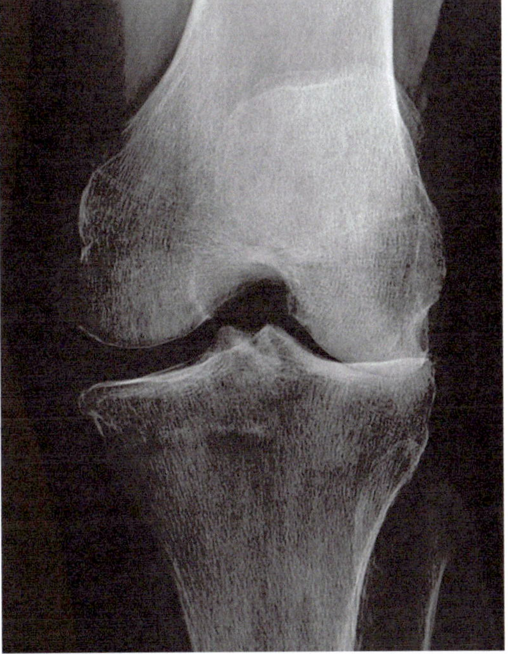

Fig. 10.2 45-Degree weight-bearing PA X-ray in the same patient as in Fig. 10.1, demonstrating severe posterolateral OA

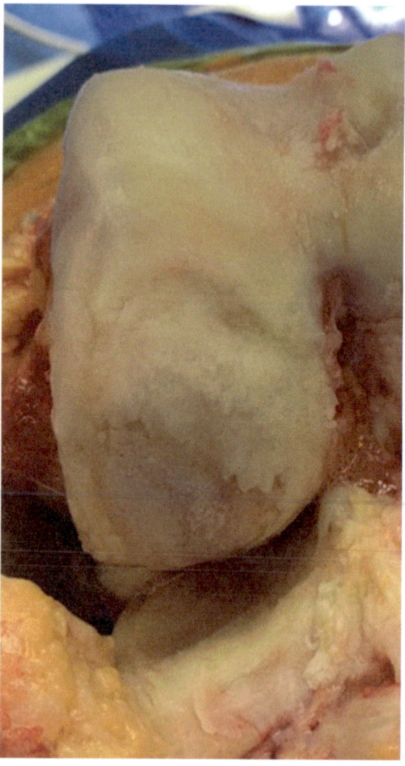

Fig. 10.3 Intraoperative findings in the same patient as in Figs. 10.1 and 10.2, confirming isolated posterolateral OA

contact pressure and area in the lateral compartment better than a correction to neutral [30]. It should be noted, however, that this cadaveric study did not record the effects of overcorrection on the medial side, which may be significant. Further studies have supported the overcorrection argument, showing good clinical outcomes by restoring the mechanical axis to 40–41% of the tibial plateau [20, 31]. Whilst the DFVO is recognised as the workhorse for the correction of the valgus knee, the tibia can also be targeted to correct valgus malalignment. Certainly, if the valgus deformity is <12° or the posterior slope is <10° a proximal tibial osteotomy has been shown to be effective [26]. If an HTO is performed outside these parameters, the knee is seen to gradually subluxate laterally [32] and the femur appears to fall off the medial tibial plateau [2]. Within these values, it would seem logical that if the valgus deformity is localised to the tibia (as a result of meniscectomy or trauma for example), then correction at the tibia is appropriate [33]. Tibial osteotomy options for the valgus knee will be discussed in the next section.

10.4 Surgical Options

To correct the valgus malaligned knee, the surgeon has four options in the form of osteotomy: medial closing-wedge distal femoral osteotomy (MCWDFO), lateral opening-wedge distal femoral osteotomy (LOWDFO), medial closing-wedge high tibial osteotomy (MCWHTO) and lateral opening-wedge high tibial osteotomy (LOWHTO).

When evaluating the optimal osteotomy for the valgus knee it is very important to understand that a valgus deformity is most commonly a flexion disease.

The aetiology of the valgus knee has two primary causes. Firstly, genu valgum which is typically congenital results in the mechanical axis passing through the lateral side of the knee. This overloads the knee primarily in extension resulting in distal femoral articular cartilage loss. The more common aetiology is post-traumatic OA secondary to an extensive lateral meniscal tear.

the limb can then be calculated as a percentage across the tibial plateau, assuming that the medial edge is 0% and the lateral edge is 100%. Anything beyond 56% can be regarded as valgus [20]. Once valgus malalignment is confirmed, the amount of correction can be calculated. The correction angle is defined as the angle between the mechanical axis of the femur (a line drawn from the centre of the femoral head to the centre of the tibial plateau) and the mechanical axis of the tibia (a line drawn from the centre of the tibial plateau to the centre of the talar dome), as succinctly demonstrated by Olivero et al. [13]. The exact amount of correction, particularly in the case of DFVO, remains controversial. Some studies suggest that a DFVO should aim to restore the mechanical axis to 48–50% from medial to lateral across the tibial plateau [28], and that overcorrection is contraindicated [2, 29]. More recent biomechanical research, however, has indicated that overcorrection by up to 5° normalises the

Biomechanically the knee acts in a medial pivot fashion whereby there is minimal translation of the medial compartment of the knee with flexion whilst the lateral compartment rolls posteriorly predominantly driven by the convex shape of the lateral tibial plateau. The lateral meniscus acts as a bumper controlling the lateral roll back and protecting the articular cartilage of the posterior lateral tibial plateau. An extensive posterior lateral meniscal tear removes the bumper resulting in a significant load increase in the posterior lateral compartment. Articular cartilage loss occurs in the posterior aspect of the lateral femoral condyle and the posterior lateral femoral condyle (Fig. 10.1). Hence with these patients the weight-bearing AP X ray typically shows a relatively normal joint space whilst the 45° weight-bearing PA view shows significant joint space reduction.

To summarise genu valgum as the primary pathology results in lateral compartment extension disease like medial compartment OA whilst post-meniscectomy lateral compartment OA is a flexion disease.

The different articular cartilage wear patterns are thus best treated differently. A distal femoral varus osteotomy will primarily affect the extension gap. For those of you who perform knee arthroplasty you will be well aware that the distal femoral cut only affects the extension gap whilst the flexion gap is determined by the posterior femoral condylar resections. So, the distal femoral varus osteotomy will alter the alignment primarily in extension so is best suited to the congenital genu valgum knee. In contrast, a tibial osteotomy will affect both the flexion and extension gap so it is better suited to the post-traumatic valgus knee.

10.4.1 Distal Femoral Osteotomy

In relation to DFO, it has been suggested by some authors that if the correction is up to $10°–12°$, then a lateral opening wedge is preferred, whilst if it is over $12°$ then a medial closing wedge should be performed [16]. Others, however, consider surgical preference and technique experience to be more important in DFVO choice [17, 20]. Current literature does not suggest superiority of one technique over another [13]. Good clinical outcomes of MCWDFO out to 10 years have been shown, with survival rates of up to 89.9% [34], whilst others report rates ranging from 64% at 10 years [35] to 45% at 15 years [36]. This trend has been supported by a review article by Chahla et al., confirming significantly higher failure rates in follow-up over 10 years [37]. Indeed, the review paper by Wylie et al. demonstrated a higher conversion rate to arthroplasty in the medial closing-wedge osteotomy patients; however this is most likely due to their longer follow-up [7] in comparison to LOWDFO.

Good outcomes have also been reported with LOWDFO, with survival rates ranging from 74% to 100% at 5 years [18, 29, 38], with Zarrouk et al. showing significant improvements in three independent knee scores [18]. Studies out to 10 years are limited; however Ekeland et al. have shown survival rates of 74% in 24 opening-wedge DFVOs [39]. Use of an adapted lateral distal femoral 'V' osteotomy has shown promising results out to 11 years, with good/excellent patient-reported outcomes using a modified Knee Society Rating System (KSS) [40]. As demonstrated, proving superiority between surgical techniques is problematic, and as such choice will remain largely down to surgical preference until longer follow-up data is available.

The other consideration with the LOWDFO is the filling of the bone gap post-correction. Puddu suggests that any gap >7.5 mm should be filled (with either autologous, allogenic or synthetic graft) and that smaller gaps can be left unfilled [2]. Rates of non-union are significantly lower when using autograft (2.6%) compared to allograft and synthetic graft (4.6% and 4.5%, respectively) [41]. It should however be noted that the use of synthetic graft and allografts allows large quantities to be used with specific gap-filling shapes [8], and does not involve donor-site morbidity.

What perhaps is more interesting in relation to DFVO is the surgical fixation method. It is widely accepted that some form of rigid internal fixation is paramount in producing good outcomes [42]. Rigid fixation options consist primarily of either an angled blade plate configuration or a locking compression plate. Puddu's locking plate design, with the associated technique [2], acts as a tension band construct. This has been shown to have clear mechanical advantages when compared to a standard medial plate alone [8], with improved patient outcomes at 7 years and reduced plate intolerance [2, 8, 38]. Similar patient outcomes and mechanical advantages have been found using locking compression plates, such as TomoFix® (Synthes) [43, 44]; however some have found a delayed healing with this plate and a high incidence of plate intolerance (86%) [45].

The use of an angled blade plate is also documented in the literature. Its use in the paediatric population shows good union rates and provides excellent stability in the cerebral palsy population [46]. More recently the use of this implant in the adult population has been compared to fixation with the locking compression plates discussed previously. Kazemi et al. compared 20 DFOs fixed with locking compression plates to those fixed with angled blade plates and found an improved valgus angle and mechanical lateral distal femoral angle in the angled blade patient subgroup. In addition, non-union rates at 9 months were 0%, compared to 20% in the locking plate group. Whilst this was not found to be statistically significant, the trend is clear and further research is recommended. Furthermore, biomechanical testing has shown the blade plate to be stiffer and more stable; however whether this has any clinical significance was not addressed [47].

10.4.2 Proximal Tibial Osteotomy

High tibial osteotomy (HTO) is a relatively common surgical treatment for varus malalignment of the knee. Proximal tibial osteotomies to correct valgus deformity, however, are far less common, with most being performed in the distal femur [7, 40, 48]. When small valgus corrections are required, of $12°$ or less in the anteroposterior plane and $10°$ or less in the sagittal, a MCWHTO or LOWHTO can be performed [49]. Surgery out with these parameters results in lateral tibial sub-

luxation and anteroposterior instability and should be avoided [2, 26, 50]. The advantage, however, of HTO for valgus malalignment is that the joint is unloaded in both extension and flexion. A DFO, in comparison, only unloads the joint in extension [51]. Even adhering to these restrictions however can produce variable results. Failure rates of up to 52% at medium-term follow-up (4.3 years) have been reported [52], whilst others show excellent outcomes in relation to kinetics and kinematics [53]. A more recent study looking at MCWHTO has shown short-term improvements in patient-reported outcomes such as function, pain and quality of life [54]. This study also highlighted an associated MCL laxity performed pre- and post-operation using instrumented laxity measurements. Coventry previously described this phenomenon and recognised that by removing a medial wedge from the proximal tibia, the superficial medial collateral ligament (sMCL) becomes lax, and a surgical reefing procedure should be performed to address this [26, 55]. A recent retrospective study on over 100 patients addressing medial laxity in MCWHTO concluded that medial reefing should be performed only in selected cases. MCWHTO provided good results in relation to survivorship (80%) and patient satisfaction out to 4.5 years [56]. Up to 25% however reported instability, which was found to significantly correlate with worse outcomes. MCL reefing may therefore improve outcomes in patients with increased MCL laxity intraoperatively. This should therefore be tested if a MCWHTO is being performed. However, it is our opinion that medial reefing is not necessary as long as care is taken not to detach the tibial insertion of the deep MCL. More extensive experience with medial opening-wedge HTO for the varus knee has shown that complete detachment of the superficial MCL does not result in medial laxity if the deep MCL remains intact.

A lateral opening-wedge high tibial osteotomy (LOWHTO) is another option for the valgus knee. In addition to providing a familiar exposure, instability can be corrected by tightening of lateral ligamentous structures, without affecting the medial stabilisers of the knee. Unlike in a

MCWHTO, the medial structures are not weakened and therefore instability is not reported [50]. In this particular study, the majority of patients were post-traumatic. Despite this, none were found to have progression of their arthritis, 88% had good/excellent results and non-union rate was 0% [50]. Of note, a transient peroneal nerve palsy rate of 9% was reported, which was similar to other studies [57, 58], and fibula osteotomies were performed in all cases at the mid-shaft level. More recent research has found similar results, with significant improvements in patient-reported outcomes as well as maintenance of both radiographic and gait improvements [33]. Survivorship at 4.3 years was found to be 91%, which is comparable to HTOs being performed for varus malalignment. Of interest, all patients in this cohort had a normal mechanical lateral distal femoral angle (mLDFA), confirming that the valgus malalignment was due to tibial deformity and fibular osteotomies were not performed in small corrections. Peroneal nerve palsy was not noted in any patients. It is therefore recommended that LOWHTO is a valid treatment option when the deformity is within the parameters suggested by Coventry, and the deformity is localised to the tibia.

It is our opinion that a tibial osteotomy should be confined to patients who have a post-traumatic posterior articular cartilage wear pattern. The resultant tibial varus should not be more than 10° of varus in extension. On a long leg X-ray the coronal tibial angle is measured. The correction angle combined with the coronal tibial angle should be <=10° of varus. This correction does not require a fibula osteotomy (Fig. 10.4).

10.5　Operative Techniques

In this section, the main surgical techniques for the correction of valgus malalignment of the knee will be briefly described. In addition to these techniques, it is widely accepted that knee arthroscopy should be performed before embarking on osteotomy surgery [2, 13, 33, 49]. This

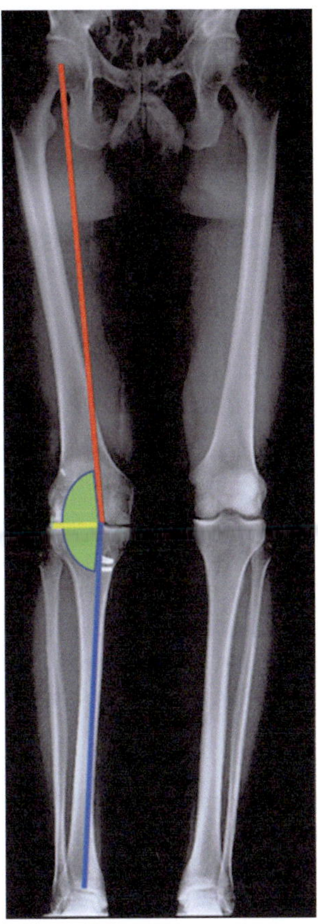

Fig. 10.4 Osteotomy planning. The red and blue lines represent the mechanical axis of the femur and tibia, respectively. The yellow line represents the coronal tibial angle and the green angle represents the angle between the tibial and femoral mechanical axes, allowing the correction angle to be calculated

allows the rest of the knee to be thoroughly examined, ensuring no medial/patellofemoral degeneration and to perform any other intra-articular procedures [47]. In addition, regardless of osteotomy type, the patient is positioned supine, ensuring that adequate intraoperative images can be taken by fluoroscopy. It has been recommended that the entire limb is exposed, including the iliac crest, to allow the axis of the limb to be assessed intraoperatively [16] and autograft to be taken if required. The use of a foam wedge to elevate the limb may also aid intraoperative imaging.

10.5.1 Distal Femoral Medial Closing-Wedge Osteotomy

On the medial side of the knee a skin incision is made either 2 cm distal to the medial epicondyle [13] or just proximal to the adductor tubercle [2] and should extend around 15 cm proximally on the anteromedial cortex of the femur. The vastus medialis fascia is incised and retracted laterally and anteriorly and the periosteum incised to access the femoral shaft. Once exposure has been achieved, an optional Kirschner wire (K-wire) can be placed under X-ray guidance, parallel to the articular joint line to guide the first osteotomy cut [17]. The first distal osteotomy cut can then be performed, ensuring that posterior structures are protected using an appropriate retractor such as a Hohmann. Both the anterior and posterior leg of this osteotomy should stop approximately 10 mm or 1/3 the diameter of the tibia leaving the lateral cortex intact [2, 13]. A second osteotomy, using the same technique, is then performed more proximally depending on the amount of desired correction. Fixation can then be performed, using either a 90° angled blade plate or a locking compression plate. The former option allows a tibiofemoral angle of 0° to be achieved by positioning the blade parallel to the joint line and the plate parallel to the medial femoral cortex, as described by McDermott et al. [59]. If a locking compression plate is preferred, bone cuts can be made using the technique developed by Healy et al. utilising pins in the distal femur to guide the osteotomy saw cuts [60], or a dedicated jig on the anterior tibia to check that alignment can be used as described by Learmonth [61].

10.5.2 Distal Femoral Lateral Opening-Wedge Osteotomy

A 12–15 cm skin incision is made, starting from the lateral epicondyle and extending proximally up the femur. The iliotibial band is identified and incised, allowing visualisation of vastus lateralis which is elevated from the intramuscular septum. Any branches from the profunda femoris should be identified and coagulated at this stage. If any open intra-articular procedures are required, such as a lateral femoral condyle cartilage procedure, these can be performed by extending the approach to a lateral parapatellar one [16].

At this stage, blunt retractors should be placed around the posterior aspect of the distal femur to protect the neurovascular structures. With the knee in extension, a K-wire is placed, under fluoroscopic guidance, 2–3 finger breadths above the lateral epicondyle aiming for the medial epicondyle, with an inclination of around 20° [2]. A mark on the cortex above and below the anticipated osteotomy helps to assess any rotation of the femur [16]. The osteotomy is then performed in line with the K-wire, again stopping 10 mm short of the medial cortex which should not be breached. This can be performed either with an oscillating saw or with osteotomes and should be regularly checked with fluoroscopy. Some advocate flexing the knee during this stage, to reduce tension on the neurovascular structures and help minimise iatrogenic injury [16]. The osteotomy can then be opened to the desired amount using either stacked osteotomes or a dedicated wedge/jack opener under X-ray guidance by hinging around the medial cortex. If a large correction is required, small drill hole perforations can be performed in the medial cortex to allow a controlled opening [16]. Fixation can either be in the form of a Puddu T-plate, which has the advantage of encompassing a 'tooth' which is the same size as the wedge, or a locking compression plate and bone graft [16, 20, 45]. Bone graft is recommended in any correction greater than 7.5 mm [2], and whilst autograft remains the gold standard, the recognised donor-site morbidity encourages the use of bone substitutes [13].

10.5.3 Proximal Tibial Medial Closing-Wedge Osteotomy

An antero-medial skin incision is made and the pes anserinus is identified and partially detached. The superficial layers of the MCL are divided and the proximal tibial metaphysis is exposed. The distal insertion of the patellar tendon should be identified and protected and the osteotomy site confirmed under fluoroscopic guidance. A K-wire is then inserted from medial to lateral and distal to proximal above the tibial tuberosity aiming for the fibular head [2]. A second K-wire can then be used more proximally, its placement depending on the amount of correction required. The osteotomies are started with the oscillating saw, which can be used for completion, or osteotomes can be utilised. Care should be taken to protect the posterior neurovascular structure with blunt retraction. Ideally around 10 mm of lateral tibial cortex should be left to act as a hinge and to ensure stability [49]. Final alignment should be checked, ensuring that the mechanical axis of the limb passes through the midpoint of the knee. Historically, fixation was often performed using staples [2]; however medial tibial locking plates are now more commonly used [49].

In addition, some surgeons advocate a biplanar osteotomy [56, 62] for tibial osteotomies. The approach remains the same as discussed above; however two osteotomies are utilised to create a biplanar osteotomy. A transverse osteotomy should run across the posterior two-thirds of the bone, leaving the anterior third intact for performing a second, ascending osteotomy in the coronal plane (Fig. 10.5). Of note, the anterior osteotomy should be complete and include the opposite cortex. The subsequent steps of the osteotomy are as previously described.

Patient-specific instrumentation (PSI) is also available for use in osteotomy surgery. As mentioned previously, posterior tibial slope (PTS) management is important to preserve biomechanics [64, 65]. In order to maintain PTS, anterior opening has been found to be equal to 67% of the medial opening [66]. Clearly this evaluation is complex and challenging to perform during surgery, and it is suggested that PSI may be a useful adjunct to manage both the sagittal and frontal plane corrections during surgery [67, 68]. Several recent studies on small patient series have suggested good accuracy and reliability of the procedure [67–69], especially when multiplanar corrections are required. Additionally, PSI is available for DFO surgery, such as the Activmotion DFO PSI® [70]. In this environment, PSI aids optimal bony cuts and plate posi-

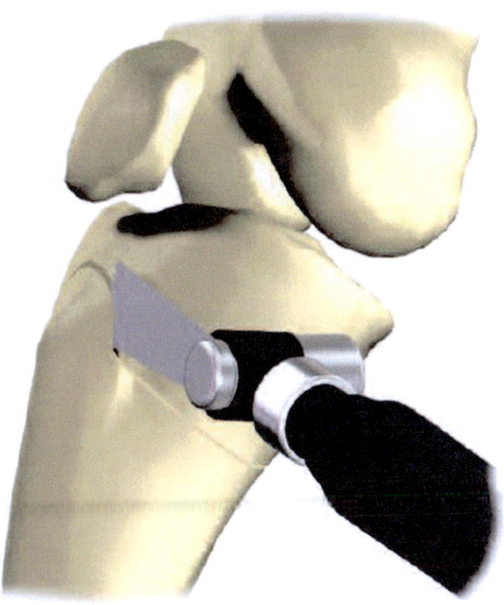

Fig. 10.5 Diagram showing biplanar tibial osteotomy. Taken, with permission, from the TomoFix® operative technique manual, DePuy Synthes [63]

tioning, reducing unwanted sagittal plane modifications as is the case with traditional cutting guides [71]. It should however be recognised that preoperative CT scans are required for PSI production, thus incurring an increased cost and radiation exposure. Menetrey et al. have however shown that the use of PSI reduces the use of intraoperative fluoroscopy and reduces surgical time [72]. The decision to use PSI for osteotomy surgery will likely come down to surgeon preference and experience, with recognition given to its use in multiplanar corrections.

10.5.4 Proximal Tibial Lateral Opening-Wedge Osteotomy

A 6–8 cm anterolateral longitudinal incision is made lateral to the tibial tuberosity, extending distally from Gerdy's tubercle. Full-thickness skin flaps should be used and fascia should be incised in line with the skin incision. Anterior compartment muscles are elevated off and retracted posteriorly. The patellar tendon and posterior soft tissues should be identified and protected with blunt retraction. The tibial osteotomy starts with the placement of a K-wire around 2 cm distal to the tibial joint surface and proximal to the tibial tuberosity under fluoroscopic guidance. The osteotomy is initiated with a microsurgical saw, which can be used for completion, or osteotomes can be used depending on surgical preference. The osteotomy should stop 10 mm from the medial cortex, which will act as a hinge. Again, if large corrections are required, the medial cortex may require drill perforation. Spreading or stacked osteotomes can then be inserted followed by a jack or wedge opener to achieve the desired correction. Once correction is confirmed by fluoroscopy, bone graft can be inserted according to surgical preference and fixation achieved with the appropriate locking compression plate [33, 50]. This procedure is technically more difficult than a medial opening-wedge osteotomy as the exposure is compromised by the anterior musculature which requires retraction, presence of the fibula and reduced surface area of the lateral cortex of the tibia which is much smaller than the medial.

10.6 Post-operative Care

Post-operative treatment is variable and highly surgeon dependant. It can be divided into treatment for opening-wedge osteotomies and that for closing-wedge osteotomies. Post-operative care for closing-wedge osteotomies, regardless of the fixation method, is immobilisation in a functional brace with an unlimited range of motion (ROM). Most research suggests that weight bearing is restricted for 6–8 weeks based on callus formation on X-rays [17, 35, 36, 49, 59], after which time partial weight bearing (PWB) can be introduced. Full weight bearing (FWB) is then advised after 3 months [36, 60]. More recently however it has been shown that reducing these times does not affect clinical outcome. Forkel et al. initiated PWB immediately post-operatively, with a full ROM [31], whilst Tirico et al. allowed toe-touch weight bearing (TTWB) immediately for 2 weeks, followed by PWB for a further 4 weeks [17], without adverse results. It would therefore seem appropriate to partially restrict weight bearing during the initial 6-week post-operative period, with weight-bearing status increasing thereafter.

Debate also exists with opening-wedge osteotomies of both the tibia and femur for the valgus-aligned knee. As with closing-wedge osteotomies, the use of a functional ROM brace is advised for the initial 4–6-week period by some; however we have not used a brace for the last 20 years. It is our opinion that adequate stability of the osteotomy is achieved by the internal fixation. A brace is cumbersome to wear and is likely to reduce restoration of knee flexion and quadricep strength. During this time, it is suggested that patients should remain NWB for 4–6 weeks [38, 40, 48], and begin PWB thereafter. More recent research has again suggested that reducing this restricted weight-bearing period does not affect outcome [29, 39], allowing TTWB immediately post-operatively, progressing to PWB or FWB at 6 weeks. Taking this further, Brinkman et al. have shown that FWB as tolerated, immediately post-operation, has no adverse effects and that the same outcomes can be achieved as in a restricted weight-bearing osteotomy population, but in a shorter time [73]. Collins et al. have also shown good outcomes with TTWB for 2 weeks, followed by FWB as tolerated [33]. Both studies used the TomoFix® (Synthes) implant, and no comparison was made between different implant options. With the post-operative advantages of newer implants being considered, the ultimate decision regarding rehabilitation remains with the operating surgeon.

10.7 Complications

General surgical complications will not be discussed here, and instead specific complications related to DFOs and HTOs for valgus malalignment will be addressed.

Perhaps the most severe complication associated with DFO is that of injury to the popliteal neurovascular bundle. Thankfully, the risk of injury is low [2], providing careful attention if paid to correct retractor placement. Further fresh frozen cadaveric work by Kim et al. has shown that the neurovascular structures are farther from the tibia with the knee flexed to 90° [74]; therefore most surgeons would suggest performing the osteotomy with the knee flexed, with blunt retractors posteriorly [2, 16, 20].

The risk of intraoperative fracture is also a recognised complication [13, 19, 39], and usually a result of either failure to divide the posterior/anterior cortex, too little medial bone hinge being left or guide pin being positioned too close to the joint line [2]. This can result in uncontrolled propagation of the osteotomy, through either the articular surface or the medial cortex. This can be prevented by ensuring that the pin placement is sufficiently distal, thus leaving an appropriately sized medial hinge, before starting the osteotomy. If medial hinge integrity is lost, this can be fixed using a contralateral screw or staple [13].

Non-union rates are also variable throughout the literature, ranging from 25 to 50% [42, 45]. Jacobi et al. reported the highest non-union rate of 6 months (50%) with an opening-wedge DFO, leading them to adopt a closing-wedge technique [45]. More recent literature, however, suggests that this trend is decreasing. Forkel et al. reported a reoperation rate for delayed or non-union of only 5% [31], whilst Ekeland et al. found a union rate of 75% at 3 months and 100% at 6 months [39]. The factors affecting this significant improvement remain unclear. The dubiety however is less pronounced when it comes to closing-wedge DFO, with most authors reporting a lower non-union rate [29, 31, 39].

Hardware intolerance, specifically in opening-wedge DFO, is a relatively frequent complication, with up to 76% requiring removal [29]. This appears to be related to the type of fixation used, with the Puddu plate removal rate being almost half that of locking compression plates such as TomoFix [39]. Despite being larger and more stable than the Puddu plate, it clearly also gives more soft-tissue irritation, thus increasing the likelihood of removal. This, in combination with the Young's modulus mismatch and reported improved Oxford Knee Scores (OKS) [75], means we routinely remove the hardware.

The deep vein thrombosis risk has been found to be similar to that of knee joint arthroplasty [8], with the highest incidence being within the first 3–4 days and ranging from 0 to 10.8% [76]. As a result, thromboprophylaxis is recommended.

HTO shares similar complications to those of DFVO, such as fracture risk and its link to correct guide pin placement. It is therefore advised that correct pin placement, pre-osteotomy, is achieved as with DFO. In addition, the risk of DVT is again similar to that of primary joint arthroplasty and should be addressed as such. Additionally, a frequently cited criticism of HTO for the valgus knee is that it creates joint-line obliquity. As previously mentioned, it is recommended that a DFVO should be performed if there is >12° of valgus or more than 10° of tibial slope [26, 60]. Indeed, Shoji and Insall have shown that medial subluxation of the femur on the tibia occurs if >15° of tibial slope is created [32]. It is therefore recommended that to avoid such complications, tibial osteotomies for the valgus malaligned knee should be reserved where small degrees of correction are required [2, 51] or the deformity is localised to the tibia [33].

Specific to MCWHTO is the issue of medial joint laxity, due to de-functioning of the sMCL. As previously discussed however, this can be prevented keeping the deep MCL attachment intact. This complication is clearly not present during a LOWHTO as the lateral ligamentous structures around the knee are tightened and the medial structures not weakened [50]. The LOWHTO does however move the patella slightly more distally and has been shown to have higher rates of non-union [76], probably due to the increased stability and metaphyseal bone-to-bone compression achieved during a MCWHTO. Certainly, if the osteotomy is performed distal to the tibial tubercle, the non-union rate is increased due to the low healing rate of the bone below the metaphysis [77].

Perhaps one of the most commonly quoted complications associated with LOWHTO is that of transient peroneal nerve palsy [42, 50, 57]. In Marti et al.'s series, transient peroneal nerve palsies were noted in 9% of patients, despite performing a mid-shaft fibula osteotomy in an attempt to reduce this complication. More recently however, it has been suggested that for small corrections, such as those recommended to be performed in the proximal tibia, no fibular osteotomy is required [33]. Instead, a proximal tibio-fibular joint arthrotomy is suggested, thus negating the need to common peroneal nerve exploration, fibular osteotomy and potential iatrogenic nerve injury. Retrospective review of the patients in this paper revealed no common peroneal nerve injuries.

Lastly, infection is a recognised complication associated with osteotomy surgery. In relation to tibial osteotomy surgery, systematic review suggests that superficial infections occur in 1–9% and deep infections in 0.5–4.7% of all HTOs [78]. No significant differences have been found between open- and closed-wedged HTO with respect to deep or superficial infections [79]. In relation to implant type, a meta-analysis by Anagnostakos et al. found no statistical difference between internal fixation options [80]; however external fixation options were found to significantly increase infection rates, most likely due to pin-site infection [78, 81].

Similarly, in DFO surgery, infection rates are noted to be higher if external fixators are used [8]. Whilst the research available on infection in DFO surgery is limited, the literature suggests that infection rates are around 1% [29], and that this does not differ between OWDFO and CWDFO [19].

10.8 Conclusions

Tibial and femoral osteotomies have been used for over a century to correct angular deformities [33]. Despite this, osteotomies have fallen out of favour, with improvements in total and unicompartmental arthroplasty [82–84]. Over the last decade the success of total-knee arthroplasty has continued [85] with increased implant survivorship. A recent paper in Lancet looking at almost 300,000 TKRs from pooled registry data showed 82.3% survival at 25 years [86]; however this age is dependent on all national joint registries showing a much higher failure rate in patients under the age of 55 [6, 87, 88]. This is particularly the case with UKAs with the Australian registry showing a 27% failure rate at 18 years [89]. The combination of this, and the increasing numbers of unicompartmental arthroplasty [90], most likely explains the decreased number of osteotomies being performed [82]. In relation to the valgus knee, genu valgum is considerably less common than genu varum, and thus the incidence of surgical correction and associated research is low [7]. Despite this however, it is widely accepted that the patient selection is essential in providing good clinical outcomes [2, 13]. After consideration of the current literature, the ideal osteotomy patient is an active patient, in good health under the age of 55 [2, 8, 16, 17]. In addition any joint degeneration or osteoarthritic change should be isolated to the lateral joint space [13]. As eluded, whether PFJ OA is a contraindication to osteotomy is debatable. Whilst some authors consider PFJ OA to be an absolute [17] or relative [16, 19] contraindication, good results have been demonstrated in patients with both PFJ OA and lateral compartment OA [18]. It is suggested therefore that whilst severe PFJ OA may be contraindicated for osteotomy, mild to moderate may not [13]. Further contraindications include nicotine use, osteoporosis and obesity, all of which are associated with poor outcomes [13, 20, 27, 55]. Significant knee instability, confirmed by tibial subluxation of >1 cm combined with severe valgus deformity (>20°), is considered an absolute contraindication [2, 13].

Evidence for the valgus malaligned patient with ACL insufficiency is scarce. In the varus knee this provides a unique and technically challenging situation. By combining an osteotomy with ACL reconstruction, the malalignment problem can be addressed as well as the resolution of instability [21, 22]. Such studies have shown good results, without an increase in complications; however others recommend alignment correction with HTO before considering ACL reconstruction [24, 25] due to high ACL re-rupture rates (75%) [25]. Whether any of these results are transferable to the valgus, ACL-deficient knee remains to be seen. The decision whether to proceed to combined or staged surgery therefore remains at the discretion of the surgeon and patient.

Assessment of the osteotomy patient should include weight-bearing anteroposterior and lateral views of the whole limb, skyline patella, Rosenberg views [8] and an MRI to assess the integrity of the medial compartment. After valgus malalignment is confirmed, correction planning should be performed as described by Olivero et al. [13]. If the primary valgus deformity is >12°, located within the femur, or shows a posterior slope that is >10° then a DFO is recommended [2, 13]. HTOs should be considered if the deformity is <12° or the posterior slope is <10° [26] and originates within the tibia [33].

The surgical osteotomy options include LOWDFO, MCWDFO, MCWHTO and LOWHTO. Independent from these techniques, it is advisable to perform knee arthroscopy before embarking on osteotomy surgery [2, 47].

In relation to DFO, current literature does not suggest superiority of medial closing wedge over lateral opening wedge [13]. MCWDFO has shown survival rates of up to 89.9% [34] at 10 years, with a decline to 45% recognised at 15 years [36]. Despite higher reported union rates [29, 31, 39], a higher conversion rate to arthroplasty in MCWDFO patients has been demonstrated; however this is most likely due to their longer follow-up [7] when compared to LOWDFO. LOWHTO also shows good outcomes, with survival rates ranging from 74% to 100% at 5 years [18, 29, 38] and 74% at 10 years [39]. They have the advantage of allowing the surgeon to fine-tune the deformity correction, whilst the MCWDFO is very surgeon reliant being technically challenging and requiring accurate preoperative planning and bony resections [19]. Bone graft is recommended in gaps >7.5 mm [2], with autograft providing the lowest non-union rate [41]. It should however be noted that the use of synthetic graft allows large quantities to be used with specific gap-filling shapes [8], and avoids donor-site morbidity. As expected bone grafting is more often required in the LOWDFO population [19]. Surgical technique therefore remains largely down to surgical pref-

erence until longer follow-up data is available [7, 13, 37].

In relation to fixation, it is accepted that rigid internal fixation is essential in producing good outcomes [42]. The use of non-rigid fixation options such as staples can carry complication rates of up to 70% [91]. Locking compression plates have shown good patient outcomes and mechanical advantages, regardless of plate type [2, 8, 38, 43, 44]. This is likely due to the long femoral lever arm requiring a more stable plate configuration in comparison to HTOs [19]. Plate intolerance is however a recognised complication in both LOWDFO (86%) and MCWDFO (70%) [19], and removal is recommended [45]. The other rigid fixation option is that of the angled blade plate. Recent research of the MCWDFO has suggested improved valgus angle and mechanical lateral distal femoral angle when compared to the locking compression plate, as well as a lower non-union rate at 9 months (0% vs. 20%, respectively). Whilst this was not found to be statistically significant (due to a small sample size), the trend is clear and further research is recommended. Furthermore, biomechanical testing has shown the blade plate to be stiffer and more stable; however whether this has any clinical significance was not addressed [47]. Future research should therefore be directed at which form of rigid internal fixation provides superior long-term results.

Osteotomy complications in general will be summarised later; however specific to DFOs is the risk of popliteal neurovascular bundle injury. The literature has reported this to be a relatively low risk of <0.01% [2, 92]; however the morbidity and mortality associated with such injuries are significant. The neurovascular structures are known to be farther from the tibia with the knee flexed to 90° [74]; thus it is suggested that DFOs are performed with the knee flexed and blunt retractors placed posteriorly [2, 16, 20].

Proximal tibial osteotomies to correct valgus deformity are uncommon, with most being performed in the distal femur [7, 40, 48]. When small valgus corrections are required, of 12° or less in the anteroposterior plane and 10° or less in the coronal, a MCWHTO or LOWHTO can be performed [49]. Surgery out with these parameters should be avoided [2, 26, 50]. The advantage of HTO for valgus malalignment is that the joint is unloaded in both extension and flexion. A DFO, in comparison, only unloads the joint in extension [51].

In relation to MCWHTOs, despite good patient-reported outcomes in up to 72% of patients out to 10 years [51], failure rates vary from 52% at medium-term follow-up (4.3 years) [52] to 77% at 9.4 years [26]. More recent studies have favoured Coventry's results, showing short-term improvements in patient-reported outcomes such as function, pain and quality of life [54]. This study also highlighted associated MCL laxity. A recent retrospective study on over 100 patients addressing medial laxity in MCWHTO concluded that medial reefing should be performed only in selected cases, when MCL laxity is confirmed intraoperatively [56].

In contrast, the LOWHTO provides a familiar exposure and instability can be corrected by tightening of lateral ligamentous structures, without affecting the medial stabilisers of the knee [50]. Up to 88% had good/excellent results and the non-union rate was 0% [50]. Whilst transient peroneal nerve palsies are reported [50, 57, 58], if the need for fibula osteotomy is negated, this rate can be reduced significantly [33] with the maintenance of improvements in patient-reported outcomes, and radiographic and gait improvements. It is therefore recommended that LOWHTO is a valid treatment option when the deformity is within the parameters suggested by Coventry [26], and the deformity is localised to the tibia [50]. The research would suggest that a fibular osteotomy should be considered in larger deformities with the acceptance of the recognised transient peroneal nerve palsy risk. Each tibial osteotomy therefore has its own pros and cons. Which surgical option to undertake will likely depend on surgeon preference, experience and consideration of the associated risks and complications.

Whilst generic surgical complications will not be discussed here, many surgical complications are specific to both tibial and femoral osteotomies. Intraoperative fracture [13, 19, 39] through uncontrolled propagation of the osteotomy can be prevented by ensuring the accurate pin placement and leaving an appropriately sized bone hinge before starting the osteotomy. Hardware intolerance is common, and timely removal is recommended. The deep vein thrombosis risk has been found to be similar to that of knee joint arthroplasty [8], with the highest incidence being within the first 3–4 days [76]. As a result, a thromboprophylaxis protocol similar to knee arthroplasty is recommended.

Post-operative treatment is variable and highly surgeon dependant. For closing-wedge osteotomies, regardless of the fixation method, research suggests that weight bearing is restricted (either PWB or TTWB) for 6–8 weeks based on callus formation on X-rays [17, 31]; however many surgeons would keep patients NWB for this period [17, 35, 36, 49, 59]. The majority agree that the knee should be immobilised in a functional brace with an unlimited range of motion (ROM) for this period; however we have not used a brace since adopting locked plates and have no complications from stopping brace use. Thereafter, either FWB or PWB can be introduced depending on surgical preference. In relation to opening-wedge osteotomies, the use of a functional ROM brace is again advised for the initial 4–6-week period. The weight-bearing status during this period is again controversial. Whilst older studies suggested NWB for 4–6 weeks [38, 40, 48] more recent research has suggested that TTWB or even FWB immediately post-operatively has no adverse outcomes [29, 33, 39, 73]. The latter two studies were noted to use the TomoFix® (Synthes) implant; therefore outcomes with other implants and immediate FWB require further research. It is likely however that with the use of such implants, post-operative WB status can be increased without detrimental effect and improve patient acceptance.

Osteotomy for the correction of the valgus knee therefore remains a good surgical option for the correct patient. Whilst no clear superiority exists between surgical techniques, the choice between tibial and femoral osteotomy should be based on the aetiology of the lateral compartment OA. It is our opinion that if the patient has OA secondary to lateral meniscal loss the arthritis will be posterior not distal; thus a tibial osteotomy will unload this arthritic area whilst a distal femoral osteotomy will not. Another important factor is the correction required. If the angle of correction combined with the tibial mechanical axis is greater than 10° the resultant increase in tibial mechanical axis introduces the risk of joint subluxation. Therefore, if the combined correction angle is greater than 10° or the patient has congenital genu valgum with distal chondral loss a DFVO is recommended.

References

1. Sharma L, et al. The role of knee alignment in disease progression and functional decline in knee osteoarthritis. JAMA. 2001;286(2):188–95.
2. Puddu G, et al. Which osteotomy for a valgus knee? Int Orthop. 2010;34(2):239–47.
3. Scott CE, et al. Predicting dissatisfaction following total knee replacement: a prospective study of 1217 patients. J Bone Joint Surg Br. 2010;92(9):1253–8.
4. Scott CE, et al. Predicting dissatisfaction following total knee arthroplasty in patients under 55 years of age. Bone Joint J. 2016;98-b(12):1625–34.
5. Noble PC, et al. Does total knee replacement restore normal knee function? Clin Orthop Relat Res. 2005;431:157–65.
6. Association, N.Z.O. The New Zealand Joint Registry. 2019.
7. Wylie JD, et al. Distal femoral osteotomy for the valgus knee: medial closing wedge versus lateral opening wedge: a systematic review. Arthroscopy. 2016;32(10):2141–7.
8. Rosso F, Margheritini F. Distal femoral osteotomy. Curr Rev Musculoskelet Med. 2014;7(4):302–11.
9. Felson DT, et al. Valgus malalignment is a risk factor for lateral knee osteoarthritis incidence and progression: findings from the multicenter osteoarthritis study and the osteoarthritis initiative. Arthritis Rheum. 2013;65(2):355–62.
10. Duivenvoorden T, et al. Comparison of closing-wedge and opening-wedge high tibial osteotomy for medial compartment osteoarthritis of the knee: a randomized controlled trial with a six-year follow-up. J Bone Joint Surg Am. 2014;96(17):1425–32.
11. Lu J, et al. Clinical outcomes of closing- and opening-wedge high tibial osteotomy for treatment of anteromedial unicompartmental knee osteoarthritis. J Knee Surg. 2019;32(8):758–63.
12. Bonasia DE, et al. Medial opening wedge high tibial osteotomy for medial compartment overload/arthritis in the varus knee: prognostic factors. Am J Sports Med. 2014;42(3):690–8.
13. Olivero M, et al. Femoral osteotomies for the valgus knee. Ann Joint. 2017;2(6)
14. Ozcan C, et al. Prospective comparative study of two methods for fixation after distal femur corrective osteotomy for valgus deformity; retrograde intramedullary nailing versus less invasive stabilization system plating. Int Orthop. 2016;40(10):2121–6.
15. Youm Y-S, et al. Bilateral hypoplasia of the medial and lateral menisci. Knee Surg Relat Res. 2017;29(2):150–2.
16. O'Malley MP, et al. Distal femoral osteotomy: lateral opening wedge technique. Arthrosc Tech. 2016;5(4):e725–30.
17. Tírico LEP, et al. Medial closing-wedge distal femoral osteotomy: fixation with proximal tibial locking plate. Arthrosc Tech. 2015;4(6):e687–95.
18. Zarrouk A, et al. Distal femoral varus osteotomy outcome: is associated femoropatellar osteoarthritis consequential? Orthop Traumatol Surg Res. 2010;96(6):632–6.
19. Kim YC, et al. Distal femoral varus osteotomy for valgus arthritis of the knees: systematic review of open versus closed wedge osteotomy. Knee Surg Relat Res. 2018;30(1):3–16.
20. Mitchell JJ, et al. Varus-producing lateral distal femoral opening-wedge osteotomy. Arthrosc Tech. 2016;5(4):e799–807.
21. Bonasia DE, et al. Opening wedge high tibial osteotomy and anterior cruciate ligament reconstruction or revision. Arthrosc Tech. 2017;6(5):e1735–41.
22. Willey M, et al. Complications associated with realignment osteotomy of the knee performed simultaneously with additional reconstructive procedures. Iowa Orthop J. 2010;30:55–60.
23. Dejour H, et al. Anterior cruciate reconstruction combined with valgus tibial osteotomy. Clin Orthop Relat Res. 1994;299:220–8.
24. Herman BV, Giffin JR. High tibial osteotomy in the ACL-deficient knee with medial compartment osteoarthritis. J Orthop Traumatol. 2016;17(3):277–85.
25. Lattermann C, Jakob RP. High tibial osteotomy alone or combined with ligament reconstruction in anterior cruciate ligament-deficient knees. Knee Surg Sports Traumatol Arthrosc. 1996;4(1):32–8.
26. Coventry MB. Proximal tibial varus osteotomy for osteoarthritis of the lateral compartment of the knee. J Bone Joint Surg Am. 1987;69(1):32–8.
27. Floerkemeier S, et al. Does obesity and nicotine abuse influence the outcome and complication rate after open-wedge high tibial osteotomy? A retrospective evaluation of five hundred and thirty-three patients. Int Orthop. 2014;38(1):55–60.
28. Dugdale TW, Noyes FR, Styer D. Preoperative planning for high tibial osteotomy. The effect of lateral tibiofemoral separation and tibiofemoral length. Clin Orthop Relat Res. 1992;274:248–64.
29. Saithna A, et al. Opening wedge distal femoral varus osteotomy for lateral compartment osteoarthritis in the valgus knee. Knee. 2014;21(1):172–5.

30. Quirno M, et al. Distal femoral varus osteotomy for unloading valgus knee malalignment: a biomechanical analysis. Knee Surg Sports Traumatol Arthrosc. 2017;25(3):863–8.
31. Forkel P, et al. Midterm results following medial closed wedge distal femoral osteotomy stabilized with a locking internal fixation device. Knee Surg Sports Traumatol Arthrosc. 2015;23(7):2061–7.
32. Shoji H, Insall J. High tibial osteotomy for osteoarthritis of the knee with valgus deformity. JBJS. 1973;55(5):963–73.
33. Collins B, et al. A case series of lateral opening wedge high tibial osteotomy for valgus malalignment. Knee Surg Sports Traumatol Arthrosc. 2013;21(1):152–60.
34. Sternheim A, Garbedian S, Backstein D. Distal femoral varus osteotomy: unloading the lateral compartment: long-term follow-up of 45 medial closing wedge osteotomies. Orthopedics. 2011;34(9):e488–90.
35. Finkelstein JA, Gross AE, Davis A. Varus osteotomy of the distal part of the femur. A survivorship analysis. J Bone Joint Surg Am. 1996;78(9):1348–52.
36. Backstein D, et al. Long-term follow-up of distal femoral varus osteotomy of the knee. J Arthroplast. 2007;22(4 Suppl 1):2–6.
37. Chahla J, et al. Opening- and closing-wedge distal femoral osteotomy: a systematic review of outcomes for isolated lateral compartment osteoarthritis. Orthop J Sports Med. 2016;4(6):2325967116649901.
38. Dewilde TR, et al. Opening wedge distal femoral varus osteotomy using the Puddu plate and calcium phosphate bone cement. Knee Surg Sports Traumatol Arthrosc. 2013;21(1):249–54.
39. Ekeland A, et al. Good functional results of distal femoral opening-wedge osteotomy of knees with lateral osteoarthritis. Knee Surg Sports Traumatol Arthrosc. 2016;24(5):1702–9.
40. Andrade MAPD, et al. Distal femoral varusing for osteoarthritis of valgus knee: a long-term follow-up. Rev Brasil Ortopedia. 2015;44(4):346–50.
41. Lash NJ, et al. Bone grafts and bone substitutes for opening-wedge osteotomies of the knee: a systematic review. Arthroscopy. 2015;31(4):720–30.
42. Mathews J, et al. Distal femoral osteotomy for lateral compartment osteoarthritis of the knee. Orthopedics. 1998;21(4):437–40.
43. Staubli AE, et al. TomoFix: a new LCP-concept for open wedge osteotomy of the medial proximal tibia-early results in 92 cases. Injury. 2003;34(Suppl 2):B55–62.
44. Elattar O, et al. Open wedge distal femoral osteotomy: accuracy of correction and patient outcomes. HSS J. 2017;13(2):128–35.
45. Jacobi M, et al. Distal femoral varus osteotomy: problems associated with the lateral open-wedge technique. Arch Orthop Trauma Surg. 2011;131(6):725–8.
46. Rutz E, et al. Distal femoral osteotomy using the LCP pediatric condylar 90-degree plate in patients with neuromuscular disorders. J Pediatr Orthop. 2012;32(3):295–300.
47. Brinkman JM, et al. Axial and torsional stability of an improved single-plane and a new bi-plane osteotomy technique for supracondylar femur osteotomies. Knee Surg Sports Traumatol Arthrosc. 2011;19(7):1090–8.
48. Haviv B, et al. The results of corrective osteotomy for valgus arthritic knees. Knee Surg Sports Traumatol Arthrosc. 2013;21(1):49–56.
49. Sherman C, Cabanela ME. Closing wedge osteotomy of the tibia and the femur in the treatment of gonarthrosis. Int Orthop. 2010;34(2):173–84.
50. Marti RK, et al. Proximal tibial varus osteotomy: indications, technique, and five to twenty-one-year results. JBJS. 2001;83(2):164.
51. Chambat P, Selmi T, Du Jour D, Denoyers J. Varus tibial osteotomy. Oper Tech Sports Med. 2000;8:44–7.
52. Mirouse G, et al. Failure of high tibial varus osteotomy for lateral tibio-femoral osteoarthritis with <10 degrees of valgus: outcomes in 19 patients. Orthop Traumatol Surg Res. 2017;103(6):953–8.
53. van Egmond N, et al. Gait analysis before and after corrective osteotomy in patients with knee osteoarthritis and a valgus deformity. Knee Surg Sports Traumatol Arthrosc. 2017;25(9):2904–13.
54. van Lieshout WAM, et al. Medial collateral ligament laxity in valgus knee deformity before and after medial closing wedge high tibial osteotomy measured with instrumented laxity measurements and patient reported outcome. J Exp Orthop. 2018;5(1):49.
55. Coventry MB. Upper tibial osteotomy for osteoarthritis. J Bone Joint Surg Am. 1985;67(7):1136–40.
56. van Lieshout WAM, et al. Medial closing wedge high tibial osteotomy for valgus tibial deformities: good clinical results and survival with a mean 4.5 years of follow-up in 113 patients. Knee Surg Sports Traumatol Arthrosc. 2020;28(9):2798–807.
57. Bettin D, et al. Time-dependent clinical and roentgenographical results of Coventry high tibial valgisation osteotomy. Arch Orthop Trauma Surg. 1998;117(1–2):53–7.
58. Takahashi T, et al. Dome-shaped proximal tibial osteotomy using percutaneous drilling for osteoarthritis of the knee. Arch Orthop Trauma Surg. 2000;120(1–2):32–7.
59. McDermott AG, et al. Distal femoral varus osteotomy for valgus deformity of the knee. J Bone Joint Surg Am. 1988;70(1):110–6.
60. Healy WL, et al. Distal femoral varus osteotomy. J Bone Joint Surg Am. 1988;70(1):102–9.
61. Learmonth ID. A simple technique for varus supracondylar osteotomy in genu valgum. J Bone Joint Surg Br. 1990;72(2):235–7.
62. Kyung HS, et al. Biplanar open wedge high tibial osteotomy in the medial compartment osteoarthritis of the knee joint: comparison between the Aescula and TomoFix plate. Clin Orthop Surg. 2015;7(2):185–90.
63. DepuySynthes A. Comprehensive Plating System for Stable Fixation of Osteotomies Around the Knee TOMOFIX® Osteotomy System Surgical Technique.
64. Rodner CM, et al. Medial opening wedge tibial osteotomy and the sagittal plane: the effect of increasing

tibial slope on tibiofemoral contact pressure. Am J Sports Med. 2006;34(9):1431–41.

65. Akamatsu Y, et al. Usefulness of long tibial axis to measure medial tibial slope for opening wedge high tibial osteotomy. Knee Surg Sports Traumatol Arthrosc. 2016;24(11):3661–7.

66. Song EK, Seon JK, Park SJ. How to avoid unintended increase of posterior slope in navigation-assisted open-wedge high tibial osteotomy. Orthopedics. 2007;30(10 Suppl):S127–31.

67. Munier M, et al. Can three-dimensional patient-specific cutting guides be used to achieve optimal correction for high tibial osteotomy? Pilot study. Orthop Traumatol Surg Res. 2017;103(2):245–50.

68. Victor J, Premanathan A. Virtual 3D planning and patient specific surgical guides for osteotomies around the knee. Bone Joint J. 2013;95-B(11_Supple_A):153–8.

69. Donnez M, et al. Are three-dimensional patient-specific cutting guides for open wedge high tibial osteotomy accurate? An in vitro study. J Orthop Surg Res. 2018;13(1):171.

70. NewClip lateral opening wedge distal femoral osteotomy using patient specific cutting guide. 2018.

71. Jacquet C, et al. More accurate correction using "patient-specific" cutting guides in opening wedge distal femur varization osteotomies. Int Orthop. 2019;43(10):2285–91.

72. Menetrey J, Duthon V, Fritschy D. Computer-assisted open-wedge high tibial osteotomy. Oper Tech Orthop. 2008;18(3):210–4.

73. Brinkman J-M, et al. Early full weight bearing is safe in open-wedge high tibial osteotomy. Acta Orthop. 2010;81(2):193–8.

74. Kim J, Allaire R, Harner CD. Vascular safety during high tibial osteotomy: a cadaveric angiographic study. Am J Sports Med. 2010;38(4):810–5.

75. Goshima K, et al. Plate removal without loss of correction after open-wedge high tibial osteotomy is possible when posterior cortex bone union reaches osteotomy gap center even in incompletely filled gaps. Knee Surg Sports Traumatol Arthrosc. 2019;28(6):1827–34.

76. Vena G, D'Adamio S, Amendola A. Complications of osteotomies about the knee. Sports Med Arthrosc Rev. 2013;21(2):113–20.

77. Tunggal JAW, Higgins GA, Waddell JP. Complications of closing wedge high tibial osteotomy. Int Orthop. 2010;34(2):255–61.

78. Anagnostakos K, Mosser P, Kohn D. Infections after high tibial osteotomy. Knee Surg Sports Traumatol Arthrosc. 2013;21(1):161–9.

79. Smith TO, et al. Opening- or closing-wedged high tibial osteotomy: a meta-analysis of clinical and radiological outcomes. Knee. 2011;18(6):361–8.

80. Reischl N, et al. Infections after high tibial open wedge osteotomy: a case control study. Arch Orthop Trauma Surg. 2009;129(11):1483–7.

81. Geiger F, et al. External fixation in proximal tibial osteotomy: a comparison of three methods. Int Orthop. 1999;23(3):160–3.

82. Niinimäki TT, et al. Incidence of osteotomies around the knee for the treatment of knee osteoarthritis: a 22-year population-based study. Int Orthop. 2012;36(7):1399–402.

83. Mont MA, et al. Different surgical options for mono-compartmental osteoarthritis of the knee: high tibial osteotomy versus unicompartmental knee arthroplasty versus total knee arthroplasty: indications, techniques, results, and controversies. Instr Course Lect. 2004;53:265–83.

84. Nwachukwu BU, et al. Unicompartmental knee arthroplasty versus high tibial osteotomy: United States practice patterns for the surgical treatment of unicompartmental arthritis. J Arthroplast. 2014;29(8):1586–9.

85. Kurtz S, et al. Prevalence of primary and revision total hip and knee arthroplasty in the United States from 1990 through 2002. J Bone Joint Surg Am. 2005;87(7):1487–97.

86. Evans JT, et al. How long does a knee replacement last? A systematic review and meta-analysis of case series and national registry reports with more than 15 years of follow-up. Lancet. 2019;393(10172):655–63.

87. Julin J, et al. Younger age increases the risk of early prosthesis failure following primary total knee replacement for osteoarthritis. A follow-up study of 32,019 total knee replacements in the Finnish arthroplasty register. Acta Orthop. 2010;81(4):413–9.

88. Jorgensen NB, et al. Major aseptic revision following total knee replacement: a study of 478,081 total knee replacements from the Australian Orthopaedic Association National Joint Replacement Registry. J Bone Joint Surg Am. 2019;101(4):302–10.

89. Association, A.O. Australian Orthopaedic Association National Joint Replacement Registry. Australian Orthopaedic Association; 2019.

90. Koskinen E, et al. Unicondylar knee replacement for primary osteoarthritis: a prospective follow-up study of 1,819 patients from the Finnish Arthroplasty Register. Acta Orthop. 2007;78(1):128–35.

91. Edgerton BC, Mariani EM, Morrey BF. Distal femoral varus osteotomy for painful genu valgum. A five-to-11-year follow-up study. Clin Orthop Relat Res. 1993;288:263–9.

92. Georgoulis AD, et al. Nerve and vessel injuries during high tibial osteotomy combined with distal fibular osteotomy: a clinically relevant anatomic study. Knee Surg Sports Traumatol Arthrosc. 1999;7(1):15–9.

Role of the Meniscus in Cartilage Injury: Basic Science

11

Bhargavi Maheshwer, Brady T. Williams,
Evan M. Polce, Robert F. LaPrade,
and Jorge Chahla

11.1 Introduction

In the United States, approximately one half of all adults will experience knee pain at some point during their lifetimes, with the majority of these cases stemming from underlying osteoarthritis (OA) [1, 2]. One of the most common factors contributing to the progression of knee OA are tears of the meniscus [3]. If left untreated, meniscal tears can often lead to articular cartilage degeneration and functional impairment [4, 5]. During load bearing, the native menisci are capable of transforming axial forces into "hoop" stresses along the circumferential fibers of the menisci, effectively increasing the total contact area, while decreasing focal loading. The menisci also serve as biological shock absorbers to mitigate impact stresses and protect the tibial and femoral articular cartilage from damage [6]. Furthermore, the medial and lateral menisci provide support against anterior-posterior translation and internal-external rotation for joint stability [4].

Historically, meniscal tears were often treated with partial or total meniscectomy with the goal of achieving short-term benefits; however, recent literature has resulted in a renewed focus on the benefit of meniscal repair techniques and interventions. Studies with long-term follow-up indicate that meniscal repairs result in reduced rates of osteoarthritis and reoperations as well as higher functional patient-reported outcome scores relative to meniscectomy [7, 8]. As such, preservation of native meniscal structure and function when possible is critical for future joint health and functionality.

The purpose of this chapter is to describe the [1] pertinent anatomy of the menisci with a focus on the anatomic root attachments; [2] microstructure and embryology of meniscal tissue; and [3] in vivo biomechanics and biomechanical properties of meniscal tissue.

11.2 Anatomy

The medial and lateral menisci are crescent-shaped wedges that function as shock absorbers and load distributors in the knee joint. The wedge shape of the menisci allows for maximum space filling between the convex and flat surfaces of the femoral and tibial condyles, respectively, which increases contact areas and decreases axial stress during load bearing [9]. At the periphery, the outermost third (referred to as the red zone)

B. Maheshwer · B. T. Williams · E. M. Polce
J. Chahla (✉)
Midwest Orthopedics at Rush, Rush University
Medical Center, Chicago, IL, USA
e-mail: jorge.chahla@rushortho.com

R. F. LaPrade
Twin Cities Orthopedics, Edina, MN, USA

© ISAKOS 2021
A. J. Krych et al. (eds.), *Cartilage Injury of the Knee*,
https://doi.org/10.1007/978-3-030-78051-7_11

constitutes the vascularized portion of the menisci, whereas the innermost third (referred to as the white zone) represents the avascular region. The menisci are securely anchored to the anterior and posterior aspects of the tibia by their respective root attachments.

The medial meniscus is composed of semilunar fibrocartilage and is located at the junction of the medial femoral condyle and medial tibial plateau (Fig. 11.1). With an average width of 9–10 mm and average thickness of 3–5 mm [10], the medial meniscus constitutes up to 60% of the articular surface of the medial tibial condyle and is crucial for distributing weight-bearing loads in the medial compartment of the knee. Relative to the lateral meniscus, the medial meniscus is more rigidly held in place with stabilizing attachments to nearby structures, including the medial collateral ligament (MCL) and posteromedial capsule.

In contrast, the lateral meniscus is an oblong, circular shape that measures slightly larger than the medial meniscus on average at 10–12 mm wide and 4–5 mm thick (Fig. 11.1). Consequently, the lateral meniscus covers a greater percentage of the articular surface relative to the medial meniscus and distributes up to 70% of the load bearing on the lateral compartment of the knee [11]. The lateral meniscus is separated from the fibular collateral ligament (FCL) laterally by the popliteus tendon.

The structural integrity and stability of the menisci are supplemented by various secondary attachments. The medial and lateral menisci are connected anteriorly by a fibrous band of tissue referred to as the anterior intermeniscal ligament. The coronary ligaments function to connect the meniscotibial capsular margins of the menisci to the tibia. The decreased mobility of the medial meniscus may be explained in part by these coronary ligaments, which more strongly anchor the medial meniscus compared to the lateral meniscus to the tibia. Finally, the meniscofemoral ligaments (MFLs) originate from the posterior horn of the lateral meniscus and insert on the lateral side of the medial femoral condyle (Fig. 11.2) [12]. The MFLs function as stabilizers of the lateral meniscus and are comprised of two distinct structures: the ligaments of Humphrey and Wrisberg (Fig. 11.2), which flank the posterior cruciate ligament (PCL) on the anterior and posterior aspects, respectively. The incidence of the MFLs is variable in the literature. Anatomical evidence has suggested that both MFLs are present in 46% of cadaver specimens with the incidence of single Humphrey and Wrisberg ligaments reported at 23% and 31%, respectively [13].

The negative consequences of impaired meniscal root function on joint pressures and

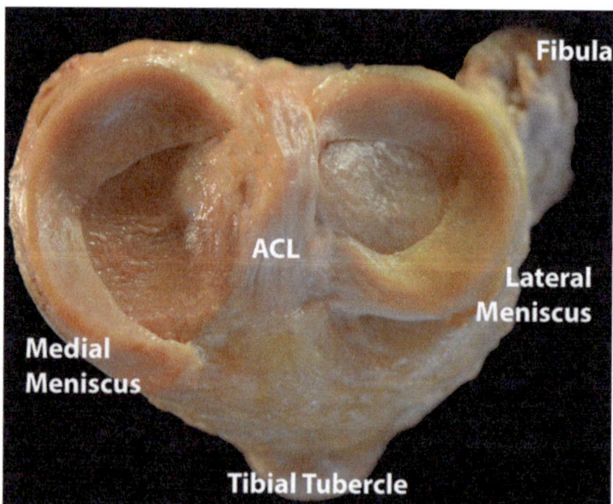

Fig. 11.1 Axial view of cadaveric right knee illustrating the anatomy of the medial meniscus and lateral meniscus in relation to the anterior cruciate ligament (ACL), tibial tubercle, and fibula

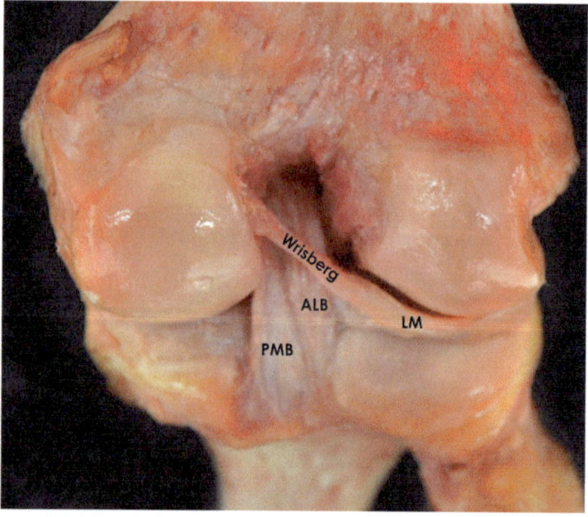

Fig. 11.2 Anterior view of cadaveric right knee demonstrating the ligament of Wrisberg originating from the posterior horn of the lateral meniscus (LM). Also pictured are the anterolateral bundle (ALB) and posteromedial bundle (PMB)

kinematics have been well documented in the literature. Allaire et al. [14] demonstrated that a medial meniscus posterior root (MPR) tear resulted in a 25% increase in peak contact pressure relative to the native intact state. LaPrade et al. [15] reported that lateral meniscus posterior root (LPR) tears or radial tears adjacent to the lateral meniscus posterior root attachment (LPRA) site caused significantly increased contact pressures and decreased contact area in the lateral compartment. Ellman et al. [16] investigated several biomechanical properties of the four meniscal roots and demonstrated that both the dense, central fibers and peripheral, supplementary fibers contribute to the structural integrity of the meniscal roots. The authors found that the native (i.e., central and supplementary fibers intact) anterior medial, posterior medial, and posterior lateral roots had significantly larger attachment areas, stiffness, and ultimate failure strength compared to the sectioned roots (meniscal roots with central roots intact but all supplementary fibers dissected). The findings of these and similar studies corroborate the notion that complete root tears impair the ability of the menisci to withstand tibiofemoral loads and distribute hoop stresses [14, 15, 17]. Accordingly, complete root tear knee states are thought to be functionally equivalent to a total meniscectomy and often progress rapidly to degenerative states of osteoarthritis [18].

One of the keys for a surgeon to successfully and safely perform meniscal root repairs is a comprehensive knowledge of the anatomical landmarks and precise attachment locations of the four roots. Johannsen et al. [19] quantitatively described the location of the MPRA and LPRA attachment sites in relation to anatomical landmarks in the joint. The authors demonstrated that the MPRA attachment can be reproducibly found 9.6 mm posterior and 0.7 mm lateral to the medial tibial eminence (MTE) apex (Fig. 11.3). Two secondary landmarks for identifying the MPRA include the medial articular cartilage inflection point (3.5 mm medial in relation to the MPRA) and the tibial attachment

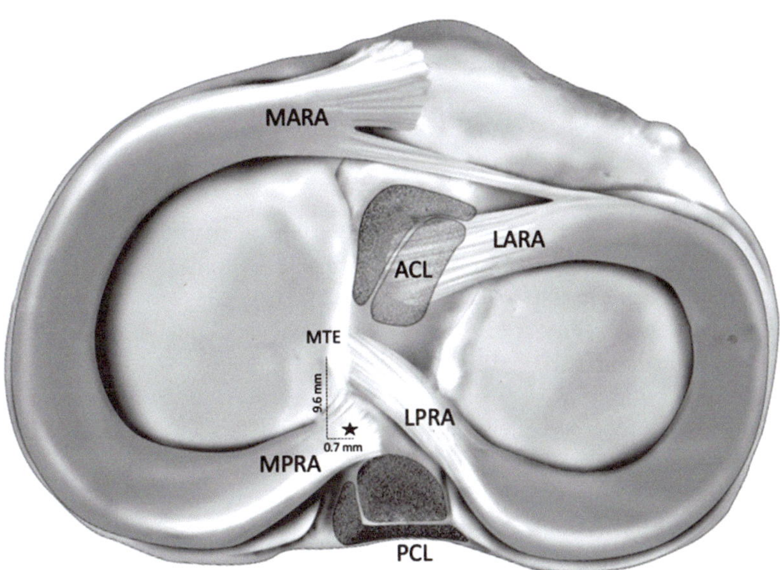

Fig. 11.3 Superior axial view of the pertinent anatomical landmarks used to identify the medial meniscus posterior root (MPRA) attachment site. *ACL* anterior cruciate ligament, *LARA* lateral meniscus anterior root attachment, *LPRA* lateral meniscus posterior root attachment, *MARA* medial meniscus anterior root attachment, *MTE* medial tibial eminence, *PCL* posterior cruciate ligament. 1. Aman ZS, DePhillipo NN, Storaci HW, et al. Quantitative and Qualitative Assessment of Posterolateral Meniscal Anatomy: Defining the Popliteal Hiatus, Popliteomeniscal Fascicles, and the Lateral Meniscotibial Ligament. The American Journal of Sports Medicine. 2019;47(8):1797–1803. https://doi.org/10.1177/0363546519849933

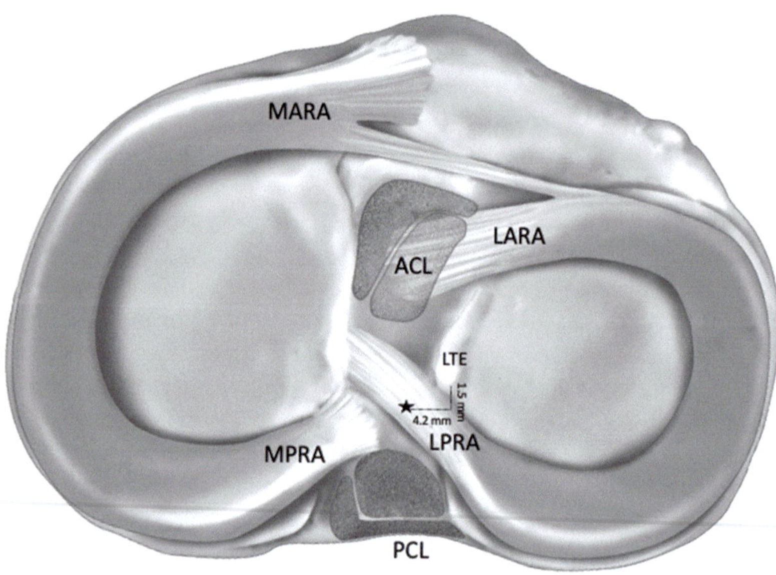

Fig. 11.4 Superior axial view of the pertinent anatomical landmarks used to identify the lateral meniscus posterior root (LPRA) attachment site. *ACL* anterior cruciate ligament, *LARA* lateral meniscus anterior root attachment, *MARA* medial meniscus anterior root attachment, *MPRA* medial meniscus posterior root attachment, *MTE* medial tibial eminence, *PCL* posterior cruciate ligament. 1. Aman ZS, DePhillipo NN, Storaci HW, et al. Quantitative and Qualitative Assessment of Posterolateral Meniscal Anatomy: Defining the Popliteal Hiatus, Popliteomeniscal Fascicles, and the Lateral Meniscotibial Ligament. The American Journal of Sports Medicine. 2019;47(8):1797–1803. https://doi.org/10.1177/0363546519849933

margin of the PCL (8.2 mm posterolateral in relation to the MPRA).

The osseous landmark consistently used to identify the LPRA was the lateral tibial eminence (LTE) (Fig. 11.4). When split into its directional components based on the anatomical axes of the knee, the LPRA was 4.2 mm medial and 1.5 mm posterior to the LTE. Other reliable anatomical landmarks for identifying the center of the LPRA include the nearest articular cartilage margin of the lateral tibial plateau (4.3 mm lateral in relation to the LPRA) and the most proximal margin of PCL tibial attachment (12.7 mm posteromedial in relation to the LPRA).

Similarly, LaPrade et al. [20] described the location of the medial meniscus anterior root attachment (MARA) and lateral meniscus anterior root attachment (LARA) relative to anatomical and arthroscopic landmarks. The tibial tuberosity and medial tibial eminence were found to be 27.0 mm lateral and distal and 27.5 mm posterior to the central MARA site. The central points of the anterior cruciate ligament (ACL) and lateral tibial eminence were found to be 5.0 mm posteromedial and 14.4 mm posterolateral to the central LARA site. It is important for surgeons to understand and recognize the anatomical location of the meniscal root attachments because previous literature has demonstrated the risk of iatrogenic root tears due to malposition of tibial tunnels during ACL [21–23] and PCL [24] reconstruction.

11.3 Embryology

Early during fetal development, normal menisci differentiate within the limb bud from mesenchymal tissue [25]. Normal menisci are defined during the eighth week of gestation and mature into their anatomic shape by week 14 [26]. As menisci mature, their peripheral blood supply recedes and the central third of the meniscus is avascular by 9 months of life. Clark and Ogden examined medial and lateral menisci from 109 fetuses ranging from 14 to 34 weeks' gestation and menisci from cadavers whose postnatal ages ranged from 3 months to 14 years old. They observed changes in the menisci that accommodated changes in the tibiofemoral contact areas. Additionally, the lateral meniscus tended to have more developmental variation. Throughout meniscal growth, the ratios of the area of each meniscus to the area of the corresponding tibial plateau and area of medial meniscus to lateral meniscus were fairly consistent, implying that there is relatively uniform growth of the menisci.

11.3.1 Congenital Malformations of the Meniscus

Congenital malformations of the meniscus are rare; however, one of the most studied disorders includes congenital discoid meniscus. There are many patients who have congenital discoid menisci and are asymptomatic; however, the reported incidence of discoid meniscus ranges from 0.4% to 17% for the lateral meniscus and 0.1% to 0.3% for the medial meniscus [27–30]. Discoid lateral menisci are most common in the Japanese population with an approximately 15% prevalence [31]. However, the true incidence and prevalence of discoid menisci are likely not known due to the many asymptomatic cases that are only diagnosed intraoperatively [32]. Regarding etiology, it has been supported by case reports that the discoid meniscus is an anatomical variant and suggests that increased shear stress causes meniscocapsular separation and secondary hypermobility [25].

The clinical presentation of discoid meniscus varies depending on the type of discoid meniscus, location, and presence of associated meniscal tear [25, 32, 33]. If a discoid meniscus is stable, it can be asymptomatic and only found incidentally. The most common tear pattern associated with discoid meniscus is a degenerative horizontal cleavage tear [32, 33]. An unstable discoid meniscus produces the characteristic "snapping knee." This is defined as an audible snap on terminal extension along with pain, swelling, and locking of the knee

in the absence of trauma. These snaps often occur spontaneously as the knee moves from flexion into extension, causing temporary pain and apprehension [32]. The snapping is usually asymptomatic in young children (ages 3–4 years old), versus in older children who may experience pain with activity. A lateral joint-line bulge may be present on physical exam, and a large "clunk" may be elicited with a McMurray's test due to subluxation of the unstable lateral meniscus [32]. It is important to examine both knees equally in patients suspected to have a discoid meniscus, as it can occasionally it can sometimes present bilaterally.

In contrast, stable discoid menisci have more variable presentations and often present in older children who have mechanical knee symptoms suggestive of a meniscal tear [32]. Stable discoid menisci are more susceptible to tearing because of their increased thickness and abnormal vascularity [26].

There have been many classification systems described for a discoid meniscus [31, 34, 35], but the most commonly used classification method was described by Watanabe and colleagues [36]. Three major meniscal abnormalities were described based on the arthroscopic appearance. Type I discoid meniscus is a complete disc-shaped meniscus and the tibial plateau is covered with a thin center. Type II is an incomplete, semilunar shaped meniscus with partial coverage of the tibial plateau. Type I and type II discoid menisci generally have normal peripheral attachments and are stable to probing [32]. Type III is described as a hypermobile meniscus due to deficient posterior tibial attachments, consequently producing the common "snapping knee" syndrome. It appears to be a normal meniscus except for a thickened posterior horn and a lack of posterior meniscocapsular attachments (including the meniscotibial ligament) [32].

11.4 Microstructure

The meniscus is composed of roughly 70% water and 30% organic matter [37]. The water contained in the meniscal tissue is greater in the posterior areas compared to the central and anterior portions of the meniscus [38]. The organic matter is comprised of 75% collagen, while the remainder consists of non-collagenous proteins [39, 40]. Overall, type I collagen fibers provide the primary structural framework of the meniscus. Three collagen fiber layers are arranged specifically in a superficial to deep manner to convert compressive loads into circumferential stresses [37]. In the superficial layer, collagen fibers course radially in order to resist shearing forces. In the middle layer, collagen fibers run parallel to the contour of the meniscus to resist circumferential stress during weight bearing. The deep layer of collagen is aligned in parallel to the periphery of the meniscus [37].

11.4.1 Histology

Histologically, the meniscus has been studied in great detail. Chevrier et al. analyzed the meniscus structure in humans, sheep, and rabbit [41]. In the human meniscus, blood vessels were only found in the outer portion of the meniscal body. The distribution of various types of collagen was also evaluated. Collagen I was present throughout the matrix of most human menisci, and collagen II was detected in the inner main body of menisci. Collagen VI was found throughout the meniscus as well as the adipose-rich tissue in the periphery of the meniscus. On a cellular level, the meniscus includes fibrochondrocytes distributed through the extracellular matrix [37]. Fibrochondrocytes create and maintain the extracellular matrix, thus exhibiting properties of both chondrocytes and fibroblasts [42].

Proteoglycans are another component of the meniscus microstructure located within the collagen fibrils. Proteoglycans are large hydrophilic molecules contributing 1–2% of the dry weight of the meniscus [43]. Within the extracellular matrix, proteoglycans are responsible for hydration and provide the tissue with the ability to resist compressive loads [44]. This is largely attributed to proteoglycans' specialized structure, charge-charge repulsion forces, and high charge density. The major proteoglycan found in human

menisci is aggrecan, which is responsible for the meniscus' viscoelastic compressive properties [44]. Other smaller proteoglycans include fibromodulin, biglycan, and decorin [45, 46]. The precise function of these smaller proteoglycans within the meniscus is not clear.

The meniscal cartilage contains a wide range of matrix glycoproteins. The functions of these molecules are still being investigated. A subgroup of the matrix glycoproteins are the adhesive glycoproteins. These molecules are in part responsible for binding with other matrix molecules [44].

11.4.2 Response to Injury

The meniscal vascular response to injury has been extensively studied in various animal models. Arnoczky et al. analyzed the normal vascular anatomy of menisci in a canine model [47]. Two weeks following complete transverse sectioning of the medial meniscus, the small gap formed between the anterior and posterior meniscal segments was filled with an organized fibrin clot. Vessels from the perimeniscal capillary plexus proliferated through the fibrin scaffold, and proliferation of mesenchymal cells was also observed [47]. Such proliferation continued until 6 weeks post-transection, at which time the gap between the meniscal segments was entirely filled by fibrovascular scar tissue. A vascular pannus was also visualized over the fibrovascular scar, appearing to be a proliferation of the synovium adjacent to the lesion. Vessels from the synovial proliferation extended over both the tibial and femoral articular surfaces and penetrated the scar to anastomose with vessels from the perimeniscal capillary plexus. By 10 weeks post-resection, the scar remodeled to depict a normal meniscal contour. The vascular proliferation from adjacent soft tissues within the knee joint seems vital to the reparative response of the meniscus [47].

Arnoczky et al. also evaluated the healing of a longitudinal meniscal lesion by creating a vascular access channel [47]. Two weeks after creating a vascular access channel to connect the longitudinal incision (located within the avascular portion of the meniscus) to the vascular meniscal tissues, a fibrin clot formed and extended throughout a majority of the incision. Similarly seen in the transverse lesion, the perimeniscal capillary vessels proliferated into the clot and synovial fringe extended over the vascular access channel. By 4 weeks, the fibrovascular scar tissue was seen proliferating within the longitudinal lesion. The synovial fringe remained limited to the area over the vascular access channel. The importance of a vascular access channel was emphasized after no healing was observed in those menisci with a longitudinal incision and no vascular access channel.

11.4.3 Stages of Healing

Meniscal healing is thought to be dependent on an adequate blood supply [48]. The biological limitations of meniscal healing were discovered in 1936 [49]. In this study examining canine menisci, King demonstrated that meniscal lesions could heal spontaneously as long as the lesion communicated with peripheral synovial blood supply. He also found that isolated lesions within the avascular portion of the meniscus failed to heal. The potential roles for blood flow in the meniscal healing process include the delivery of nutrients and oxygen, the infiltration of the affected site with cells pertinent to tissue repair (neutrophils, macrophages, and lymphocytes), and the formation of blood clots and release of tissue remodeling mediators [48].

Bray et al. performed a study on adult rabbits to investigate the effects of immobilization on the vascular response of the meniscus to injury [48]. They found that the healing response of the meniscus may be affected by the location of the injury, lower perfusion, lower vascular index, and immobilization. Specifically, knee immobilization inhibited the normal increase in blood flow seen in response to meniscal injury. This correlation could help explain the association between immobilization and reduced healing. In addition, meniscal healing may be affected by decreased synovial fluid production and decreased tissue nutrition [48]. The findings by Bray et al. are in

accordance with the results of the study performed by Huang et al. [50]. They used a rabbit model to study the healing potential and histologic characteristics of injured menisci and found that immobilization in flexion did not affect the rate of healing, but instead resulted in degenerative changes in the menisci compared to controls. In another study performed by Ochi et al., they found that degenerative changes in the deep zones of normal rabbit menisci after 6–8 weeks of immobilization did not reverse after 4 weeks of joint remobilization [51]. Dowdy et al. examined the effect of cast immobilization on repaired meniscal lesions in canine menisci and found a decrease in collagen formation after 10 weeks of immobilization compared to non-immobilized controls [52]. The cumulative results from these studies emphasize the importance of joint mobilization and adequate blood flow in order to promote long-term healing of the meniscus.

11.5 Biomechanical Properties

The menisci are complex structures that must respond to a wide variety of physiologic loads and stresses, including compression, shear, and tension. The regional and layered variability in the biochemical composition of the menisci discussed previously is reflective of the variety of loads and stresses observed by the menisci [53].

Similar to other soft tissues, the biomechanical properties of the meniscus can be described in terms of quantifiable tissue characteristics including viscoelasticity, creep and stress relaxation, permeability, shear stiffness, and ultimate tensile strength. Overall, viscoelasticity refers to materials that exhibit both viscous and elastic properties when deformed. The viscous properties are due to the fluid phase (water, interstitial electrolytes), while the elastic properties are attributable to the meniscal matrix composed largely of collagen and proteoglycans with some other minor non-collagen proteins [54]. These properties are observed in a time-dependent manner over the course of load application. The meniscal tissue initially behaves elastically in its resistance to an applied load; however, with continued application of load, the porous-permeable nature of the tissue results in fluid flow through the matrix of the menisci during the viscous phase [38, 55, 56]. The duration and characteristics of the viscous phase are largely dependent on the permeability of the meniscus, which determines how easily fluid flows through the meniscal matrix. With slow-controlled flow, the compressive forces are accommodated and distributed, without excessive deformation, displacement, or loss of shape of the meniscus [57–61]. In comparison to articular cartilage, the meniscus has a lower fluid permeability resulting in a slower rate of fluid flow, and preservation of the meniscal shape during loading [38, 57, 62].

Due to the viscoelastic properties, the menisci demonstrate both creep and stress relaxation with loading [57]. Creep refers to continued deformation, such as elongation, with the continued application of a given load, while stress relaxation refers to the observed reduction in force or tension over time when a tissue is held at a fixed displacement or compression [55, 57]. In the context of the meniscus, creep is observed during the application of a compressive force. When the force is initially applied, the meniscus resists deformation elastically; however, with continued application of the force, additional displacement is observed. In contrast, stress relaxation is observed when the meniscus is compressed or stretched and held at a fixed displacement, and over time the observed compressive force or tension decreases as the tissue relaxes with continued displacement being observed through the viscous or fluid phase.

In addition, there are other changes that are observed in response to axial loading of the meniscus including redistribution of the applied axial load through meniscal "hoop stresses." [9, 63–66] As the name would suggest, these are circumferential tension forces that are observed in line with the circumferential fibers of the meniscus. These forces are dependent on the integrity of the "hoop," and therefore disruption of the continuity of these fibers, such as in cases of radial tears or tears of the meniscal roots, results in the loss of these hoop stresses. In the context of posteromedial meniscectomy, Seitz et al. reported no differences in hoop strains in all tested flexion angles with 50% partial medial meniscectomy [67]. However, with sufficient injury and in the absence of hoop stresses, additional radial extrusion of the menisci is observed [68, 69]. Meniscal root tears are a common clinical scenario in which this is demonstrated [70]. With disrupted hoop stresses, the meniscus extrudes to a point that equates to a functionally meniscectomized state [9, 14, 66]. Extrusion, in turn, reduces the force-distributing capabilities of the meniscus, resulting in altered tibiofemoral contact profiles including increased mean and peak pressures and decreased contact areas [14].

The other primary forces that are observed include shear and tension. Shear forces refer to instances in which the applied force is parallel to the cross-sectional area of the meniscus. The meniscus has a relatively low shear stiffness compared to other tissues of the knee, such as bone and cartilage. This means that the meniscus is deformed more easily in response to these forces, allowing the meniscus to adapt and maintain congruency with the femur throughout a range of motion and loading profiles [55]. Tension refers to stretching forces exerted on the meniscus which elongates the relatively relaxed collagen fibers; however, the capacity of the meniscus to resist tensile forces (e.g., ultimate failure load and stiffness) exhibits regional variability within the meniscus.

11.5.1 Motion and Stability

In vivo, the meniscus serves multiple functions; however, biomechanically these roles can be broadly categorized into load distribution and joint stability [71, 72]. The summation of the biomechanical properties outlined in the previous section allows the menisci to distribute loads and decrease peak and mean contact pressures. In addition, the menisci have stabilizing roles, functioning as secondary stabilizers primarily to anterior-posterior translation. Yet, the menisci must also be sufficiently mobile to be able to adapt and serve these functions throughout a range of motion.

Historically, the load-distributing capacity of the meniscus has been demonstrated based on clinical observations, primarily through the progressive narrowing of joint space following meniscectomy [64]. These load-distributing roles have subsequently been quantified in the lab via pressure mapping studies that demonstrate the function of the intact menisci, the consequence of various injuries and meniscectomies, and the ability of repair to restore meniscal function and contact pressure profiles [72–75]. Compared to the intact state, Ahmed et al. demonstrated a 50–70% decrease in contact area following medial meniscectomy, resulting in increased peak contact pressures [73]. Lee et al. investigated the impact of serial posteromedial meniscectomies of increasing size, demonstrating decreasing contact areas, and increasing mean contact stresses with increasing meniscectomy percentage [76]. Other investigations looking at smaller percentages of resection, including the study by Seitz et al., have suggested that a 20% partial posteromedial meniscectomy can be performed without compromising contact profiles [67]. The same authors suggested that 50% meniscectomy may not significantly impact contact pressures and areas in and near full extension (0 and 30°). In the context of medial meniscus root tears, Padalecki et al. demonstrated 36–37% decrease in contact areas and 59–78% increase in mean contact pressure for medial root avulsion and varying medial root tear locations. Following transtibial pullout repair, contact areas and pressures were restored to the intact states [77]. Additional investigations have also demonstrated the consequences of nonanatomic repair. LaPrade et al. reported that a nonanatomic transtibial root repair resulted in a 44% decrease in contact area and a 67% increase in contact pressure compared to the intact state, demonstrating the importance of restoring the native meniscal anatomy [78].

The menisci also have a secondary role in stabilization. The medial meniscus is a significant secondary restraint to anterior translation, which is primarily accomplished by the more stable posterior horns of the menisci [57, 71, 79–82]. This is most apparent in ACL-deficient knees; however, with a sufficient percentage of meniscectomy (46%), investigators have demonstrated significant differences in anterior-posterior stability [80]. In the setting of ACL deficiency this is accentuated, in which the medial meniscus, particularly the posterior horn, becomes the primary anterior stabilizer [81–84]. This lends credence to the notion that the ACL serves as a protector of the meniscus. Overburdened with the role of resisting anterior translation in the setting of ACL tears, the menisci may be more susceptible to injury and tears [83]. Similarly, in the context of ACL injuries, multiple biomechanical studies indicate that the integrity of the posterolateral meniscal root may play a role in anterior-posterior in addition to internal rotation stability [85, 86].

However, in addition to restricting translation as a secondary stabilizer, the medial and lateral menisci must also be highly mobile, and move reciprocally with respect to each other, to maintain the congruency of the articulation and function throughout a range of motion. In this regard, the lateral meniscus is much more mobile, with a magnitude of translation that is two times or more than that of the medial meniscus [87–90]. The viscoelastic properties of the meniscus also allow for motion of the horns of the menisci with respect to each other. For example, in extension, a greater anterior-posterior dimension of the condyles forces the horns of the menisci apart. In contrast, in deeper flexion, a smaller area of the posterior condyles is in contact with the tibia, and therefore the horns of the menisci are closer together [90].

Although the menisci are paired structures, there are important biomechanical differences between the medial and lateral tibiofemoral joints and menisci that have clinical implications. Foremost, the geometric differences of the medial and lateral plateaus have implications for the roles of the meniscus. The medial plateau is more concave, theoretically resulting in greater bony stability and congruity. In contrast the lateral plateau is more convex, and as a consequence may have greater reliance on the lateral meniscus to maintain joint congruity throughout a range of motion. Clinically, patients with lateral meniscal injury and deficiency do worse than those with medial deficiency [5, 91]. The lateral meniscus, as stated previously, is also much more mobile and observes greater loads compared to the medial meniscus [6].

11.6 Conclusion

The meniscus is a vital component for the normal function and long-term health of the knee joint. The menisci increase stability to femorotibial articulation, distribute axial load, absorb shock, and provide lubrication to the knee joint. Understanding the menisci on a molecular and biomechanical level enables greater knowledge and awareness of their preservation and protection from injury.

References

1. Baker P, et al. Knee disorders in the general population and their relation to occupation. Occup Environ Med. 2003;60(10):794–7.
2. Grover M. Evaluating acutely injured patients for internal derangement of the knee. Am Fam Phys. 2012;85(3):247–52. ISSN 0002-838x
3. Badlani JT, et al. The effects of meniscus injury on the development of knee osteoarthritis: data from the osteoarthritis initiative. Am J Sports Med. 2013;41(6):1238–44. ISSN 0363-5465
4. Räber DA, Friederich NF, Hefti F. Discoid lateral meniscus in children. Long-term follow-up after total meniscectomy. J Bone Joint Surg Am. 1998;80(11):1579–86. ISSN 0021-9355
5. Mcnicholas MJ, et al. Total meniscectomy in adolescence. A thirty-year follow-up. J Bone Joint Surg Br. 2000;82(2):217–21. ISSN 0301-620X
6. Messner K, Gao J. The menisci of the knee joint. Anatomical and functional characteristics, and a rationale for clinical treatment. J Anat. 1998;193(Pt 2):161–78. ISSN 0021-8782
7. Hoser C, et al. Long-term results of arthroscopic partial lateral meniscectomy in knees without associated damage. J Bone Joint Surg Br. 2001;83(4):513–6. ISSN 0301-620X
8. Stein T, et al. Long-term outcome after arthroscopic meniscal repair versus arthroscopic partial meniscectomy for traumatic meniscal tears. Am J Sports Med. 2010;38(8):1542–8. ISSN 1552-3365
9. Mcdermott ID, AMIS AA. The consequences of meniscectomy. J Bone Joint Surg Br. 2006;88(12):1549–56. ISSN 0301-620X (Print)
10. Laprade RF, et al. The menisci: a comprehensive review of their anatomy, biomechanical function and surgical treatment. Berlin: Springer; 2017.
11. Seedhom BB, Dowson D, Wright V. Proceedings: functions of the menisci. A preliminary study. Ann Rheum Dis. 1974;33(1):111. ISSN 0003-4967
12. Poynton AR, et al. The meniscofemoral ligaments of the knee. J Bone Joint Surg Br. 1997;79(2):327–30. ISSN 0301-620X
13. Kusayama T, et al. Anatomical and biomechanical characteristics of human meniscofemoral ligaments. Knee Surg Sports Traumatol Arthrosc. 1994;2(4):234–7. ISSN 0942-2056
14. Allaire R, et al. Biomechanical consequences of a tear of the posterior root of the medial meniscus. Similar to total meniscectomy. J Bone Joint Surg Am. 2008;90(9):1922–31. ISSN 1535-1386 (Electronic)
15. Laprade CM, et al. Altered tibiofemoral contact mechanics due to lateral meniscus posterior horn root avulsions and radial tears can be restored with in situ pull-out suture repairs. J Bone Joint Surg Am. 2014;96(6):471–9. ISSN 1535–1386 (Electronic)
16. Ellman MB, et al. Structural properties of the meniscal roots. Am J Sports Med. 2014;42(8):1881–7. ISSN 1552–3365
17. Bhatia S, et al. A novel repair method for radial tears of the medial meniscus: biomechanical comparison of Transtibial 2-tunnel and double horizontal mattress suture techniques under cyclic loading. Am J Sports Med. 2016;44(3):639–45. ISSN 1552–3365
18. Vyas D, Harner CD. Meniscus root repair. Sports Med Arthrosc Rev. 2012;20(2):86–94. ISSN 1538–1951
19. Johannsen AM, et al. Qualitative and quantitative anatomic analysis of the posterior root attachments of the medial and lateral menisci. Am J Sports Med. 2012;40(10):2342–7. ISSN 1552–3365
20. Laprade CM, et al. Anatomy of the anterior root attachments of the medial and lateral menisci: a quantitative analysis. Am J Sports Med. 2014;42(10):2386–92. ISSN 1552–3365
21. Laprade CM, et al. Anterior medial meniscal root avulsions due to malposition of the tibial tunnel during anterior cruciate ligament reconstruction: two case reports. Knee Surg Sports Traumatol Arthrosc. 2014;22(5):1119–23. ISSN 1433–7347
22. Karakasli A, et al. Iatrogenic lateral meniscus anterior horn injury in different tibial tunnel placement techniques in ACL reconstruction surgery - a cadaveric study. Acta Orthop Traumatol Turc. 2016;50(5):514–8. ISSN 2589–1294
23. Laprade CM, et al. Posterior lateral meniscal root tear due to a malpositioned double-bundle anterior cruciate ligament reconstruction tibial tunnel. Knee Surg Sports Traumatol Arthrosc. 2015;23(12):3670–3. ISSN 1433–7347
24. Kennedy NI, et al. Iatrogenic meniscus posterior root injury following reconstruction of the posterior cruciate ligament: a report of three cases. JBJS Case Connect. 2014;4(1 Suppl 6):e20–e6. ISSN 2160–3251
25. Yaniv M, Blumberg N. The discoid meniscus. J Child Orthop. 2007;1(2):89–96. ISSN 1863–2521
26. Clark CR, Ogden JA. Development of the menisci of the human knee joint. Morphological changes

and their potential role in childhood meniscal injury. J Bone Joint Surg Am. 1983;65(4):538–47. ISSN 0021–9355

27. Ikeuchi H. Arthroscopic treatment of the discoid lateral meniscus. Technique and long-term results. Clin Orthop Relat Res. 1982;167:19–28. ISSN 0009–921X

28. Kini SG, Walker P, Bruce W. Bilateral symptomatic discoid medial meniscus of the knee: a case report and review of literature. Archiv Trauma Res. 2015;4(1):e27115.

29. Kelly BT, Green DW. Discoid lateral meniscus in children. Curr Opin Pediatr. 2002;14(1):54–61. ISSN 1040–8703

30. Silverman JM, Mink JH, Deutsch AL. Discoid menisci of the knee: MR imaging appearance. Radiology. 1989;173(2):351–4. ISSN 0033–8419

31. Jordan MR. Lateral meniscal variants: evaluation and treatment. J Am Acad Orthop Surg. 1996;4(4):191–200. ISSN 1067–151X

32. Kramer DE, Micheli LJ. Meniscal tears and discoid meniscus in children: diagnosis and treatment. J Am Acad Orthop Surg. 2009;17(11):698–707. ISSN 1067–151X

33. Atay ÖA, et al. Management of discoid lateral meniscus tears: observations in 34 knees. Arthroscopy. 2003;19(4):346–52. ISSN 0749–8063

34. Young RB. The external semilunar cartilage as a complete disc. Memoirs and memoranda in anatomy; 1889.

35. Kaplan EB. Discoid lateral meniscus of the knee joint. J Bone Joint Surg. 1957;39:77–87.

36. Watanabe M, Takeda S, Ikeuchi H. Atlas of arthroscopy. Berlin: Springer; 1979. ISBN 3540076743

37. Brindle T, Nyland J, Johnson DL. The meniscus: review of basic principles with application to surgery and rehabilitation. J Athl Train. 2001;36(2):160.

38. Proctor CS, et al. Material properties of the normal medial bovine meniscus. J Orthop Res. 1989;7(6):771–82. ISSN 0736-0266

39. Peters TJ, Smillie ES. Studies on the chemical composition of the menisci of the knee joint with special reference to the horizontal cleavage lesion. Clin Orthop Relat Res (1976–2007). 1972;86:245–52.

40. McDevitt CA, Webber RJ. The ultrastructure and biochemistry of meniscal cartilage. Clin Orthop Relat Res. 1990;252:8–18. ISSN 0009-921X

41. Chevrier A, et al. Meniscus structure in human, sheep, and rabbit for animal models of meniscus repair. J Orthop Res. 2009;27(9):1197–203. ISSN 0736-0266

42. Mow C. Structure and function relationships of the menisci of the knee. Knee Meniscus: Basic and Clinical Foundations; 1992.

43. Ghosh P, Taylor TK. The knee joint meniscus. A fibrocartilage of some distinction. Clin Orthop Relat Res. 1987;224:52–63. ISSN 0009-921X

44. Fox AJS, Bedi A, Rodeo SA. The basic science of human knee menisci: structure, composition, and function. Sports Health. 2011;4(4):340–51. https://doi.org/10.1177/1941738111429419. Acesso em: 2020/04/03. ISSN 1941-7381

45. Nakano T, Dodd CM, Scott PG. Glycosaminoglycans and proteoglycans from different zones of the porcine knee meniscus. J Orthop Res. 1997;15(2):213–20. ISSN 0736-0266

46. Scott PG, Nakano T, Dodd CM. Isolation and characterization of small proteoglycans from different zones of the porcine knee meniscus. Biochim Biophys Acta. 1997;1336(2):254–62. ISSN 0304-4165

47. Arnoczky SP, Warren RF. The microvasculature of the meniscus and its response to injury: an experimental study in the dog. Am J Sports Med. 1983;11(3):131–41. ISSN 0363-5465

48. Bray RC, et al. Vascular response of the meniscus to injury: effects of immobilization. J Orthop Res. 2001;19(3):384–90. ISSN 0736-0266

49. King D. The healing of the semilunar cartilages. J Bone Joint Surg. 1936;18:333–42.

50. Huang TL, et al. Healing potential of experimental meniscal tears in the rabbit. Preliminary results. Clin Orthop Relat Res. 1991;267:299–305. ISSN 0009-921X

51. Ochi M, et al. Changes in the permeability and histologic findings of rabbit menisci after immobilization. Clin Orthop Relat Res. 1997;334:305–15. ISSN 0009-921X

52. Dowdy PA, et al. The effect of cast immobilization on meniscal healing: an experimental study in the dog. Am J Sports Med. 1995;23(6):721–8. ISSN 0363-5465

53. Fox AJ, Bedi A, Rodeo SA. The basic science of human knee menisci: structure, composition, and function. Sports Health. 2012;4(4):340–51. ISSN 1941-0921

54. Bursac P, et al. Influence of donor age on the biomechanical and biochemical properties of human meniscal allografts. Am J Sports Med. 2009;37(5):884–9. ISSN 0363-5465

55. Andrews S. Meniscus structure and function. Calgary, AB: University of Calgary; 2013.

56. Fithian DC, Kelly MA, Mow C. Material properties and structure-function relationships in the menisci. Clin Orthop Relat Res. 1990;252:19–31. ISSN 0009-921X (Print)

57. McDermott ID, Masouros SD, Amis AA. Biomechanics of the menisci of the knee. Curr Orthop. 2008;22(3):193–201. ISSN 0268-0890

58. Spilker RL, Donzelli PS, Mow C. A transversely isotropic biphasic finite element model of the meniscus. J Biomech. 1992;25(9):1027–45. ISSN 0021-9290

59. Sweigart MA, et al. Intraspecies and interspecies comparison of the compressive properties of the medial meniscus. Ann Biomed Eng. 2004;32(11):1569–79. ISSN 0090–6964 (Print)

60. Joshi MD, et al. Interspecies variation of compressive biomechanical properties of the meniscus. J Biomed Mater Res. 1995;29(7):823–8. ISSN 0021-9304 (Print).

61. Hacker S, et al. Compressive properties of the human meniscus. Tran Annu Meet Orthop Res Soc. 1992;627

62. Favenesi J, Shaffer J, Mow V. Biphasic mechanical properties of knee meniscus. Trans Orthop Res Soc. 1983;8:57.

63. Shrive NG, O'Connor JJ, Goodfellow JW. Load-bearing in the knee joint. Clin Orthop Relat Res. 1978;131:279–87. ISSN 0009-921X

64. Fairbank TJ. Knee joint changes after meniscectomy. J Bone Joint Surg Br. 1948;30B(4):664–70. ISSN 0301-620X

65. Bullough PG, et al. The strength of the menisci of the knee as it relates to their fine structure. J Bone Joint Surg Br. 1970;52(3):564–7. ISSN 0301-620X

66. Jones RS, et al. Direct measurement of hoop strains in the intact and torn human medial meniscus. Clin Biomech (Bristol, Avon). 1996;11(5):295–300. ISSN 0268-0033

67. Seitz AM, et al. Effect of partial meniscectomy at the medial posterior horn on tibiofemoral contact mechanics and meniscal hoop strains in human knees. J Orthop Res. 2012;30(6):934–42. ISSN 0736-0266

68. Kummer B. 38. Anatomie und Biomechanik des Kniegelenksmeniscus. Langenbecks Archiv für. Chirurgie. 1987;372(1):241–6. ISSN 0023-8236

69. Kenny C. Radial displacement of the medial meniscus and Fairbank's signs. Clin Orthop Relat Res. 1997;339:163–73. ISSN 0009-921X (Print)

70. Lerer DB, et al. The role of meniscal root pathology and radial meniscal tear in medial meniscal extrusion. Skeletal Radiol. 2004;33(10):569–74. ISSN 0364-2348 (Print)

71. Vedi V, et al. Meniscal movement. An in-vivo study using dynamic MRI. J Bone Joint Surg Br. 1999;81(1):37–41. ISSN 0301-620X

72. Walker PS, Erkman MJ. The role of the menisci in force transmission across the knee. Clin Orthop Relat Res. 1975;109:184–92. ISSN 0009-921X (Print)

73. Ahmed AM, Burke DL. In-vitro measurement of static pressure distribution in synovial joints—Part I: Tibial surface of the knee. J Biomech Eng. 1983;105(3):216–25. ISSN 0148-0731 (Print)

74. Fukubayashi T, Kurosawa H. The contact area and pressure distribution pattern of the knee. A study of normal and osteoarthrotic knee joints. Acta Orthop Scand. 1980;51(6):871–9. ISSN 0001-6470 (Print)

75. Ihn JC, Kim SJ, Park IH. In vitro study of contact area and pressure distribution in the human knee after partial and total meniscectomy. Int Orthop. 1993;17(4):214–8. ISSN 0341-2695 (Print)

76. Lee SJ, et al. Tibiofemoral contact mechanics after serial medial meniscectomies in the human cadaveric knee. Am J Sports Med. 2006;34(8):1334–44. ISSN 0363–5465 (Print)

77. Padalecki JR, et al. Biomechanical consequences of a complete radial tear adjacent to the medial meniscus posterior root attachment site: in situ pull-out repair restores derangement of joint mechanics. Am J Sports Med. 2014;42(3):699–707. ISSN 0363-5465

78. Laprade CM, et al. Biomechanical consequences of a nonanatomic posterior medial meniscal root repair. Am J Sports Med. 2015;43(4):912–20. ISSN 0363-5465

79. Bargar WL, et al. In vivo stability testing of post-meniscectomy knees. Clin Orthop Relat Res. 1980;150:247–52. ISSN 0009-921X

80. Arno S, et al. The effect of arthroscopic partial medial meniscectomy on tibiofemoral stability. Am J Sports Med. 2013;41(1):73–9. ISSN 1552-3365

81. Levy IM, Torzilli PA, Warren RF. The effect of medial meniscectomy on anterior-posterior motion of the knee. J Bone Joint Surg Am. 1982;64(6):883–8. ISSN 0021-9355

82. Markolf KL, Mensch JS, Amstutz HC. Stiffness and laxity of the knee--the contributions of the supporting structures. A quantitative in vitro study. J Bone Joint Surg Am. 1976;58(5):583–94. ISSN 0021-9355 (Print)

83. Allen CR, et al. Importance of the medial meniscus in the anterior cruciate ligament-deficient knee. J Orthop Res. 2000;18(1):109–15. ISSN 0736-0266

84. Shoemaker SC, Markolf KL. The role of the meniscus in the anterior-posterior stability of the loaded anterior cruciate-deficient knee. Effects of partial versus total excision. J Bone Joint Surg Am. 1986;68(1):71–9. ISSN 0021-9355 (Print)

85. Forkel P, et al. Repair of the lateral posterior meniscal root improves stability in an ACL-deficient knee. Knee Surg Sports Traumatol Arthrosc. 2018;26(8):2302–9. ISSN 0942-2056

86. Tang X, et al. Lateral meniscal posterior root repair with anterior cruciate ligament reconstruction better restores knee stability. Am J Sports Med. 2019;47(1):59–65. ISSN 0363-5465

87. Bylski-Austrow DI, et al. Displacements of the menisci under joint load: an in vitro study in human knees. J Biomech. 1994;27(4):421425–3431. ISSN 0021-9290

88. Aagaard H, Verdonk R. Function of the normal meniscus and consequences of meniscal resection. Scand J Med Sci Sports. 1999;9(3):134–40. ISSN 0905-7188

89. Brantigan OC, Voshell AP. The mechanics of the ligaments and menisci of the knee joint. J Bone Joint Surg Am. 1941;23:44–66.

90. Thompson WO, et al. Tibial meniscal dynamics using three-dimensional reconstruction of magnetic resonance images. Am J Sports Med. 1991;19(3):210–5. discussion 215-6. ISSN 0363-5465

91. Raber DA, Friederich NF, Hefti F. Discoid lateral meniscus in children. Long-term follow-up after total meniscectomy. J Bone Joint Surg Am. 1998;80(11):1579–86. ISSN 0021-9355 (Print)

Concomitant Meniscus Repair for Cartilage Treatment

12

Faiz S. Shivji and Tim Spalding

Chondral lesions have been found to be present in 69% of patients undergoing arthroscopic partial meniscectomy (APM) [1]. Patients with unstable chondral lesions who undergo APM have a poorer functional outcome than those without chondral lesions [2]. Hence, the presence of a functioning meniscus in patients with chondral damage is important to preserve function, reduce pain, and reduce the risk of arthritis. In those meniscal tears amenable to repair, a variety of techniques are available, which are discussed. The role of partial restoration of lost meniscal tissue is explained. Finally, the evidence behind the use of biological augmentation is presented. The repair of ramp and root lesions is discussed in separate chapters.

12.1 Importance of Meniscal Repair

A UK study into the long-term outcomes of 834,393 patients undergoing APM showed that these patients were ten times more likely to undergo arthroplasty surgery than the general population and three times more likely when compared to their normal contralateral knee [3]. In a separate case-control study, meniscal injury was found to be associated with a 15 times higher risk for requiring total-knee arthroplasty (TKA) [4]. Lateral total or subtotal meniscectomy increases the peak contact and shear stresses by double the amount when compared with a medial meniscectomy [5]. Hence it is no surprise that the rate of OA after lateral meniscectomy is higher than medial [6].

The menisci are crucial in resisting forces such as shear and compression. They also distribute load across the knee, reducing stress on the articular cartilage. They provide lubrication and nutrition to the avascular cartilage and add to knee stability. Due to the deleterious effects of the loss or defunctioning of either meniscus, any patient undergoing cartilage repair must have meniscal integrity confirmed and/or restored to have the best chance of an optimal outcome.

12.2 Assessment of Tear Repairability

12.2.1 Tear Factors

12.2.1.1 Tear Location

As can be seen from Fig. 12.1, a description of tear location has been proposed by the European Society for Sports Traumatology, Knee Surgery and Arthroscopy (ESSKA), based on the original work of Cooper et al. [7, 8]. The traditional description of red-red (vas-

F. S. Shivji · T. Spalding (✉)
University Hospitals of Coventry & Warwickshire,
Coventry, UK
e-mail: tim.spalding@uhcw.nhs.uk

© ISAKOS 2021
A. J. Krych et al. (eds.), *Cartilage Injury of the Knee*,
https://doi.org/10.1007/978-3-030-78051-7_12

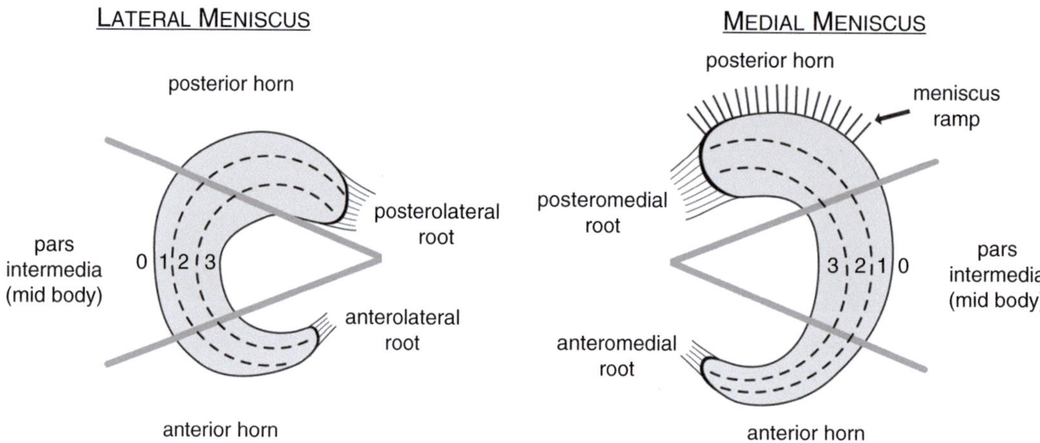

Fig. 12.1 Proposed classification for meniscal tear location. (Reproduced with permission from Kopf et al. 2020 [8])

cularized area 0–3 mm from the rim), red-white (intermediate area 3–5 mm from the rim), and white-white (inner avascular area 5–7 mm from the rim) was used to explain the likelihood of tears healing [9]. However, the blood supply of the menisci has subsequently been found to change throughout life and is difficult to assess intraoperatively, hence the change in proposed description to Zones 0–3 [8, 10]. Tears in Zones 1 and 2 have good reported healing rates of 64–91% with tears in Zone 1 (87–91%) much better than Zone 2 (59–79%) [8]. Intraoperatively, this equates to 4 mm or less from the rim to demarcate the extent of repairable tears. The anteroposterior location of the tear does not influence repairability. There is also no difference in failure rates of medial versus lateral repairs.

12.2.1.2 Tear Orientation

As shown in Fig. 12.2, tears can be vertical, horizontal, radial, or a combination. Vertical tears can be simple peripheral tears with minimal displacement or larger bucket handle types, and both disrupt the radial fibers. The orientation of these tears makes them amenable to repair with excellent results [11].

Horizontal tears occur within the meniscus parallel to the joint surface. They do not disrupt the radial or circumferential fibers and hence leave contact pressures unchanged. However,

they are associated with parameniscal cyst formation. Traditionally, these tears were treated with resection of the inferior leaflet. However, cadaveric studies of the effects of this in both medial and lateral meniscal tears have shown reduced contact area post-resection of the inferior leaflet [12, 13]. A systematic review of 98 repaired tears showed a healing rate of 77.8% [14]. Therefore, in non-degenerative horizontal tears, repair may be preferable to resection, albeit with limited evidence.

Radial tears are vertically orientated but pass in the direction across the Zones 0–3, defunctioning the meniscus if the tear extends through all zones. In such tears, repair should be attempted to heal the disrupted circumferential fibers. In tears which have an intact peripheral rim, a partial resection of the unstable inner edges can be performed.

12.2.1.3 Tear Length

The evidence of the relationship between tear length and repairability is unclear. There is evidence that leaving lateral tears that are less than 10 mm long does not lead to subsequent reoperations suggesting that these can be left untreated. However, this has not been replicated for medial tears [16]. Due to conflicting evidence, it is suggested that if a tear is otherwise amenable to repair, it seems sensible to proceed with repair no matter what the length.

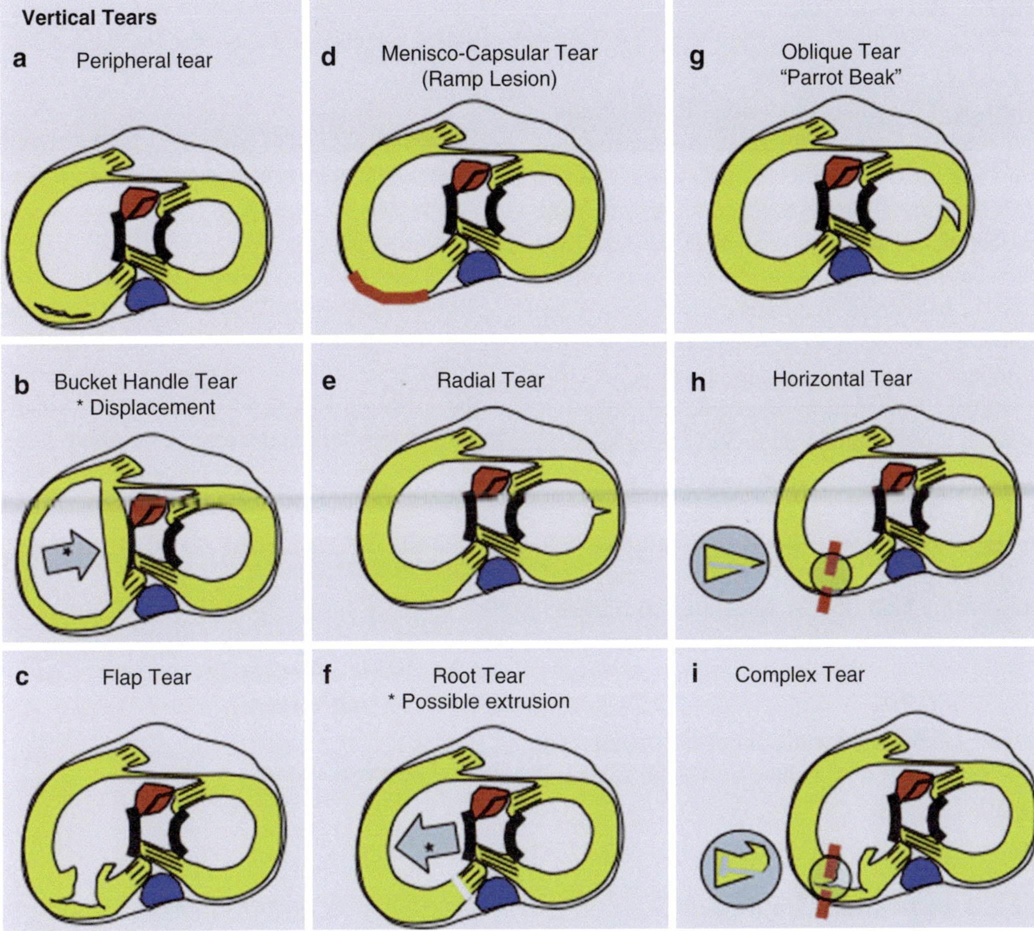

Fig. 12.2 Descriptive classification of meniscal tears based on tear orientation and meniscal fiber disruption shown on a superior view of a right knee. Anterior cruciate ligament insertion shown in red. Posterior cruciate ligament insertion shown in blue. *MM* medial meniscus (left), *LM* lateral meniscus (right). Tear types: (**a**) vertical longitudinal peripheral tear (posterior horn of MM); (**b**) vertical longitudinal displaced "bucket handle" tear (of MM); (**c**) vertical longitudinal flap tear (posterior horn of MM); (**d**) vertical longitudinal menisco-capsular tear (of MM); (**e**) vertical radial tear (body of LM); (**f**) meniscal root tear (posterior root of MM); (**g**) vertical oblique "parrot beak" tear (body of LM); (**h**) horizontal tear (posterior horn MM), with the horizontal component shown on the inset sagittal image; (**i**) complex tear (posterior horn of MM) with the vertical flap component shown on the superior view and the horizontal and flap components shown on the inset sagittal view [15]. (Reproduced with permission from Lawton et al. 2019)

12.2.1.4 Age of Tear

There is no evidence to suggest that the time between trauma and repair influences healing. A study of 238 meniscal repairs found no difference between those treated within 2 weeks, 2–12 weeks, and over 12 weeks of injury [17]. A different study of 25 patients undergoing surgery at a mean 27 months post-injury showed that 21 patients healed post-repair [18]. A further study of 24 patients with bucket handle medial meniscal tears treated at a mean 10 months post-injury showed that 20 healed [19]. However, with increasing time larger tears may undergo deformation making repair more challenging.

12.2.2 Patient Factors

12.2.2.1 Age, BMI, Sex

The age of the patient does not affect the healing potential of tears. Two studies comparing outcomes in those over and under 40 years found no difference in failure rates [20, 21]. A systematic review of 1141 menisci treated in 1063 patients showed that there was no difference in failure rates in patients at age thresholds of above and below 25, 30, 35, and 40 years [22]. However, with increasing age the likelihood of preexisting meniscal degeneration rises; hence this may have an adverse effect on healing. Any signs of macroscopic degeneration should be sought intraoperatively.

The BMI of the patient does not seem to influence failure rates of meniscal repair [23]. However, a high BMI is associated with meniscal degeneration which may influence outcomes. Women have been found to have a significantly lower failure rate in a systematic review of bucket handle meniscal repairs but this has not been replicated across all meniscal repairs [24, 25].

12.2.3 Indications for Repair

Patients should be considered for meniscal repair if they have had a traumatic event leading to mechanical symptoms (e.g., locked, locking, catching), if they have pain associated with the location of the meniscal tear, or if they are amenable to repair during a cartilage procedure.

Meniscal repair in the presence of OA should be avoided. Other factors to consider include the following:

1. Vascularity: Cooper Zones 0–1 are ideal with Zone 3 having a low chance of healing. Zone 2 tear can be repaired if other factors are in favor.
2. Pattern and location: Partial-thickness, oblique, parrot-beak, and complex tears are often not amenable to repair. Vertical tears and radial tears affecting the peripheral rim should be repaired. Horizontal tears are usually degenerate but can be repaired as stated above.
3. Tear length and age: No evidence to prohibit repair.
4. Patient: Age, sex, and BMI do not appear to affect the outcome.

12.3 Which Repair Technique to Use When

12.3.1 Radial Tears

Radial tears that do not extend into the peripheral zone can be resected. However, those that do extend should be repaired using a "tie-grip" or "rip-stop" technique (Fig. 12.3). This method involves using two inside-out sutures placed either side of the tear in a vertical mattress orientation to anchor the meniscus to the capsule. 3–4 horizontal mattress sutures are then placed from one side to another over the top of the vertical sutures. The vertical sutures prevent the horizon-

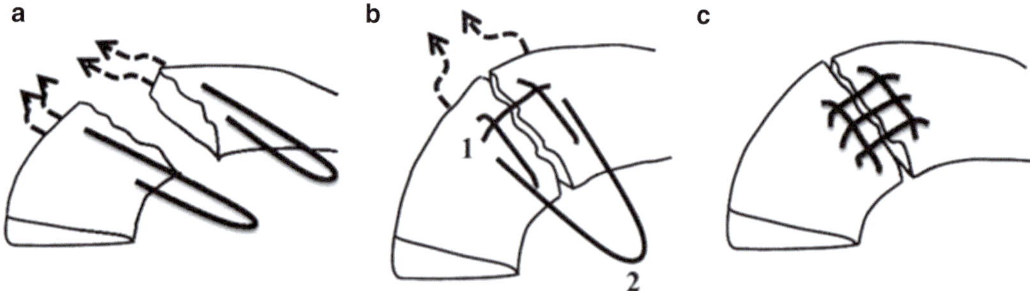

Fig. 12.3 The "tie-grip" suture technique. (**a**). Vertical sutures inserted to stop subsequent sutures pulling through meniscus. (**b**). Horizontal sutures inserted over the top of the virital loops. (**c**). final configuration of sutures, tied over the periperal capsuse. (Reproduced with permission from Tsuji et al. 2018 [30])

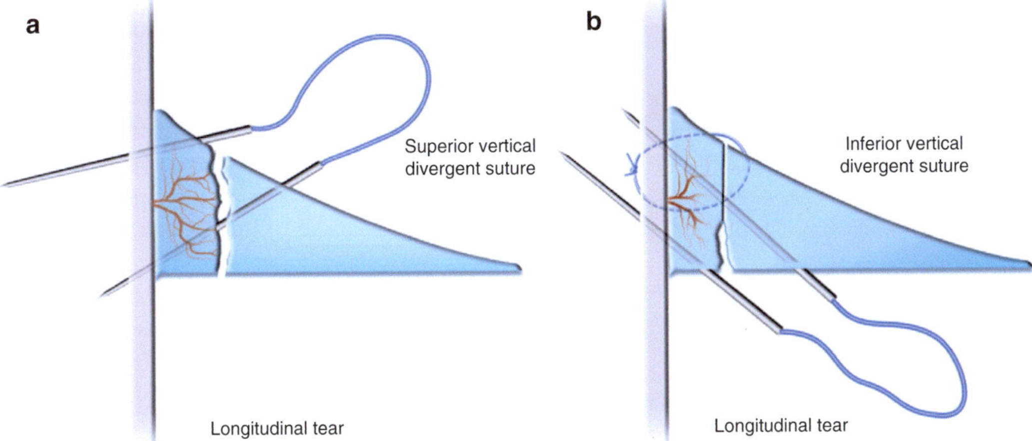

Fig. 12.4 Double-stacked vertical suture pattern used in the repair of longitudinal meniscus tears. (**a**) The superior sutures are placed first to close the superior gap and to reduce the meniscus to its bed. (**b**) Then, the inferior suture is placed through the tear to close the inferior gap.

(Reproduced with permission from Noyes' Knee Disorders: Surgery, Rehabilitation, Clinical Outcomes, Noyes FR, Barber-Westin SD, Meniscus tears: diagnosis, repair techniques, clinical outcomes, p692, Copyright Elsevier, 2016)

tal sutures cutting out due to sliding along the circumferential meniscal fibers, and are known as "rip-stop" sutures [26, 27].

12.3.2 Vertical and Bucket Handle Tears

For long vertical tears that extend from posterior to anterior, the authors prefer to use a hybrid technique of inside-out and all-inside sutures. Inside-out sutures may be used in the lateral meniscus to repair any section of the tear that lies in front of the popliteal hiatus. The posterior horn can then be repaired using all-inside sutures [28]. Similarly, the mid-body and anterior horn of the medial meniscus can be fixed using inside-out sutures, and the posterior horn using all-inside sutures. Anterior horn tears can also be repaired using outside-in sutures [29]. This combination reduces the expense by using fewer all-inside devices and also prevents the need for exposure of the posterior capsule and the protection of neurovascular structures by not using inside-out sutures posteriorly. As shown in Fig. 12.4, a combination of superior and under-surface sutures is required to close the gap, fully opposing the tear.

12.3.3 Horizontal Tears

For horizontal tears in younger (<50 years) patients without preexisting arthritis, repair can be performed. All-inside sutures can be placed along the length of the tear at 5 mm intervals. The sutures should start at the meniscocapsular junction above the superior leaflet and finish vertically below the inferior leaflet again at the meniscocapsular junction. These sutures provide uniform circumferential compression on both leaflets [31] (Fig. 12.5).

12.4 Partial Meniscus Restoration

In those patients where repair is impossible and resection is carried out, options exist to replace the segmental loss. Where the bulk of the meniscus is removed or is defunctioned following an irreparable full radial tear, then meniscal allograft transplantation is indicated. This is not covered in this chapter.

Options for segmental reconstruction include the Collagen Meniscus Implant (CMI, Stryker, USA) made from a bovine type 1 collagen matrix and Actifit (Orteq, London, UK) which is poly-

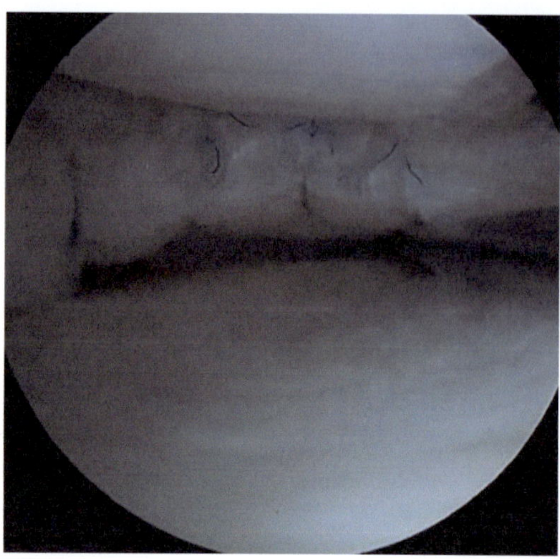

Fig. 12.5 Arthroscopic image viewing from the antero-medial portal with the probe inserted from the anterolateral portal showing repair of a horizontal cleavage meniscus tear in a left knee using circumferential compression stitches. (Reproduced with permission from Woodmass et al. 2017)

urethane based. The CMI is intended to be a resorbable scaffold (12–18 months) consisting of collagen fibers enriched with glycosaminoglycans in which native meniscal tissue grows, as opposed to a prosthesis, although the evidence for this is limited. Recent histology has shown a more fibrous tissue and fibroblast-like cells, although a previous study did show the presence of some meniscus-like tissue [32, 33]. Actifit has a synthetic porous scaffold which degrades over the course of 4–6 years and is intended to act as a scaffold for growth. Histological analysis of Actifit has shown a paucity of fibrochondrocytes when compared to normal meniscal tissue and cartilage-like appearances consisting of chondroblasts [33, 34].

To use either implant, the area of previous resection is prepared to achieve a stable 2–3 mm vascular rim and sharp 90° defect edges. The implant is cut to a size slightly larger than the defect and inserted into the gap. It is sutured in place using all-inside, inside-out, or a hybrid technique.

The indication for partial meniscus restoration (PMR) is a patient with pain in a knee compartment with a previous partial meniscectomy and an absence of OA (ICRS <4) or untreated cartilage lesions. Although PMR has been used in the acute setting for irreparable meniscal tears, a RCT showed no difference in outcomes when used acutely, but a significant difference when used in the chronic setting [32]. Prerequisites for PMR use are intact meniscal roots and meniscal rim with neutral limb alignment and a stable joint.

Both types of scaffold have shown improvement in pain and function when used in either the medial or the lateral meniscus, albeit in limited patient numbers. Patients generally improve over the course of 12 months with a typical improvement of 30 points on Lysholm and 3.5 points on VAS scores [35]. Seventeen male patients who had a CMI had a reduction in pain and improvement in IKDC scores when compared to 16 patients who had partial medial meniscectomy with follow-up of at least 10 years [36]. A further 22 patients with a minimum follow-up of 10 years showed a mean Lysholm score of 87.5 compared with 59.9 preoperatively [37]. These results have been replicated in case series elsewhere [38, 39].

At 2-year follow-up, 54 patients with post-meniscectomy syndrome treated with Actifit implants in the lateral meniscus showed a significant improvement in pain, IKDC, and KOOS scores [40]. Similar results have been reported both in the lateral and medial meniscus [41, 42]. A systematic review comparing CMI (311 patients) and Actifit (347 patients) at a mean 45-month follow-up showed a failure rate of 9.9% in the Actifit cohort and 6.7% in the CMI cohort suggesting that both have similar outcomes in terms of failure [43]. A meta-analysis of 613 patients (444 CMI, 169 Actifit) stated that both groups had an improvement in mean Lysholm, IKDC, VAS, and Tegner scores with an overall complication rate of 12.6%. Complications included pain, infection, non-integration or tear of the scaffold, and suture problems [44].

In summary, PMR certainly has a role in the select group of patients with persistent pain post-partial meniscectomy. Long-term outcomes and poor prognostic factors are unknown, but in the short term improvements in pain and function can be expected. In addition, the cost and availability of such implants make them an attractive option.

12.5 Biologic Augmentation

The use of natural substances to improve the healing rate of meniscal tears is a growing field of interest. Several methods have been described and the techniques and evidence of each are broadly outlined below.

12.5.1 Synovial Abrasion/ Trephination

Synovial abrasion involves roughening the synovium adjacent to the tear as well as the tear itself, commonly using a diamond rasp, to stimulate a healing response. It has been proposed that this upregulates chondrocytes to produce cytokine and growth factors which attract vascularized synovial tissue to the area to increase healing [45]. This process has been showed to occur in rabbit models [46, 47]. Trephination is performed using either a 19G needle to pierce through the skin, synovium, and meniscal rim or a spinal needle from inside through the meniscus and synovium. This aims to create vascular channels from the synovium to the avascular meniscus with evidence of this occurring in canines [48]. The clinical evidence for synovial abrasion and trephination is limited [45, 49]. In 47 patients undergoing rasping without suture repair with a second-look arthroscopy to review healing at a mean 21-month follow-up, 71% had complete healing and 21% incomplete healing. However, 67% of these patients had concomitant ACL reconstruction and tears varied in orientation, location, and thickness [50]. A case-control study of 191 patients with peripheral, vertical, non-displaceable (into the notch) medial meniscal tears treated with trephination alone at the time of ACL reconstruction had no functional difference with the control group who had no tears found during ACL surgery, suggesting that trephination may be all that is required in some patients [51]. In a series of 332 lateral meniscal tears, 43 were

treated with trephination and abrasion and 289 left in situ during ACL reconstruction, with no difference in clinical outcomes [52]. The conclusion regarding trephination and abrasion is that although the evidence is limited, there appears to be minimal disadvantage to attempting either technique.

12.5.2 Marrow Stimulation and Stem Cells

Bone marrow stimulation is generally performed by using a microfracture awl to penetrate the cortex in the notch at the time of meniscal repair or at tunnel creation during cruciate ligament reconstruction. The aim is to release mesenchymal stem cells which can differentiate into a variety of cells, including chondrocytes, and attract other proteins responsible for healing. In addition to stem cells, there are also reports of increased platelet-derived and vascular endothelial growth factors in knee joint fluid after ACL reconstruction which could improve meniscal healing [53, 54]. Alternative ways to harvest stem cells include bone marrow aspiration or processing of adipose tissue (to create a stromal vascular fraction). All techniques produce unpredictable amounts of stem cells but adipose tissue appears to produce more than bone marrow aspirate (4737 cells/mL of tissue to 1,550,000 cells/mL of tissue versus 1–30 to 317,400 cells/mL, respectively) [55].

There are few studies regarding the use of any stem cell technique and meniscal repair in clinical practice, but animal studies suggest a potential benefit. Marrow stimulation via drilling of the notch in rabbits showed a nonsignificant increase in meniscal healing [56]. A study of meniscal repair in goats comparing repair with and without microfracture showed that 65% of meniscal tears performed with microfracture were completely healed, compared to 12% of menisci without microfracture [57]. A further study sutured adipose-derived stem cells into meniscal tears in rabbits which increased the odds of healing [58]. Injection of synovial stem cells in rabbits also led to increased healing of a meniscal defect when compared with a control group [59].

The majority of recent literature has concentrated on the use of scaffolds seeded with stem cells and growth factors to deliver enhanced healing at the site of the tear. The use of a stromal vascular fraction seeded hydrogel to augment the repair of a radial tear in goats led to increased healing and less osteochondral degeneration when compared to those treated with suturing alone [60]. Bone marrow aspirate seeded into a collagen scaffold has been tested for safety in five humans with further trials ongoing [61]. A study reporting on a 3D printed scaffold seeded with stem cells and implanted in rabbits with total meniscectomies found growth of fibrochondrocytes and collagen and reduced cartilage degeneration compared to the control group [62]. Similar results were found in a nanofibrous scaffold seeded with stem cells used to repair 5 mm radial defects in rabbits. These scaffolds prevented meniscal extrusion and provided chondroprotection when compared to the scaffold alone or no treatment [63].

In summary, although evidence is limited, bone marrow stimulation may aid healing without significant morbidity. Clinical trials regarding stem cell-seeded scaffolds are awaited. There does not appear to be sufficient evidence currently for intra-articular injection of stem cells, especially when cost and morbidity are considered.

12.5.3 Fibrin Clot

Fibrin/blood clots interposed in the repaired meniscal tear provide growth and healing factors at the site. The technique is as follows (P. Myers, personal communication):

1. Withdraw 60 mL blood from peripheral venepuncture, and empty into kidney dish.
2. Stir with a glass rod for 15 min to allow clot to form on the rod.
3. Place the clot onto swab and clean with 2–3 drops of saline.

4. Place meniscal repair inside-out sutures in the meniscus, but do not tighten.
5. Shape and cut the clot to size and introduce into the joint using a grasper. An arthroscopic portal cannula device, or sutures on the clot, may aid introduction.
6. Position the clot under or in the meniscal tear and tighten sutures.
7. Once stable, additional sutures can be added as necessary.

Clinical evaluation of fibrin clots is limited to case series. 18 of 24 degenerative medial meniscal tears treated with autologous fibrin clot had clinical healing at a mean follow-up of 39.3 months [64]. Forty-one heterogenous tears treated using a fibrin clot were reviewed at a second-look arthroscopy at mean 8.3 months post-surgery with 39 found to have healed [65]. It appears that the use of a fibrin clot may aid healing and due to the minimal cost and morbidity of the procedure it is a useful option. However, it is technically challenging.

12.5.4 Platelet-Rich Plasma

Platelet-rich plasma (PRP) is simple to access for most clinicians. It is produced using autologous blood taken from the periphery which is then centrifuged to separate the PRP from whole blood. The potential benefit of PRP is the local delivery of growth factors and cytokines to the meniscal tear. However, the exact constituents in each PRP preparation differ due to different separation techniques and patients. Broadly speaking, PRP preparations can be leukocyte rich or poor, contain activated or inactivated platelets, and have a higher or lower concentration of platelets. It is still unknown which preparation works best in each situation [66].

In a retrospective study of 15 isolated meniscal repairs augmented (tear sutured over the PRP) with PRP versus 20 without, there was no difference in reoperation or function at 2-year follow-up [67]. Similar findings of no difference in function or failure with the use of PRP were reported in another retrospective study of 14 PRP versus 15 control in discoid lateral menisci [68]. A prospective RCT compared 20 menisci repaired using PRP augmentation versus a control group of 18 menisci. The primary endpoint was evidence of healing on MRI or second-look arthroscopy at 18 weeks. There was a significant difference in the healing rate of 85% in the PRP group versus 47% in the control. At 42 months after surgery, patients with PRP augmentation had significantly improved IKDC scores [69]. Interestingly, a previous study performed a post hoc power calculation and suggested that 153 patients with PRP and 219 without PRP would need to be included to demonstrate a difference using IKDC [67].

In summary, there is little evidence that PRP has any effect on meniscal healing, failure, or functional outcomes [70]. In addition, there is still confusion as to what constitutes the correct formulation of PRP. Therefore, it is currently hard to recommend this augmentation strategy.

12.5.5 Growth Factor

Growth factor injections aim to improve angiogenesis and cell formation around a meniscal tear. The use of a platelet-derived growth factor/hepatocyte growth factor-enhanced collagen gel led to organized meniscal tissue growth in vitro [71]. Transforming growth factor-β1 (TGF-β1) was found to increase cell proliferation in repaired meniscal explants from pigs. However, it did not affect the strength of the repair [72]. TGF-β1 was also found to stimulate healing of meniscal defects in rabbits with fibrous tissue (type 2 collagen) [73]. Gelatin hydrogels containing fibroblast growth factor-2 significantly stimulated proliferation, enhancing meniscal repair in a rabbit model [74]. As of yet there has been no translation of such research into clinical trials, but it remains an area of promise.

12.6 Rehabilitation

There is insufficient evidence to recommend any particular rehabilitation protocol [75]. Restricted protocols (limiting weight bearing and range of movement) have been compared to accelerated protocols (immediate weight bearing and full range of movement) with no difference found in complication rate or function. The authors of this chapter prefer to use differing protocols depending on the tear orientation:

1. Vertical tear: Immediate weight bearing (WB) in brace locked in extension for 4 weeks. 0–90° range of movement (ROM) allowed immediately when non-weight bearing. From 4 weeks, the brace is removed, and full WB allowed with 0–90° ROM. Squatting beyond 90° and cutting sports allowed after 4 months.
2. Radial tear: Non-WB for 6 weeks with 0–90° ROM in brace. Remove brace and increase weight bearing as tolerated thereafter. Squatting beyond 90° and cutting sports allowed after 4 months.
3. Partial Meniscal Restoration: Non-WB for 1 week, then partial WB for 5 weeks, then full. Brace to control ROM at 0–60° for 4 weeks, then 0–90 for 2 weeks, then full. No squatting beyond 90° or cutting sports until 6 months.

References

1. Guermazi A, Niu J, Hayashi D, Roemer FW, Englund M, Neogi T, et al. Prevalence of abnormalities in knees detected by MRI in adults without knee osteoarthritis: population based observational study (Framingham Osteoarthritis Study). BMJ. 2012;345:e5339. Available from: https://www.bmj.com/content/345/bmj.e5339.
2. Bisson LJ, Kluczynski MA, Wind WM, Fineberg MS, Bernas GA, Rauh MA, et al. How does the presence of unstable chondral lesions affect patient outcomes after partial meniscectomy? The ChAMP randomized controlled trial. Am J Sports Med. 2018;46(3):590–7.
3. Abram SGF, Judge A, Beard DJ, Carr AJ, Price AJ. Long-term rates of knee arthroplasty in a cohort of 834 393 patients with a history of arthroscopic partial meniscectomy. Bone Joint J. 2019;101-B(9):1071–80.
4. Khan T, Alvand A, Prieto-Alhambra D, Culliford DJ, Judge A, Jackson WF, et al. ACL and meniscal injuries increase the risk of primary total knee replacement for osteoarthritis: a matched case–control study using the Clinical Practice Research Datalink (CPRD). Br J Sports Med. 2019;53(15):965–8.
5. Peña E, Calvo B, Martinez MA, Palanca D, Doblaré M. Why lateral meniscectomy is more dangerous

than medial meniscectomy. A finite element study. J Orthop Res. 2006;24(5):1001–10.

6. Papalia R, Del Buono A, Osti L, Denaro V, Maffulli N. Meniscectomy as a risk factor for knee osteoarthritis: a systematic review. Br Med Bull. 2011;99:89–106.

7. Cooper DE, Arnoczky SP, Warren RF. Arthroscopic meniscal repair. Clin Sports Med. 1990; 9(3):589–607.

8. Kopf S, Beaufils P, Hirschmann MT, Rotigliano N, Ollivier M, Pereira H, et al. Management of traumatic meniscus tears: the 2019 ESSKA meniscus consensus. Knee Surg Sports Traumatol Arthrosc. 2020; https://doi.org/10.1007/s00167-020-05847-3.

9. Arnoczky SP, Warren RF. Microvasculature of the human meniscus. Am J Sports Med. 1982;10(2):90–5.

10. Petersen W, Tillmann B. Age-related blood and lymph supply of the knee menisci. A cadaver study. Acta Orthop Scand. 1995;66(4):308–12.

11. Lutz C, Dalmay F, Ehkirch FP, Cucurulo T, Laporte C, Le Henaff G, et al. Meniscectomy versus meniscal repair: 10 years radiological and clinical results in vertical lesions in stable knee. Orthop Traumatol Surg Res. 2015;101(8 Suppl):S327–31.

12. Koh JL, Yi SJ, Ren Y, Zimmerman TA, Zhang L-Q. Tibiofemoral contact mechanics with horizontal cleavage tear and resection of the medial meniscus in the human knee. J Bone Joint Surg Am. 2016;98(21):1829–36.

13. Koh JL, Zimmerman TA, Patel S, Ren Y, Xu D, Zhang L-Q. Tibiofemoral contact mechanics with horizontal cleavage tears and treatment of the lateral meniscus in the human knee: an in vitro cadaver study. Clin Orthop Relat Res. 2018;476(11):2262–70.

14. Kurzweil PR, Lynch NM, Coleman S, Kearney B. Repair of horizontal meniscus tears: a systematic review. Arthroscopy. 2014;30(11):1513–9.

15. Lawton R, Thompson P, Spalding T. Meniscal repair and replacement. Orthop Trauma. 2019;33(2):109–18.

16. Duchman KR, Westermann RW, Spindler KP, Reinke EK, Huston LJ, Amendola A, et al. The fate of meniscus tears left in situ at the time of anterior cruciate ligament reconstruction: a 6-year follow-up study from the MOON cohort. Am J Sports Med. 2015;43(11):2688–95.

17. van der Wal RJP, Thomassen BJW, Swen J-WA, van Arkel ERA. Time interval between trauma and arthroscopic meniscal repair has no influence on clinical survival. J Knee Surg. 2016;29(5):436–42.

18. Popescu D, Sastre S, Caballero M, Lee JWK, Claret I, Nuñez M, et al. Meniscal repair using the FasT-fix device in patients with chronic meniscal lesions. Knee Surg Sports Traumatol Arthrosc. 2010;18(4):546–50.

19. Espejo-Reina A, Serrano-Fernández JM, Martín-Castilla B, Estades-Rubio FJ, Briggs KK, Espejo-Baena A. Outcomes after repair of chronic bucket-handle tears of medial meniscus. Arthroscopy. 2014;30(4):492–6.

20. Poland S, Everhart JS, Kim W, Axcell K, Magnussen RA, Flanigan DC. Age of 40 years or older does not affect meniscal repair failure risk at 5 years. Arthroscopy. 2019;35(5):1527–32.

21. Everhart JS, Magnussen RA, Poland S, DiBartola AC, Blackwell R, Kim W, et al. Meniscus repair five-year results are influenced by patient pre-injury activity level but not age group. Knee. 2020;27(1):157–64.

22. Rothermel SD, Smuin D, Dhawan A. Are outcomes after meniscal repair age dependent? A systematic review. Arthroscopy. 2018;34(3):979–87.

23. Sommerfeldt MF, Magnussen RA, Randall KL, Tompkins M, Perkins B, Sharma A, et al. The relationship between body mass index and risk of failure following meniscus repair. J Knee Surg. 2016;29(8):645–8.

24. Ardizzone CA, Houck DA, McCartney DW, Vidal AF, Frank RM. All-inside repair of bucket-handle meniscal tears: clinical outcomes and prognostic factors. Am J Sports Med. 2020;48:3386–93.

25. Lyman S, Hidaka C, Valdez AS, Hetsroni I, Pan TJ, Do H, et al. Risk factors for meniscectomy after meniscal repair. Am J Sports Med. 2013;41:2772–8. Available from: https://journals.sagepub.com/doi/10.1177/0363546513503444.

26. Buckley PS, Kemler BR, Robbins CM, Aman ZS, Storaci HW, Dornan GJ, et al. Biomechanical comparison of 3 novel repair techniques for radial tears of the medial meniscus: the 2-tunnel transtibial technique, a "hybrid" horizontal and vertical mattress suture configuration, and a combined "hybrid tunnel" technique. Am J Sports Med. 2019;47(3):651–8.

27. Nakata K, Shino K, Kanamoto T, Mae T, Yamada Y, Amano H, et al. New technique of arthroscopic meniscus repair in radial tears. In: Doral MN, editor. Sports injuries: prevention, diagnosis, treatment and rehabilitation. Berlin: Springer; 2012. p. 305–11. https://doi.org/10.1007/978-3-642-15630-4_41.

28. Turman KA, Diduch DR, Miller MD. All-inside meniscal repair. Sports Health. 2009;1(5):438–44.

29. Thompson SM, Spalding T, Church S. A novel and cheap method of outside-in meniscal repair for anterior horn tears. Arthrosc Tech. 2014;3(2):e233–5.

30. Tsujii A, Amano H, Tanaka Y, Kita K, Uchida R, Shiozaki Y, et al. Second look arthroscopic evaluation of repaired radial/oblique tears of the midbody of the lateral meniscus in stable knees. J Orthop Sci. 2018;23(1):122–6.

31. Woodmass JM, Johnson JD, Wu IT, Saris DBF, Stuart MJ, Krych AJ. Horizontal cleavage meniscus tear treated with all-inside circumferential compression stitches. Arthrosc Tech. 2017;6(4):e1329–33.

32. Rodkey WG, DeHaven KE, Montgomery WH, Baker CL, Beck CL, Hormel SE, et al. Comparison of the collagen meniscus implant with partial meniscectomy. A prospective randomized trial. J Bone Joint Surg Am. 2008;90(7):1413–26.

33. Bulgheroni E, Grassi A, Campagnolo M, Bulgheroni P, Mudhigere A, Gobbi A. Comparative study of collagen versus synthetic-based meniscal scaffolds in

treating meniscal deficiency in young active population. Cartilage. 2016;7(1):29–38.
34. Pereira H, Fatih Cengiz I, Gomes S, Espregueira-Mendes J, Ripoll PL, Monllau JC, et al. Meniscal allograft transplants and new scaffolding techniques. EFORT Open Rev. 2019;4(6):279–95.
35. de Caro F, Perdisa F, Dhollander A, Verdonk R, Verdonk P. Meniscus scaffolds for partial meniscus defects. Clin Sports Med. 2020;39(1):83–92.
36. Zaffagnini S, Marcheggiani Muccioli GM, Lopomo N, Bruni D, Giordano G, Ravazzolo G, et al. Prospective long-term outcomes of the medial collagen meniscus implant versus partial medial meniscectomy: a minimum 10-year follow-up study. Am J Sports Med. 2011;39(5):977–85.
37. Monllau JC, Gelber PE, Abat F, Pelfort X, Abad R, Hinarejos P, et al. Outcome after partial medial meniscus substitution with the collagen meniscal implant at a minimum of 10 years' follow-up. Arthroscopy. 2011;27(7):933–43.
38. Bulgheroni E, Grassi A, Bulgheroni P, Marcheggiani Muccioli GM, Zaffagnini S, Marcacci M. Long-term outcomes of medial CMI implant versus partial medial meniscectomy in patients with concomitant ACL reconstruction. Knee Surg Sports Traumatol Arthrosc. 2015;23(11):3221–7.
39. Hirschmann MT, Keller L, Hirschmann A, Schenk L, Berbig R, Lüthi U, et al. One-year clinical and MR imaging outcome after partial meniscal replacement in stabilized knees using a collagen meniscus implant. Knee Surg Sports Traumatol Arthrosc. 2013;21(3):740–7.
40. Bouyarmane H, Beaufils P, Pujol N, Bellemans J, Roberts S, Spalding T, et al. Polyurethane scaffold in lateral meniscus segmental defects: clinical outcomes at 24 months follow-up. Orthop Traumatol Surg Res. 2014;100(1):153–7.
41. Warth RJ, Rodkey WG. Resorbable collagen scaffolds for the treatment of meniscus defects: a systematic review. Arthroscopy. 2015;31(5):927–41.
42. De Coninck T, Huysse W, Willemot L, Verdonk R, Verstraete K, Verdonk P. Two-year follow-up study on clinical and radiological outcomes of polyurethane meniscal scaffolds. Am J Sports Med. 2013;41(1):64–72.
43. Houck DA, Kraeutler MJ, Belk JW, McCarty EC, Bravman JT. Similar clinical outcomes following collagen or polyurethane meniscal scaffold implantation: a systematic review. Knee Surg Sports Traumatol Arthrosc. 2018;26(8):2259–69.
44. Filardo G, Di Matteo B, Di Martino A, Merli ML, Cenacchi A, Fornasari P, et al. Platelet-rich plasma intra-articular knee injections show no superiority versus viscosupplementation: a randomized controlled trial. Am J Sports Med. 2015;43(7):1575–82.
45. Ghazi Zadeh L, Chevrier A, Farr J, Rodeo SA, Buschmann MD. Augmentation techniques for meniscus repair. J Knee Surg. 2018;31(1):99–116.
46. Okuda K, Ochi M, Shu N, Uchio Y. Meniscal rasping for repair of meniscal tear in the avascular zone. Arthroscopy. 1999;15(3):281–6.
47. Ochi M, Uchio Y, Okuda K, Shu N, Yamaguchi H, Sakai Y. Expression of cytokines after meniscal rasping to promote meniscal healing. Arthroscopy. 2001;17(7):724–31.
48. Gershuni DH, Skyhar MJ, Danzig LA, Camp J, Hargens AR, Akeson WH. Experimental models to promote healing of tears in the avascular segment of canine knee menisci. J Bone Joint Surg Am. 1989;71(9):1363–70.
49. Anz AW. Biological augmentation of meniscal repairs. In: LaPrade RF, Arendt EA, Getgood A, Faucett SC, editors. The menisci: a comprehensive review of their anatomy, biomechanical function and surgical treatment. Berlin: Springer; 2017. p. 137–46. https://doi.org/10.1007/978-3-662-53792-3_13.
50. Uchio Y, Ochi M, Adachi N, Kawasaki K, Iwasa J. Results of rasping of meniscal tears with and without anterior cruciate ligament injury as evaluated by second-look arthroscopy. Arthroscopy. 2003;19(5):463–9.
51. Shelbourne KD, Benner RW, Nixon RA, Gray T. Evaluation of peripheral vertical nondegenerative medial meniscus tears treated with trephination alone at the time of anterior cruciate ligament reconstruction. Arthroscopy. 2015;31(12):2411–6.
52. Shelbourne KD, Heinrich J. The long-term evaluation of lateral meniscus tears left in situ at the time of anterior cruciate ligament reconstruction. Arthroscopy. 2004;20(4):346–51.
53. de Girolamo L, Galliera E, Volpi P, Denti M, Dogliotti G, Quaglia A, et al. Why menisci show higher healing rate when repaired during ACL reconstruction? Growth factors release can be the explanation. Knee Surg Sports Traumatol Arthrosc. 2015;23(1):90–6.
54. Galliera E, De Girolamo L, Randelli P, Volpi P, Dogliotti G, Quaglia A, et al. High articular levels of the angiogenetic factors VEGF and VEGF-receptor 2 as tissue healing biomarkers after single bundle anterior cruciate ligament reconstruction. J Biol Regul Homeost Agents. 2011;25(1):85–91.
55. Vangsness CT, Sternberg H, Harris L. Umbilical cord tissue offers the greatest number of harvestable mesenchymal stem cells for research and clinical application: a literature review of different harvest sites. Arthroscopy. 2015;31(9):1836–43.
56. Driscoll MD, Robin BN, Horie M, Hubert ZT, Sampson HW, Jupiter DC, et al. Marrow stimulation improves meniscal healing at early endpoints in a rabbit meniscal injury model. Arthroscopy. 2013;29(1):113–21.
57. Howarth WR, Brochard K, Campbell SE, Grogan BF. Effect of microfracture on meniscal tear healing in a goat (*Capra hircus*) model. Orthopedics. 2016;39(2):105–10.
58. Ruiz-Ibán MÁ, Díaz-Heredia J, García-Gómez I, Gonzalez-Lizán F, Elías-Martín E, Abraira V. The

effect of the addition of adipose-derived mesenchymal stem cells to a meniscal repair in the avascular zone: an experimental study in rabbits. Arthroscopy. 2011;27(12):1688–96.

59. Hatsushika D, Muneta T, Horie M, Koga H, Tsuji K, Sekiya I. Intraarticular injection of synovial stem cells promotes meniscal regeneration in a rabbit massive meniscal defect model. J Orthop Res. 2013;31(9):1354–9.

60. Rothrauff BB, Sasaki H, Kihara S, Overholt KJ, Gottardi R, Lin H, et al. Point-of-care procedure for enhancement of meniscal healing in a goat model utilizing infrapatellar fat pad-derived stromal vascular fraction cells seeded in photocrosslinkable hydrogel. Am J Sports Med. 2019;47(14):3396–405.

61. Whitehouse MR, Howells NR, Parry MC, Austin E, Kafienah W, Brady K, et al. Repair of torn avascular meniscal cartilage using undifferentiated autologous mesenchymal stem cells: from in vitro optimization to a first-in-human study. Stem Cells Transl Med. 2017;6(4):1237–48.

62. Zhang Z-Z, Wang S-J, Zhang J-Y, Jiang W-B, Huang A-B, Qi Y-S, et al. 3D-Printed poly(ε-caprolactone) scaffold augmented with mesenchymal stem cells for total meniscal substitution: a 12- and 24-week animal study in a rabbit modelss. Am J Sports Med. 2017;45:1497–511. Available from: https://journals.sagepub.com/doi/10.1177/0363546517691513.

63. Shimomura K, Rothrauff BB, Hart DA, Hamamoto S, Kobayashi M, Yoshikawa H, et al. Enhanced repair of meniscal hoop structure injuries using an aligned electrospun nanofibrous scaffold combined with a mesenchymal stem cell-derived tissue engineered construct. Biomaterials. 2019;192:346–54.

64. Nakayama H, Kanto R, Kambara S, Iseki T, Onishi S, Yoshiya S. Successful treatment of degenerative medial meniscal tears in well-aligned knees with fibrin clot implantation. Knee Surg Sports Traumatol Arthrosc. 2020;28:3466–73.

65. Jang SH, Ha JK, Lee DW, Kim JG. Fibrin clot delivery system for meniscal repair. Knee Surg Relat Res. 2011;23(3):180–3.

66. Wang D, Rodeo SA. Platelet-rich plasma in orthopaedic surgery: a critical analysis review. JBJS Rev. 2017;5(9):e7.

67. Griffin JW, Hadeed MM, Werner BC, Diduch DR, Carson EW, Miller MD. Platelet-rich plasma in meniscal repair: does augmentation improve surgical outcomes? Clin Orthop Relat Res. 2015;473(5):1665–72.

68. Dai W-L, Zhang H, Lin Z-M, Shi Z-J, Wang J. Efficacy of platelet-rich plasma in arthroscopic repair for discoid lateral meniscus tears. BMC Musculoskelet Disord. 2019;20:113. Available from: https://www.ncbi.nlm.nih.gov/pmc/articles/PMC6421692/.

69. Kaminski R, Kulinski K, Kozar-Kaminska K, Wielgus M, Langner M, Wasko MK, et al. A prospective, randomized, double-blind, parallel-group, placebo-controlled study evaluating meniscal healing, clinical outcomes, and safety in patients undergoing meniscal repair of unstable, complete vertical meniscal tears (bucket handle) augmented with platelet-rich plasma. Biomed Res Int. 2018;2018:9315815. Available from: https://www.ncbi.nlm.nih.gov/pmc/articles/PMC5866900/.

70. Haunschild ED, Huddleston HP, Chahla J, Gilat R, Cole BJ, Yanke AB. Platelet-rich plasma augmentation in meniscal repair surgery: a systematic review of comparative studies. Arthroscopy. 2020;36:1765–74.

71. Bhargava MM, Hidaka C, Hannafin JA, Doty S, Warren RF. Effects of hepatocyte growth factor and platelet-derived growth factor on the repair of meniscal defects in vitro. In Vitro Cell Dev Biol Anim. 2005;41(8):305–10.

72. Riera KM, Rothfusz NE, Wilusz RE, Weinberg J, Guilak FL, McNulty A. Interleukin-1, tumor necrosis factor-alpha, and transforming growth factor-beta 1 and integrative meniscal repair: influences on meniscal cell proliferation and migration. Arthritis Res Ther. 2011;13(6):R187.

73. Chen C, Song J, Qiu J, Zhao J. Repair of a meniscal defect in a rabbit model through use of a thermosensitive, injectable, in situ crosslinked hydrogel with encapsulated bone mesenchymal stromal cells and transforming growth factor β1. Am J Sports Med. 2020;48(4):884–94.

74. Narita A, Takahara M, Sato D, Ogino T, Fukushima S, Kimura Y, et al. Biodegradable gelatin hydrogels incorporating fibroblast growth factor 2 promote healing of horizontal tears in rabbit meniscus. Arthroscopy. 2012;28(2):255–63.

75. Spang RC III, Nasr MC, Mohamadi A, DeAngelis JP, Nazarian A, Ramappa AJ. Rehabilitation following meniscal repair: a systematic review. BMJ Open Sport Exerc Med. 2018;4(1):e000212. Available from: https://www.ncbi.nlm.nih.gov/pmc/articles/PMC5905745/.

Meniscus Root Tear and Its Treatment

13

Matthew D. LaPrade, Lucas K. Keyt, and Aaron J. Krych

13.1 Meniscus Root Tear Introduction

Meniscus tears are quite common in the general public and represent approximately one-eighth of all orthopedic visits involving the knee [1, 2]. The meniscus is an important structure in the knee that provides the joint with shock absorption and support, and is crucial for joint preservation [3, 4]. Meniscus root tears, defined as avulsions or radial tears within 1 cm of the meniscus root attachment (Figs. 13.1 and 13.2), occur in up to 10–20% of patients undergoing arthroscopic meniscectomy [1, 3, 5–7]. Meniscus roots are crucial to the stability of the meniscus, and loss of the root attachment has been shown to significantly alter knee mechanics, increase joint contact pressures, and ultimately lead to the rapid development of osteoarthritis [1, 8].

Increased understanding regarding the rapid development of osteoarthritis following meniscus root tears has shifted how surgeons treat root tears [1]. Most meniscus tears occur in the fourth or fifth decade of life, so meniscus root tears were often treated nonoperatively or with partial meniscectomy [9]. However, it is now well accepted that

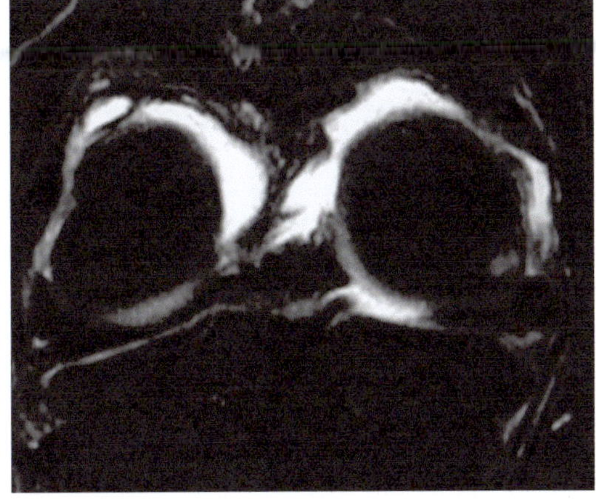

Fig. 13.1 Coronal MRI image demonstrating a radial tear near the root of the medial meniscus posterior root, as well as medial meniscus extrusion

meniscectomy leads to progressive degenerative changes including joint-space narrowing and flattening of the femoral condyles [1]. There has been a recent shift to repairing root tears to better preserve the joint cartilage and prevent the need for total-knee arthroplasty (TKA) at an early age [1, 9]. Meniscus root repair has shown promising results regarding the improvement of knee contact pressures, kinematics, and patient-reported outcome scores [1, 5, 9–11]. This chapter focuses on the state-of-the-art treatment of meniscus root tears with special consideration of the impact that root tears have on the articular cartilage.

M. D. LaPrade · L. K. Keyt · A. J. Krych (✉)
Department of Orthopedic Surgery and Sports
Medicine, Mayo Clinic, Rochester, MN, USA
e-mail: lapr0012@umn.edu;
Krych.Aaron@mayo.edu

© ISAKOS 2021
A. J. Krych et al. (eds.), *Cartilage Injury of the Knee*,
https://doi.org/10.1007/978-3-030-78051-7_13

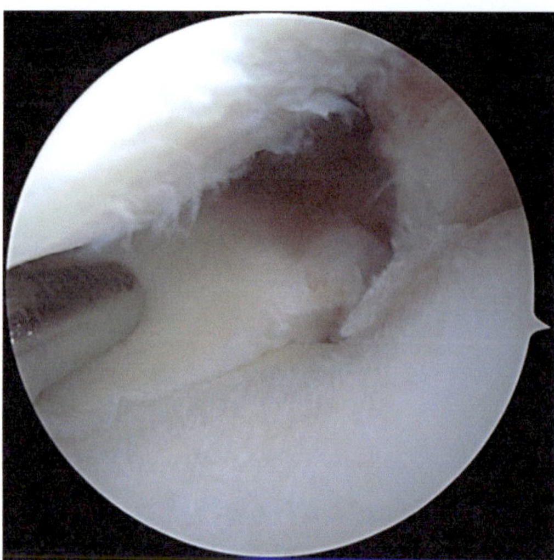

Fig. 13.2 Intraoperative arthroscopic view of a posterior medial meniscus root tear

Meniscus Root and Articular Cartilage Anatomy

The menisci are composed of fibrocartilage, which is primarily composed of dense collagen type I fibers and helps with shock absorption, stability, and load transmission [12]. The meniscus roots anchor the menisci in place and are critical to maintaining the stability and function of the menisci [13]. There are four distinct meniscus root attachments, with an anterior and posterior attachment on the medial and lateral menisci, respectively [13].

13.1.1 Anterior Roots

The anterior root of the medial meniscus has the largest attachment area and inserts on the anterior intercondylar crest of the tibia [1, 13]. The center of the medial meniscus anterior root is 18.2 mm anteromedial from the center of the ACL insertion [14]. Of note, anatomic reaming for intramedullary tibial nails was found to significantly damage the anterior root of the medial meniscus in smaller female cadaver knees [15].

The anterior root of the lateral meniscus inserts deeply beneath the ACL on the tibia, with 63% of the root attachment overlapped by the ACL attachment [16]. The center of the anterior root of the lateral meniscus is 5 mm anteromedial from the center of the ACL and is susceptible to iatrogenic injury during anatomic single-bundle ACL reconstruction [14, 17].

13.1.2 Posterior Roots

The posterior root of the medial meniscus is located posterior from the medial tibial eminence apex and anteromedial in relation to the PCL attachment [16]. The center of the posterior root of the medial meniscus is 8.2 mm from the nearest PCL edge [16].

The posterior root of the lateral meniscus is located anterolateral from the posterior root of the medial meniscus and anterior to the PCL [16]. The center of the posterior root of the lateral meniscus is located 12.7 mm from the nearest edge of the PCL, and 10.1 mm from the posterior edge of the anterior root of the lateral meniscus [16].

13.1.3 Articular Cartilage

Unlike the meniscus, articular cartilage is composed of hyaline cartilage made up from type II collagen fibers which provides the joint with a smooth, lubricated surface for articulation [18]. Articular cartilage injuries can cause significant pain and morbidity and are common, with an estimated 2/3 of patients undergoing knee arthroscopy having articular cartilage injuries [19–21]. The articular cartilage can be injured in the setting of a meniscus root injury. For a medial meniscus root tear, often diffuse degeneration of the medial compartment articular cartilage can be observed. For lateral root tears, which typically occur in younger patients with ACL tears, posterior cartilage damage to the lateral femoral condyle is observed. Similarly to the meniscus, articular cartilage is avascular and has little capacity to heal and repair itself [18, 22]. Occasionally, articular cartilage defects are replaced with fibrocartilage, which is less suited to withstand repetitive cyclical and compressive forces. In summary, articular cartilage injuries are common, have little ability to heal, and are a predisposing factor for the development of osteoarthritis [18, 19, 23].

13.2 Clinical Presentation and Diagnosis of Root Tears

The clinical diagnosis of meniscus root tears can be difficult because root tears often lack the telltale signs of meniscus body injuries, such as locking, catching, or giving way [4]. The most common positive physical exam findings are joint-line tenderness, a positive McMurray sign, and posterior knee pain with deep flexion [4]. Pain while performing a varus stress test with complete knee extension has been reported to be a clinical sign of a posterior root avulsion of the medial meniscus [24].

Meniscus tears can occur as traumatic, acute events or in a degenerative manner [1]. Traumatic root tears more commonly affect the lateral meniscus and are associated with concomitant cartilage and ligamentous injuries. Compared to degenerative tears, traumatic root tears are more commonly associated with patients who are younger and male and have a lower BMI and fewer degenerative changes at the time of arthroscopy [25]. Degenerative root tears more commonly affect the medial roots [25], and have been reported to represent 70% of all posterior root tears [26]. These degenerative tears typically occur without a recognizable injury and are thought to be caused by minor trauma, such as getting up from a chair or deep squatting [26]. Rarely, patients may present with root tears bilaterally [25]. Physicians should be suspicious of meniscus root tears in patients with knee pain that started without an identifiable event, especially medial meniscus root tears.

13.3 Imaging

MRI is the preferred imaging method to diagnose meniscus root tears [1, 4]. Root injuries are best visualized on T2-weighted MRI [27, 28]. Important visual cues can be used to suggest that a meniscus root tear is present. They include (1)

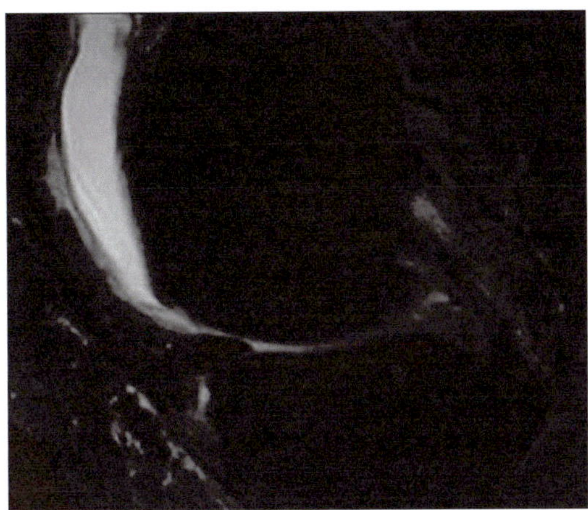

Fig. 13.3 Sagittal MRI image demonstrating a "ghost sign" appearance in the posterior compartment, consistent with medial meniscus posterior horn root tear

a "ghost sign," where a portion of the meniscus is not identifiable on sagittal or coronal imaging (Fig. 13.3); (2) a "cleft sign," where a linear/vertical high signal is present through the meniscus on sagittal or coronal imaging; and (3) a "truncation sign," where there is an abrupt ending of the triangular meniscus root on sagittal or coronal imaging [1, 28]. Even with improved quality of MRIs, recent studies have shown that a large proportion of posterior root tears are missed on MRI [29]. Krych et al. found that up to 67% of lateral meniscus posterior root tears were missed on preoperative MRI and recommended that radiologists report that "the root is poorly visualized" to ensure that surgeons investigate the root more thoroughly in the operative room [29].

13.4 Root Tear Classification and Meniscal Extrusion

Root tears have been classified based on tear morphologies to aid in the diagnosis and treatment of these tears. The LaPrade classification is the most widely used classification system for meniscus root tears [8]. Type 1 tears were defined as partial root tears that are stable (7.0%), type 2 tears are complete radial tears <9 mm from the root attachment (67.6%), type 3 are bucket handle tears with root detachments (5.6%), type 4 tears are complete oblique tears <9 mm from the root attachment

(9.9%), and type 5 tears are avulsion fractures at the root attachment (9.9%) [8]. Type 2 tears were further subclassified into three categories based on the location of the complete radial tear in relation to the root, with type 2A tears located <3 mm from the root, type 2B tears located between 3 and <6 mm to the root, and type 2C tears located 6–9 mm from the root attachment [8].

Meniscus extrusion and association with meniscus root tears have become increasingly recognized in the literature. Meniscus extrusion has been defined as displacement of the meniscus beyond the tibial plateau margins on MRI [30, 31]. Previous studies have found that extrusion is associated with posterior meniscus root tears; however, it is unclear whether root tears lead to extrusion, or the other way around [30–32]. It is clear, however, that meniscus extrusion is associated with the development of arthritis, and that anatomic root repair alone is unable to completely correct extrusion [30, 33]. Meniscus centralization, where the mid-body of the meniscus is "centralized" by stabilizing it onto the rim of the tibial plateau, has been proposed as a method to reduce meniscus extrusion [34]. It is hoped that centralization will better protect the articular cartilage and restore near-normal contact pressures compared to root repair alone.

13.5 Natural History

Unsurprisingly, the natural history of meniscus root tears is relatively poor. As described above, meniscus root tears are considered to be functionally equivalent to complete meniscectomy [5], which leads to rapid development of osteoarthritis without treatment. It has been reported that up to 28% of patients with unrepaired meniscus root tears underwent TKA at an average of 3.2 years from the initial diagnosis [1].

13.5.1 Subchondral Insufficiency Fractures of the Knee (SIFK)

Notably, increased contact pressures from root tears may predispose the knee to subchondral insufficiency fractures of the knee (SIFK), which were originally thought to be idiopathic and were referred to as spontaneous insufficiency fractures of the knee (SONK) [1, 35, 36]. SIFK have been found to be highly associated with posterior meniscus tears, with SIFK estimated to occur in 50–100% of patients with posterior meniscus tears [35, 36].

13.5.2 Articular Cartilage Damage

Damage to the articular cartilage can occur concomitantly with acute meniscus root tears, or can occur progressively over time due to altered contact pressures in the knee compartment. Articular cartilage injuries can cause significant pain and morbidity and are common with meniscus injuries [19, 23].

Acute, small cartilage defects can be treated with a variety of cartilage restoration procedures such as chondroplasty, microfracture, and osteochondral autograft transfer; however, these are outside the scope of this chapter [19]. Surgeons should be aware of patients with acute cartilage defects that may be amenable to treatment at the time of meniscus root treatment [19]. Progressive deterioration of the articular cartilage following an articular cartilage defect is an important mechanism surrounding the development of widespread knee osteoarthritis.

13.6 Clinical Outcomes

The main goals of meniscus root treatments are to prevent, or delay, the development of progressive osteoarthritis of the knee and to help the patient return to activity. As described above, meniscectomy or nonoperative treatment was the historical treatment for symptomatic meniscus root tears. More recently, several studies have demonstrated that partial meniscectomy is a significant risk factor for the development of osteoarthritis [4, 5, 37, 38]. Meniscectomy has become less commonly used to treat root tears as the research has become stronger to support the hypothesis that root repairs outperform meniscectomy and nonoperative treatment [9].

Early studies of the efficacy of meniscus root repair in delaying the progression of generalized osteoarthritis and TKA have been promising [9, 30, 38]. Chung et al. found that patients who underwent root repairs for medial meniscus posterior root tears had significantly less arthritis (measured by change in Kellgren-Lawrence (K-L) grade) grade progression, medial joint-space narrowing, and progression to TKA compared to patients who underwent partial meniscectomy at a follow-up of at least 5 years [10]. More recently, Bernard et al. found that patients undergoing root repair had significantly less K-L progression of osteoarthritis and progression to arthroplasty compared to matched cohorts of patients undergoing nonoperative and partial meniscectomy treatments at a mean follow-up period of 74 months [38]. Chung et al. found that 0% of repair patients underwent arthroplasty compared to 35% of partial meniscectomy patients at 6-year follow-up [10]. Similarly, Bernard et al. found that 0% of patients who underwent root repair progressed to arthroplasty, compared to 40% of partial meniscectomy and 27% of nonoperative patients [38].

Our understanding of root tears and the associated risk factors for repair failure has increased greatly over the past 20 years; however, there remain several unsolved questions [6]. Obesity and malalignment ≤5° place additional stress on the meniscus and are risk factors for potential repair failure [39]. Root repair has been shown to slow the progression of development of osteoarthritis; however, extrusion has also been found to be an important predictor of osteoarthritis progression [30, 33, 40]. In a recent comparative root repair study, Chung et al. found that patients with less meniscus extrusion had significantly less joint-space narrowing and significantly better K-L grades and clinical scores compared to patients with more meniscus extrusion at 1-year follow-up [30]. Interestingly, postoperative clinical scores improved significantly across both groups compared to their respective preoperative scores [10]. Meniscus centralization has been proposed as a way to correct extrusion and hope-

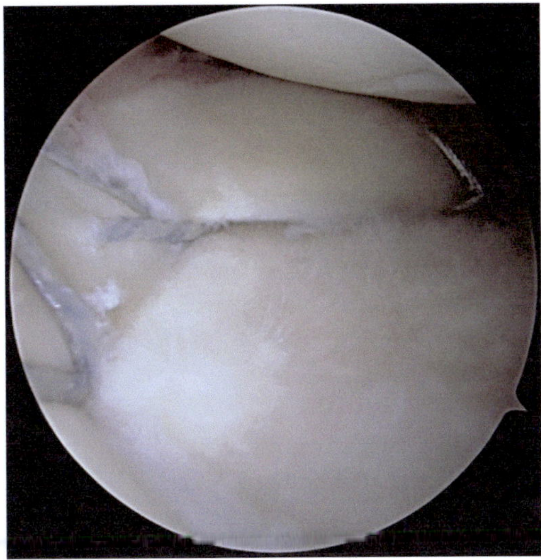

Fig. 13.4 Arthroscopic image of centralization sutures in the body of the medial meniscus performed concomitantly with a transtibial meniscus root repair

fully restore normal contact pressures (Fig. 13.4) [34]. Early reports regarding meniscus centralization are limited, yet promising, with further studies currently underway [33, 41–43].

13.7 Repair Options

Our group believes that repairs should be performed in young patients with otherwise healthy knees. It is very important to correct underlying issues at the time of repair, such as malalignment and ligamentous/cartilage injuries, in order to prevent repair failures and progression to osteoarthritis. Patients with generalized osteoarthritis and varus malalignment >5° are unlikely to benefit from repair [1, 6]. Obesity and malalignment ≤5° both place additional stress on the meniscus and are risk factors for potential repair failure [39]. Our group has strict inclusion criteria for patients undergoing root repair, because not all patients are good candidates for repair. Contraindications include K-L grade ≥3 on X-ray, grade 3 chondromalacia or worse at the time of arthroscopy, subchondral bone collapse, or varus malalignment >5°.

13.7.1 Transtibial Pull-Through Repair

The transtibial pull-through method requires drilling a transtibial bone tunnel to facilitate passing of a transosseous suture that is used to fix the meniscus root to the tibial insertion [1, 4]. The suture is then tied over a button on the tibia [4]. Our preferred technique for transtibial pull-through repair will be described further in Sect. 13.8 of this chapter.

13.7.2 Suture Anchor Repair

The suture anchor technique was designed to alleviate the need for drilling of tibial bone tunnels in the setting of patients with concomitant ligament reconstruction [4]. Engelsohn et al. first described the suture anchor technique, where an arthroscopic approach was used to repair the meniscus root tear [44]. The suture anchor technique is challenging, requires the use of a posterior portal that is near the neurovascular bundle, and uses a specialized, curved guide [45].

13.8 Author's Preferred Operative Technique: Transtibial Pull-Through

Repair of meniscal root tears has been described using sutures pulled through a transtibial tunnel and also using direct fixation with suture anchors. Although published outcomes support the efficacy of both suture anchor and transtibial constructs, with satisfactory and comparable structural healing and patient-reported outcome scores, the suture anchor technique is technically challenging, requires a posterior portal adjacent to the neurovascular structures, and uses specialized, curved suture-passing devices for constrained passing within the knee. Given this, the authors are proponents of transtibial fixation using standard and familiar arthroscopy portals, which has an established record of positive mid-term to long-term results [10, 46, 47].

Our preferred technique of meniscal root repairs has previously been described in detail [1, 48]. Standard knee arthroscopy portals are used, including a portal ipsilateral to the tear to allow for direct visualization of the posterior root. The attachment of the meniscal horn is inspected and palpated with a probe, which is of clinical significance because of the high rate of incomplete tear visualization on preoperative MRI [29]. In cases where it is difficult to obtain adequate visualization of the posterior meniscal roots and their respective compartments, we recommend consideration of (reverse) notchplasty or pie crusting of the medial collateral ligament to provide satisfactory arthroscopic access [49]. Given that meniscal root tears are challenging to identify preoperatively, including in the setting of both primary and revision ACL reconstruction, surgeons must always thoroughly inspect the meniscal attachments and be ready to repair detected root tears. For this reason, we recommend having meniscal suture-passing devices specialized for root repair available at the time of all knee cases.

After establishment of optimal portals and working space, attention is turned to tibial socket preparation. Given the importance of anatomic socket location, our preference is to use a root-specific tibial guide placed through the ipsilateral arthroscopy portal and centered on the meniscal root footprint. However, this can also be achieved with a standard ACL guide and drill. Subsequently, a 6 mm all-in-one guide pin/reamer is introduced into the joint through an incision on the proximal and medial tibia and deployed so that a shallow 6 mm socket is formed to provide fixation access to healing vascular subchondral bone. This can also be achieved with the standard 6 mm drill; however, this leads to greater bone loss along the length of the entire tibial tunnel compared with selective inside-out drilling with all-in-one instrumentation.

For meniscal fixation, a free No. 0 nonabsorbable suture is passed through the torn meniscus in a simple cinch configuration using a self-retrieving suture-passing device (Fig. 13.5). A total of 2–3 locking sutures are placed, depending on the tissue size and quality, and then individually tightened, with the knee cycled to remove creep from

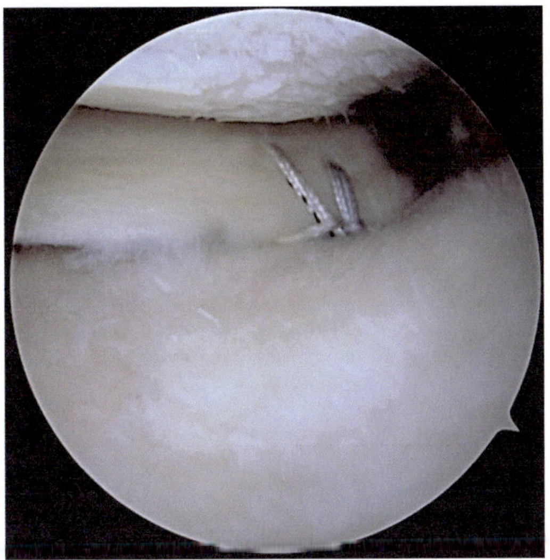

Fig. 13.5 Intraoperative view of a completed transtibial root repair for a medial meniscus posterior root tear

the system. Subsequently, the sutures are tensioned through the tibial socket to reduce the meniscal root back to the native bony root attachment. Tibial fixation is subsequently obtained using a 5.5 mm anchor or, as classically described, a tibial button, with the knee in 90° of flexion.

13.9 Postoperative Care

The postoperative period after meniscus root repair is crucial to the success of the operation. Healing of the meniscus best occurs when the knee is not loaded, especially in deep flexion, for the first several months. The postoperative care guidelines described below are for a patient undergoing an isolated root repair. Other concomitant procedures or ligamentous reconstructions (i.e., ACL reconstruction) can impact the timelines for root repair patients, and should be individualized based on surgeon and physical therapist recommendations.

In the early stages postoperatively, weight bearing is limited to toe-touch weight bearing in full knee extension while wearing a brace for the first 6 weeks. In addition, knee flexion is restricted beyond 90° for the first 6 weeks.

After 6 weeks, patients are allowed to progressively increase weight bearing and are no longer required to wear their brace. Patients are also encouraged to exercise their knee through full range of motion when the joint is unloaded; however, deep flexion beyond 90° is restricted until at least 4 months postoperatively.

The resumption of sporting activities is dictated by the postoperative timeline and the clinical readiness of the patient. After 3 months, patients are able to gradually increase physical activities. Patients with normal strength and symmetric gaits are allowed to gently ease into basic sporting activities between 4 and 6 months postoperatively. Patients with isolated root repairs are typically given a 6–9-month timeline to return to full sporting activities.

13.10 Controversies

Currently, there is controversy regarding whether meniscus root repairs are chondroprotective or not [1]. It is unclear whether repairing root tears protects the articular cartilage and prevents the development of OA. A recent study by Bernard et al. found that patients undergoing root repair have a significantly lower rate of progression to osteoarthritis compared to partial meniscectomy or nonoperative treatment [38]. This suggests that root repairs are likely improving the situation but not making it normal. Meniscus extrusion is not corrected with anatomic root repair [30, 33] and extrusion is associated with the development of osteoarthritis [30, 33]. Centralization has therefore been proposed as a way to correct meniscus extrusion at the time of repair, and has shown promising preliminary results [33, 41, 43]. However, further research is needed to determine the effectiveness of the centralization technique on chondroprotection.

Acknowledgments This study was partially funded by the following: National Institute of Arthritis and Musculoskeletal and Skin Diseases for the Musculoskeletal Research Training Program (T32AR56950). Its contents are solely the responsibility of the authors and do not necessarily represent the official views of the NIH.

References

1. Krych AJ, Hevesi M, Leland DP, Stuart MJ. Meniscal root injuries. J Am Acad Orthop Surg. 2020;28:491–9.
2. Majewski M, Susanne H, Klaus S. Epidemiology of athletic knee injuries: a 10-year study. Knee. 2006;13:184–9.
3. Papalia R, Vasta S, Franceschi F, D'Adamio S, Maffulli N, Denaro V. Meniscal root tears: from basic science to ultimate surgery. Br Med Bull. 2013;106:91–115.
4. Bhatia S, LaPrade CM, Ellman MB, LaPrade RF. Meniscal root tears: significance, diagnosis, and treatment. Am J Sports Med. 2014;42(12):3016–30.
5. Allaire R, Muriuki M, Gilbertson L, Harner CD. Biomechanical consequences of a tear of the posterior root of the medial meniscus. Similar to total meniscectomy. J Bone Joint Surg Am. 2008;90(9):1922–31.
6. Krych AJ. Editorial commentary: Knee medial meniscus root tears: "you may not have seen it, but it's seen you". Arthroscopy. 2018;34(2):536–7.
7. Kim SB, Ha JK, Lee SW, Kim DW, Shim JC, Kim JG, et al. Medial meniscus root tear refixation: comparison of clinical, radiologic, and arthroscopic findings with medial meniscectomy. Arthroscopy. 2011;27(3):346–54.
8. LaPrade CM, James EW, Cram TR, Feagin JA, Engebretsen L, LaPrade RF. Meniscal root tears: a classification system based on tear morphology. Am J Sports Med. 2015;43(2):363–9.
9. Faucett SC, Geisler BP, Chahla J, Krych AJ, Kurzweil PR, Garner AM, et al. Meniscus root repair vs meniscectomy or nonoperative management to prevent knee osteoarthritis after medial meniscus root tears: clinical and economic effectiveness. Am J Sports Med. 2019;47(3):762–9.
10. Chung KS, Ha JK, Yeom CH, Ra HJ, Jang HS, Choi SH, et al. Comparison of clinical and radiologic results between partial meniscectomy and refixation of medial meniscus posterior root tears: a minimum 5-year follow-up. Arthroscopy. 2015;31(10):1941–50.
11. LaPrade CM, LaPrade MD, Turnbull TL, Wijdicks CA, LaPrade RF. Biomechanical evaluation of the transtibial pull-out technique for posterior medial meniscal root repairs using 1 and 2 transtibial bone tunnels. Am J Sports Med. 2015;43(4):899–904.
12. Fox AJ, Wanivenhaus F, Burge AJ, Warren RF, Rodeo SA. The human meniscus: a review of anatomy, function, injury, and advances in treatment. Clin Anat. 2015;28(2):269–87.
13. Koenig JH, Ranawat AS, Umans HR, Difelice GS. Meniscal root tears: diagnosis and treatment. Arthroscopy. 2009;25(9):1025–32.
14. LaPrade CM, Ellman MB, Rasmussen MT, James EW, Wijdicks CA, Engebretsen L, et al. Anatomy of the anterior root attachments of the medial and lateral menisci: a quantitative analysis. Am J Sports Med. 2014;42(10):2386–92.
15. LaPrade MD, LaPrade CM, Hamming MG, Ellman MB, Turnbull TL, Rasmussen MT, et al. Intramedullary tibial nailing reduces the attachment area and ultimate load of the anterior medial meniscal root: a potential explanation for anterior knee pain in female patients and smaller patients. Am J Sports Med. 2015;43(7):1670–5.
16. Johannsen AM, Civitarese DM, Padalecki JR, Goldsmith MT, Wijdicks CA, LaPrade RF. Qualitative and quantitative anatomic analysis of the posterior root attachments of the medial and lateral menisci. Am J Sports Med. 2012;40(10):2342–7.
17. LaPrade CM, Smith SD, Rasmussen MT, Hamming MG, Wijdicks CA, Engebretsen L, et al. Consequences of tibial tunnel reaming on the meniscal roots during cruciate ligament reconstruction in a cadaveric model, part 1: the anterior cruciate ligament. Am J Sports Med. 2015;43(1):200–6.
18. Sophia Fox AJ, Bedi A, Rodeo SA. The basic science of articular cartilage: structure, composition, and function. Sports Health. 2009;1(6):461–8.
19. Camp CL, Stuart MJ, Krych AJ. Current concepts of articular cartilage restoration techniques in the knee. Sports Health. 2014;6(3):265–73.
20. Aroen A, Loken S, Heir S, Alvik E, Ekeland A, Granlund OG, et al. Articular cartilage lesions in 993 consecutive knee arthroscopies. Am J Sports Med. 2004;32(1):211–5.
21. Curl W, Krome J, Gordon S, Rushing J, Paterson B, Poehling G. Cartilage injuries: a review of 31,516 knee arthroscopies. Arthroscopy. 1997;13:456–60.
22. Patil S, Tapasvi SR. Osteochondral autografts. Curr Rev Musculoskelet Med. 2015;8(4):423–8.
23. Heir S, Nerhus TK, Rotterud JH, Loken S, Ekeland A, Engebretsen L, et al. Focal cartilage defects in the knee impair quality of life as much as severe osteoarthritis: a comparison of knee injury and osteoarthritis outcome score in 4 patient categories scheduled for knee surgery. Am J Sports Med. 2010;38(2):231–7.
24. Seil R, Duck K, Pape D. A clinical sign to detect root avulsions of the posterior horn of the medial meniscus. Knee Surg Sports Traumatol Arthrosc. 2011;19(12):2072–5.
25. Krych AJ, Bernard CD, Kennedy NI, Tagliero AJ, Camp CL, Levy BA, et al. Medial vs. lateral meniscus root tears: is there a difference in injury presentation, treatment decisions, and surgical repair outcomes? Arthroscopy. 2020;36:1135–41.
26. Pache S, Aman ZS, Kennedy MI, Nakama G, Moatshe G, Ziegler C, et al. Meniscal root tears: current concepts review. Arch Bone Jt Surg. 2018;6:250–9.
27. Lee SY, Jee WH, Kim JM. Radial tear of the medial meniscal root: reliability and accuracy of MRI for diagnosis. AJR Am J Roentgenol. 2008;191(1):81–5.
28. Harper KW, Helms CA, Lambert HS 3rd, Higgins LD. Radial meniscal tears: significance, incidence, and MR appearance. AJR Am J Roentgenol. 2005;185(6):1429–34.
29. Krych AJ, Wu IT, Desai VS, Murthy NS, Collins MS, Saris DBF, et al. High rate of missed lateral meniscus posterior root tears on preoperative magnetic resonance imaging. Orthop J Sports Med. 2018;6(4):2325967118765722.

30. Chung KS, Ha JK, Ra HJ, Nam GW, Kim JG. Pullout fixation of posterior medial meniscus root tears: correlation between meniscus extrusion and midterm clinical results. Am J Sports Med. 2017;45(1):42–9.

31. Krych AJ, Bernard CD, Leland DP, Camp CL, Johnson AC, Finnoff JT, et al. Isolated meniscus extrusion associated with meniscotibial ligament abnormality. Knee Surg Sports Traumatol Arthrosc. 2020;28:3599–605.

32. Krych AJ, Johnson NR, Mohan R, Hevesi M, Stuart MJ, Littrell LA, et al. Arthritis progression on serial MRIs following diagnosis of medial meniscal posterior horn root tear. J Knee Surg. 2018;31(7):698–704.

33. Daney BT, Aman ZS, Krob JJ, Storaci HW, Brady AW, Nakama G, et al. Utilization of transtibial centralization suture best minimizes extrusion and restores tibiofemoral contact mechanics for anatomic medial meniscal root repairs in a cadaveric model. Am J Sports Med. 2019;47(7):1591–600.

34. Koga H, Muneta T, Yagishita K, Watanabe T, Mochizuki T, Horie M, et al. Arthroscopic centralization of an extruded lateral meniscus. Arthrosc Tech. 2012;1(2):e209–12.

35. Robertson DD, Armfield DR, Towers JD, Irrgang JI, Maloney WJ, Harner CD. Meniscal root injury and spontaneous osteonecrosis of the knee: an observation. J Bone Joint Surg Am. 2009;91-B(2):190–5.

36. Hussain ZB, Chahla J, Mandelbaum BR, Gomoll AH, LaPrade RF. The role of meniscal tears in spontaneous osteonecrosis of the knee: a systematic review of suspected etiology and a call to revisit nomenclature. Am J Sports Med. 2019;47(2):501–7.

37. Salata MJ, Gibbs AE, Sekiya JK. A systematic review of clinical outcomes in patients undergoing meniscectomy. Am J Sports Med. 2010;38(9):1907–16.

38. Bernard CD, Kennedy NI, Tagliero AJ, Camp CL, Saris DBF, Levy BA, et al. Medial meniscus posterior root tear treatment: a matched cohort comparison of nonoperative management, partial meniscectomy, and repair. Am J Sports Med. 2020;48(1):128–32.

39. Krych AJ, Johnson NR, Mohan R, Dahm DL, Levy BA, Stuart MJ. Partial meniscectomy provides no benefit for symptomatic degenerative medial meniscus posterior root tears. Knee Surg Sports Traumatol Arthrosc. 2018;26(4):1117–22.

40. Kim SJ, Choi CH, Chun YM, Kim SH, Lee SK, Jang J, et al. Relationship between preoperative extrusion of the medial meniscus and surgical outcomes after partial meniscectomy. Am J Sports Med. 2017;45(8):1864–71.

41. Koga H, Muneta T, Watanabe T, Mochizuki T, Horie M, Nakamura T, et al. Two-year outcomes after arthroscopic lateral meniscus centralization. Arthroscopy. 2016;32(10):2000–8.

42. Ozeki N, Koga H, Matsuda J, Kohno Y, Mizuno M, Katano H, et al. Biomechanical analysis of the centralization procedure for extruded lateral menisci with posterior root deficiency in a porcine model. J Orthop Sci. 2020;25(1):161–6.

43. Ozeki N, Muneta T, Kawabata K, Koga H, Nakagawa Y, Saito R, et al. Centralization of extruded medial meniscus delays cartilage degeneration in rats. J Orthop Sci. 2017;22(3):542–8.

44. Engelsohn E, Umans H, Difelice GS. Marginal fractures of the medial tibial plateau: possible association with medial meniscal root tear. Skelet Radiol. 2007;36(1):73–6.

45. Lee SK, Yang BS, Park BM, Yeom JU, Kim JH, Yu JS. Medial meniscal root repair using curved guide and soft suture anchor. Clin Orthop Surg. 2018;10(1):111–5.

46. Chung KS, Noh JM, Ha JK, Ra HJ, Park SB, Kim HK, et al. Survivorship analysis and clinical outcomes of transtibial pullout repair for medial meniscus posterior root tears: a 5- to 10-year follow-up study. Arthroscopy. 2018;34(2):530–5.

47. Woodmass JM, Mohan R, Stuart MJ, Krych AJ. Medial meniscus posterior root repair using a transtibial technique. Arthrosc Tech. 2017;6(3):e511–e6.

48. Hevesi M, Stuart MJ, Krych AJ. Medial meniscus root repair: a transtibial pull-out surgical technique. Oper Techniq Sports Med. 2018;26(3):205–9.

49. Bert JM. First, do no harm: protect the articular cartilage when performing arthroscopic knee surgery! Arthroscopy. 2016;32(10):2169–74.

Cartilage Debridement of Symptomatic Lesions

14

John G. Lane and Macarena Morales Yañez

14.1 Introduction to Cartilage Debridement

Cartilage debridement or chondroplasty is the process of removing all unstable or detached cartilage fragments, in order to obtain a uniform and stable defect with vertical walls, which will help transfer the load to the articulating cartilage surface. This procedure was first described by Magnuson in 1941 as an open procedure with synovectomy, meniscectomy, osteophyte resection, and at times patellectomy. Currently, this is a much less invasive procedure that is performed arthroscopically in an attempt to preserve as much cartilage tissue as possible [1]. It still remains one of the most frequently used procedures in knee arthroscopy [2].

14.1.1 Epidemiology and Demographics

Most patients undergoing a cartilage procedure are young, 35 ± 11 years, with a BMI of 26 ± 4 DS [3]. Cartilage defects are widespread and can be found in as many as 34–62% [2, 4, 5] of all knee arthroscopies. Full-thickness lesions can be encountered in 10–19% [2, 4], which can rise to 36% in athletes [6]. The most frequent type of lesion is a traumatic injury with a grade II cartilage lesion by Outerbridge classification (41%). Many patients have multiple cartilage lesions (28%), with the patella being the most common site in 56%, followed by the medial femoral condyle in 34% [7]. However, the medial femoral condyle has been described as the most frequent site for a full-thickness isolated lesion in 50–58% of patients [2, 4, 5]. Approximately 32% are associated with other joint injuries, with a medial meniscus tear being the most commonly affected in 57%, followed by anterior cruciate ligament injury in 36% of injuries [2–4, 7].

14.1.2 Conservative Management

Unless there are significant mechanical symptoms, conservative management should be the initial approach before deciding to perform arthroscopic surgery. Physical therapy, weight loss, muscle strengthening, and oral supplements may be used in tandem to manage pain prior to surgery. In addition, injections such as cortisone or hyaluronan are appropriate options [8, 9]. Only if these treatments fail and the lesion continues to be symptomatic should surgery be considered.

J. G. Lane (✉)
Musculoskeletal and Joint Research Foundation,
University of California San Diego,
San Diego, CA, USA
e-mail: jglane@san.rr.com

M. M. Yañez
Department of Orthopaedic and Trauma Surgery,
Mataro Hospital, Mataró, Barcelona, Spain

© ISAKOS 2021
A. J. Krych et al. (eds.), *Cartilage Injury of the Knee*,
https://doi.org/10.1007/978-3-030-78051-7_14

14.1.3 Surgical Debridement

Chondral debridement is one of the most frequently performed procedures in arthroscopy [10]. It is a fast, effective, and easy-to-perform procedure to remove loose fragments and contour the remaining cartilage defect. The goal is to create a smooth articular surface with stable cartilage margins that may provide pain relief. It is also part of the preparation for other cartilage-resurfacing procedures such as matrix autologous chondrocyte implantation (MACI), BMAC, PJAC, and augmented microfracture-type procedures.

The use of debridement is still a matter of debate in patients with OA. Several studies have compared placebo, lavage, and debridement, without finding any statistically significant difference between osteoarthritic patient groups [11]. A Cochrane review by Spahn concluded that in the setting of osteoarthritis, debridement had no beneficial outcomes when compared to lavage [12, 13]. Consequently, the cornerstone of having a successful outcome will be selecting the correct patient with the right chondral lesion.

14.2 General Evaluation

14.2.1 Patient Characteristics

A complete patient history should be obtained to determine if an acute traumatic event or chronic exposure has occurred, causing a symptomatic chondral injury. Additionally, any history of additional meniscal or ligamentous injury or surgical intervention should be recorded. Early osteoarthritis risk factors such as meniscal root tear, partial or subtotal meniscectomy, ACL tear, and altered joint biomechanics should be carefully examined as this will determine the prognosis for the future (Table 14.1).

14.2.1.1 Establishing Desired Activity Level

It is imperative to understand the limitations of chondroplasty in order to achieve good results and patient satisfaction. The first consideration is

Table 14.1 Chondral treatment checklist

Patient characteristics	Lesion characteristics
BMI	Size (in cm^2)
Alignment	Depth
Meniscus	Location (weight bearing vs. non-WB)
Stability	Acute vs. overuse
Subchondral bone	ICRS scale

the patient's goals. One must correlate the patient's desires for activity with the treatment of various types and sizes of lesions. One needs to take into consideration the timing of the procedure to be performed and the recovery.

14.2.1.2 Level of Osteoarthritis at the Time of Surgery

As discussed previously, debridement in the setting of advanced osteoarthritis is not recommended. Various studies reported the lack of efficacy of debridement, even in cases of mild osteoarthritis, or where mechanical symptoms are present. This was described by Kirkley et al., in a randomized study in which arthroscopic treatment was compared to nonoperative and physical therapy treatments. In the study, subgroups were divided by different Kellgren and Lawrence levels of osteoarthritis, as well as the presence or absence of mechanical symptoms (i.e., locking or catching). At 1- and 2-year follow-ups, no differences were observed when comparing WOMAC scores, physical function, pain, or health-related quality of life between the groups and subgroups [11, 14]. Therefore, a cautious approach should be applied when treating these patients.

14.2.1.3 Status of the Meniscus

An intact meniscus is very important for proper knee biomechanics; once injured, it becomes a risk factor in the development of early osteoarthritis. If the resultant alterations in knee biomechanics are not appropriately addressed, the degenerative changes will progress over time. When performing osteochondral debridement in the context of partial meniscectomy, studies have not determined any differences in outcome whether chondroplasty was performed or not. This information must be analyzed carefully—the lack of data regarding the correct indications for meniscectomy and the status of the meniscus must be taken into account. Performance of chondral debridement in the setting of various types of degenerative meniscus tears may result in osteoarthritis, and it might result in limited benefit. The study by Bisson et al. suggests that there is no benefit to arthroscopic debridement of unstable chondral lesions encountered during arthroscopic partial meniscectomy (APM), and it is recommended that these lesions be left in situ [13]. In an acute setting, meniscal repair in combination with the debridement of a small osteochondral defect, which is less than 2 cm^2, results in outcomes which are significantly better than meniscectomy alone. Thus, each injury must be characterized individually and addressed appropriately. The key point is meniscal preservation and repair when possible [15].

14.2.1.4 Pain and Mobility

There are no specific signs or symptoms when cartilage defects are present. The various patient-reported outcome scales could be used, including KOOS, which is simple and quick, and patients can complete it on their own [16].

14.2.2 Lesion Characteristics and Classification

Identifying the lesion characteristics is crucial in treatment selection. Determining lesion location, size in cm^2, as well as relative size to the surrounding surfaces and depth of the defect are the most important considerations. These classifications, such as Outerbridge or the International Cartilage Regeneration and Joint Preservation Society (ICRS), should be used as a guide and not as an exact measure (Table 14.1).

14.2.2.1 Anatomic Location

Determining lesion location is a crucial first step in considering treatment algorithms. Biomechanically the medial femoral condyle transfers 53–92% of the total body load. This is the reason why chondral lesions are more frequent in the medial compartment. The same-size lesions are not as well tolerated in the medial femoral condyle compared to the lateral femoral condyle and progress more rapidly; as a result, the indications for debridement will only be more restricted [17]. For documentation purposes of the lesion location, the ICRS has developed the articular cartilage mapping system, which divides both condyles into quadrants: the anterior, central, posterior, and trochlea (Fig. 14.1) [18]. The importance of this method of documentation relies on the fact that a lesion located in the medial femoral condyle in the weight-bearing area will have much more pressure force than a non-weight-bearing location (Fig. 14.2) [19, 20].

14.2.2.2 Size

Classically, debridement is a preferred treatment option for defects up to 1.5–2 cm^2; this is based on the "critical size defect" concept [21]. A critical size defect references the fact that the size of a defect lacks sufficient width to have an effect on the success of the treatment even if the defect cannot heal spontaneously. At this threshold, it has been shown in animal models that there is a negative effect on the surrounding cartilage, causing a rapid exponential progression with even very small increments in the diameter of the lesion [21]. Flanigan et al. described in a bovine model that the critical size of full-thickness cartilage lesions that produces significant contact of the subchondral bone within the defect is 1.61 cm^2 for the medial femoral condyle, and 0.73 cm^2 for the lateral femoral condyle [22]. In cadaveric human knees, Papanaiau et al. recorded a significant pressure threshold in lesions >0.75 cm^2, with no statistically significant change between 0.75 and 2 cm^2 [23]. Contact pressure and critical size are subjective measures because the pressure is correlated with other mechanical parameters acting on the cartilage surface, such as the meniscus and synovial fluid. Thus the failure and development of osteoarthritis will also depend on its surrounding structures. At present, none of these models can reproduce the in vivo setting accurately.

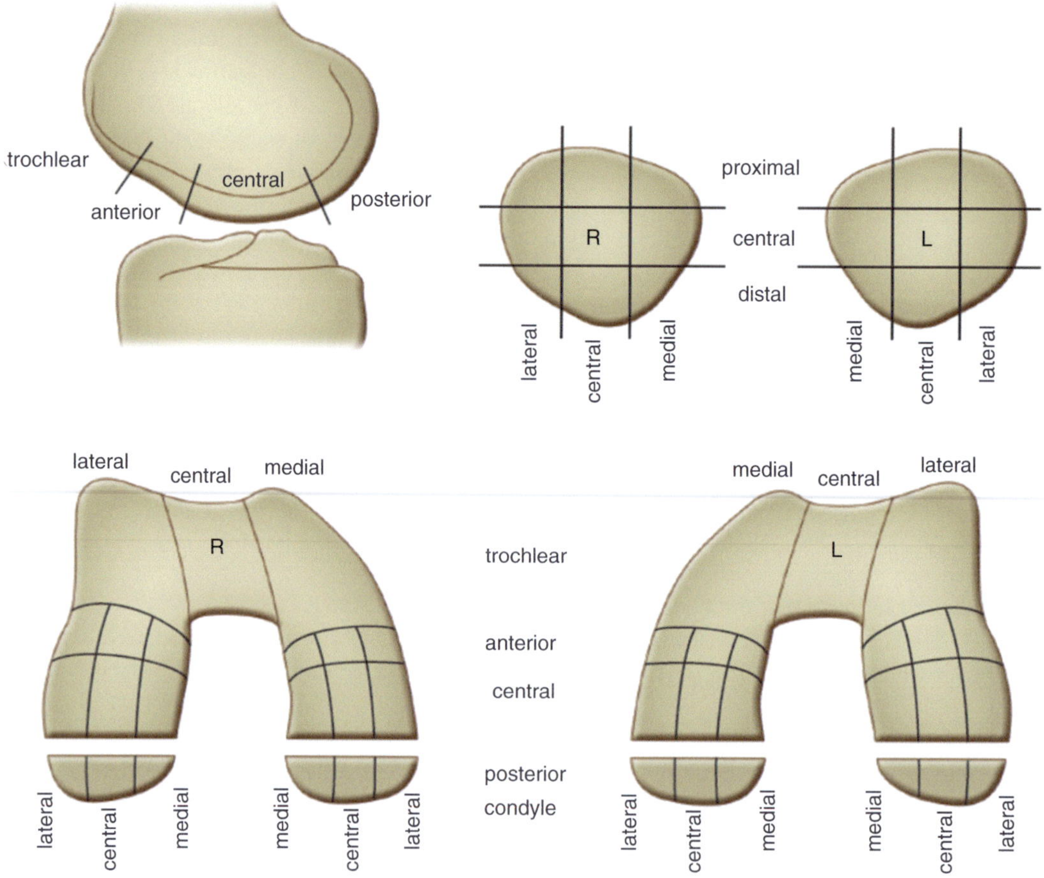

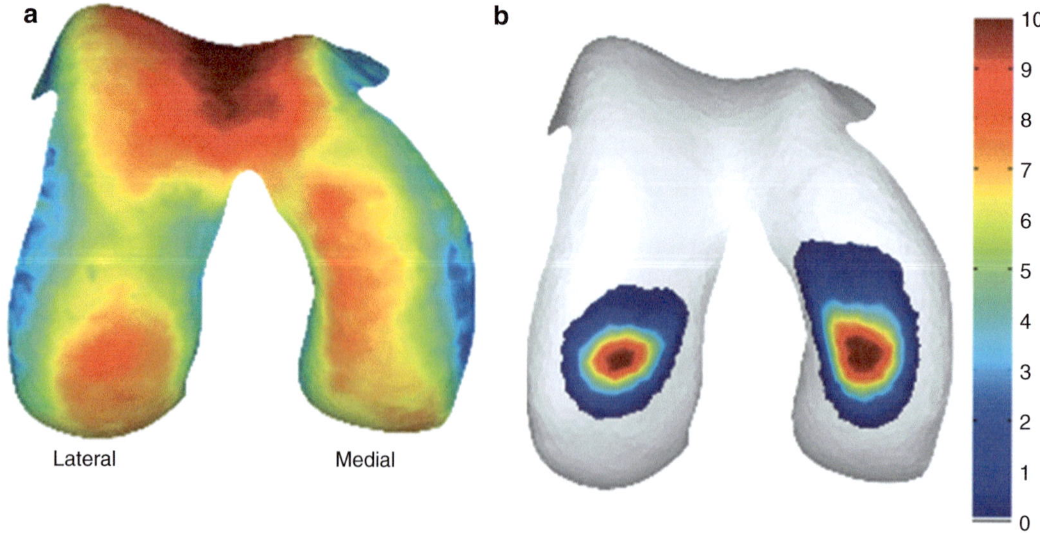

Fig. 14.1 ICRS—Articular cartilage injury mapping system. (Reproduced with permission from Mats Brittberg et al. (2000). Based on data from Ref. [18])

Fig. 14.2 Local correlations between cartilage pressure and thickness. (**a**) Average thickness distribution of all subjects. (**b**) Average pressure map. (Based on data from Ref. [19]. Reproduced with permission from Sam Van Rossom et al. (2017))

14.2.2.3 Depth

Depth can be described as partial-thickness <50% or full-thickness chondral lesion, and can be divided into IV stages according to Outerbridge or ICRS classification. Regarding partial-thickness injuries, after the initial injury, a zone of necrosis adjacent to the margins of the wound is created, followed by a period of mitotic activity and matrix synthesis. Still, this activity ceases with no progression of healing over time. These lesions usually remain stable and rarely progress to osteoarthritis.

Full-thickness lesions grade IV ICRS violate the subchondral plate. The healing process is stimulated by subchondral bone filling, first with a fibrin clot. Initially, it may have type II collagen, but later in the process, it is mostly composed of type I collagen with decreased content of proteoglycans. By 6–12 months, it creates a fibrocartilage matrix, which is biomechanically weaker with fibrillation over time that subsequently undergoes degeneration.

Most of the time, this tissue does not integrate well with the native cartilage and may be separated by a gap, which precipitates micromotion and degenerative changes. In conclusion, the most critical factor when classifying the depth of the chondral lesion is to determine if there is a violation of the tidemark.

14.2.2.4 Subchondral Bone Involvement

Special care must be taken when assessing the state of subchondral bone before considering a surgical decision. The presence of subchondral cysts or bone marrow lesions has been associated with chondral damage next to the lesion, even though the exact mechanism of development remains unknown. It has been associated with acute traumatic lesions, chronic osteoarthritis, and rheumatoid arthritis [24]. They should be identified with magnetic resonance imaging (MRI) as X-rays are not sensitive enough to detect small cysts and bone marrow edema [25]. We must carefully evaluate the need for core decompression in cases of significant bone marrow edema or other biologic treatments when a cyst or lesion extends to the subchondral bone

[26, 27]. For this reason, it is important to report the bony proportion of the defect as an independent depth. Another critical factor to take into account is that for certain bone marrow lesions, such as spontaneous osteonecrosis, a minimum of 4–6 weeks have to pass in order to see changes in MRI [28]; this can be a confounding factor during the surgery or if MRI is repeated after surgery.

14.3 Treatment

Debridement should be performed for select patients; frequently, it may be performed in conjunction with other procedures. The goal will be to preserve as much viable cartilage as possible; in order to accomplish that, the limits of the lesion must be carefully defined in width and depth. Loose flaps should be carefully resected rather than delaminated. A cartilage-sparing technique should be used, and afterwards, the underlying cause of the chondral damage has to be carefully addressed (Table 14.2).

14.3.1 Surgical Techniques

Two primary types of debridement have been described: mechanical and radiofrequency, which can be further divided into thermal and nonthermal. There is still controversy regarding which one is the best method; the main goal will be to stabilize cartilage margins and remove any loose fragments, preserving as much native cartilage as possible.

14.3.1.1 Mechanical Debridement

Mechanical debridement includes oscillating shavers and other handpieces like curettes, bas-

Table 14.2 Main indications and contraindications to debridement

Indication	Relative contraindication
1 cm² to <1.5 cm²	>2 cm
II–III Outerbridge	IV Outerbridge
In season athlete	Osteoarthritis II–IV
Pain	Asymptomatic

kets, and rongeurs. The dilemma is to create a stable articular surface without taking more cartilage than is needed.

Histologic analysis after shaving demonstrates that the remaining cartilage has a fissured and fibrillated surface, with chondrocyte death adjacent to the debrided regions [29, 30]. In contrast to other methods, it does not imply a chemical reaction; thus, it does not liberate energy, making the process somewhat safer for the remaining cartilage.

14.3.1.2 Radiofrequency Debridement

Radiofrequency devices are thought to contour the cartilage surface smoothly. The rationale supporting the radiofrequency use is that it purportedly seals the fibrillated cartilage surface, and it has been hypothesized that it may delay the degenerative process of cartilage delamination and fraying. However, it is debatable as to whether or not these techniques minimize the inflammatory cascade [31].

Thermal Radiofrequency

Thermal radiofrequency was introduced in 1990 based on the application of modulated thermal energy to produce a compact and uniform "biological scar." It creates a more effective removal of impaired cartilage compared to mechanical debridement with a precise approach to margins, avoiding fragmentation of tissue.

There are two main types of thermal debridement, monopolar and bipolar. There is no consensus established that supports the use of technology [32, 33].

Radiofrequency has been associated with a (low) risk of producing subchondral osteonecrosis, although causality has not been conclusively established, especially in light of other risk factors that a patient could have [34].

Nonthermal Radiofrequency

Nonthermal radiofrequency is also known as coblation (controlled ablation), or plasma radiofrequency. It is a bipolar wand, set in the ablation mode, with active control of temperature below 50 °C. Soft-tissue dissolution occurs from a plasma-like layer produced by a conductive medium, such as saline. The bipolar wand disassociates saline into sodium and chloride ions. Highly energized ions form a plasma field which is sufficiently strong to break organic molecular bonds within soft tissue causing its debridement. When used correctly, there is no contact from the probe to the soft tissue, so the thermal penetration is thought to be minimal [35].

Historically when radiofrequency has been compared to mechanical debridement, several clinical and histological studies reported good short-term outcomes in favor of radiofrequency [5, 36–38]. In 2016 Spahn et al. conducted a long-term randomized controlled trial, concluding that there were no meaningful clinical differences after 10 years. With the new advancement of technology and the use of confocal microscopy, the histological results were less clear. Both coblation and thermal radiofrequency have been shown to produce as much as twice the maximum depth of chondrocyte death compared with mechanical debridement 3 months after the procedure [39–42]. Edwards et al., in an equine model, compared these treatment modalities, and results showed that monopolar radiofrequency had significantly less chondral damage than the coblation system. The authors hypothesized that the thermal radiofrequency probe had less surface area, producing local coagulation without penetrating into deeper layers [29] (Fig. 14.3).

There is much to be discussed and clarified about the different methods for debriding. Until now, these differences have lacked clinical relevance. For any chosen device, it is essential to know its limits and correct way of usage.

14.3.1.3 Quality of Cartilage in a Defect

Cartilage generally lacks the ability to regenerate after a chondroplasty, and peripheral chondrocytes have a limited capacity to migrate or regenerate the defect [43]. The lesion will fill with fibrocartilage tissue high in type I collagen, which possesses inferior properties and diminished load transference, and increased probability of failure [44, 45]. Therefore, even if studies have shown excellent short-term outcomes, it

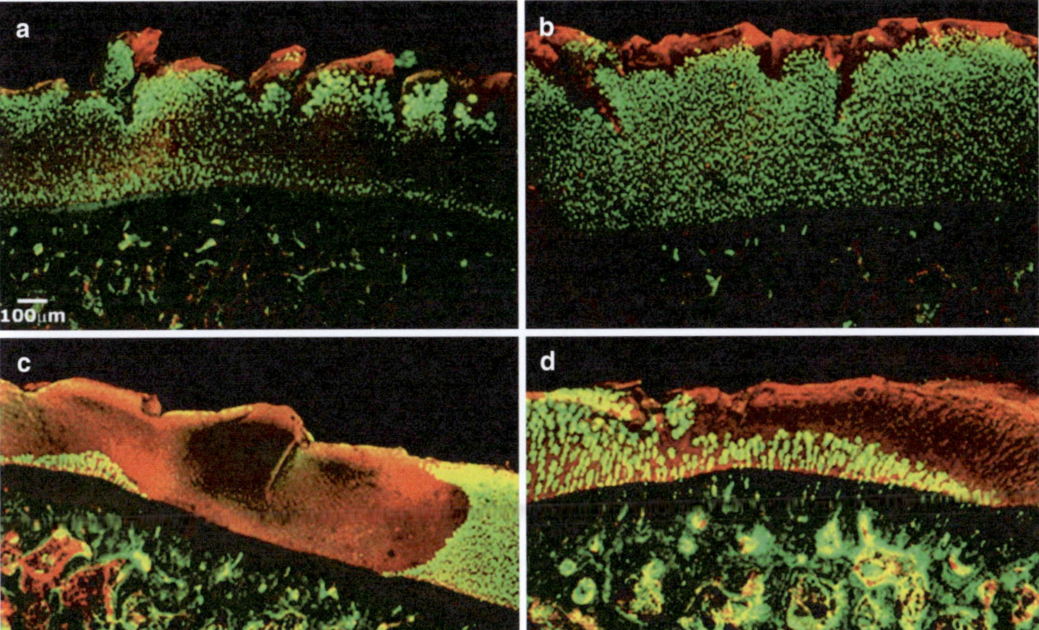

Fig. 14.3 Confocal laser microscopy images demonstrating increased cell death for both monopolar and bipolar radiofrequency, compared to control and mechanical debridement. Green dots are viable cells, and red dots are dead cells. (**a**) Control; (**b**) mechanical debridement; (**c**) nonthermal debridement; (**d**) thermal debridement [27]. (Reprinted from [39] Edwards RB, Lu Y, Uthamanthil RK, Bogdanske JJ, Muir P, Athanasiou KA, et al. Comparison of mechanical debridement and radiofrequency energy for chondroplasty in an in vivo equine model of partial thickness cartilage injury. Osteoarthr Cartil. 2007 Feb 1;15(2):169–78. With permission from Elsevier)

would be necessary to consider cartilage-reparative techniques such as MACI, OATS, or osteochondral allograft depending on the patient's expectations and lesion characteristics.

When there are no other treatment options, debridement can provide a fibrocartilage layer, which, regardless of its inferior biomechanical properties and earlier failure, helps to protect the subchondral bone. However, our objective is to recommend the preservation of the subchondral bone tidemark.

14.3.1.4 Concomitant Procedures

As previously discussed, it is imperative to manage the knee as a complex dynamic system. If the leading cause of the chondral defect is not addressed, the surgical procedure is doomed to fail. Other factors to consider are limb or patellar alignment, instability, and meniscal pathology.

Debridement can also be used as preparation for other procedures such as MACI. It is desirable to obtain stable vertical walls of healthy cartilage up to the edge of the defect and to maintain integrity of the subchondral bone and the calcified cartilage layer within the defect site. An overly aggressive debridement will cause damage to the subchondral bone and bleeding. On the other hand, an incomplete debridement will leave unstable cartilage with partial- or full-thickness defects. Drobnič et al. compared different techniques for the preparation of chondral defects before ACI implantation. He observed that when debriding lesions with margins perpendicular to the subchondral plate and removing the calcified cartilage layer open or arthroscopically assisted, manual curettage was better than the mechanical shaving or bipolar-electrode technique [46].

14.3.2 Clinical Outcomes and Follow-Up

The surgical outcome will be directly related to all the points discussed above, such as lesion characteristics, patients' characteristics, and association with other lesions of the knee.

14.3.2.1 Evolution of Osteochondral Lesion After Debridement

Most patients with focal chondral grade II–III lesions demonstrate improved clinical symptoms post-debridement. This debridement becomes less predictable when combined with other procedures like meniscectomy [15]. It is reported that approximately 80% of patients will remain pain free at 1 year post-chondroplasty, and 50% at 5 years, but symptoms will not always correlate with the severity of the chondral lesion [47, 48]. As a result, a close follow-up should be maintained for a possible increase in structural damage.

14.3.2.2 Rehabilitation

After surgery, the goal will be to maintain continuous active or passive motion and weight bearing as tolerated. Early articular movement has been demonstrated to have anti-inflammatory effects [49, 50], preventing adhesions and erosions. The patient should understand that chondral damage is a precursor of osteoarthritis in the future and therefore adopt a lifestyle that results in lower BMI, muscle strengthening for joint unloading, and lower impact rehabilitation exercises and workouts, and should know when to seek medical attention. When initiating physical therapy, exercises should be focused on balancing muscle function.

14.4 Summary and Conclusions

Cartilage debridement has been used as a treatment for articular cartilage defects since described by Magnuson in 1941. Care has to be taken to consider the shape and orientation of the defect and its relationship to the opposing articular surface. Also, while absolute size is generally reported, size should also be considered relative to the overall dimensions of the joint surface. While this procedure does not allow anatomical cartilage restoration, it can provide good pain relief with smaller defects. Mechanical debridement was noted to cause a limited degree of injury in the adjacent cartilage margins as a consequence of the debridement procedure. In my experience, a significant number of patients undergoing initial cartilage biopsy for a secondary procedure with stabilization of the margins of the cartilage defects experience substantial improvement and therefore do not elect to pursue additional cartilage repair procedures, at least in the short and midterm. A well-done debridement procedure does not preclude additional cartilage restoration options because it allows for subchondral bone preservation. Use of radiofrequency and thermal energy has been touted as possible ways of stimulating repair of cartilage lesions; however, this remains controversial. The concept of the procedure has evolved from a more extensive debridement with removal of cartilage surfaces with even mild changes and penetration of the subchondral bone to more of a stabilization procedure with removal of only loose and unstable fragments and preservation of the underlying bone surfaces. Smaller defects, less than 1.5 cm^2, can often be treated with debridement alone with good results. Therefore, debridement procedures remain a useful tool in the overall continuum of care for cartilage injury patients.

References

1. Magnuson PB. The classic: joint debridement: surgical treatment of degenerative arthritis. Clin Orthop Relat Res. 1974;101:4–12.
2. Curl WW, Krome J, Gordon ES, Rushing J, Smith BP, Poehling GG. Cartilage injuries: a review of 31,516 knee arthroscopies. Arthroscopy. 1997;13(4):456–60. Available from: https://linkinghub.elsevier.com/retrieve/pii/S0749806397901249.
3. Conley C, Mcnicholas M, Biant L. The ICRS patient registry annual report February 2019 1st annual report. 2019. p. 1–28.
4. Åroøen A, Løken S, Heir S, Alvik E, Ekeland A, Granlund OG, et al. Articular cartilage lesions in 993

consecutive knee arthroscopies. Am J Sports Med. 2004;32(1):211–5. Available from: http://journals.sagepub.com/doi/10.1177/0363546503259345.

5. Hjelle K, Solheim E, Strand T, Muri R, Brittberg M. Articular cartilage defects in 1,000 knee arthroscopies. Arthroscopy. 2002;18(7):730–4.

6. Flanigan DC, Harris JD, Trinh TQ, Siston RA, Brophy RH. Prevalence of chondral defects in athletes' knees: a systematic review. Med Sci Sports Exerc. 2010;42(10):1795–801. Available from: http://journals.lww.com/00005768-201010000-00001.

7. Widuchowski W, Widuchowski J, Trzaska T. Articular cartilage defects: study of 25,124 knee arthroscopies. Knee. 2007;14(3):177–82.

8. Strauss EJ, Hart JA, Miller MD, Altman RD, Rosen JE. Hyaluronic acid viscosupplementation and osteoarthritis: current uses and future directions. Am J Sports Med. 2009;37(8):1636–44. Available from: http://www.ncbi.nlm.nih.gov/pubmed/19168804.

9. Hepper CT, Halvorson JJ, Duncan ST, Gregory AJM, Dunn WR, Spindler KP. The efficacy and duration of intra-articular corticosteroid injection for knee osteoarthritis: a systematic review of level I studies. J Am Acad Orthop Surg. 2009;17(10):638–46.

10. Bonazza NA, Smuin DM, Joshi R, Ba D, Liu G, Leslie DL, et al. Surgical trends in articular cartilage injuries of the knee, analysis of the Truven Health MarketScan commercial claims database from 2005-2014. Arthrosc Sport Med Rehab. 2019;1(2):e101–7.

11. Bruce Moseley J, O'Malley K, Petersen NJ, Menke TJ, Brody BA, Kuykendall DH, et al. A controlled trial of arthroscopic surgery for osteoarthritis of the knee. N Engl J Med. 2002;347(2):81–8. Available from: http://www.nejm.org/doi/abs/10.1056/NEJMoa013259.

12. Spahn G, Kahl E, Mückley T, Hofmann GO, Klinger HM. Arthroscopic knee chondroplasty using a bipolar radiofrequency-based device compared to mechanical shaver: results of a prospective, randomized, controlled study. Knee Surg Sport Traumatol Arthrosc. 2008;16(6):565–73. Available from: http://www.ncbi.nlm.nih.gov/pubmed/18327566.

13. Bisson LJ, Kluczynski MA, Wind WM, Fineberg MS, Bernas GA, Rauh MA, et al. Patient outcomes after observation versus debridement of unstable chondral lesions during partial meniscectomy the chondral lesions and meniscus procedures (ChAMP) randomized controlled trial. J Bone Joint Surg Am. 2017;99(13):1078–85.

14. Kirkley A, Birmingham TB, Litchfield RB, Giffin JR, Willits KR, Wong CJ, et al. A randomized trial of arthroscopic surgery for osteoarthritis of the knee. N Engl J Med. 2008;359(11):1097–107. Available from: http://www.nejm.org/doi/abs/10.1056/NEJMoa0708333.

15. Weißenberger M, Heinz T, Boelch SP, Niemeyer P, Rudert M, Barthel T, et al. Is debridement beneficial for focal cartilage defects of the knee: data from the German Cartilage Registry (KnorpelRegister DGOU). Arch Orthop Trauma Surg. 2020;140(3):373–82. https://doi.org/10.1007/s00402-020-03338-1.

16. Collins NJ, Prinsen CAC, Christensen R, Bartels EM, Terwee CB, Roos EM. Knee injury and osteoarthritis outcome score (KOOS): systematic review and meta-analysis of measurement properties. Osteoarthritis Cartil. 2016;24:1317–29.

17. Kumar D, Manal KT, Rudolph KS. Knee joint loading during gait in healthy controls and individuals with knee osteoarthritis. Osteoarthr Cartil. 2013;21(2):298–305.

18. Brittberg M. Evaluation of cartilage injuries and cartilage repair. Osteologie. 2000;9(1):17–25.

19. Harris JD, Siston RA, Pan X, Flanigan DC. Autologous chondrocyte implantation: a systematic review. J Bone Joint Surg A. 2010;92:2220–33. Available from: http://journals.lww.com/00004623-201009150-00012.

20. Everhart JS, Siston RA, Flanigan DC. Tibiofemoral subchondral surface ratio (SSR) is a predictor of osteoarthritis symptoms and radiographic progression: data from the osteoarthritis initiative (OAI). Osteoarthr Cartil. 2014;22(6):771–8.

21. Katagiri H, Mendes LF, Luyten FP. Definition of a critical size osteochondral knee defect and its negative effect on the surrounding articular cartilage in the rat. Osteoarthr Cartil. 2017;25(9):1531–40.

22. Flanigan DC, Harris JD, Brockmeier PM, Siston RA. The effects of lesion size and location on subchondral bone contact in experimental knee articular cartilage defects in a bovine model. Arthroscopy. 2010;26(12). Available from: https://linkinghub.elsevier.com/retrieve/pii/S0749806310005074.

23. Papaioannou G, Demetropoulos CK, King YH. Predicting the effects of knee focal articular surface injury with a patient-specific finite element model. Knee. 2010;17(1):61–8. Available from: https://linkinghub.elsevier.com/retrieve/pii/S0968016009000830.

24. Crema MD, Roemer FW, Zhu Y, Marra MD, Niu J, Zhang Y, et al. Subchondral cystlike lesions develop longitudinally in areas of bone marrow edema-like lesions in patients with or at risk for knee osteoarthritis: detection with MR imaging—the MOST study. Radiology. 2010;256(3):855–62.

25. Zanetti M, Bruder E, Romero J, Hodler J. Bone marrow edema pattern in osteoarthritic knees: correlation between MR imaging and histologic findings. Radiology. 2000;215(3):835–40.

26. Hernigou P, Flouzat-Lachaniette CH, Delambre J, Poignard A, Allain J, Chevallier N, et al. Osteonecrosis repair with bone marrow cell therapies: state of the clinical art. Bone. 2015;70:102–9.

27. Li X, Xu X, Wu W. Comparison of bone marrow mesenchymal stem cells and core decompression in treatment of osteonecrosis of the femoral head: a meta-analysis. Int J Clin Exp Pathol. 2014;7(8):5024–30.

28. Nakamura T, Matsumoto T, Nishino M, Tomita K, Kadoya M. Early magnetic resonance imaging and histologic findings in a model of femoral head necrosis. Clin Orthop Relat Res. 1997;334:68–72. Available from: http://www.ncbi.nlm.nih.gov/pubmed/9005897.

29. Edwards RB, Lu Y, Cole BJ, Muir P, Markel MD. Comparison of radiofrequency treatment and mechanical debridement of fibrillated cartilage in an equine model. Vet Comp Orthop Traumatol. 2008;21(01):41–8.

30. Tew SR, Kwan AP, Hann A, Thomson BM, Archer CW. The reactions of articular cartilage to experimental wounding: role of apoptosis. Arthritis Rheum. 2000;43(1):215–25. Available from: http://www.ncbi.nlm.nih.gov/pubmed/10643718.

31. Peng L, Li Y, Zhang K, Chen Q, Xiao L, Geng Y, et al. The time-dependent effects of bipolar radiofrequency energy on bovine articular cartilage. J Orthop Surg Res. 2020;15(1):106. Available from: https://josr-online.biomedcentral.com/articles/10.1186/s13018-020-01626-5.

32. Huber M, Eder C, Mueller M, Kujat R, Roll C, Nerlich M, et al. Temperature profile of radiofrequency probe application in wrist arthroscopy: monopolar versus bipolar. Arthroscopy. 2013;29(4):645–52.

33. Cook JL, Kuroki K, Kenter K, Marberry K, Brawner T, Geiger T, et al. Bipolar and monopolar radiofrequency treatment of osteoarthritic knee articular cartilage. J Knee Surg. 2004;17(2):99–108. Available from: http://www.thieme-connect.de/DOI/DOI?10.1055/s-0030-1248205.

34. Rocco P, Lorenzo DB, Guglielmo T, Michele P, Nicola M, Vincenzo D. Radiofrequency energy in the arthroscopic treatment of knee chondral lesions: a systematic review. Br Med Bull. 2016;117(1):149–56.

35. Belov SV. Use of high-frequency cold plasma ablation technology for electrosurgery with minimized invasiveness. Biomed Eng (NY). 2004;38(2):80–5. Available from: http://link.springer.com/10.1023/B:BIEN.0000035727.52535.11.

36. Kang RW, Gomoll AH, Nho SJ, Pylawka TK, Cole BJ. Outcomes of mechanical debridement and radiofrequency ablation in the treatment of chondral defects. J Knee Surg. 2008;21(2):116–21.

37. Owens BD, Stickles BJ, Balikian P, Busconi BD. Prospective analysis of radiofrequency versus mechanical debridement of isolated patellar chondral lesions. Arthroscopy. 2002;18(2):151–5.

38. Stein DT, Ricciardi CA, Viehe T. The effectiveness of the use of electrocautery with chondroplasty in treating chondromalacic lesions: a randomized prospective study. Arthroscopy. 2002;18(2):190–3.

39. Edwards RB, Lu Y, Uthamanthil RK, Bogdanske JJ, Muir P, Athanasiou KA, et al. Comparison of mechanical debridement and radiofrequency energy for chondroplasty in an in vivo equine model of partial thickness cartilage injury. Osteoarthr Cartil. 2007;15(2):169–78.

40. Lu Y, Edwards RB, Kalscheur VL, Nho S, Cole BJ, Markel MD. Effect of bipolar radiofrequency energy on human articular cartilage: comparison of confocal laser microscopy and light microscopy. Arthroscopy. 2001;17(2):117–23. Available from: https://linkinghub.elsevier.com/retrieve/pii/S0749806301675133.

41. Buckup K. Pruebas clínicas para patología ósea, articular y muscular. Pruebas clínicas para Patol ósea, Articul y muscular. 2007.

42. Caffey S, McPherson E, Moore B, Hedman T, Vangsness CT. Effects of radiofrequency energy on human articular cartilage: an analysis of 5 systems. Am J Sports Med. 2005;33(7):1035–9. Available from: http://journals.sagepub.com/doi/10.1177/0363546504271965.

43. Hunziker EB, Quinn TM. Surgical removal of articular cartilage leads to loss of chondrocytes from cartilage bordering the wound edge. J Bone Joint Surg A. 2003;85-A:85–92.

44. Saris DBF, Vanlauwe J, Victor J, Almqvist KF, Verdonk R, Bellemans J, et al. Treatment of symptomatic cartilage defects of the knee: characterized chondrocyte implantation results in better clinical outcome at 36 months in a randomized trial compared to microfracture. Am J Sports Med. 2009;37(1_Suppl):10S–9S.

45. Steadman JR, Rodkey WG, Briggs KK. Microfracture to treat full-thickness chondral defects: surgical technique, rehabilitation, and outcomes. J Knee Surg. 2002;15:170–6.

46. Drobnič M, Radosavljevič D, Cör A, Brittberg M, Stražar K. Debridement of cartilage lesions before autologous chondrocyte implantation by open or transarthroscopic techniques. J Bone Joint Surg Br. 2010;92-B(4):602–8. Available from: http://online.boneandjoint.org.uk/doi/10.1302/0301-620X.92B3.22558.

47. Grieshober JA, Stanton M, Gambardella R. Debridement of articular cartilage: the natural course. In: Sports medicine and arthroscopy review, vol. 24. Philadelphia, PA: Lippincott Williams and Wilkins; 2016. p. 56–62. Available from: http://content.wkhealth.com/linkback/openurl?sid=WKPTLP:landingpage&an=00132585-201606000-00006.

48. Messner K, Maletius W. The long-term prognosis for severe damage to weight-bearing cartilage in the knee: a 14-year clinical and radiographic follow-up in 28 young athletes. Acta Orthop Scand. 2009. Available from: https://www.tandfonline.com/action/journalInformation?journalCode=iort20.

49. Ferretti M, Srinivasan A, Deschner J, Gassner R, Baliko F, Piesco N, et al. Anti-inflammatory effects of continuous passive motion on meniscal fibrocartilage. J Orthop Res. 2005;23(5):1165–71.

50. Xu Z, Buckley MJ, Evans CH, Agarwal S. Cyclic tensile strain acts as an antagonist of IL-1β actions in chondrocytes. J Immunol. 2000;165(1):453–60.

Robert L. Parisien, Nathan L. Grimm, and James L. Carey

15.1 Introduction

Since Franz König first described and coined the term osteochondritis dissecans (OCD) [1, 2], much has been learned. Our early understanding of OCD began with initial confusion regarding the pathoanatomy and etiology with suspicion of *inflammation* as a cause, hence the suffix "*-itis*" in the name. Although this language does not capture the unknown etiology of OCD, its name has prevailed in the literature nonetheless. In an attempt to standardize language for discussing OCD lesions, the Research in Osteochondritis Dissecans of the Knee (ROCK) Group [3] has defined the term osteochondritis dissecans as a focal, idiopathic alteration of subchondral bone with risk for instability and disruption of adjacent articular cartilage that may result in premature osteoarthritis [4].

R. L. Parisien
University of Pennsylvania, Philadelphia, PA, USA

N. L. Grimm
Idaho Sports Medicine Institute, Boise, ID, USA

J. L. Carey (✉)
Orthopaedic Surgery, Perelman School of Medicine at the University of Pennsylvania, Philadelphia, PA, USA

Penn Center for Advanced Cartilage Repair and Osteochondritis Dissecans Treatment, Philadelphia, PA, USA
e-mail: James.Carey@pennmedicine.upenn.edu

Currently, there is no conclusive agreement on the exact cause of OCD. Several etiological hypotheses have been suggested and include occult or repetitive microtrauma [5–8], inflammatory causation [1, 9], and vascular abnormalities [10, 11] as well as a genetic predisposition [12–15]. In the sports medicine literature, there is pervasive support for repetitive microtrauma as the likely etiology, which may account for the increased incidence of medial femoral condyle lesions of the knee given the location's proximity to the tibial eminence [16]. Unfortunately, this hypothesis fails to explain the etiologic development of OCD in other locations.

Linden has been credited with performing the first true epidemiological analysis of knee OCD in Malmö, Sweden [17]. Linden showed the highest incidence occurred between the ages of 10 and 20, which was found to be approximately 18/100,000 for women and 28/100,000 for men [17]. More recently in the United States, Kessler et al. [18] performed an epidemiological analysis utilizing a large, diverse cohort of over 1 million individuals aged 2–19 years old showing 9.5/100,000 overall with a higher risk for boys than girls (15.4/100,000 vs 3.3/100,000). Furthermore, when stratified by race, this study revealed that African Americans had the highest odds ratio of knee OCD [18].

Understanding the behavior of OCD lesions is paramount to determining the most appropriate treatment. OCD lesions may occur on a

A. J. Krych et al. (eds.), *Cartilage Injury of the Knee*,
https://doi.org/10.1007/978-3-030-78051-7_15

spectrum and can be categorized into *stable* and *unstable* lesions with the assistance of classification schemes. Classification of OCD in the knee is further broken down by lesion location, characterization of the lesion (in situ vs ex situ), status of the overlying cartilage, and skeletal maturity. These variables are elucidated with the use of radiographs, MRI and direct visualization through arthroscopy and/or open arthrotomy in certain cases. The ROCK group has developed novel classification schemes for X-ray [19], arthroscopy [20], and MRI to help further characterize and categorize OCD lesions of the knee. These lesions have been categorized into two distinct groups representing mobile and immobile progeny fragments. Arthroscopic features of the immobile group are further classified as a *cue ball*, representing no abnormality, *a shadow*, indicating intact cartilage with subtle demarcation, or a *wrinkle*, indicating demarcated articular cartilage with the presence of a fissure or a wrinkle. In comparison, mobile lesions are further classified as a *locked door*, indicating cartilage fissuring at the periphery of the progeny fragment that is *unable* to be hinged open, a *trapped door*, indicating peripheral cartilage fissure that is *able* to be hinged open, or a *crater*, representing an exposed subchondral bone defect [20]. In an effort to determine which progeny fragments are most appropriate to retain, they are further characterized as either *salvageable* or *unsalvageable*. A salvageable lesion is one in which there is bone present on the deep surface, the lesion is a single fragment and consists mostly of normal articular cartilage. Conversely, an unsalvageable lesion consists solely of cartilage without the presence of bone or may be comprised of multiple fragments with damaged or absent articular cartilage [21].

The purpose of this chapter is to provide a detailed review of the treatment of osteochondritis dissecans of the knee. Special attention will be given to *reparative* and *restorative* treatment. The concepts for these categories will be described in detail below.

15.2 Natural History

In 1985, Bernard Cahill makes a clear distinction between the successful outcomes of juvenile OCD (JOCD) and the adult form (AOCD) stating, "JOCD and [AOCD] are distinct conditions. The former has a much more favorable prognosis than the latter" [22]. Perhaps the most important factor on prediction of healing is the status of the distal femoral physis. Skeletally immature OCD lesions have shown to yield far better results compared to skeletally mature OCD lesions [16]. This suggests that perhaps the natural history of the skeletally immature OCD lesion differs from that of the skeletally mature OCD lesion.

In attempt to determine healing rates following nonoperative management of stable OCD lesions in the skeletally immature, Wall et al. [23] developed a nomogram using normalized lesion length, width, and associated clinical symptoms. Of note, the nomogram has not proven predictive in skeletally mature OCD lesions. Although there is a lack of corroborating literature with regard to exact duration, a trial of at least 3–6 months of nonoperative management is the primary approach to knee OCD in the skeletally immature. Such management may include immobilization in the form of a brace or splint, modified weightbearing and activity restriction. A review by Kocher et al. [24] describes a three phase protocol in which the authors recommend 4–6 weeks of knee immobilization with partial weightbearing during the first phase. Phase 2 consists of progression to weightbearing as tolerated without immobilization for 6–12 week with the initiation of a low-impact quadriceps and hamstring strengthening program. Phase 3 may then begin at 3–4 months with signs of clinical and radiographic healing. A gradual return to sports is allowed in the absence of knee symptoms. In the archetypal location of the medial femoral condyle, literature suggests that up to 67% of OCD lesions in the skeletally immature may demonstrate successful healing given 12 months of nonoperative management [23, 25]. However, atypical lesions of the lateral femoral condyle and patellofemoral joint are more likely to be unstable with less predictable healing potential [26, 27].

However, it is believed that skeletally mature OCD lesions may simply be the result of a persistent lesion that was present during childhood [16, 24, 28]. Hughes et al. [29] evaluated the natural history of skeletally immature OCD lesions using clinical and MRI criteria over an extended period of time. In this cohort, despite subchondral bone changes on MRI, 95% of cases with intact overlying cartilage improved with conservative treatment [29]. In contrast, skeletally mature OCD lesions have been shown to have poor results with conservative treatment [16, 30]. It is the senior author's recommendation that all symptomatic, skeletally mature OCD lesions be treated surgically for optimal results.

15.3 Reparative Management

The purpose of *reparative* management of OCD lesions is to facilitate healing of the progeny fragment to the parent bone and to maintain articular congruity. The two primary *reparative* approaches to OCD leasions are arthroscopic drilling and internal fixation. Both will be discussed in further detail here.

15.3.1 Drilling

The operative method of arthroscopic drilling is typically utilized for OCD lesions in the skeletally immature that remain symptomatic and fail to demonstrate radiographic healing following at least 3–6 months of nonoperative management. Upon careful arthroscopic evaluation via direct probing, lesions amenable to drilling are classified as immobile, per the ROCK classification, and may be described as a cue ball, shadow, or wrinkle in the rug. Furthermore, these lesions are determined salvageable given they are non-fragmented with bone present on the deep surface and consist mostly of normal articular cartilage [21]. Arthroscopic drilling is a technique performed in attempt to restore devitalized vascular channels via subchondral marrow stimulation. This may be done with a transarticular or retro-articular approach.

Transarticular drilling is performed under direct arthroscopic visualization and involves distal to proximal transchondral drilling from the articular surface into the femoral epiphysis. Standard arthroscopic portals are utilized for the majority of lesions although situational accessories portals may be required. A drill sleeve or small cannula is inserted through the portal to protect the soft-tissue. One or two sutures may also be placed through one portal and removed through a second portal on either side of the patella tendon with both ends clamped together with a hemostat to facilitate retraction of the fat pad. A 0.062 in. (1.6 mm) K-wire is advanced into the joint through drill sleeve or cannula and orthogonally positioned with relation to the lesion. The archetypal location along the lateral aspect of the medial femoral condyle may best be accessed via the anterolateral arthroscopic portal. Central focal lesions located on the distal aspect of the lateral femoral condyle (LFC) may be approached orthogonally from the anterolateral portal with the knee in variable degrees of flexion. The K-wire is then advanced into the articular cartilage penetrating the subchondral bone with care not to violate the distal femoral physis. The return of fat droplets indicates adequate penetration of the cancellous bone. Drill holes are to be repeated about 3–5 mm apart, covering the entire diameter of the lesion. The arthroscopic inflow may then be turned off with visualization of blood and marrow elements seeping into the joint.

Retro-articular drilling is an alternative method requiring intra-operative fluoroscopic assistance to accurately target the lesion and avoid joint penetration. It is important to position the fluoroscopy machine in such a manner to allow unobstructed access to the femur. A small longitudinal incision is made distal to the growth plate followed by insertion of a 0.062 in. (1.6 mm) K-wire. Under fluoroscopic visualization, the wire is advanced into the center of the lesion with care taken not to violate the articular surface. The wire may be left in place to allow for parallel placement of additional wires or a parallel wire guide may be utilized. In this manner, drill holes are to be repeated about 3–5 mm apart, covering the entire diameter of the lesion.

Postoperative management involves protected weightbearing for 6 weeks without motion limitation. Impact and sport-specific activities may resume at 12 weeks. Return to play is allowed with demonstration of radiographic healing as well as the achievement of normal ROM, near-normal strength and pain-free sport-specific activities.

In evaluation of clinical outcomes of transarticular versus retro-articular drilling of stable OCD lesions in the skeletally immature, Gunton et al. [31] performed a systematic review of 12 studies and reported no difference in patient-oriented outcomes. Transarticular drilling resulted in radiographic healing of 91% of lesions at 4.5 months while retro-articular drilling demonstrated radiographic healing in 86% of lesions at 5.6 months. There were no complications identified via either technique.

It is the senior author's opinion that the ideal candidate for drilling has an OCD lesion that is immobile and salvageable. These patients are almost always skeletally immature.

15.3.2 Internal Fixation

The operative method of internal fixation may be achieved via open or arthroscopic approaches. Upon careful evaluation, lesions amenable to internal fixation are classified as mobile and may be described as a locked door or trapped door per the ROCK classification. These particular lesions may be determined as salvageable if they are non-fragmented with bone present on the deep surface and consist mostly of normal articular cartilage [21]. A locked door lesion is described as cartilage fissuring at the periphery that is unable to be hinged open upon probing [20]. In comparison, a trapped door progeny fragment exhibits fissuring of the articular cartilage at the periphery of the lesion with the ability to hinge the fragment open, thus providing access to the subchondral bone. Such mobile but salvageable

progeny fragments may be amenable to fixation with or without bone grafting. In vitro studies have demonstrated that compression results in friction between the progeny and parent bone improving stability and resisting shear [32].

In the case of a trapped door lesion, an open arthrotomy is typical to facilitate access for bone grafting. A standard parapatellar arthrotomy is utilized allowing for adequate visualization of the unstable but salvageable progeny fragment. The fragment is hinged open with care taken not to disrupt the remaining articular connection. The base of the lesion is then meticulously debrided with removal of fibrous tissue and sclerotic bone. A microfracture awl or 0.062 in. (1.6 mm) drill may be utilized to facilitate marrow stimulation at the margins of the parent bone. The senior author prefers to harvest autogenous cancellous bone graft from the proximal aspect of the ipsilateral tibia. Sharp dissection is performed 25 mm distal to the anteromedial joint line at the midpoint between the tibial crest and posteromedial border of the tibia near the typical ACL tibial tunnel starting point. The cortical bone is then penetrated with a curette and serially dilated with larger currettes until a arthroscopy grasper can access the cancellous bone. If the patient is skeletally immature, great care is taken to avoid the proximal tibial physis during bone graft harvest. With use of the arthroscopic grasper, the bone graft is placed into a sterile cup, which may then be placed into the bone defect. Care must to taken so as not to overstuff the lesion, thus allowing for the door to be easily closed resulting in restoration of articular congruence.

Fixation may be achieved with use of various forms of either metal or bioabsorbable devices. Disadvantages of metallic implants include MRI interference, loosening and a second surgery for removal [33]. Although a single surgery may be a benefit of bioabsorbable implant use, they are associated with significant complications including osteolysis, synovitis, nonunion and screw breakage [31, 34]. In evaluation of 61 biodegradable screws utilized for fixation of 30 skeletally immature OCD lesions, Camathias et al. [35] reported a 23% incidence of screw breakage.

The authors of this chapter prefer the following fixation methods depending on the robustness of the progeny bone fragment. If <3 mm thick, fixation is achieved with 1.5 mm solid screws, which require removal at about 8 weeks postoperatively. If the progeny bone fragment is >3 mm thick, fixation is achieved with variable pitch metallic screws, which do not require subsequent removal. The progeny fragment is typically fixed with two or more screws to maximize compression and rotational stability (Fig. 15.1). A screw that is 24 mm in length will capture sufficient parent bone without threatening the distal femoral physis. Once adequate fixation has been achieved, a formal "approach and withdraw" technique is utilized via fluoroscopy to ensure there is no screw prominence in relation to the subchondral bone.

Postoperative management consists of protected weightbearing for 6 weeks without motion limitation. Activity and muscle strengthening may increase at 12 weeks with resumption of impact activity at 18 weeks. Return to play is allowed with demonstration of radiographich healing and when the patient achieves normal motion, near-normal strength and pain-free sport-specific activities.

It is the senior author's opinion that the ideal candidate for internal fixation and bone grafting has an OCD lesion that is mobile yet salvageable. Although these patients are typically skeletally mature, internal fixation may be utilized in skeletally mature patients as well. As a rule of thumb, a progeny fragment should be retained when it possesses the aforementioned characteristics.

15.4 Restorative Management

In contrast to *reparative* techniques, *restorative* management of OCD lesions can be thought of as restoring the normal geometry and articular surface with new materials. Such materials may come from adjacent, less utilized areas as is the case of osteochondral autograft transfer. Another readily utilized graft material is via osteochondral allograft transfer from a donor with matching articular surface geometry. More advanced techniques allow us to develop de novo materials from the patient's own chondrocyte cell lineage, such as with autologous chondrocyte implantation (ACI) techniques. The following will describe each of the aforementioned techniques with the author's recommendations for indications, surgical pearls and a discussion of outcomes.

15.4.1 Osteochondral Grafts

Osteochondral grafting consists of autograft or allograft transfer. D'Aubigne first described a technique of osteochondral autograft transfer in 1945 with the technique being later refined by Outerbridge [36] Regarding osteochondral autograft transfers, the surgeon should keep in mind its limitations. Lesions larger than 1–2 cm in diameter (2–4 cm^2) should be considered outside the indications of this technique and one should consider alternative methods (e.g., osteochondral allograft or ACI with bone grafting) [37]. This limitation in size is due to availability of donor site volume, especially in the pediatric population or with smaller adults. For example, Sherman et al. report that although the indications for treatment may be lesions <1 cm, it is important to take this into context in individuals with smaller condyles as a lesion <1 cm may be proportionally large [37].

During autograft transfer surgery, at least 8–10 mm of subchondral bone should be harvested. A technical pearl to avoid fracture of the osteochondral plug during retrieval is to be careful not to toggle the graft retrieval tube once the desired depth is met. Following this, a 90° twist of the harvester should be performed to circumferentially detach the subchondral parent bone from the graft plug. Difficulties with achieving donor graft congruency to the native surrounding cartilage are not uncommon with both autograft and allograft transfers. This can lead to an articular height mismatch between the graft and the surrounding articular cartilage. Articular incongruency can be mitigated by taking care to place the graft delivery tube perpendicular to the recipient site bed, slow and meticulous delivery and

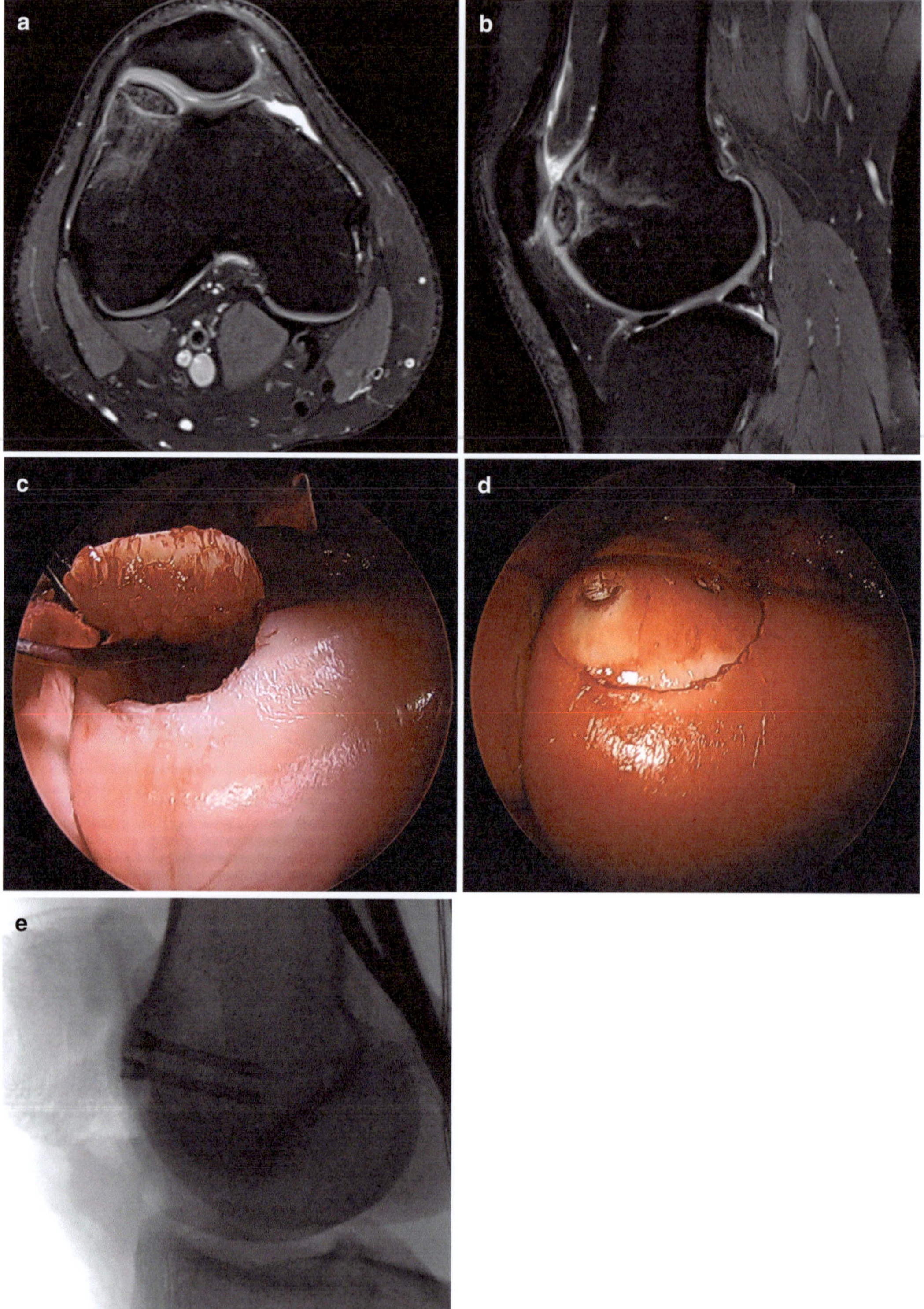

Fig. 15.1 Showing large OCD lesion of the proximal, lateral trochlear ridge on T2-weighted MRI, axial (**a**) and sagittal (**b**) slices. Intraoperative view of a trapped door lesion being hinged open illustrating adequate subchondral bone on progeny fragment for fixation (**c**) and after securing lesion with two variable-pitch screws (**d**). Fluoroscopic lateral showing screw placement for fixation (**e**)

gentle tamping can be performed to achieve a final seating of the donor graft as appropriate.

Grafts that are congruent or countersunk up to 1 mm fare well (Fig. 15.2), however, those that are countersunk >1 mm or that remain proud have been shown to demonstrate higher failure rates [38, 39]. With larger defects, two overlapping fresh osteochondral allografts can also be considered for treatment—the so called "Snowman" or "Mastercard" Technique [40]. A K-wire may be placed in the first osteochondral allograft for stability prior to creation of the secondary overlapping recipient site to prevent displacement of the initial graft.

Postoperative management involves protected weightbearing for the first 6 weeks with a hinged brace locked in extension. The patient can increase weightbearing as tolerated after 6 weeks with progession to light jogging and running at 9 months. Return to play is allowed with demonstration of radiographic healing and when the patient achieves normal motion, near-normal strength and pain-free sport-specific activities.

Although autografts provide utilization of the patients own tissue, limitations of their use involve donor site morbidity, lack of donor cartilage thickness and difficulty to restore the normal condylar contour. Outcomes of osteochondral autografts for the treatment of OCD have been shown to favor smaller lesions and those of the medial femoral condyle. In evaluation of 61 OCD lesions treated with osteochondral augtografts, Ollat et al. [41] reported 72.5% good or excellent results with 8-year follow-up. An additional study by Gudas et al. [42] reported on 10 year outcomes of osteochondral defects of the knee treated with either microfracture or OATS in 60 athletes. The OATS group demonstrated better outcomes as compared to microfracture with only 4 failures at 10 years. With regard to osteochondral allograft utilization, mid- and long-term outcomes for full-thickness osteochondral defects have demonstrated favorable results. In a large series of mostly OCD cases, Levy et al. [43] reported an 82% survivorship at 10 years, 74% at 15 years and 66% at 20 years.

It is the senior author's opinion that the ideal candidate for osteochondral autograft has a nar-

row unsalvageable OCD lesion <2 cm^2 while the ideal candidage for an allograft has an unsalvageable lesion >2 cm^2 that is a circular-shaped defect on the extension surface of the femoral condyle in an adult.

15.4.2 Cell-Based Therapy

Autologous chondrocyte implantation in its first-generation form was initially described in the early 1990s [44]. The third generation ACI technique and implant has been FDA approved in the US since late 2016 [45]. This is the first product approved by the FDA that employs tissue engineering to grow autologous articular cartilage cells on a scaffold. ACI has been described in the management of various osteochondral lesion types and locations. This treatment is indicated for medium to large, full-thickness cartilage defects in the knee [46].

During tissue harvest, concomitant intra-articular pathology can be addressed and the lesion can be comprehensively evaluated under direct arthroscopic visualization. Therefore, a careful arthroscopic evaluation of meniscal pathology, ligament stability, patella maltracking, and intra-articular loose bodies should be addressed during this stage. Tissue harvest for cell growth is typically obtained from non-weightbearing regions of the knee such as the intercondylar notch, far-medial or far-lateral aspects of the trochlea. A technical pearl of the tissue harvest involves running a curette or curved gouge to free the cartilage biopsy at one end while leaving it still attached at the other end as a flap, as loss of the tissue culture intra-operatively can be problematic. This may allow ease of retrieval with an arthroscopic grasper or pituitary rongeur. The biopsy specimen is then sent to a private company where the chondrocytes are extracted and expanded via proprietary technology. The cells are then seeded onto a Type I/III collagen membrane with a density of 500,000–1,000,000 per cm^2. At the time of the second procedure, the expanded autologous chondrocytes are ready for implantation. The joint is accessed via an arthrotomy to expose the articular cartilage

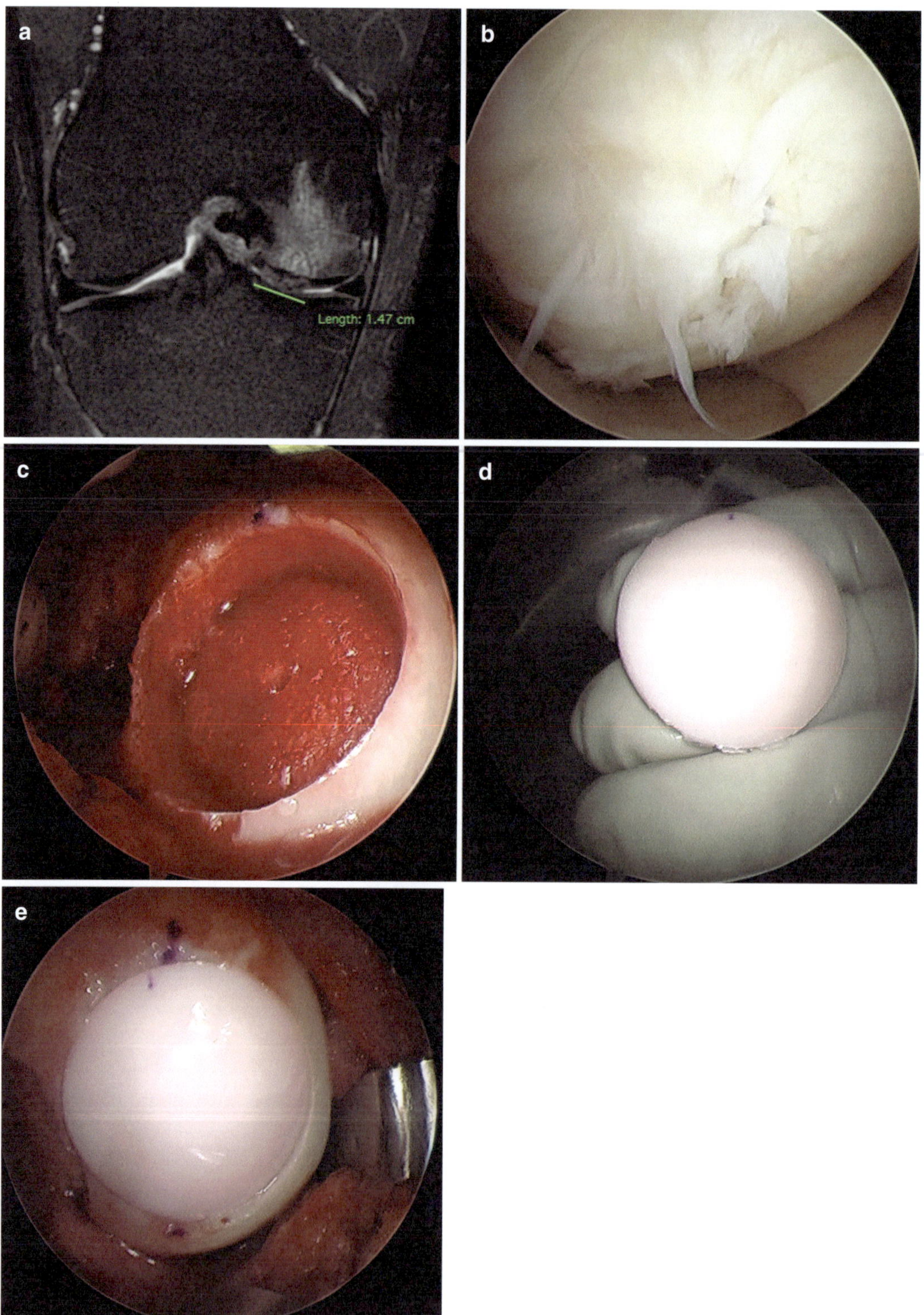

Fig. 15.2 Showing large osteochondral lesion of the medial femoral condyle on T2-weighted coronal MRI (**a**). Intraoperative view of lesion with overlying cartilage dam-age (**b**). Preparation of recipient site for osteochondral allograft (**c**), creation of size-matched osteochondral allograft plug (**d**) and final placement of graft in recipient site (**e**)

defect. The defect is then prepared by removing the calcified layer of cartilage, thus exposing the healthy subchondral bone plate (Fig. 15.3). A scalpel is utilized to create sharp, well-defined articular borders. The senior author's preferred method of implant templating involves utilization of the suture packaging by placing it over the articular defect, creating an exact imprint. The appropriately sized suture packaging is then taped to a Tegaderm™ (3M; St. Paul, MN) transparent film dressing to provide a solid base on which to place and cut the collagen membrane. The collagen memberane is carefully removed from its container with forceps and placed over the sized suture packaging. The collagen membrane is then cut to size and carefully transferred to the surgical field. The collagen membrane is placed into the defect and secured via fibrin sealant, with or without peripheral suture fixation as needed.

It is important to note that uncontained lesions or lesions with subchondral bone loss can be treated with ACI. For bone loss greater than 6 mm in depth, more specialized techniques such as the "sandwich technique" [47] may need to be employed. Sclerotic bone must be removed from the base of the lesion and the depth carfully measured. Autogenous bone graft can be harvested from a number of locations. The original description of the sandwich technique involved harvest through a bone window proximal to the condyle where the arthrotomy was performed [47]. The senior author prefers to harvest autogenous cancellous bone graft from the proximal aspect of the ipsilateral tibia. Sharp dissection is performed 25 mm distal to the anteromedial joint line at the midpoint between the tibial crest and posteromedial border of the tibia near the typical ACL tibial tunnel starting point. The cortical bone is then penetrated with a curette and serially dilated with larger currettes until a arthroscopy grasper can access the cancellous bone. If the patient is skeletally immature, great care is taken to avoid the proximal tibial physis during bone graft harvest. With use of the arthroscopic grasper, the bone graft is placed into a sterile cup, which may then be placed into the bone defect. The bone graft is typically covered with a collagen membrane that is secured with a few very small anchors and fibrin sealant. Routine ACI is then performed on top of the bone graft and membrane.

Postoperative management involves protected weightbearing for the first 6 weeks with a hinged brace locked in extension. The patient can increase weightbearing as tolerated after 6 weeks with progession to light jogging and running at 9 months. Beyond 9 months or so, return to play is allowed when the patient achieves normal motion, near-normal strength, and pain-free sport-specific activities.

Outcomes of ACI for appropriately indicated OCD lesions has demonstrated favorable results. In evaluation of 55 patients with 61 unsalvageable OCD lesions at median follow-up of 19 years, Carey et al. [48] demonstrated that 13% required revision ACI with only 3% undergoing total knee arthroplasty. The authors further report ACI survivorship for OCD as 87% at 10 years, 85% at 15 years, and 82% at 20 years.

It is the senior author's opinion that the ideal candidate for autologous chondrocyte implantation has an unsalvageable OCD lesion >2 cm^2.

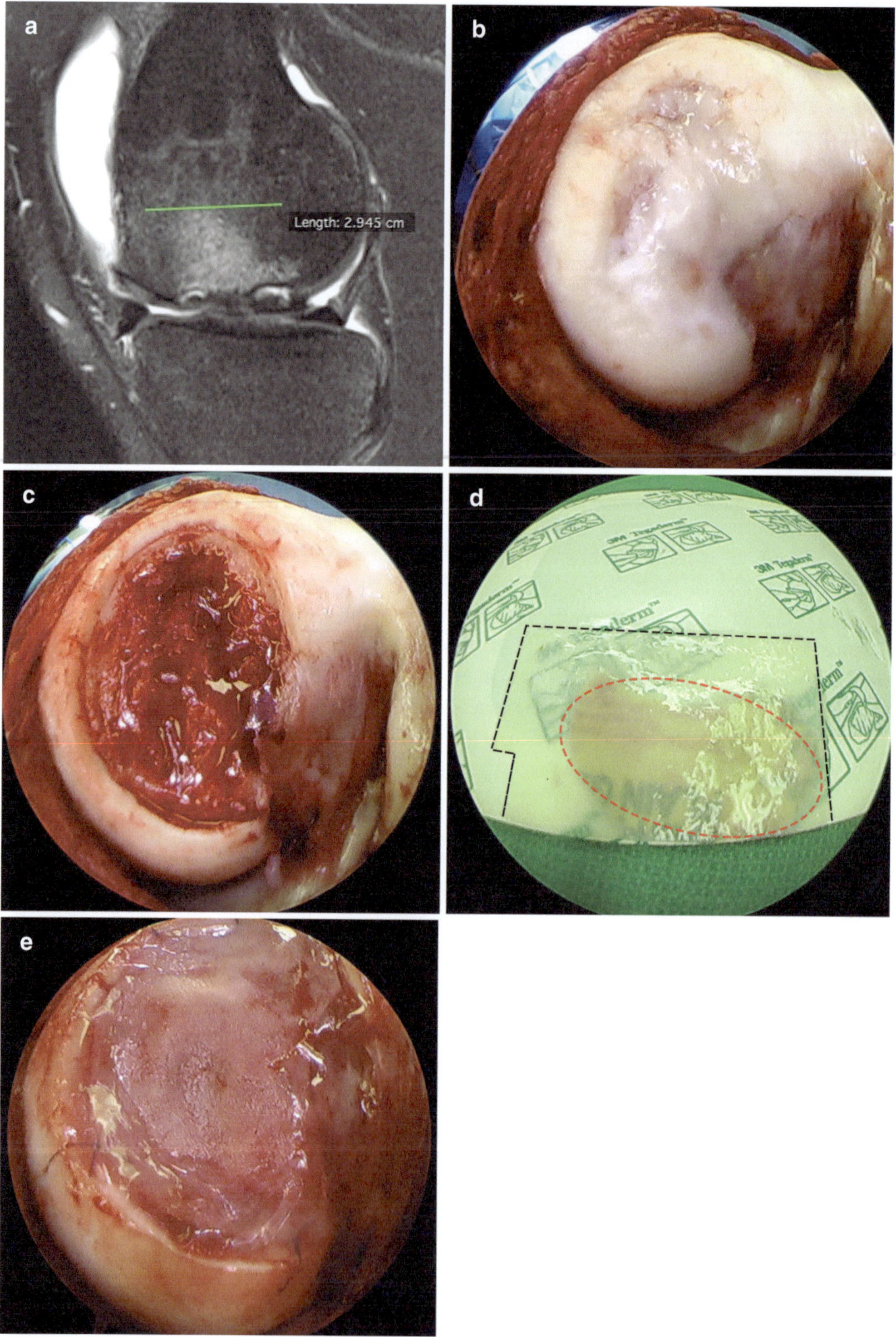

Fig. 15.3 Showing large osteochondral lesion of the medial femoral condyle on T2-weighted sagittal MRI (**a**). Intraoperative view of *oval-shaped* lesion with overlying cartilage damage (**b**), preparation of lesion bed and healthy shouldered cartilage (**c**), creation of size-specific, oval graft using foil template from lesion bed (red outline) with graft (black outline) lying on Tegaderm to provide support while cutting the shape (**d**) and final placement of graft over recipient site with layer of fibrin glue (**e**)

References

1. Konig F. Uber freie Körper in den Gelenken. Dtsch Z Klin Chir. 1887;27:90–109.
2. Brand RA. Biographical sketch: Franz Konig, MD 1832-1910. Clin Orthop Relat Res. 2013;471:1116–7.
3. Research in Osteochondritis Dissecans of the Knee (ROCK) Group. OCD of the knee. https://kneeocd.org/patient-education/ocd-knee/. Accessed 21 May 2020
4. Edmonds EW, Shea KG. Osteochondritis dissecans: editorial comment. Clin Orthop Relat Res. 2013;471:1105–6.
5. Conway FM. Osteochondritis dissecans. description of the stages of the condition and its probable traumatic etiology. Am J Surg. 1937;38:691–9.
6. Crawford DC, Safran MR. Osteochondritis dissecans of the knee. J Am Acad Orthop Surg. 2006;14:90–100.
7. Detterline AJ, Goldstein JL, Rue JP, Bach BR Jr. Evaluation and treatment of osteochondritis dissecans lesions of the knee. J Knee Surg. 2008;21:106–15.
8. Smillie IS. Treatment of osteochondritis dissecans. J Bone Joint Surg Br. 1957;39-B:248–60.
9. Schenck RC Jr, Goodnight JM. Osteochondritis dissecans. J Bone Joint Surg Am. 1996;78:439–56.
10. Campbell CJ, Ranawat CS. Osteochondritis dissecans: the question of etiology. J Trauma. 1966;6:201–21.
11. Linden B, Telhag H. Osteochondritis dissecans. A histologic and autoradiographic study in man. Acta Orthop Scand. 1977;48:682–6.
12. Andrew TA, Spivey J, Lindebaum RH. Familial osteochondritis dissecans and dwarfism. Acta Orthop Scand. 1981;52:519–23.
13. Kozlowski K, Middleton R. Familial osteochondritis dissecans: a dysplasia of articular cartilage? Skelet Radiol. 1985;13:207–10.
14. Phillips HO, Grubb SA. Familial multiple osteochondritis dissecans. Report of a kindred. J Bone Joint Surg Am. 1985;67:155–6.
15. Stougaard J. Familial occurrence of osteochondritis dissecans. J Bone Joint Surg Br. 1964;46:542–3.
16. Cahill BR. Osteochondritis dissecans of the knee: treatment of juvenile and adult forms. J Am Acad Orthop Surg. 1995;3:237–47.
17. Linden B. The incidence of osteochondritis dissecans in the condyles of the femur. Acta Orthop Scand. 1976;47:664–7.
18. Kessler JI, Hooman N, Shea KG, Jacobs JC, Bedchuk JD, Weiss JM. The demographics and epidemiology of osteochondritis dissecans of the knee in children and adolescents. Am J Sports Med. 2014;42(2):320–6.
19. Wall EJ, Polousky JD, Shea KG, et al. Novel radiographic feature classification of knee osteochondritis dissecans: a multicenter reliability study. Am J Sports Med. 2015;43:303–9.
20. Carey JL, Wall EJ, Grimm NL, et al. Novel arthroscopic classification of osteochondritis dissecans of the knee: a multicenter reliability study. Am J Sports Med. 2016;44:1694–8.
21. Shea KG, Carey JL, Brown GA, Murray JN, Pezold R, Sevarino KS. Management of osteochondritis dissecans of the femoral condyle. J Am Acad Orthop Surg. 2016;24:e102–4.
22. Cahill B. Treatment of juvenile osteochondritis dissecans and osteochondritis dissecans of the knee. Clin Sports Med. 1985;4:367–84.
23. Wall EJ, Vourazeris F, Myer GD, et al. The healing potential of stable juvenile osteochondritis dissecans knee lesions. Bone Joint Surg Am. 2008;90(12):2655–64.
24. Kocher MS, Tucker R, Ganley TJ, Flynn JM. Management of osteochondritis dissecans of the knee: current concepts review. Am J Sports Med. 2006;34:1181–91.
25. Krause M, Hapfelmeier A, Möller M, Amling M, Bohndorf K, Meenen NM. Healing predictors of stable juvenile osteochondritis dissecans knee lesions after 6 and 12 months of nonoperative treatment. Am J Sports Med. 2013;41(10):2384–91.
26. Samora WP, Chevillet J, Adler B, Young GS, Klingele KE. Juvenile osteochondritis dissecans of the knee: predictors of lesion stability. J Pediatr Orthop. 2012;32(1):1–4.
27. Wall EJ, Heyworth BE, Shea KG, Edmonds EW, Wright RW, Anderson AF, Eismann EA, Myer GD. Trochlear groove osteochondritis dissecans of the knee patellofemoral joint. J Pediatr Orthop. 2014;34(6):625–30.
28. Flynn JM, Kocher MS, Ganley TJ. Osteochondritis dissecans of the knee. J Pediatr Orthop. 2004;24:434–43.
29. Hughes JA, Cook JV, Churchill MA, Warren ME. Juvenile osteochondritis dissecans: a 5-year review of the natural history using clinical and MRI evaluation. Pediatr Radiol. 2003;33:410–7.
30. Jurgensen I, Bachmann G, Schleicher I, Haas H. Arthroscopic versus conservative treatment of osteochondritis dissecans of the knee: value of magnetic resonance imaging in therapy planning and follow-up. Arthroscopy. 2002;18:378–86.
31. Gunton MJ, Carey JL, Shaw CR, Murnaghan ML. Drilling juvenile osteochondritis dissecans: Retro- or Transarticular? Clin Orthop Relat Res. 2013;471:1144–51.
32. Morelli M, Poitras P, Grimes V, Backman D, Dervin G. Comparison of the stability of various internal fixators used in the treatment of osteochondritis dissecans: a mechanical model. J Orthop Res. 2007;25(4):495–500.
33. Guhl JF. Arthroscopic treatment of osteochondritis dissecans. Clin Orthop Relat Res. 1982;167:65–74.
34. Alford JW, Cole BJ. Cartilage restoration, part 2: techniques, outcomes, and future directions. Am J Sports Med. 2005;33(3):443–60.
35. Camathias C, Gögüs U, Hirschmann MT, Rutz E, Brunner R, Haeni D, Vavken P. Implant failure after biodegradable screw fixation in osteochondritis dissecans of the knee in skeletally immature patients. Arthroscopy. 2015;31(3):410–5.

36. Barber FA, Chow JC. Arthroscopic chondral osseous autograft transplantation (COR procedure) for femoral defects. Arthroscopy. 2006;22:10–6.
37. Sherman SL, Thyssen E, Nuelle CW. Osteochondral autologous transplantation. Clin Sports Med. 2017;36:489–500.
38. Patil S, Tapasvi SR. Osteochondral autografts. Curr Rev Musculoskelet Med. 2015;8(4):423–8.
39. Huang FS, Simonian PT, Norman AG, Clark JM. Effects of small incongruities in a sheep model of osteochondral grafting. Am J Sports Med. 2004;32(8):1842–8.
40. Pisanu G, Cottino U, Rosso F, et al. Large osteochondral allografts of the knee: surgical technique and indications. Joints. 2018;6:42–53.
41. Ollat D, Lebel B, Thaunat M, Jones D, Mainard L, Dubrana F, Versier G, French Arthroscopy Society. Mosaic osteochondral transplantations in the knee joint, midterm results of the SFA multicenter study. Orthop Traumatol Surg Res. 2011;97(8 Suppl):S160–6.
42. Gudas R, Gudaite A, Pocius A, Gudiene A, Cekanauskas E, Monastyreckiene E, Basevicius A. Ten-year follow-up of a prospective, randomized clinical study of mosaic osteochondral autologous transplantation versus microfracture for the treatment of osteochondral defects in the knee joint of athletes. Am J Sports Med. 2012;40(11):2499–508.
43. Levy YD, Gortz S, Pulido PA, McCauley JC, Bugbee WD. Do fresh osteochondral allografts successfully treat femoral condyle lesions? Clin Orthop Relat Res. 2013;471:231–7.
44. Brittberg M, Lindahl A, Nilsson A, Ohlsson C, Isaksson O, Peterson L. Treatment of deep cartilage defects in the knee with autologous chondrocyte transplantation. N Engl J Med. 1994;331(14):889–95.
45. FDA approves scaffold to repair knee cartilage. Lippincott's Bone and Joint Newsletter. 2017;23(4):45.
46. Hinckel BB, Gomoll AH. Autologous chondrocytes and next-generation matrix-based autologous chondrocyte implantation. Clin Sports Med. 2017;36(3):525–48.
47. Bartlett W, Gooding CR, Carrington RW, Skinner JA, Briggs TW, Bentley G. Autologous chondrocyte implantation at the knee using a bilayer collagen membrane with bone graft. A preliminary report. J Bone Joint Surg Br. 2005;87:330–2.
48. Carey JL, Shea KG, Lindahl A, Vasiliadis HS, Lindahl C, Peterson L. Autologous chondrocyte implantation as treatment for unsalvageable osteochondritis dissecans: 10 to 25 year follow up. Am J Sports Med. 2020;48(5):1134–40.

Managing Concomitant Cartilage Injury with ACL Tears

Michael James McNicholas and Eran Beit-ner

16.1 ACL Anatomy and Biomechanics

There are six main structures responsible for joint stability: the ACL, posterior cruciate ligament, medial collateral ligament, lateral collateral ligament, posterolateral and posteromedial corners. The ACL is the primary restraint to anterior translation of the tibia on the femur. Its length within the joint is 22–41 mm (avg. 32–33 mm) [1]; its width averages 10–11 mm (7–17 mm). The cross-sectional area varies throughout its course as well as through the flexion arc with an average thickness of 3.9 mm [2]. The ACL originates from the medial surface of the lateral femoral condyle. It is extrasynovial but intracapsular. The ACL has an oblique course within the knee joint from posterior-lateral to anterior-medial. It inserts into a broad and irregular area of the anterior central tibial plateau between the tibial eminences. In 1938, Ivan Palmer [3] first described the ACL as being divided into two bundles: a posterior-lateral bundle and an anteromedial bundle. In 1975, Girgis described their different functions [4], leading to the development of double-bundle reconstruction techniques. With only limited biomechanical advantages, meta-analyses have not found any long-term clinical advantage [5]. Over the past 15 years, the description of the ACL as one or two ropes has been questioned. Smigielski stated that the ACL anatomy resembles a ribbon [6], with a "C-shape" tibial insertion along the medial tibial spine (Fig. 16.1) and two types of insertion to the origin site were identified: direct and an indirect (with a fan-like insertion) [7]. Siebold confirmed these findings and concluded that the ACL should be described as consisting of fibers, rather than bundles [8] and a technique addressing this concept has recently been published [9]. Early clinical results are encouraging for this technique, but medium- and long-term results are awaited.

16.1.1 Functional Biomechanics of the ACL

The ACL is the primary restraint to anterior translation of the tibia on the femur and to hyperextension. It also serves as a secondary restraint to varus and valgus movements at full extension, and at nearly full extension resists internal and external rotation [10].

Traditionally, the ACL is divided into two bundles—anteromedial (AM) and posterolateral (PL). The AM bundle is larger and stronger than

M. J. McNicholas (✉)
Liverpool University Hospitals, Liverpool, UK
e-mail: mike@mcnicholaskneeclinic.com

E. Beit-ner
Department of Trauma and Orthopaedic Surgery,
University of Manchester, Manchester, UK

© ISAKOS 2021
A. J. Krych et al. (eds.), *Cartilage Injury of the Knee*,
https://doi.org/10.1007/978-3-030-78051-7_16

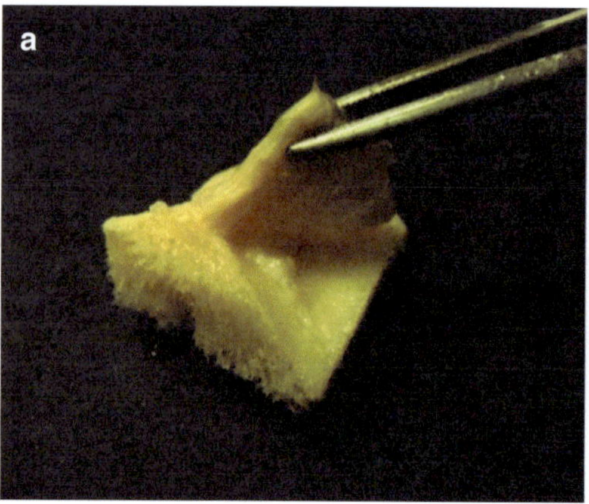
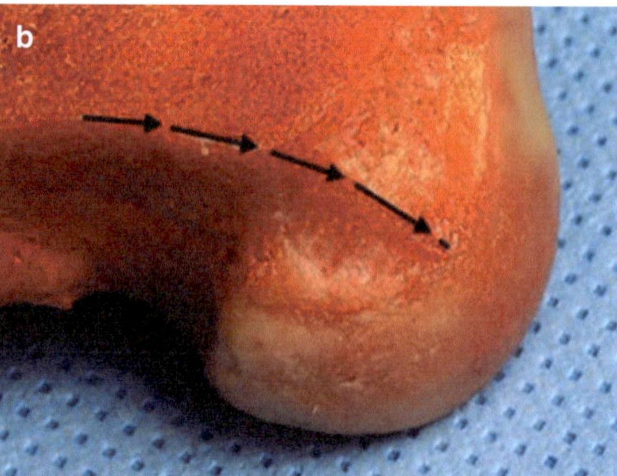

Fig. 16.1 (**a, b**) The direct insertion of the ribbon-like ACL fibers is in continuity of the posterior femoral cortex. (From Smigielski R et al.: Ribbon-like appearance of the midsubstance fibers of the anterior cruciate ligament close to its femoral insertion site: a cadaveric study including 111 knees. Knee Surg Sports Traumatol Arthrosc (2015) 23:3143–3150. DOI https://doi.org/10.1007/s00167-014-3146-7. Published under the Creative Commons Attribution 4.0 International (CC BY) https://creativecommons.org/licenses/by/4.0/)

the PL band, and it is more important for knee stabilization. However, the two bundles work and tense in a reciprocal manner. In flexion, the AM band tights while the PL band lax. In extension, an opposite pattern is observed as the PL tightens because the AM becomes less tense.

16.1.2 The Menisci

The menisci are commonly injured in ACL injuries. Their preservation is to be encouraged with many previously resected tear patterns now being successfully repaired. This will hopefully reduce the incidence of osteoarthritis (OA) in the long term after ACL injury.

16.2 ACL Injuries

16.2.1 General

ACL tears are the most common athletic injury [11]. The age- and sex-adjusted annual incidence of ACL tears is 68.6 per 100,000 person-years [12]. In the USA, over 120,000 ACL injuries occur annually [13]. The prevalence of ACL injuries is higher in males with 72% [14] of the cases in the UK. However, female athletes are more predisposed to these injuries compared to male

[15], attributed to anatomic, hormonal, biomechanical differences. ACL injuries hugely impact both patients and health systems. They may still end a professional athlete's career and cause early OA in the majority of all those affected.

16.2.2 Injury Patterns and Mechanisms

Injury patterns can be divided into contact (direct) and non-contact (indirect) mechanisms. Direct mechanisms are inevitable risk when participating in a contact sport or trauma. 61% of injuries have a non-contact mechanism [16]. Consequently, clinical research has focused on their prevention.

16.2.3 Overview of Treatment Options

Due to the high incidence of ACL injuries among athletes, both recreational and professional, preventative measures are the first step of addressing these injuries. Preventative rehabilitation programs, initially described by Silvers and Mandelbaum [17], have been widely adopted, such as the FIFA11+ program [18] and have reduced the incidence of ACL injuries.

For a diagnosed ACL injury, treatment options may be either non-surgical or surgical. Conservative management consists of progressive rehabilitation, aiming to improve muscular strength and balance [19], life style change, adjustment of performed physical activity, and use of braces. Surgical options include a variety of techniques from simple repair of the ligament to one of many anterior cruciate ligament reconstruction (ACLR) techniques [19]. When deciding on treatment, surgeons must address to patients' characteristics, their injury pattern, and functional needs. Non-surgical management is more appropriate for older, low demand patients. A surgical approach is more suitable for the young active patients with higher functional needs and elite and professional athletes.

ACL repair avoids donor site morbidity associated with autologous graft harvest [20] and may maintain native biomechanics, proprioception, and gait patterns. However, it has been shown to have a high failure rate, especially in younger and more active patients [21]. Nonetheless, there has been a recent resurgence in interest in ACL repair [22]. With varying results reported, a current technique of ACL repair using independent suture tape reinforcement has been described by Mackay [23]. However, it is the current view in the UK that this is a technique that maybe of merit, but its specific indications are not yet fully defined.

ACLR has been the gold standard for the past 50 years and remains so today. ACLR via either open or arthroscopic approaches uses a graft. These may be autologous, allograft, or synthetic. Hamstring tendons (most commonly semitendinosus and gracilis from the injured limb) and bone-patella tendon-bone (BPTB) graft are most commonly used [24].

16.3 Concomitant Injuries

16.3.1 Introduction

The incidence of associated cartilage and meniscal pathology with ACL tears varies widely in the literature. Approximately 50% of primary ACL ruptures and over 90% of failed reconstructions have coexisting cartilage and/or meniscal pathology [25]. Concomitant chondral lesions are seen in 15–46% of the ACL injuries [26]. This inconsistency may be due to the variability in grading and chronicity of different reports. Slauterbeck et al. [27] geographically mapped meniscal and cartilage lesions in ACL reconstruction (ACLR) patients: 43% had femoral chondral lesions; age affected the number and severity of lesions. Patients over the age of 25 were more likely to have multiple cartilage lesions: 7.7% versus 1.3% in younger patients, as well as isolated medial femoral condyle lesions: 24.2% versus 13.3%. Males had higher grade MFC lesions (grade 3–4) compared to females 49% compared with 35%.

16.3.2 Influence of Isolated ACL Tear on the Articular Cartilage

ACL injuries are associated with an early OA [28], knee joint laxity, concomitant meniscal and chondral injuries, reduced quadriceps strength, and changes in load balance. An isolated ACL tear can affect the articular cartilage in two patterns: acute and chronic. Acute injury results from the primary trauma and impact, leading to bone bruise and hemarthrosis, followed by cartilage healing or permanent defect. Primary impact may produce inflammatory changes, which potentially damage the hyaline cartilage. The chronic pattern, attributed to ongoing instability, is associated with higher risk of concomitant medial meniscal and chondral injury [25, 29].

The incidence of concomitant injuries in an untreated ACL tear increase over time, even when concomitant injuries were absent initially. Delayed surgical reconstruction increases the risk of both meniscal tears and chondral lesions, emphasizing the protective role of reconstruction.

Intact menisci and cartilage were associated with better surgical outcomes for both acute and chronic ACL tears and instability [30].

16.3.3 The Influence of Concomitant ACL and Meniscal Tears on the Articular Cartilage

Meniscal tears double the likelihood of articular cartilage damage in symptomatic ACL-deficient patients [25]. Medial meniscus tears, in particularly, were associated with chondral lesions of weightbearing areas [31]. Delay in ACLR increased the risk and severity of chondral lesions in the adult knee [27, 32]. Granan et al. examined the Norwegian Knee Ligament Registry (NKLR) and found that the odds for an adult knee cartilage lesion increased by nearly 1% for each month that passed from the time of injury until the surgery. Articular cartilage lesions were nearly twice as frequent if there was a meniscal tear and vice versa [32]. Surgical delay of more than 1 year drastically increases the risk for chondral lesions (60% compared with 47% for all others). It also increases the proportion of large and grade-3 lesions of the lateral femoral condyle [27].

16.3.4 Injuries Associated with Hyperlaxity and Instability

The medial collateral ligament (MCL) provides the knee stability in the coronal plane. It is the primary restraint to valgus stress and helps the ACL stabilize the knee in different directions and loads. Over 75% of grade III MCL injuries coexist with an ACL injury [33, 34]. Forces absorbed by the MCL are amplified when the ACL is insufficient. When both the MCL and ACL are damaged valgus rotation increase dramatically with significant resultant instability. Concomitant ACL-MCL injury can be managed surgically or non-surgically: grade I and II MCL injuries are usually treated non-surgically; concomitant grade III may be addressed by multiple ligament reconstruction [35].

The lateral collateral ligament (LCL) is the knee's primary varus stabilizer, preventing external rotation and posterior displacement of the tibia as part of the PLC complex [36]. 57% of grade III LCL injuries are associated with ACL tears.

The posterior cruciate ligament (PCL) provides knee stability in the sagittal plane and limits excessive posterior translation. It also plays a crucial role in the rollback mechanism of the knee during flexion. PCL injuries are commonly presented as part of multiligamentous injuries with only 3.5–15% of the cases are isolated injuries [37, 38]. When identified as part of a multi-

ligamentous injury, PCL repair, or reconstruction are advised [39].

The posteromedial corner (PMC) is a complex that consists of five major structures: posterior oblique ligament (POL), semimembranosus tendon, oblique popliteal ligament (OPL), postero-medial joint capsule, and the posterior horn of the medial meniscus. The PMC acts to control and restrict valgus stress, excessive anterior translation, and external rotation of the tibia, commonly referred to as anteromedial rotational instability (AMRI). In extension, the PMC appears to participate in restraining tibial internal rotation and valgus [40].

The posterolateral corner (PLC) primarily consists of the LCL, the popliteus tendon (PLT) and popliteofibular ligament and includes secondary static and dynamic stabilizers [41]. It holds several roles including control and restrain of external tibial rotation, varus restraint, and limitation of posterior tibial translation [42]. PLC injury plays an important role in the ACL-deficient knee. PLC injuries account for up to 16% of all knee ligament injuries. With only 28% of all PLC injuries are isolated, PLC injuries are commonly associated with cruciate ligament injuries. Studies showed that a missed PLC injury diagnosis is a common cause for ACLR failure attributed to an increased tension of the graft. Combined acute PLC and ACL injury necessitates reconstruction or a combined hybrid repair [43].

16.4 Treatment

16.4.1 Introduction

Optimal management of concomitant injury of ACL tear and chondral damage remains controversial [44, 45]. Many surgeons advise early intervention in these injuries as the risk of future OA in adolescents and young adults substantially increased following ACL injury [46]. This association was supported by evidence of increased biomarkers of cartilage turnover after ACL injury [47]. Concomitant injuries may further increase this risk with some reports of radiographic evidence of OA in up to 80% of the cases at

5–15 years after the initial injury. Athletes were shown to have an even higher risk. Furthermore, delay in ACLR increased the risk and severity of chondral lesions in the adult knee [27, 32]. On the other hand, other studies did not find any difference in long-term outcomes following ACLR in patients with and without concomitant asymptomatic chondral damage [37]. Progression to OA following ACL injury is probably multifactorial and can be contributed to primary cartilage, meniscal or ligamentous concomitant injury, or to secondary injury due to the evolving instability and kinematic changes.

Concomitant injuries can be managed by: non-surgical treatment for both the ACL and the chondral injury; partial surgical approach and a concomitant surgery for both. Conservative management usually consists of a progressive rehabilitation program to improve muscular strength, balance, adjustment of the performed physical activity and bracing [19].

Partial surgical approaches focus on repairing or reconstructing the ACL with initial arthroscopic assessment of the joint space, followed by debridement. Concomitant articular cartilage damage negatively affects ACLR's long-term outcomes [30]. However, this has been questioned in cases with asymptomatic chondral defects [44].

The combined surgical approach, first described by Matsusue et al. [48], uses known techniques for treating both conditions during the same surgery.

Gudas et al. [49] compared the outcomes of osteochondral autograft transfer (OAT), microfracture (MFx), and debridement performed during concomitant ACLR. All were beneficial at 3 years, with better IKDC score in OAT-ACLR group. OAT-ACLR was inferior to ACLR without concomitant chondral injury. Stability at 3 years was not significantly affected by the modality.

MFx has been found to be beneficial to symptomatic patients with ACL instability and a single small cartilage lesion (≤ 2 cm^2), even if deep (ICRS 3–4), with excellent short-term clinical and functional improvement with high levels of return to pre-injury sport activity level [50]. Higher chondral defects correlated with worse subjective outcomes and reduction in sport activity.

Symptomatic full-thickness articular cartilage defects (ICRS 3–4, mean area 3.5 cm^2) that were associated with ACL instability showed favorable outcomes after simultaneous ACLR (bone patellar tendon-bone—BPTB graft) and OATs [51].

Imade et al. [52] compared drilling and OATs for chondral damage during ACLR. Second-look arthroscopy revealed important differences in the cartilage appearance. 50% of the drilling group showed improved cartilage, 17% had deterioration, compared to 100% improvement after OATs. There were no differences in IKDC score and PROMs. 64% of the OAT-ACLR group returned to pre-injury levels of sports compared to 37% of the patients in the drilling group.

Peterson et al. assessed the outcomes of ACLR and (autologous chondrocyte implantation) ACI for concomitant ACL and moderate to large (1.3–12.0 cm^2) full-thickness femoral condyle chondral defects. Most had prior knee interventions. These patients showed good clinical outcomes on PROMs. 75% showed significant improvement during second-look arthroscopy [53].

Pike et al. reported moderate long-term improvement in pain and function after combined ACI for large chondral defects (mean 8.4 cm^2) and ACLR. Despite high revision rate (50%), patient showed some improvement. They concluded this approach remains a good option for treating these challenging cases [54].

Some surgeons advocate harvest cartilage when identifying chondral lesion, enabling a potential future use of these cells as part of an ACI, but this would not be commonly practiced in the UK.

16.4.2 ACLR Techniques

Despite the recent resurgence in interest and potential advantages of ACL repair [23], due to the reports of high failure rate [21] and the lack of well-defined indications, it is the current view in the UK that ACLR remains the gold standard for the treatment of ACL tears. Whether being performed in an open or arthroscopic approach, intra-articular ACLR consists of several fundamental stages: graft selection, placement, tensioning, fixation, and postoperative rehabilitation. ACL graft sources may be either autologous or allograft. Synthetic ligament substitutes are also available. During graft selection surgeons must assess the patient's characteristics, injury pattern, and functional needs. Younger age, increased activity level, higher demands have all been identified as risk factors for graft failure. The use of allograft in these patients was found to increase the risk for failure [55]. Hamstring tendons graft (most commonly ipsilateral semitendinosus and gracilis) and BPTP construct are the most commonly used autografts. Many studies have tried to compare the two with no difference in outcome shown [24]. Quadriceps tendon autograft has been suggested as an alternative for these grafts with more predictable outcomes and less donor site morbidity [56]. Current data are insufficient to prove superiority. The variety of allograft choices includes tibialis anterior and posterior, Achilles, hamstrings, and patellar tendons. While no donor site morbidity exists with allograft tissue, there are concerns about the potential of viral and bacterial disease transmission and immunogenic graft-host reaction. Graft processing and preparation may affect reconstruction failure rates [55]. The use of synthetic grafts is unpopular due to early failure. Newer generations of synthetic graft continue to develop, which potentially make them future alternatives. The influence of ACL graft selection on the outcome of combined cartilage injury treatment has not been studied. Most surgeons will not change their graft selection or technique according to the presence of chondral injury.

16.4.3 Bone Bruising

The mechanism by which ACL injury occur associated with major forces that lead to powerful impact between tibial and femoral articular cartilage. These forces are transferred to bones and commonly result in a bone bruise [57]. Bone bruising is diagnosed by MRI with sensitivity over 80% and specificity over 95%. Fluid-sensitive T2-weighted sequences present increased signal intensity in the injured area while on T1-weighted images the area demonstrates a decreased signal. Short tau inversion recovery (STIR) sequence can increase the sensitivity of the MRI by suppressing the signal from the normal medullary fat [58]. Bone bruising correlated to injury severity and was with persisting and progressive chondral damage, suggesting an association with early OA development [59]. Bone bruises are associated with poorer short-term clinical outcomes. Their appearance on pre-op MRI was associated with lower return to sport rates after ACLR. Severity and location affect the ACLR outcomes. Lateral distribution was associated with higher instability and ROM limitation while medial distribution correlated with higher pain [58]. Figure 16.2 presents bone bruise distribution.

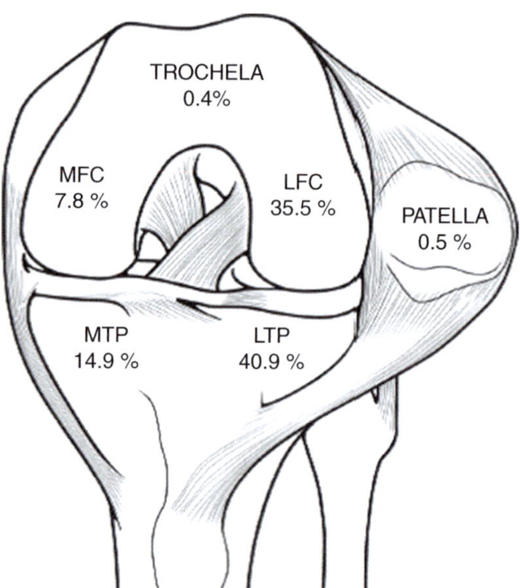

Fig. 16.2 Percentage of bone bruise distribution in the affected anatomic bone locations. *LTP* lateral tibial plateau, *LFC* lateral femoral condyle, *MTP* medial tibial plateau, *MFC* medial femoral condyle. (From Filardo G. et al.: Bone bruise in anterior cruciate ligament rupture entails a more severe joint damage affecting joint degenerative progression. Knee Surgery, Sports Traumatology, Arthroscopy (2019) 27:44–59. https://doi.org/10.1007/s00167-018-4993-4. Published under the Creative Commons Attribution 4.0 International (CC BY) https://creativecommons.org/licenses/by/4.0/)

16.4.4 Principles of Combined Injury Treatment

One's philosophy will influence the approach joint restoration one uses. Current literature does not favor a specific approach or technique. We believe that the biomechanics of the knee must be addressed before its biology. Krych et al. showed the most common reason for failure of cartilage restoration surgery was untreated malalignment [60]. To improve cartilage restoration technique outcomes, we recommend addressing the subject as follows:

Biomechanics:

Alignment—correcting malalignment by osteotomy

Stability—reconstruction of the ACL and other injured ligaments

Significant meniscal deficiency—meniscus allograft transplantation or other advanced treatments.

Biology:

Articular cartilage—may now be addressed.

Preferred Method of ACL Reconstruction

Operation steps:

- Under general anesthetic, an ultrasound-guided adductor canal block and IV antibiotics are given.
- Full examination under anesthetic performed. ACL status confirmed by anterior drawer, Lachman examination, and pivot shift tests. Other ligament laxities are assessed including PLC status.
- Thigh holder over uninflated tourniquet.
- Diagnostic arthroscopy
  - A high anterolateral portal for arthroscopic camera insertion. The anteromedial portal is marked under vision with a white needle, just medial to the fat pad, close to the upper meniscal surface. All knee compartments viewed.
  - Menisci are fully probed and damage addressed.
  - All articular cartilage surfaces are fully visualized and probed, any unstable lesions debrided to a stable edge.
  - Assess the intercondylar notch ACL tear confirmed arthroscopically prior to graft harvest. ACL stump debrided by powershaver via the medial portal. Notchplasty performed if required.
  - Femoral tunnel placement is marked with a 45° microfracture awl approximately 5 mm anterior to the over the top position, 10:30 in a right or 1:30 on the left knee. Satisfactory placement confirmed by viewing from the medial portal.
- Four bundled semitendinosus and gracilis harvested, sutured with 5 ethibond and then presoaked in Vancomycin solution [61] during pretensioning.
- The tibial tunnel is drilled from outside with an elbow aimer at 55°. The tip is placed in the back of the ACL tibial footprint, with the elbow lying against the PCL. The 2.4 mm guide pin drilled until its tip protrudes 5 mm into the joint. The knee is then fully extended while that tip is visualized to ensure its position is central and just inside the apex of the notch.
- Landmarks to guide the correct tunnel placement are the medial tibial eminence and intermeniscal ligament [62]. The anterior horn of the lateral meniscus serves as its lateral and partially anterior borders [63].
- Indelible felt-tip pen marks the graft at the tunnel length and 5 mm beyond. Graft pulled into femoral socket, markings visually confirming fully seated, when the second marked band is at the tunnel mouth. Then the flipping suture pulled to flip the endobutton. Once that has deployed then retrograde pull on the graft sutures from the anterior tibia will mean the first marked band on the graft seen at the mouth of the socket.

- The knee is then put through a full ROM, cycled ten times, while manual maximum tension is applied to the graft trailing sutures, ensuring appropriate graft tension. While reducing the tibia backward onto the intact PCL with the knee in full extension an interference screw is inserted over a guide wire placed between the four graft limbs until the round end is just at the cortex ensuring aperture fixation. The graft is kept under full tension throughout to avoid the screw cutting it.
- Images captured via the anterolateral portal confirming no impingement of intra-articular graft with the knee at 90° and full extension.
- Confirm normalization of Lachman, anterior drawer, and pivot tests.
- Portals and donor site sutured.

tions dictated by the location or size of the cartilage lesion treated protect the articular surfaces from excessive compressive or shearing forces [71]. Tibiofemoral lesions require a minimum period of 6 weeks touch-weightbearing, then progressing to full-weightbearing [72]. OATs, particularly when several osteochondral plugs have been used for larger defects require a short period of non-weightbearing [71]. Patellofemoral cartilage surgery patients, with the knee in a brace locked in extension during ambulation, need a 2-week period of partial-weightbearing, before full-weightbearing is permitted [73]. From 8 weeks, the brace is unlocked and CKC strengthening exercises can be introduced within a range that does not engage the lesion, as identified intra-operatively. Following MFx, a graduated running program can be commenced from 4 months [73]. Timeframes for OAT and ACI are more variable [74, 75]. Time to return to play after combined ACLR and OAT is delayed by the ACLR time-based criterion [76].

16.5 Rehabilitation

Pre-rehabilitation is recommended before ACLR as pre-operative full range of motion (ROM) and a between-limb strength deficit of <20% is associated with improved postoperative patient outcomes and lower complication rates [64]. Postoperatively, practice guidelines recommend three criterion-based phases of rehabilitation [65]: impairment-based; sport-specific training and return to play. The impairment-based phase focuses on controlling pain and effusion, restoring knee ROM, voluntary quadriceps control, and a normal gait pattern. While for Immediate full-weightbearing is recommended following ACLR concomitant chondral restoration requires a period of protected ROM and weightbearing [66, 67]. Chondral debridement does not alter the above rehabilitation plan [68]. While continuous passive motion (CPM) following isolated ACLR [69] demonstrates no long-term benefits, its use immediately after combined ACLR and articular cartilage surgery promotes healing and reduces arthrofibrosis risk [70]. Weightbearing restric-

16.6 Conclusions

Cartilage injuries are common findings in ACL-deficient knees which can result from the primary trauma and impact or from the chronic instability in the damaged knee. The incidence of associated cartilage and meniscal pathology with ACL tears varies widely in the literature, partly because the high percentage of asymptomatic chondral damage and for the increased incidence over time in knees with untreated tears. Nevertheless, these conditions can affect the diagnosis, the treatment, and prognosis of each other.

The optimal management of concomitant injury of ACL tear and chondral damage remains unclear as there are some inconsistencies regarding the long-term effects of cartilage injury in the ACL-deficient knee. It was shown that ACL injury predisposes the young healthy knee to early OA. Several studies have showed that concomitant injuries may further increase this risk. While some showed that this is true even after ACL reconstruction, others have shown that in the case of asymptomatic chondral defects, the presence of the latter did not affect the long-time outcomes. However, as delays in ACLR increased the risk and severity of chondral lesions in the adult knee, a surgical approach is more suitable for the young active patients with higher functional needs and elite and professional athletes. A combined surgical approach which addresses both conditions during the same surgery is usually the treatment of choice.

While current literature does not favor a specific approach or technique. We suggest addressing the biomechanics of the knee addressed before its biology. This includes correction of any existing malalignment, reconstruction of the ACL, and any other laxity in order to achieve stability and treating meniscal injuries and deficiencies before treating the chondral damages in one of the common methods. In combination with appropriate physical therapy and guidance before and after the surgery, patients would benefit and regain functionality. However, it is important to remember that even after optimal treatment these injuries may be devastating, potentially ending a professional athlete's career and cause long-term disability.

References

1. Amis AA, Dawkins GP. Functional anatomy of the anterior cruciate ligament. Fibre bundle actions related to ligament replacements and injuries. J Bone Joint Surg Br. 1991;73(2):260–7.
2. Kraeutler MJ, Wolsky RM, Vidal AF, Bravman JT. Anatomy and biomechanics of the native and reconstructed anterior cruciate ligament: surgical implications. J Bone Joint Surg Am. 2017;99(5):438–45.
3. Palmer I. On the injuries to the ligaments of the knee joint: a clinical study. 1938. Clin Orthop Relat Res. 2007;454:17–22; discussion 14.
4. Girgis FG, Marshall JL, Monajem A. The cruciate ligaments of the knee joint. Anatomical, functional and experimental analysis. Clin Orthop Relat Res. 1975;106:216–31.
5. Tiamklang T, Sumanont S, Foocharoen T, Laopaiboon M. Double-bundle versus single-bundle reconstruction for anterior cruciate ligament rupture in adults. Cochrane Database Syst Rev. 2012;11:CD008413.
6. Śmigielski R, Zdanowicz U, Drwięga M, Ciszek B, Ciszkowska-Łysoń B, Siebold R. Ribbon like appearance of the midsubstance fibres of the anterior cruciate ligament close to its femoral insertion site: a cadaveric study including 111 knees. Knee Surg Sports Traumatol Arthrosc. 2015;23(11):3143–50.
7. Iwahashi T, Shino K, Nakata K, Otsubo H, Suzuki T, Amano H, et al. Direct anterior cruciate ligament insertion to the femur assessed by histology and 3-dimensional volume-rendered computed tomography. Arthroscopy. 2010;26(9):S13–20.
8. Siebold R. Flat ACL anatomy: fact no fiction. Knee Surg Sports Traumatol Arthrosc. 2015;23(11):3133–5.
9. Fink C, Smigielski R, Siebold R, Abermann E, Herbort M. Anterior cruciate ligament reconstruction using a ribbon-like graft with a C-shaped tibial bone tunnel. Arthrosc Tech. 2020;9(2):e247–62.
10. Woo SL, Debski RE, Withrow JD, Janaushek MA. Biomechanics of knee ligaments. Am J Sports Med. 1999;27(4):533–43.
11. Majewski M, Susanne H, Klaus S. Epidemiology of athletic knee injuries: a 10-year study. Knee. 2006;13(3):184–8.
12. Sanders TL, Maradit Kremers H, Bryan AJ, Larson DR, Dahm DL, Levy BA, et al. Incidence of anterior cruciate ligament tears and reconstruction: a 21-year population-based study. Am J Sports Med. 2016;44(6):1502–7.
13. Gornitzky AL, Lott A, Yellin JL, Fabricant PD, Lawrence JT, Ganley TJ. Sport-specific yearly risk and incidence of anterior cruciate ligament tears in high school athletes: a systematic review and meta-analysis. Am J Sports Med. 2016;44(10):2716–23.
14. The National Ligament Registry. The fifth annual report. 2019. Available from: https://www.uknlr.co.uk/pdf/annual-report-2019.pdf.
15. Beynnon BD, Vacek PM, Newell MK, Tourville TW, Smith HC, Shultz SJ, et al. The effects of level of competition, sport, and sex on the incidence of first-time noncontact anterior cruciate ligament injury. Am J Sports Med. 2014;42(8):1806–12.
16. Kobayashi H, Kanamura T, Koshida S, Miyashita K, Okado T, Shimizu T, et al. Mechanisms of the anterior cruciate ligament injury in sports activities: a twenty-year clinical research of 1,700 athletes. J Sports Sci Med. 2010;9(4):669–75.
17. Silvers HJ, Mandelbaum BR. Preseason conditioning to prevent soccer injuries in young women. Clin J Sport Med. 2001;11(3):206.
18. Sadigursky D, Braid JA, De Lira DNL, Machado BAB, Carneiro RJF, Colavolpe PO. The FIFA 11+ injury prevention program for soccer players: a systematic review. BMC Sports Sci Med Rehabil. 2017;9(1):18.
19. Monk AP, Davies LJ, Hopewell S, Harris K, Beard DJ, Price AJ. Surgical versus conservative interventions for treating anterior cruciate ligament injuries. Cochrane Database Syst Rev. 2016;4(4):CD011166. Available from: http://doi.wiley.com/10.1002/14651858.CD011166.pub2.
20. Gagliardi AG, Carry PM, Parikh HB, Traver JL, Howell DR, Albright JC. ACL repair with suture ligament augmentation is associated with a high failure rate among adolescent patients. Am J Sports Med. 2019;47(3):560–6.

21. Strand T, Mølster A, Hordvik M, Krukhaug Y. Long-term follow-up after primary repair of the anterior cruciate ligament: clinical and radiological evaluation 15-23 years postoperatively. Arch Orthop Trauma Surg. 2005;125(4):217–21.

22. Taylor SA, Khair MM, Roberts TR, DiFelice GS. Primary repair of the anterior cruciate ligament: a systematic review. Arthroscopy. 2015;31(11):2233–47.

23. Heusdens CHW, Hopper GP, Dossche L, Roelant E, Mackay GM. Anterior cruciate ligament repair with independent suture tape reinforcement: a case series with 2-year follow-up. Knee Surg Sports Traumatol Arthrosc. 2019;27(1):60–7.

24. Mohtadi NG, Chan DS, Dainty KN, Whelan DB. Patellar tendon versus hamstring tendon autograft for anterior cruciate ligament rupture in adults. Cochrane Database Syst Rev. 2011;(9):CD005960. Available from: http://doi.wiley.com/10.1002/14651858.CD005960.pub2.

25. Pike AN, Patzkowski JC, Bottoni CR. Meniscal and chondral pathology associated with anterior cruciate ligament injuries. J Am Acad Orthop Surg. 2019;27(3):75–84.

26. Brophy RH, Zeltser D, Wright RW, Flanigan D. Anterior cruciate ligament reconstruction and concomitant articular cartilage injury: incidence and treatment. Arthroscopy. 2010;26(1):112–20.

27. Slauterbeck JR, Kousa P, Clifton BC, Naud S, Tourville TW, Johnson RJ, et al. Geographic mapping of meniscus and cartilage lesions associated with anterior cruciate ligament injuries. J Bone Joint Surg Am. 2009;91(9):2094–103.

28. Allen CR, Livesay GA, Wong EK, Woo SL. Injury and reconstruction of the anterior cruciate ligament and knee osteoarthritis. Osteoarthr Cartil. 1999;7(1):110–21.

29. Kluczynski MA, Marzo JM, Bisson LJ. Factors associated with meniscal tears and chondral lesions in patients undergoing anterior cruciate ligament reconstruction: a prospective study. Am J Sports Med. 2013;41(12):2759–65.

30. Shelbourne KD, Gray T. Results of anterior cruciate ligament reconstruction based on meniscus and articular cartilage status at the time of surgery. Five- to fifteen-year evaluations. Am J Sports Med. 2000;28(4):446–52.

31. Maffulli N, Binfield PM, King JB. Articular cartilage lesions in the symptomatic anterior cruciate ligament-deficient knee. Arthroscopy. 2003;19(7):685–90.

32. Granan L-P, Bahr R, Lie SA, Engebretsen L. Timing of anterior cruciate ligament reconstructive surgery and risk of cartilage lesions and meniscal tears: a cohort study based on the Norwegian National Knee Ligament Registry. Am J Sports Med. 2009;37(5):955–61.

33. Lee RJ, Margalit A, Nduaguba A, Gunderson MA, Ganley TJ. Risk factors for concomitant collateral ligament injuries in children and adolescents with anterior cruciate ligament tears. Orthop J Sports Med. 2018;6(11):2325967118810389.

34. Fetto JF, Marshall JL. Medial collateral ligament injuries of the knee: a rationale for treatment. Clin Orthop Relat Res. 1978;132:206–18.

35. Elkin JL, Zamora E, Gallo RA. Combined anterior cruciate ligament and medial collateral ligament knee injuries: anatomy, diagnosis, management recommendations, and return to sport. Curr Rev Musculoskelet Med. 2019;12(2):239–44.

36. Grawe B, Schroeder AJ, Kakazu R, Messer MS. Lateral collateral ligament injury about the knee: anatomy, evaluation, and management. J Am Acad Orthop Surg. 2018;26(6):e120–7.

37. Fanelli GC, Edson CJ. Posterior cruciate ligament injuries in trauma patients: part II. Arthroscopy. 1995;11(5):526–9.

38. Caldas MTL, Braga GF, Mendes SL, da Silveira JM, Kopke RM. Posterior cruciate ligament injury: characteristics and associations of most frequent injuries. Rev Bras Ortop. 2013;48(5):427–31.

39. Goyal A, Tanwar M, Joshi D, Chaudhary D. Practice guidelines for the management of multiligamentous injuries of the knee. Indian J Orthop. 2017;51(5):537–44.

40. Bonasia DE, Bruzzone M, Dettoni F, Marmotti A, Blonna D, Castoldi F, et al. Treatment of medial and posteromedial knee instability: indications, techniques, and review of the results. Iowa Orthop J. 2012;32:173–83.

41. Cooper JM, McAndrews PT, LaPrade RF. Posterolateral corner injuries of the knee: anatomy, diagnosis, and treatment. Sports Med Arthrosc Rev. 2006;14(4):213–20.

42. Norris R, McNicholas MJ. In Response to: Frog-Leg Test Maneuver for the Diagnosis of Injuries to the Posterolateral Corner of the Knee: A Diagnostic Accuracy Study. Clin J Sport Med. 2017;27(3):e33.

43. Dean RS, LaPrade RF. ACL and posterolateral corner injuries. Curr Rev Musculoskelet Med. 2020;13:123–32.

44. Widuchowski W, Widuchowski J, Koczy B, Szyluk K. Untreated asymptomatic deep cartilage lesions associated with anterior cruciate ligament injury: results at 10- and 15-year follow-up. Am J Sports Med. 2009;37(4):688–92.

45. Røtterud JH, Sivertsen EA, Forssblad M, Engebretsen L, Arøen A. Effect of meniscal and focal cartilage lesions on patient-reported outcome after anterior cruciate ligament reconstruction: a nationwide cohort study from Norway and Sweden of 8476 patients with 2-year follow-up. Am J Sports Med. 2013;41(3):535–43.

46. Simon D, Mascarenhas R, Saltzman BM, Rollins M, Bach BR, MacDonald P. The relationship between anterior cruciate ligament injury and osteoarthritis of the knee. Adv Orthop. 2015;2015:928301.

47. Svoboda SJ, Harvey TM, Owens BD, Brechue WF, Tarwater PM, Cameron KL. Changes in serum bio-

markers of cartilage turnover after anterior cruciate ligament injury. Am J Sports Med. 2013;41(9):2108–16.

48. Matsusue Y, Yamamuro T, Hama H. Arthroscopic multiple osteochondral transplantation to the chondral defect in the knee associated with anterior cruciate ligament disruption. Arthroscopy. 1993;9(3):318–21.

49. Gudas R, Gudaitė A, Pocius A, Gudienė A, Čekanauskas E, Monastyreckienė E, et al. Ten-year follow-up of a prospective, randomized clinical study of mosaic osteochondral autologous transplantation versus microfracture for the treatment of osteochondral defects in the knee joint of athletes. Am J Sports Med. 2012;40(11):2499–508.

50. Osti L, Papalia R, Del Buono A, Amato C, Denaro V, Maffulli N. Good results five years after surgical management of anterior cruciate ligament tears, and meniscal and cartilage injuries. Knee Surg Sports Traumatol Arthrosc. 2010;18(10):1385–90.

51. Klinger H-M, Baums MH, Otte S, Steckel H. Anterior cruciate reconstruction combined with autologous osteochondral transplantation. Knee Surg Sports Traumatol Arthrosc. 2003;11(6):366–71.

52. Imade S, Kumahashi N, Kuwata S, Kadowaki M, Tanaka T, Takuwa H, et al. A comparison of patient-reported outcomes and arthroscopic findings between drilling and autologous osteochondral grafting for the treatment of articular cartilage defects combined with anterior cruciate ligament injury. Knee. 2013;20(5):354–9.

53. Peterson L, Minas T, Brittberg M, Nilsson A, Sjögren-Jansson E, Lindahl A. Two- to 9-year outcome after autologous chondrocyte transplantation of the knee. Clin Orthop Relat Res. 2000;374:212–34.

54. Pike AN, Bryant T, Ogura T, Minas T. Intermediate-to long-term results of combined anterior cruciate ligament reconstruction and autologous chondrocyte implantation. Orthop J Sports Med. 2017;5(2):2325967117693591.

55. Duchman KR, Lynch TS, Spindler KP. Graft selection in anterior cruciate ligament surgery. Clin Sports Med. 2017;36(1):25–33.

56. Slone HS, Romine SE, Premkumar A, Xerogeanes JW. Quadriceps tendon autograft for anterior cruciate ligament reconstruction: a comprehensive review of current literature and systematic review of clinical results. Arthroscopy. 2015;31(3):541–54.

57. Patel SA, Hageman J, Quatman CE, Wordeman SC, Hewett TE. Prevalence and location of bone bruises associated with anterior cruciate ligament injury and implications for mechanism of injury: a systematic review. Sports Med. 2014;44(2):281–93.

58. Filardo G, Andriolo L, di Laura Frattura G, Napoli F, Zaffagnini S, Candrian C. Bone bruise in anterior cruciate ligament rupture entails a more severe joint damage affecting joint degenerative progression. Knee Surg Sports Traumatol Arthrosc. 2019;27(1):44–59.

59. Fang C, Johnson D, Leslie MP, Carlson CS, Robbins M, Di Cesare PE. Tissue distribution and measurement of cartilage oligomeric matrix protein in patients with magnetic resonance imaging-detected bone bruises after acute anterior cruciate ligament tears. J Orthop Res. 2001;19(4):634–41.

60. Krych AJ, Hevesi M, Desai VS, Camp CL, Stuart MJ, Saris DBF. Learning from failure in cartilage repair surgery: an analysis of the mode of failure of primary procedures in consecutive cases at a tertiary referral center. Orthop J Sports Med. 2018;6(5):2325967118773041.

61. Pérez-Prieto D, Torres-Claramunt R, Gelber PE, Shehata TMA, Pelfort X, Monllau JC. Autograft soaking in vancomycin reduces the risk of infection after anterior cruciate ligament reconstruction. Knee Surg Sports Traumatol Arthrosc. 2016;24(9):2724–8.

62. Ferretti M, Doca D, Ingham SM, Cohen M, Fu FH. Bony and soft tissue landmarks of the ACL tibial insertion site: an anatomical study. Knee Surg Sports Traumatol Arthrosc. 2012;20(1):62–8.

63. Kusano M, Yonetani Y, Mae T, Nakata K, Yoshikawa H, Shino K. Tibial insertions of the anterior cruciate ligament and the anterior horn of the lateral meniscus: a histological and computed tomographic study. Knee. 2017;24(4):782–91.

64. Failla MJ, Logerstedt DS, Grindem H, Axe MJ, Risberg MA, Engebretsen L, et al. Does extended preoperative rehabilitation influence outcomes 2 years after ACL reconstruction? A comparative effectiveness study between the MOON and Delaware-Oslo ACL cohorts. Am J Sports Med. 2016;44(10):2608–14.

65. van Melick N, van Cingel REH, Brooijmans F, Neeter C, van Tienen T, Hullegie W, et al. Evidence-based clinical practice update: practice guidelines for anterior cruciate ligament rehabilitation based on a systematic review and multidisciplinary consensus. Br J Sports Med. 2016;50(24):1506–15.

66. Gudas R, Gudaitė A, Mickevičius T, Masiulis N, Simonaitytė R, Cekanauskas E, et al. Comparison of osteochondral autologous transplantation, microfracture, or debridement techniques in articular cartilage lesions associated with anterior cruciate ligament injury: a prospective study with a 3-year follow-up. Arthroscopy. 2013;29(1):89–97.

67. Amin AA, Bartlett W, Gooding CR, Sood M, Skinner JA, Carrington RWJ, et al. The use of autologous chondrocyte implantation following and combined with anterior cruciate ligament reconstruction. Int Orthop (SICO). 2006;30(1):48–53.

68. Irrgang JJ, Pezzullo D. Rehabilitation following surgical procedures to address articular cartilage lesions in the knee. J Orthop Sports Phys Ther. 1998;28(4):232–40.

69. Wright RW, Haas AK, Anderson J, Calabrese G, Cavanaugh J, Hewett TE, et al. Anterior cruciate ligament reconstruction rehabilitation: MOON guidelines. Sports Health. 2015;7(3):239–43.

70. Knapik DM, Harris JD, Pangrazzi G, Griesser MJ, Siston RA, Agarwal S, et al. The basic science of continuous passive motion in promoting knee health: a systematic review of studies in a rabbit model. Arthroscopy. 2013;29(10):1722–31.

71. Tyler TF, Lung JY. Rehabilitation following osteo-chondral injury to the knee. Curr Rev Musculoskelet Med. 2012;5:72–81.
72. Ebert JR, Fallon M, Ackland TR, Janes GC, Wood DJ. Minimum 10-year clinical and radiological outcomes of a randomized controlled trial evaluating 2 different approaches to full weightbearing after matrix-induced autologous chondrocyte implantation. Am J Sports Med. 2020;48(1):133–42.
73. Hurst JM, Steadman JR, O'Brien L, Rodkey WG, Briggs KK. Rehabilitation following microfracture for chondral injury in the knee. Clin Sports Med. 2010;29(2):257–65, viii.
74. Hurley ET, Davey MS, Jamal MS, Manjunath AK, Alaia MJ, Strauss EJ. Return-to-play and rehabilitation protocols following cartilage restoration procedures of the knee: a systematic review. Cartilage. 2019;19:1947603519894733.
75. Werner BC, Cosgrove CT, Gilmore CJ, Lyons ML, Miller MD, Brockmeier SF, et al. Accelerated return to sport after osteochondral autograft plug transfer. Orthop J Sports Med. 2017;5(4):2325967117702418.
76. Krych AJ, Pareek A, King AH, Johnson NR, Stuart MJ, Williams RJ. Return to sport after the surgical management of articular cartilage lesions in the knee: a meta-analysis. Knee Surg Sports Traumatol Arthrosc. 2017;25(10):3186–96.

Marrow Stimulation: Microfracture, Drilling, and Abrasion

17

Avi S. Robinson, Jamie L. Friedman, and Rachel M. Frank

17.1 Introduction

Chondral or osteochondral lesions are present in over 60% of all knee arthroscopies, making them a commonly encountered pathology for the orthopedic surgeon [1–4]. Articular cartilage is incapable of healing on its own and is thought to clinically deteriorate over time [3]. While more severe lesions typically progress to osteoarthritis if left untreated, less is known about the natural history of asymptomatic lesions found incidentally. Until we can reliably discern which lesions will progress from those that will remain asymptomatic, the surgeon is left to decide when to intervene.

For a patient presenting with knee pain, the history and physical examination can provide important clues to the etiology. It is difficult to diagnose a cartilage defect by physical examination alone; therefore, radiographs and advanced imaging aid in identifying these lesions. However, arthroscopy remains the gold standard in the assessment of articular cartilage in the knee. When considering treatment options, factors including lesion location (e.g., patellofemoral, femoral condyle, tibial plateau), defect size and depth, and the age and activity of the patient must be considered [5–7].

There is a spectrum of treatment options for focal cartilage defects including palliative, reparative, and restorative/reconstructive procedures. Palliative treatment includes debridement/chondroplasty, which aims to reduce mechanical symptoms without stimulating cartilage healing. Reparative surgery includes marrow stimulation, commonly known as microfracture. Reparative procedures induce healing of the articular surface, but with fibrocartilaginous tissue composed of Type I collagen. This tissue has inferior mechanical properties compared to native articular hyaline cartilage (Type II collagen) [8, 9]. Restorative procedures such as matrix-associated autologous chondrocyte implantation and osteochondral autograft or allograft transplantation aim to treat chondral and osteochondral defects, with tissue indistinguishable from the surrounding healthy cartilage [10, 11]. This manuscript focuses on marrow stimulation techniques for chondral defects of the knee.

A. S. Robinson · J. L. Friedman
Department of Orthopaedic Surgery, University of Colorado School of Medicine, Aurora, CO, USA
e-mail: avi-chai.robinson@cuanschutz.edu;
jamie.friedman@cuanschutz.edu

R. M. Frank (✉)
Department of Orthopaedic Surgery, University of Colorado School of Medicine, Aurora, CO, USA

Sports Medicine, University of Colorado Athletics, Aurora, CO, USA

Cartilage Restoration, University of Colorado Athletics, Aurora, CO, USA

Shoulder Surgery, University of Colorado Athletics, Aurora, CO, USA
e-mail: rachel.frank@cuanschutz.edu

© ISAKOS 2021
A. J. Krych et al. (eds.), *Cartilage Injury of the Knee*,
https://doi.org/10.1007/978-3-030-78051-7_17

Palliative techniques were first described in the early 1940s by Haggart and Magnuson. Both were proponents of debridement, a sort of "house-cleaning" procedure, in which the aim was to remove all mechanical irritants in the knee. Magnuson theorized that mechanical irritation led to osteoarthritis and that thorough debridement might possibly prevent progression of osteoarthritis [12–15].

Pridie led the development of the first reparative technique for cartilage defects of the knee. In 1959, he described resurfacing osteoarthritic joints by drilling into the subchondral bone plate after debridement [16]. In 1989, Steadman began treating patients with high-grade focal articular cartilage defects using a microfracture technique which he developed in an animal model [17, 18]. Using this technique, Steadman recommended arthroscopic debridement and microfracture as the first-line treatment for traumatic full-thickness chondral defects of the knee [19]. These marrow stimulation techniques work by creating holes through the bottom of the subchondral bone plate allowing marrow contents to fill the debrided area. Creating a "well-shouldered" cartilage rim with vertical walls is critical to successful filling of the defect. When comparing these two marrow stimulation techniques, microfracture is thought to be superior by limiting any thermal necrosis associated with drilling. By the beginning of the twenty-first century, marrow stimulation by microfracture was considered the first-line treatment for full-thickness chondral defects [20, 21].

The inability of cartilage defects to heal is largely a consequence of its avascularity [22]. Microfracture, or the mechanical penetration into subchondral bone using an awl-like pick, disrupts the vasculature of the bone while maintaining the overall integrity of the subchondral bone plate [23]. Microfracture is a cost-effective minimally invasive procedure and was originally thought to not preclude subsequent surgery should the initial treatment fail [24–26]. Efforts to improve upon the repair tissue characteristics and long-term durability led to the investigation of strategies to augment microfracture. Microfracture augmentation techniques continue to evolve and include the addition of scaffolding, chondrocytes, hyaluronic acid, growth factors, and cytokine modulation [27, 28]. Future basic research has focused on cellular profiling, using molecular markers to identify the quality of cartilage repair between different populations of bone marrow mesenchymal signaling (stem) cells (BM-MSCs) [29].

17.2 Indications

The earliest results of both Haggart and Magnuson indicated that patients over 30 years old reported significantly worse outcomes than their younger counterparts. They also identified patient characteristics such as postoperative compliance as critical to success [12–14]. Current indications include failure of non-operative management, age less than 40 years, full-thickness lesions less than 4 cm^2, and body mass index less than 30 kg/m^2. Notably, these indications are not "set in stone" and certainly, individual patients must be evaluated and indicated for surgery on a case-by-case basis.

17.3 Contraindications

Axial malalignment, partial thickness defects, ligament instability, meniscal deficiency, and patients unwilling to follow a postoperative rehabilitation protocol are absolute contraindications [8, 24, 30]. Relative contraindications include age over 40, body mass index greater than 30 kg/m^2, an insufficient rim of cartilage, defect size greater than 4 cm^2, and bipolar lesions [21, 26].

17.4 Technique

The microfracture procedure begins with a thorough diagnostic arthroscopy of the knee. The next step is to debride the lesion using an arthroscopic shaver and various curettes (Figs. 17.1 and 17.2) to form a stable vertical wall of healthy cartilage to contain the fibrocartilage that will fill the defect (Fig. 17.3). Next, a curette is used, and care is taken to completely remove the calcium cartilage layer without disrupting the subchondral bone plate. Starting at

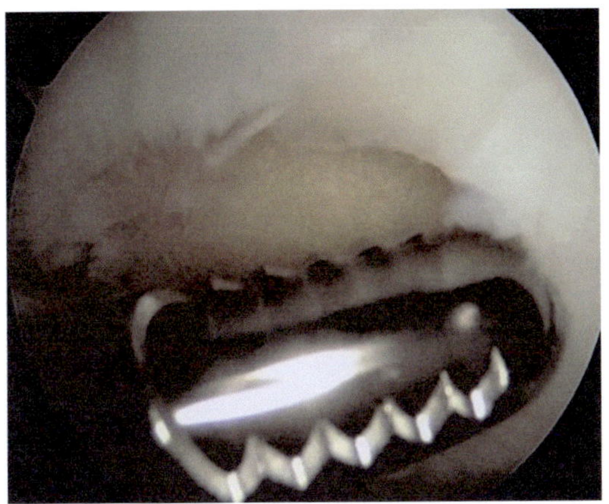

Fig. 17.1 Debridement of a focal chondral defect of the femoral condyle with an arthroscopic shaver. (Reprinted from Operative Techniques in Sports Medicine, Vol 26, Douleh, Diane and Frank, Rachel M., Marrow Stimulation: Microfracture, Drilling, and Abrasion, Pages No. 170–174, Copyright (2018), with permission from Elsevier)

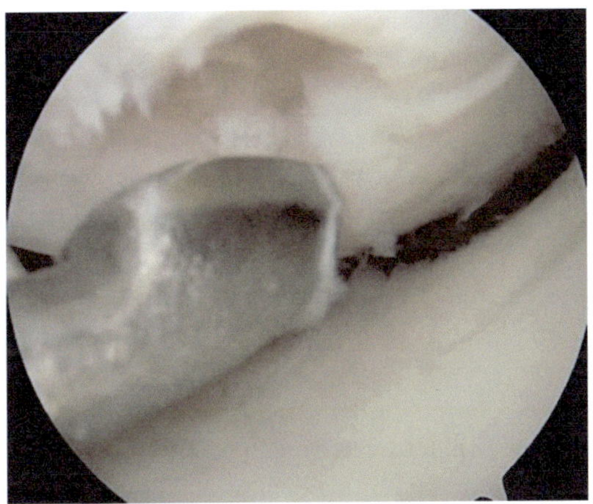

Fig. 17.2 Debridement of a focal chondral defect of the femoral condyle with a curette to create a stable rim of vertical walls around the lesion. (Reprinted from Operative Techniques in Sports Medicine, Vol 26, Douleh, Diane and Frank, Rachel M., Marrow Stimulation: Microfracture, Drilling, and Abrasion, Pages No. 170–174, Copyright (2018), with permission from Elsevier)

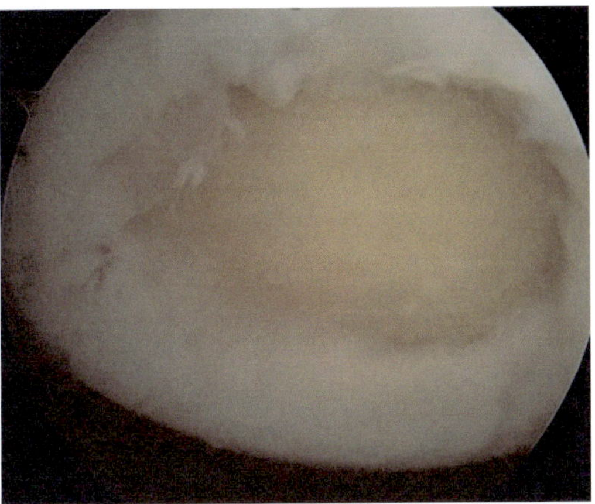

Fig. 17.3 Focal chondral defect of the femoral condyle after debridement, demonstrating a stable vertical wall around that will allow an environment optimized to hold the eventual fibrocartilage clot in place. (Reprinted from Operative Techniques in Sports Medicine, Vol 26, Douleh, Diane and Frank, Rachel M., Marrow Stimulation: Microfracture, Drilling, and Abrasion, Pages No. 170–174, Copyright (2018), with permission from Elsevier)

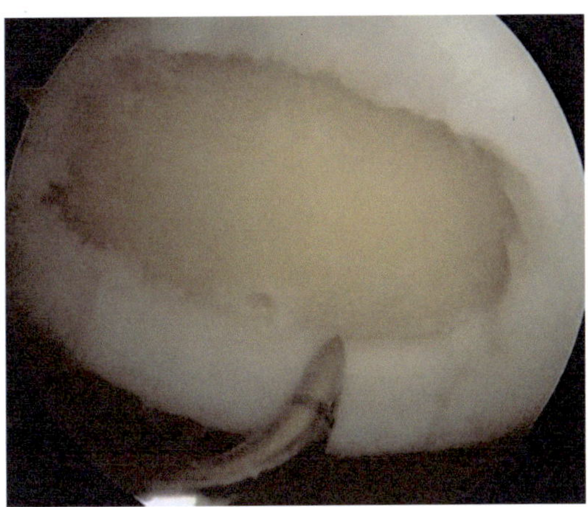

Fig. 17.4 Use of a microfracture awl to create microfracture holes through the subchondral bone plate of a focal chondral defect of the femoral condyle. (Reprinted from Operative Techniques in Sports Medicine, Vol 26, Douleh, Diane and Frank, Rachel M., Marrow Stimulation: Microfracture, Drilling, and Abrasion, Pages No. 170–174, Copyright (2018), with permission from Elsevier)

the periphery of the lesion and working towards the center, specialized awls, a micro-drill, or power-pick style drill are used to create small holes in the subchondral bone plate that are 3–4 mm apart and 2–4 mm deep (Figs. 17.4, 17.5, and 17.6). Finally, arthroscopic fluid pressure is reduced to observe fat and blood coming out of the holes to ensure marrow simulation has occurred (Fig. 17.7) [17, 25, 31]. Biologic augmentation including platelet-rich plasma and/or other scaffolds can be added to the microfracture bed as well.

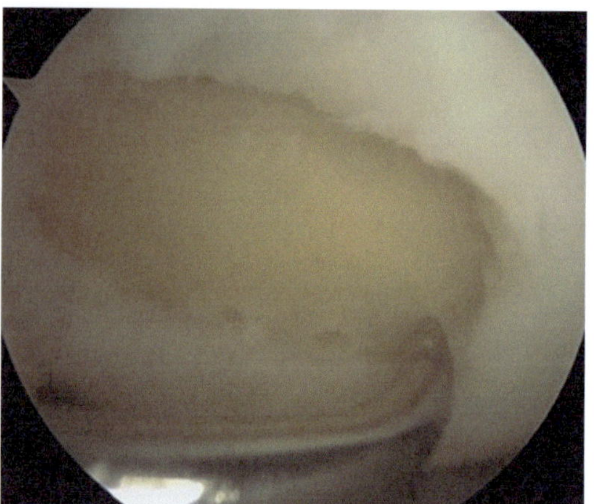

Fig. 17.5 Microfracture holes are created perpendicular to the subchondral bone, beginning along the periphery first, with subsequent holes continuing towards the center of the lesion. (Reprinted from Operative Techniques in Sports Medicine, Vol 26, Douleh, Diane and Frank, Rachel M., Marrow Stimulation: Microfracture, Drilling, and Abrasion, Pages No. 170–174, Copyright (2018), with permission from Elsevier)

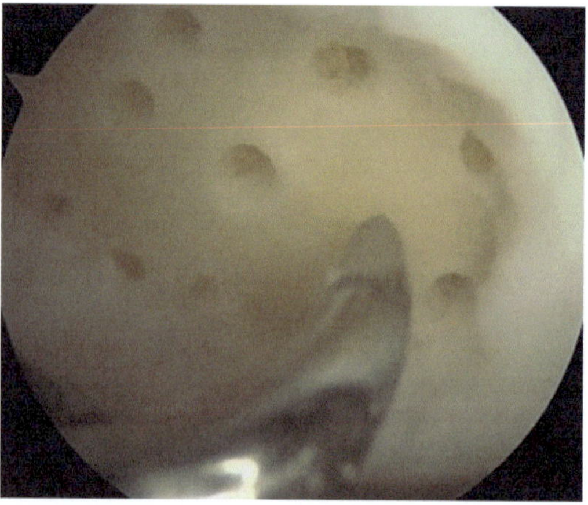

Fig. 17.6 Demonstration of microfracture holes placed approximately 3–4 mm apart, and approximately 3–4 mm deep. (Reprinted from Operative Techniques in Sports Medicine, Vol 26, Douleh, Diane and Frank, Rachel M., Marrow Stimulation: Microfracture, Drilling, and Abrasion, Pages No. 170–174, Copyright (2018), with permission from Elsevier)

17.5 Postoperative Care

Rehabilitation considerations include concomitant procedures performed as well as the location of the lesion. For a lesion of the femoral condyle

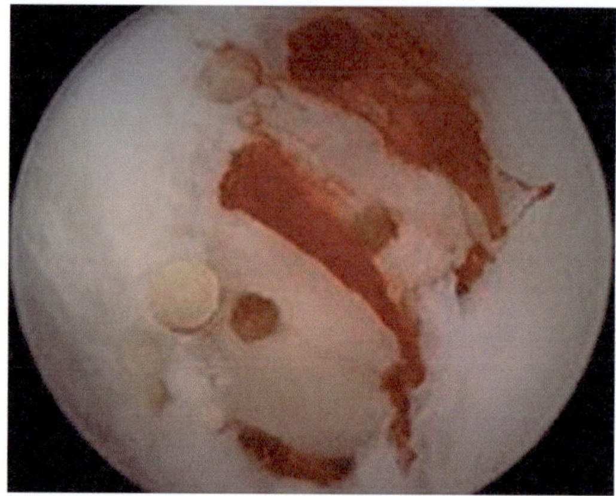

Fig. 17.7 Demonstration of blood/marrow visualized exiting out the microfracture holes from the subchondral bone after the arthroscopic fluid pressure is decreased. (Reprinted from Operative Techniques in Sports Medicine, Vol 26, Douleh, Diane and Frank, Rachel M., Marrow Stimulation: Microfracture, Drilling, and Abrasion, Pages No. 170–174, Copyright (2018), with permission from Elsevier)

or tibial plateau, the postoperative protocol includes protected weight bearing for 6–8 weeks and the use of a continuous passive motion (CPM) machine for 6–8 h per day for 6 weeks [19, 26]. Lesions of the patellofemoral compartment are not affected by weight bearing; therefore, weight bearing as tolerated with the knee locked in full extension (using a long leg knee brace) is allowed immediately after surgery [25, 26]. However, range of motion must be limited to protect formation of the fibrocartilage, so the patient is placed in a brace postoperatively with progression of 30° every 2 weeks [19]. CPM is also used in these patients but with the appropriate flexion limitations. Range of motion and weight-bearing restrictions are lifted after 8 weeks, with full return to activity expected by 6–12 months postoperatively.

17.6 Outcomes

While early results of microfracture showed a significant functional improvement over the short-term, particularly for younger athletes, long-term results were less encouraging [32]. Research suggests that restorative procedures such as autologous osteochondral transplantation

(OAT), autologous chondrocyte implantation (ACI), and osteochondral allograft transplant (OCA) may be superior to microfracture in return-to-sport time, treating patellofemoral lesions, and long-term clinical outcomes [33–38]. This may be especially true for larger lesions (>3 cm^2); however, more research is needed for clarification [39]. Currently, there is ongoing research on the effectiveness of restorative procedures following microfracture as well as the effect of concomitant procedures on outcomes of cartilage restoration surgery. There is mounting evidence that failed microfracture is an independent risk factor for failure of advanced cartilage restoration techniques such as OCA and ACI [40, 41]. This has led to a growing concern over third-party payors only reimbursing for advanced cartilage restoration procedures once microfracture has failed [42]. This reimbursement practice conflicts with the current accepted guidelines for treating cartilage injuries with microfracture for any size defect [43].

References

1. Hjelle K, Solheim E, Strand T, Muri R, Brittberg M. Articular cartilage defects in 1,000 knee arthroscopies. Arthroscopy. 2002;18(7):730–4.
2. Aroen A, Loken S, Heir S, et al. Articular cartilage lesions in 993 consecutive knee arthroscopies. Am J Sports Med. 2004;32(1):211–5.
3. Curl WW, Krome J, Gordon ES, Rushing J, Smith BP, Poehling GG. Cartilage injuries: a review of 31,516 knee arthroscopies. Arthroscopy. 1997;13(4):456–60.
4. Redler LH, Caldwell JM, Schulz BM, Levine WN. Management of articular cartilage defects of the knee. Phys Sportsmed. 2012;40(1):20–35.
5. Camp CL, Stuart MJ, Krych AJ. Current concepts of articular cartilage restoration techniques in the knee. Sports Health. 2014;6(3):265–73.
6. Behery O, Siston RA, Harris JD, Flanigan DC. Treatment of cartilage defects of the knee: expanding on the existing algorithm. Clin J Sport Med. 2014;24(1):21–30.
7. Sherman SL, Garrity J, Bauer K, Cook J, Stannard J, Bugbee W. Fresh osteochondral allograft transplantation for the knee: current concepts. J Am Acad Orthop Surg. 2014;22(2):121–33.
8. Alford JW, Cole BJ. Cartilage restoration, part 1: basic science, historical perspective, patient evaluation, and treatment options. Am J Sports Med. 2005;33(2):295–306.
9. Bae DK, Yoon KH, Song SJ. Cartilage healing after microfracture in osteoarthritic knees. Arthroscopy. 2006;22(4):367–74.
10. Gomoll AH, Farr J, Gillogly SD, Kercher J, Minas T. Surgical management of articular cartilage defects of the knee. J Bone Joint Surg Am. 2010;92(14):2470–90.
11. Vanlauwe J, Saris DB, Victor J, et al. Five-year outcome of characterized chondrocyte implantation versus microfracture for symptomatic cartilage defects of the knee: early treatment matters. Am J Sports Med. 2011;39(12):2566–74.
12. Haggart GE. Surgical treatment of degenerative arthritis of the knee joint. J Bone Joint Surg. 1940;22:717.
13. Magnuson PB. Joint debridement. Surgical treatment of degenerative arthritis. Surg Gynecol Obstet. 1941;73:1.
14. Haggart GE. Surgical treatment of degenerative arthritis of the knee joint. N Engl J Med. 1947;236:971.
15. Insall J. The Pridie debridement operation for osteoarthritis of the knee. Clin Orthop Relat Res. 1974;101:61–7.
16. Pridie KH. A method of resurfacing osteoarthritic knee joints. J Bone Joint Surg. 1959;41-B:618.
17. Steadman JR, Rodkey WG, Singleton SB, Briggs KK. Microfracture technique for full-thickness chondral defects: technique and clinical results. Oper Tech Orthop. 1997;7(4):300–4.
18. Frisbie DD, Trotter GW, Powers BE, et al. Arthroscopic subchondral bone plate microfracture technique augments healing of large chondral defects in the radial carpal bone and medial femoral condyle of horses. Vet Surg. 1999;28(4):242–55.
19. Steadman JR, Briggs KK, Rodrigo JJ, Kocher MS, Gill TJ, Rodkey WG. Outcomes of microfracture for traumatic chondral defects of the knee: average 11-year follow-up. Arthroscopy. 2003;19(5):477–84.
20. Gill TJ. The role of the microfracture technique in the treatment of full-thickness chondral injuries. Oper Tech Sports Med. 2000;8(2):138–40.
21. Steadman JR, Rodkey WG, Briggs KK. Microfracture: its history and experience of the developing surgeon. Cartilage. 2010;1(2):78–86.
22. Newman AP. Articular cartilage repair. Am J Sports Med. 1998;26(2):309–24.
23. Ghivizzani SC, Oligino TJ, Robbins PD, Evans CH. Cartilage injury and repair. Phys Med Rehabil Clin N Am. 2000;11(2):289–307, vi.
24. Kreuz PC, Steinwachs MR, Erggelet C, et al. Results after microfracture of full-thickness chondral defects in different compartments in the knee. Osteoarthr Cartil. 2006;14(11):1119–25.
25. Mithoefer K, Williams RJ 3rd, Warren RF, et al. Chondral resurfacing of articular cartilage defects in the knee with the microfracture technique. Surgical technique. J Bone Joint Surg Am. 2006;88(Suppl 1 Pt 2):294–304.
26. Mithoefer K, McAdams T, Williams RJ, Kreuz PC, Mandelbaum BR. Clinical efficacy of the microfracture technique for articular cartilage repair in the

knee: an evidence-based systematic analysis. Am J Sports Med. 2009;37(10):2053–63.

27. Strauss EJ, Barker JU, Kercher JS, Cole BJ, Mithoefer K. Augmentation strategies following the microfracture technique for repair of focal chondral defects. Cartilage. 2010;1(2):145–52.

28. Bark S, Piontek T, Behrens P, Mkalaluh S, Varoga D, Gille J. Enhanced microfracture techniques in cartilage knee surgery: fact or fiction? World J Orthop. 2014;5(4):444–9.

29. Dwivedi G, Chevrier A, Alameh MG, Hoemann CD, Buschmann MD. Quality of cartilage repair from marrow stimulation correlates with cell number, clonogenic, chondrogenic, and matrix production potential of underlying bone marrow stromal cells in a rabbit model. Cartilage. 2018; https://doi.org/10.1177/1947603518812555.

30. Steadman JR, Rodkey WG, Briggs KK. Microfracture chondroplasty: indications, techniques, and outcomes. Sports Med Arthrosc Rev. 2003;11(4):236–44.

31. Steadman JR, Rodkey WG, Rodrigo JJ. Microfracture: surgical technique and rehabilitation to treat chondral defects. Clin Orthop Relat Res. 2001;391(Suppl):S362–9.

32. Gobbi A, Nunag P, Malinowski K. Treatment of full thickness chondral lesions of the knee with microfracture in a group of athletes. Knee Surg Sports Traumatol Arthrosc. 2005;13(3):213–21.

33. Pareek A, Reardon PJ, Maak TG, Levy BA, Stuart MJ, Krych AJ. Long-term outcomes after osteochondral autograft transfer: a systematic review at mean follow-up of 10.2 years. Arthroscopy. 2016;32(6):1174–84.

34. Sherman SL, Thyssen E, Nuelle CW. Osteochondral autologous transplantation. Clin Sports Med. 2017;36(3):489–500.

35. Solheim E, Hegna J, Inderhaug E. Long-term clinical follow-up of microfracture versus mosaicplasty in articular cartilage defects of medial femoral condyle. Knee. 2017;24:1402–7.

36. Werner BC, Cosgrove CT, Gilmore CJ, et al. Accelerated return to sport after osteochondral autograft plug transfer. Orthop J Sports Med. 2017;5(4):2325967117702418.

37. Degen RM, Coleman NW, Tetreault D, et al. Outcomes of patellofemoral osteochondral lesions treated with structural grafts in patients older than 40 years. Cartilage. 2017;8(3):255–62.

38. York PJ, Wydra FB, Belton ME, Vidal AF. Joint preservation techniques in orthopaedic surgery. Sports Health. 2017;9(6):545–54.

39. Wydra FB, York PJ, Vidal AF. Allografts: osteochondral, Shell, and paste. Clin Sports Med. 2017;36(3):509–23.

40. Frank RM, Lee S, Levy D, et al. Osteochondral allograft transplantation of the knee: analysis of failures at 5 years. Am J Sports Med. 2017;45(4):864–74.

41. Muller PE, Gallik D, Hammerschmid F, et al. Third-generation autologous chondrocyte implantation after failed bone marrow stimulation leads to inferior clinical results. Knee Surg Sports Traumatol Arthrosc. 2020;28:470–7.

42. Duchman KR, Wolf BR. Editorial commentary: trends in cartilage surgery-who is steering the ship? Arthroscopy. 2019;35(1):179–81.

43. Chahla J, Stone J, Mandelbaum BR. How to manage cartilage injuries? Arthroscopy. 2019;35(10):2771–3.

Microfracture Augmentation Options for Cartilage Repair

18

Hailey P. Huddleston, Eric D. Haunschild,
Stephanie E. Wong, Brian J. Cole,
and Adam B. Yanke

18.1 Introduction

Focal chondral defects (FCD) have been reported to be present in up to 63% of knee arthroscopies [1]. When symptomatic, these lesions can cause pain and have significant deleterious effects on functional and athletic abilities. A variety of cartilage restoration and repair procedures are available for treating full-thickness cartilage defects. Historically, the algorithmic approach to treating symptomatic FCD suggested performing marrow stimulation for smaller defects (<2 cm) in less active, younger patents [2–4]. Marrow stimulation techniques result in fibrocartilage filling of the defect.

Marrow stimulation has significantly evolved from the originally proposed subchondral drilling by Pridie in 1959, to microfracture in the 1990s [5]. Recently, there has been an increasing shift toward improving microfracture techniques. Basic science and animal models have been utilized to investigate the ideal tools, location, and depth for marrow stimulation. These studies have suggested that microdrilling may provide superior preservation of the subchondral osseous architecture as long as used with cooled irrigation

to prevent heat osteonecrosis [6, 7]. Eldracher et al., for example, reported improved repair in a sheep model when utilizing a smaller trabecular sized, 1 mm diameter drill holes, instead of larger, 1.8 mm holes [8, 9]. In addition, Chen et al. suggested that traditional microfracture (large diameter awl) can cause bone compaction adjacent to the stimulation sites, obstructing the release of marrow elements [7, 10]. A similar finding was reported by Gianakos et al. who found increased subchondral architecture disruption when using large (2 mm) microfracture awls or 1.25 mm K-wires compared to a 1 mm awl in the talus [11]. These studies demonstrate that within marrow stimulation, not all techniques provide similar structural results.

From 2005 to 2014, the incidence of marrow stimulation decreased by approximately 10% [12]. While studies have suggested that marrow stimulation techniques are being used less frequently in recent years, marrow stimulation is still being performed over ten-fold more often than other cartilage restoration procedures such as osteochondral allograft transplantation (OCA) or autologous chondrocyte implantation (ACI) [13]. Marrow stimulation is a technically easier, faster, and cost-effective procedure to perform compared to other cartilage restoration procedures such as OCA but the main concern regarding marrow stimulation techniques is its durability [14–19]. Kreuz et al., for example, reported a significant decrease in International Cartilage Repair Society (ICRS)

H. P. Huddleston · E. D. Haunschild · S. E. Wong
B. J. Cole · A. B. Yanke (✉)
Rush University Medical Center, Chicago, IL, USA
e-mail: brian.cole@rushortho.com;
Adam.Yanke@RushOrtho.com

© ISAKOS 2021
A. J. Krych et al. (eds.), *Cartilage Injury of the Knee*,
https://doi.org/10.1007/978-3-030-78051-7_18

scores between 18 and 36 months postoperative in patients who underwent marrow stimulation to the trochlea, patella, or tibia [14]. Solheim et al. reported less than 60% survivorship 3 years after microfracture with a mean time to failure (knee arthroplasty or Lyscholm score <65) of 4 years [20]. This lack of durability may be attributed to the biologic differences between fibrocartilage and native hyaline cartilage, namely due to the absence of type II collagen in fibrocartilage [15, 21]. To combat these issues, surgeons are utilizing new microfracture techniques and proposing and investigating novel marrow stimulation adjuvants to improve long-term clinical outcomes.

In addition, regulatory guidelines have created an environment that is conducive to the development of new microfracture augmentation techniques. The Food and Drug Administration (FDA) formed the Tissue Reference Group (TRG) in 1997, which oversees the jurisdiction and regulation of human cells, tissues, and cellular and tissue-based products (HCT/Ps). If the product meets the 21 criteria of the TRG (i.e., the product is minimally manipulated or is only for homologous use), it is exempt from the FDA market approval pathway [22]. Because of this, investigations in the United States have mainly focused on microfracture augmentations instead of cell-based therapies to take advantage of the FDA's approval process for these products and techniques [23].

Marrow stimulation augmentation techniques, which aim to improve the quality and durability of repair tissue, fall into two main types of augmentation: scaffold and injectable adjuvants [24]. Scaffold adjuvants used in autologous matrix-induced chondrogenesis (AMIC), such as collagen-based scaffolds, address the hypothesis that a scaffold or barrier is necessary to contain subchondral marrow products to facilitate cartilage repair [21]. In contrast, injectable adjuvants, such as bone marrow aspirate concentrate (BMAC) and amniotic products, address the possibility that inferior results from marrow stimulation may be due to suboptimal levels of mesenchymal cells and cytokines released from the subchondral marrow [25–27]. This chapter will review novel marrow stimulation augmentations, their mechanism, indications, and clinical outcomes where applicable.

18.2 Autologous Matrix-Induced Chondrogenesis (AMIC)

AMIC is a commonly investigated, attractive microfracture augmentation technique. It was first introduced by Behrens et al. in the early 2000s and entails performing a type of marrow stimulation (commonly microfracture) followed by placing, and then fixating, a scaffold onto the defect. Technically, AMIC is very similar to ACI but can be performed in a one-stage procedure, avoiding a second-stage surgery associated with ACI cell culturing.

18.2.1 Indications

Similar to microfracture, the indications for an AMIC are similar to that of an ACI and include a full-thickness chondral lesion and osteochondral lesions. AMIC may not be the ideal treatment for multifocal or bipolar lesions, nor patients with diffuse degenerative changes. Patients with multifocal defects may experience inferior postoperative outcomes compared to patients with a single defect [27]. AMIC may also be preferred in younger patients (<40) with lower levels of activity [3]. Although Behrens et al. originally suggested AMIC be reserved for smaller lesion (<1.5 cm^2) and microfracture has historically been utilized and most successful in smaller lesions (<2 cm^2), clinical outcome studies have reported good results for a wide range of lesion sizes. A recent study by Bertho et al. on 13 patients with a mean defect area of 3.7 cm^2, suggested that AMIC may provide adequate outcomes in patients with large (>2 cm) osteochondral lesions (ICRS grade and 4) [28].

18.2.2 Technique

Briefly, the lesion size and severity are investigated via arthroscopy, and the site is debrided to remove any flaps and create stable, vertical edge. Marrow stimulation is then performed [29, 30]. AMIC was historically performed with awls, but given advances in the microfracture literature, a 1.1 mm K-wire is now often used for marrow stimulation at 5-mm intervals [31]. The blood clot generated by the marrow stimulation can be fixated in various ways. First, a combination of fibrin glue with autologous thrombin can be utilized to provide fixation. Alternatively, a scaffold could be utilized. A wide range of scaffolds exist for use with the AMIC technique. Historically, a collagen type scaffold is used. However, there are many novel scaffolds under clinical investigation as described in a later section. After trimming the matrix to be slightly smaller than the defect size and preparing according to manufacturer's instructions, the scaffold is fixated using allogenic fibrin glue or suturing.

18.2.3 Outcomes of AMIC

Outcomes of AMIC have been investigated in a variety of study designs and settings and are most commonly performed with a Chondro-Gide (Geistlich Pharma AG, Wolhusen, CH) scaffold, a double-layer collagen matrix scaffold. An early case series performed by Kusano et al. demonstrated significant improvements after AMIC with Chondro-Gide in patient reported outcomes—Tegner, Lysholm, International Knee Documentation Committee (IKDC), and pain visual analog scale (VAS)—at a mean of 28.8 ± 1.5 months (range, 13–51 months) [32]. Patients were indicated for AMIC if they had lesions that were >2 cm^2, ICRS grade 3 or 4. The femoral condyle osteochondral group and patellar cartilage groups demonstrated significant improvement at final follow-up on all patient reported outcomes (PROs) ($p < 0.0001–p = 0.0115$) except Tegner in the patella group. However, improvement from baseline did not reach significance for the femoral cartilage group. In addition, MRI evaluation demonstrated the presence of tissue filling within the defect for many cases; however, some cases demonstrated hypertrophy or subchondral bone abnormalities. An additional case series by Gille et al. reported on 57 patients in the AMIC Registry [33]. Patients were a mean of 37.3 years old and had a mean defect size of 3.4 cm^2. At 1-year and 2-year postoperative, patients reported a significant decrease in VAS pain ($p < 0.001$) and significant increase in Lysholm score ($p < 0.001$). Furthermore, in a subanalysis investigating lesion size, no significant differences in Lysholm ($p = 0.703$) or VAS ($p = 0.969$) were observed between groups. Similarly, Gille et al. reported on 2-year outcomes on 32 defects in 27 patients and demonstrated significant improvements on Tegner, Meyer, and ICRS scores as well reporting that 87% of patients were highly satisfied with their surgery [34]. These studies suggest AMIC provides significant clinical benefit compared to baseline.

High level evidence outcome studies for AMIC are limited. One study by Volz et al. performed a randomized control trial comparing microfracture to AMIC at 2- and 5-years follow-up [35]. Forty-seven patients were enrolled with a mean age of 37 ± 10 years and a mean defect size of 3.6 ± 1.6 cm^2 were stratified between three groups: microfracture ($n = 13$), AMIC with suture ($n = 17$), and AMIC with fibrin glue ($n = 17$). Significant improvements from baseline were reported for the mean modified Cincinnati score in all groups at 1-year, 2-years, and 5-years postoperative. For the modified ICRS score, at 5-years pain was significantly improved for both AMIC groups but had a trend to worse scores (although not statistically significant) in the microfracture group. Furthermore, a higher defect filling rate was reported in the AMIC group (over 60%) compared to the microfracture group (25%). These results suggest that AMIC may provide more durable clinical outcomes compared to microfracture. An additional randomized control trial by Ander et al. compared microfracture to AMIC at 1- and 2-years postoperative [36]. Thirty-eight patients were randomized to either microfracture ($n = 10$) or AMIC (suture [$n = 13$] or glue [$n = 15$]). Similar improvements were observed in the Modified Cincinnati score at 1-year between the three groups and all groups demonstrated significant improvements compared to baseline ($p < 0.001–p = 0.02$). These findings were maintained at 2-years postoperative. These studies support AMIC as providing comparable clinical outcomes compared to microfracture.

In addition, one randomized control trial compared AMIC to ACI. Fossum et al. randomized 41 patients to either an AMIC ($n = 20$, mean total defect size 5.2 ± 2.4 cm²) or ACI ($n = 21$, mean total defect size 4.9 ± 4.4 cm²) treatment arm [37]. The study included patients with 1 or more cartilage or osteochondral lesions of the femur and/or patella. At 2-years follow-up, significant improvements were observed on Knee Injury and Osteoarthritis Outcome Score (KOOS) and Lysholm for both groups. In addition, VAS scores had decreased to almost half of what they were at baseline (50–30.4 for ACI and 57.6–27 for AMIC). In addition, 3 patients from the ACI group underwent a second look arthroscopy during the first 2 years of follow-up (all demonstrated good defect fill) and 3 from the AMIC group (1 of 3 demonstrated sparse filling). In addition, 2 patients from the AMIC group progressed to a total knee arthroplasty (TKA). This study suggested comparable clinical outcomes between AMIC and ACI at short-term follow-up.

As discussed in detail later, orthobiologics can also be utilized to augment microfracture techniques. Furthermore, they can be utilized in conjunction with AMIC. A randomized study by de Girolamo et al. reported preliminary outcomes after AMIC and BMAC compared to standard AMIC in 24 patients [38]. Patients who had BMAC augmented AMIC demonstrated higher Lysholm scores ($p = 0.015$) and lower VAS ($p = 0.011$) compared to the AMIC group at 1-year postoperative. However, both groups maintained significantly lower VAS scores compared to baseline up to 100 months postoperative. In addition, the AMIC with BMAC group demonstrated significant improvements in IKDC 2-years follow-up ($p < 0.05$), in contrast to the AMIC group, which did not reach significance. Literature on AMIC in combination with orthobiologics remains sparse. Future studies are needed to investigate clinical outcomes in this setting.

18.2.4 Limitations of AMIC

One of the main limitations in our understanding of the performance and durability of AMIC is the lack of long-term outcome data. Generally, the available outcome studies focused on the mid-term results of AMIC at 2-year follow-up, with only a handful of papers reporting outcomes at 5-year follow-up. Furthermore, while a few studies have compared AMIC to commonly performed procedures such as microfracture and ACI, there is limited literature on the long-term survivorship of AMIC, and how this is compared to other cartilage procedures. Future long-term investigations are needed.

AMIC is also subject to similar disadvantages as microfracture. For example, a study by Beck et al. investigated the effect of microfracture and autologous matrix-induced chondrogenesis (AMIC) on subchondral bone structure and subchondral bone cyst formation in 36 sheep [39]. The sheep were stratified into three groups (control, microfracture, and AMIC) underwent analysis at either 13 weeks ($n = 6$ per group) or 26 weeks ($n = 6$ per group) postoperative. Analysis included percentage of infill, histology, histomorphology, and micro-CT (at 26 weeks only). There were no significant differences in infill between microfracture and AMIC, which was greater than in the control group. However, there was a high rate of subchondral cyst formation in both the microfracture and AMIC groups at 13 weeks (AMIC: 50%, microfracture: 33%) and 26 weeks (AMIC: 100%, microfracture 83%) postoperative. Furthermore, subchondral histological and micro-CT findings demonstrated increased bone volume and trabecular thickness associated with cyst formation. This study is a reminder that microfracture augmentation techniques, such as AMIC, are subject to similar limitations as microfracture and these disadvantages should be considered in surgical decision-making. Furthermore, when comparing AMIC to isolated microfracture, the marrow stimulation technique in both treatment groups should be considered. If small diameter drilling in an AMIC group is compared to large awl microfracture, structural and clinical outcomes may differ between groups but may be due to differences in stimulation approaches rather than the utilization of a scaffold.

An additional limitation when interpreting the available AMIC literature is the range of techniques, scaffolds, and indications that are used. For example, some studies have reported on utilizing fibrin glue while others report on suturing. Although more time intensive and technically challenging, suturing has been shown to provide more secure collagen patch fixation in in vitro models compared to fibrin glue [40, 41]. In addition, while Chondro-Gide is the most commonly cited scaffold in the outcome literature other studies have reported clinical outcomes using the Hyalofast matrix scaffold [30]. Lastly, like all novel procedures, the indications of AMIC greatly vary between studies. This is most obvious when analyzing lesion number and size. While some studies report on smaller lesions of 2–3 cm^2, others include multifocal or very large lesions, further complicating any comparisons that can be made between studies. Future clinical studies are needed to validate the use of AMIC and identify its indications.

18.3 Novel Scaffold Adjuvants

While historically a collagen matrix scaffold has been used for AMIC, multiple novel scaffolds are available and described in the clinical literature. Similar to collagen matrices, these scaffolds attempt to inhibit extravasation of mesenchymal stem cells (MSCs) into the joint, which can then be captured within the scaffold, resulting in cartilage defect filling [42]. Numerous novel scaffold types have been developed or proposed, such as poly(ethylene glycol)-based hydrogels (PEG) and porcine chondrocyte extracellular membranes. Hydrogels, a commonly investigated scaffold type, have demonstrated the ability to provide similar biocompatible properties as cartilage and allow for easy diffusion of solutes in both synthetic (e.g., hyaluronic acid or chitosan) and natural (e.g., PEG) forms [43, 44]. This section will explore novel scaffold augmentation types and associated clinical investigations.

18.3.1 ChonDux

ChonDux (Zimmer Biomet, Warsaw, IN) is chondroitin-sulfate and PEG hydrogel that is polymerized intraoperatively with UV light. Bench work demonstrated the tensile strength of this hydrogel and the ability for glycosaminoglycans and collagens to be produced within the scaffold. Specifically, the ChonDux allowed for GAG and collagen production of adjacent MSCs to double compared to those cultured without ChonDux [45, 46]. In a caprine animal model, ChonDux ($n = 6$) was compared to an isolated microfracture ($n = 6$) technique. The ChonDux group demonstrated superior mechanical properties (1.56-fold strength, $p < 0.05$) of the clot compared to microfracture [46].

In a pilot human clinical trial, 18 patients underwent ChonDux implantation for symptomatic focal chondral defects (2–4 cm^2). At MRI at 6 months, more patients had greater fill (>75%) in the ChonDux group (12 of 14 patients) versus the microfracture group (1 of 3 patients) [45]. Wolf et al. investigated these patients at 24-months follow-up [47]. On MRI, a mean 94.2% ± 16.3% fill was observed in the ChonDux group. In addition, VAS pain severity ($p < 0.05$) and frequency ($p < 0.01$) significantly decreased at 6 months follow-up compared to baseline. In addition, significant improvements were observed on IKDC at 18 months and 24 months compared to baseline ($p < 0.05$ for both). However, IKDC improvement at 3 months, 6 months, and 12 months did not reach significance. These preliminary clinical outcome studies demonstrated that ChonDux may provide similar clinical outcomes compared to isolated microfracture.

18.3.2 Chondrotissue

Chondrotissue (BioTissue AG, Switzerland) is a cell-free polyglycolic with freeze-dried acid-hyaluronan (PGA-HA) scaffold. The PGA-HA scaffold was compared to traditional microfracture techniques in a study by Erggelet et al. in 8 sheep [48]. This study suggested that the addition of HA for 14 days to the PGA scaffold-induced expression of chemotactic molecules, such as cartilage link protein, aggrecan, and type II alpha-1 collagen. In addition, the authors reported that at 3 months after surgery, only the PGA-HA group demonstrated cartilage repair.

This approach has also been combined with platelet-rich plasma (PRP) and evaluated in the clinical setting. Siclari et al. reported on 5-year follow-up in 52 patients who underwent Chondrotissue implants that were incubated in PRP for 5–10 min [49]. Clinical outcomes were evaluated with KOOS, which demonstrated significant improvements at 1-year, 2-year, and 5-year follow-up compared to baseline. Twenty-one of the 52 patients returned for MRI evaluation at 4 years follow-up and 20 of the 21 patients demonstrated excellent MOCART scores. An additional study by Enea et al. reported a case series of nine patients who underwent Chondrotissue with BMAC-augmented microfracture [50]. Clinical outcomes including IKDC, Lysholm, VAS, and Tegner significantly improved from baseline to final follow-up at a mean of 22 ± 2 months. In addition, four MRIs that were performed 8–12 months postoperatively, demonstrated defect filling, although mild bone marrow lesions were present in all cases. Despite these successful results, it remains unclear how these findings compared to PGA-HA without BMAC or PRP and to other scaffolds.

18.3.3 GelrinC

GelrinC (Regentis Biomaterials, Princeton, NJ) is composed of a synthetic polyethylene glycol di-acrylate (PEG-DA) and denatured fibrinogen. The unique formulation allows implantation of the hydrogel in liquid form on a microfractured lesion. Once implanted, UVA light is used to set the implant in place, thus removing the need to use fibrin glue or suture to adhere to the scaffold. Over 6–12-months postoperative, theoretically, the implant acts like as scaffold attracting chondrocytes and MSC. As this occurs, the GelrinC slowly disintegrates, leaving behind a filled in cartilage defect. Currently, a large-scale clinical trial of the efficacy and clinical outcomes of GelrinC for FCDs is being performed in the United States (NCT03262909). This 5-year non-randomized clinical trial will ultimately conclude in 2023 and will consist of 181 patients (age 18–50) who were selected for ether a GelrinC treatment arm or traditional microfracture control arm. Patients with multifocal lesions, high BMI (35), lesions >2.5 cm in diameter, untreated ligamentous injury, prior failed ACI or MACI, and/or microfracture surgery within 1 year of their planned surgery are excluded. The primary outcomes of this study will be an evaluation of KOOS physical function and pain scores at 2 years after surgery.

18.3.4 BST CarGel

BST CarGel (Smith and Nephew, London, UK) is based on mixing a chitosan solution (chitosan-glycerol phosphate) with patient's whole blood to create an autologous bioscaffold. Hoemann et al. was the first to investigate the efficacy of BST CarGel in 2007. In a rabbit model, BST CarGel was compared to traditional microfracture on small (3.5×4 mm) trochlear defects [51]. At 1 day after surgery, the defects were analyzed by histomorphology, while at 8 weeks the degree of repair was analyzed with histology, histomorphology, collagen type II expression, and stereology. The authors reported that the BST CarGel defects generated clots that were more resistant to retraction compared to control defects at 1-day postoperative ($p < 0.0001$). In addition, they observed a greater amount of hyaline cartilage, and greater integration in the BST CarGel group compared to isolated microfracture at 8 weeks. These findings were supported by a human clinical study by Méthot et al., which investigated the structure of BST CarGel treatments to traditional microfracture with MRI at a mean of 13-months follow-up [52]. In addition, about 50% of the patients from each group (BST CarGel: 21/41, microfracture: 17/39) underwent a second-look arthroscopy. The authors reported that BST CarGel group had superior ICRS I and II histological parameters (i.e., surface architecture, superficial assessment, cell viability, and cell distribution) ($p = 0.007$–0.042). In addition, BST CarGel demonstrated more organized repair on light microscopy ($p = 0.0003$) and superior ICRS scoring ($p = 0.0002$) on arthroscopy.

In addition, multiple clinical trials in Canada and Europe have investigated the efficacy BST CarGel. At press, this product is not available for use in the United States. One such by Shive et al. investigated 1-year MRI and clinical outcomes (WOMAC scores) in 80 patients randomized to BST CarGel ($n = 41$) versus isolated microfracture ($n = 39$) [53]. In this study, BST Cartgel, demonstrated greater lesion filling (BST CarGel: 92.8% ± 2.0% vs microfracture: 85.2% ± 2.1%, $p = 0.011$). In terms of clinical outcomes, both groups demonstrated comparable, significant improvements in WOMAC scores ($p < 0.0001$ from baseline for both groups). In addition, a continuation of this 1-year study culminated in a 5-year study of 80 patients that were randomized to either a BST CarGel or isolated microfracture group for treatment of an FCD (ICRS grade III or IV) of the knee [54]. At 5-years follow-up, MRI analysis demonstrated significant greater lesion filling in the BST CarGel group ($p = 0.017$). In addition, there were similar, significant improvements in both the BST CarGel and microfracture groups on WOMAC subscales ($p < 0.0001$). This study also demonstrated that BST CarGel had a similar safety profile to microfracture with 19.4% patients experiencing an adverse event (most commonly pain) compared to 26.9% of those in the microfracture group. BST CarGel is one of the more well-studied novel scaffold augmentations; however, how these findings are compared to other cartilage restoration procedures, such as ACI, remain unclear.

18.3.5 ArtiFilm ECM

ArtiFilm (Regenprime Co., Ltd., Korea) is a porcine chondrocyte-derived extracellular membrane. ArtiFilm takes porcine cartilage that is isolated and cultured for 3 weeks, then decellularizes and washes the extracellular matrix and chondrocyte complex to form the final ArtiFilm product. ArtiFilm was developed to combat potential complications associated with using a periosteal or traditional collagen membrane after it was demonstrated that a porcine extracellular matrix would allow for the proliferation and adhesion of chondrocytes in mice [55, 56]. In a study in beagles, Li et al. demonstrated that ArtiFilm did not result in any cytotoxicity or immune responses in vivo [57]. In addition, the thin film demonstrated a high tensile strength of 85.64 N. When compared to traditional marrow stimulation, the ArtiFilm group demonstrated a higher macroscopic ICRS grade with more hyaline cartilage at 18 weeks on histology.

Clinical investigations on the outcomes of the use of ArtiFilm are limited. One clinical prospective, non-randomized study by Chung et al. compared cartilage repair and 2-year clinical outcomes in patients who underwent microfracture with ArtiFilm ($n = 45$) to traditional microfracture ($n = 19$) [58]. In terms of MRI outcomes, 75% of patients had moderate (34–66% cartilage fill) to good (>67% cartilage fill) cartilage repair compared to 50% of patients moderate to good results in the microfracture group ($p = 0.043$). Patients in the ArtiFilm group demonstrated significant improvements on IKDC, VAS satisfaction, and VAS pain (all $p < 0.001$). In comparison, the microfracture group only demonstrated improvements on VAS satisfaction ($p = 0.015$). However, there were no significant differences in clinical outcomes between the two groups. Future randomized trials are needed to support these preliminary findings.

18.3.6 Limitations of Novel Scaffolds

Despite all of the advances in scaffolds and regenerative medicine for treating FCDs, a few large limitations still remain. The current randomized, controlled trials compare the novel scaffolds to a control group of microfracture patients. While this historically makes sense, it remains unknown how these different novel scaffolds are compared to each other and other cartilage restoration options such as ACI or MACI. In addition, the indications for novel scaffold adjuvants and how these treatment options fit into the larger FCD treatment algorithm remains unclear. Future studies are needed to evaluate differences in scaffold types, how they are compared to other mainstay cartilage procedures and their specific indications.

18.4 BioCartilage

In contrast to AMIC, the BioCartilage technique (Arthrex, Naples, FL) combines microfracture with dehydrated, micronized allogeneic cartilage, platelet-rich plasma, and fibrin glue. Prior investigations have suggested that the composition of BioCartilage is conducive to chondrocyte and MSC adherence and proteomic analysis demonstrated the presence of a variety of bioactive proteins [59, 60]. The technique allows for a single-staged surgery that does not require a collagen or alternative composition scaffold. In this approach, the lesion is prepared in standard fashion [61]. Then microfracture is performed and the BioCartilage is prepared in accordance with the manufacturer's instruction and is mixed with PRP. The resultant paste is then carefully spread over the microfractured defect so that it is slightly sunken compared to the adjacent cartilage. Lastly, fibrin glue is applied over the top of the Biocartilage. Literature on the clinical outcomes of this novel surgical approach remains limited [62]. Additional research is necessary to investigate the durability of this approach and how it compares both to two-stage approaches, such as ACI and OCA, and to other one-stage augmented microfracture techniques.

18.5 Biologic Augmentation

In addition to scaffold-based augmentation techniques, there is an array of injectable adjuncts to microfracture that have shown promise in preliminary trials. In general, these modalities introduce mediators that stimulate and proliferate chondrogenesis within microfractured defects. These factors are believed to promote differentiation of the stem cells introduced by microfracture into a more hyaline-like repair tissue than the fibrocartilage produced in traditional microfracture, which has been cited as a probable etiology of the long-term functional outcome deterioration associated with microfracture [15, 21, 63, 64]. In addition, many techniques introduce additional MSCs to the defect site, with the ambition of further promoting chondrogenesis within the repair.

18.5.1 Bone Marrow Aspirate Concentrate

One promising new injectable augmentation of microfracture is the use of BMAC. BMAC, which can be collected and processed at the time of surgery using a number of commercial centrifugation systems, is a source of MSCs, growth factors, and cytokines believed to improve tissue regeneration. In particular, BMAC has been identified to have high concentrations of transforming growth factor beta (TGF-β), bone morphogenetic protein-2 (BMP-2), vascular endothelial growth factor (VEGF), interleukin-1 receptor antagonist (IL-1RA), and interleukin-8 (IL-8) [65, 66]. The anti-inflammatory and immunomodulatory properties of these cytokines and growth factors stimulate chondrocytes to produce cartilage matrix and upregulate proteoglycan and type II collagen production needed in chondrogenesis.

To date, clinical evaluations of BMAC augmentation for microfracture of the knee remain limited. Murphy et al. prospectively investigated BMAC augmentation in microfracture of the talus, finding that those receiving BMAC had significantly lower revision rates than those with isolated microfracture at a minimum of 36 months after surgery [67]. In the knee, early investigations of BMAC and scaffold single-stage repairs have shown similar promise, demonstrating favorable outcomes at mid- to long-term follow-up when compared to traditional microfracture [68, 69]. However, the role of BMAC augmentation on microfracture itself has yet to be evaluated.

18.5.2 Platelet-Rich Plasma

PRP is another attractive adjunct being investigated for a number of orthopedic procedures, including microfracture. As with BMAC, the promise of PRP is attributed to its high concentration of chondrogenic growth factors, including platelet-derived growth factor (PDGF), TGF-β, and VEGF [70]. These modulators facilitate chondrogenesis by stimulating cartilage matrix deposition and upregulating proteoglycan and type II collagen production. In addition,

TGF-β in particular has been identified as a key modulator in the differentiation of MSCs into chondrocytes. [71] These benefits have been evident in preclinical studies using rat and sheep models, where PRP-augmented microfracture repairs displayed favorable healing when compared controls at serial histologic evaluations [72–74].

Despite its promise in facilitating a more favorable repair tissue over microfractured defects, PRP has shown mixed results in early human investigations. In a recent meta-analysis of seven studies investigating PRP augmentation of microfracture in the knee and ankle, Boffa et al. found that while augmentation did significantly improve short-term outcomes, it was to a clinically insignificant degree [75]. Notably, differing PRP preparations and injection protocols were utilized in each trial, limiting the ability to generalize results. Future investigations using standardized PRP products are needed to better assess their efficacy in microfracture augmentation.

18.5.3 Adipose-Derived Injections

Another attractive source of stem cells for microfracture repairs is adipose-derived mesenchymal stem cells (ADSCs), which can be harvested and processed at the time of microfracture [76]. In addition, adipose injectables are rich in anti-inflammatory cytokines and growth factors that may aid in tissue healing [77]. These benefits have been evaluated in small animal models, demonstrating efficacy of ADSCs in improving cartilage repair quality [78, 79]. The effect of ADSC augmentation of microfracture has also been clinically evaluated by Koh et al., who prospectively compared 40 patients receiving traditional microfracture to 40 patients receiving microfracture and ADSC injection for isolated chondral defects [26]. At 2-year follow-up evaluation, patients receiving ADSC had improved radiographic outcomes and KOOS pain and symptom scores when compared to those receiving isolated microfracture.

18.5.4 Amniotic Suspension Allograft Injections

Amniotic suspension allograft (ASA) injections present another source of high concentrations of anabolic growth factors and anti-inflammatory modulators that may aid in favorable healing of microfractured defects. ASA products have been identified to contain TGF-β, basic fibroblast growth factor, PDGF, and several interleukins including IL-8, IL-4, IL-6, and IL-10 [80]. In addition, ASA products contain high concentrations of tissue inhibitors of metalloproteinases (TIMPs) and free hyaluronic acid, whose anti-inflammatory properties may further improve joint homeostasis [81, 82]. Early preclinical studies using Lewis rat osteoarthritis models by Willett et al. and Raines et al. have demonstrated the promise of amniotic products in attenuating cartilage degeneration [83, 84]. Recently, Farr et al. completed a randomized-controlled clinical trial of ASA injections compared to hyaluronic acid and saline controls in improving osteoarthritis symptoms at 3 and 6 months after injection. They found that those receiving ASA injections had significantly greater improvements in VAS, KOOS pain, and KOOS activities of daily living at 6 months after injection, demonstrating the promise of ASA injections in symptomatic OA [81]. The effect of ASA augmentation of microfracture, however, has yet to be evaluated.

18.5.5 Other Promising Injectable Augmentation Modalities

Other injectable modalities that have been investigated for microfracture augmentation include hyaluronic acid and IL-1ra gene therapy. The therapeutic potential of IL-1ra gene therapy was investigated using an equine model by Morisset et al. [85]. In this study, horses injected in vivo with the gene therapy were found to have greater proteoglycan and type II collagen present in healed defects at 16 weeks compared to controls. Hyaluronic acid has been used for conservative management of OA and as an augmentation of microfracture due to its stimulatory effect on chondrocyte metabolism [86–88]. Despite this potential benefit, hyaluronic acid has had mixed results in preclinical and clinical evaluations of its use as an injectable and scaffold-based augmentation technique [88–91]. Further investigations are needed to evaluate its role in augmentation, particularly when considering the greater reported efficacy of other treatment modalities.

18.6 Conclusion

Over the past decade, as literature has demonstrated the lack of durability of microfracture for focal chondral defects, there has been a significant interest in techniques for microfracture augmentation. These investigations have focused on incorporating scaffolds and orthobiologics into microfracture procedures. Preliminary clinical outcomes have suggested that these approaches may provide superior defect filling than microfracture, however clinical outcomes appear to be similar. There is limited information on how these augmented microfracture techniques are compared to other cartilage surgical treatments such as OCA and ACI. Future studies are needed to compare augmented microfracture techniques to each other and to mainstay cartilage surgeries to identify proper uses and indications.

References

1. Curl WW, et al. Cartilage injuries: a review of 31,516 knee arthroscopies. Arthroscopy. 1997;13:456–60.
2. Weber AE, et al. Clinical outcomes after microfracture of the knee: midterm follow-up. Orthop J Sports Med. 2018;6:2325967117753572.
3. Kreuz PC, et al. Is microfracture of chondral defects in the knee associated with different results in patients aged 40 years or younger? Arthroscopy. 2006;22:1180–6.
4. Steadman JR, Rodkey WG, Briggs KK. Microfracture. Cartilage. 2010;1:78–86.
5. Steadman JR, Rodkey WG, Singleton SB, Briggs KK. Microfracture technique for full-thickness chondral defects: technique and clinical results. Oper Tech Orthop. 1997;7:300–4.
6. Augustin G, et al. Thermal osteonecrosis and bone drilling parameters revisited. Arch Orthop Trauma Surg. 2007;128:71–7.
7. Chen H, et al. Drilling and microfracture lead to different bone structure and necrosis during bone-marrow stimulation for cartilage repair. J Orthop Res. 2009;27:1432–8.
8. Eldracher M, Orth P, Cucchiarini M, Pape D, Madry H. Small subchondral drill holes improve marrow stimulation of articular cartilage defects. Am J Sports Med. 2014;42:2741–50.
9. Orth P, Duffner J, Zurakowski D, Cucchiarini M, Madry H. Small-diameter awls improve articular cartilage repair after microfracture treatment in a translational animal model. Am J Sports Med. 2015;44:209–19.
10. Chen H, et al. Depth of subchondral perforation influences the outcome of bone marrow stimulation cartilage repair. J Orthop Res. 2011;29:1178–84.
11. Gianakos AL, et al. The effect of different bone marrow stimulation techniques on human talar subchondral bone: a micro-computed tomography evaluation. Arthroscopy. 2016;32:2110–7.
12. Bonazza NA, et al. Surgical trends in articular cartilage injuries of the knee, analysis of the Truven Health MarketScan commercial claims database from 2005-2014. Arthrosc Sports Med Rehab Online. 2019;1:e101–7.
13. Gowd AK, et al. Management of chondral lesions of the knee: analysis of trends and short-term complications using the national surgical quality improvement program database. Arthroscopy. 2018;35:138–46.
14. Kreuz PC, et al. Results after microfracture of full-thickness chondral defects in different compartments in the knee. Osteoarthr Cartil. 2006;14:1119–25.
15. Gobbi A, Karnatzikos G, Kumar A. Long-term results after microfracture treatment for full-thickness knee chondral lesions in athletes. Knee Surg Sports Traumatol Arthrosc. 2013;22:1986–96.
16. Gudas R, et al. A prospective randomized clinical study of mosaic osteochondral autologous transplantation versus microfracture for the treatment of osteochondral defects in the knee joint in young athletes. Arthroscopy. 2005;21:1066–75.
17. Solheim E, Hegna J, Strand T, Harlem T, Inderhaug E. Randomized study of long-term (15-17 years) outcome after microfracture versus mosaicplasty in knee articular cartilage defects. Am J Sports Med. 2017;46:826–31.
18. Krych AJ, Harnly HW, Rodeo SA, Williams RJ. Activity levels are higher after osteochondral autograft transfer mosaicplasty than after microfracture for articular cartilage defects of the knee: a retrospective comparative study. J Bone Joint Surg Am. 2012;94:971–8.
19. Aae TF, Randsborg P-H, Lurås H, Årøen A, Lian ØB. Microfracture is more cost-effective than autologous chondrocyte implantation: a review of level 1 and level 2 studies with 5 year follow-up. Knee Surg Sports Traumatol Arthrosc. 2017;26:1044–52.
20. Solheim E, Hegna J, Inderhaug E. Long-term survival after microfracture and mosaicplasty for knee articular cartilage repair: a comparative study between two treat-

ments cohorts. Cartilage. 2018:1947603518783482. https://doi.org/10.1177/1947603518783482.

21. Strauss EJ, Barker JU, Kercher JS, Cole BJ, Mithoefer K. Augmentation strategies following the microfracture technique for repair of focal chondral defects. Cartilage. 2010;1:145–52.

22. Yanke AB, Chubinskaya S. The state of cartilage regeneration: current and future technologies. Curr Rev Musculoskelet Med. 2015;8:1–8.

23. Riff A, Davey A, Cole B. Joint Preserv Knee. 2019:295–319. https://doi.org/10.1007/978-3-030-01491-9_18.

24. Arshi A, et al. Can biologic augmentation improve clinical outcomes following microfracture for symptomatic cartilage defects of the knee? A systematic review. Cartilage. 2018;9:146–55.

25. Lee GW, Son J-H, Kim J-D, Jung G-H. Is platelet-rich plasma able to enhance the results of arthroscopic microfracture in early osteoarthritis and cartilage lesion over 40 years of age? Eur J Orthop Surg Traumatol. 2012;23:581–7.

26. Koh Y-G, Kwon O-R, Kim Y-S, Choi Y-J, Tak D-H. Adipose-derived mesenchymal stem cells with microfracture versus microfracture alone: 2-year follow-up of a prospective randomized trial. Arthroscopy. 2015;32:97–109.

27. Gudas R, Mačiulaitis J, Staškūnas M, Smailys A. Clinical outcome after treatment of single and multiple cartilage defects by autologous matrix-induced chondrogenesis. J Orthop Surg Hong Kong. 2019;27:2309499019851011.

28. Bertho P, Pauvert A, Pouderoux T, Robert H, Orthopaedics and Traumatology Society of Western France (SOO). Treatment of large deep osteochondritis lesions of the knee by autologous matrix-induced chondrogenesis (AMIC): preliminary results in 13 patients. Orthop Traumatol Surg Res. 2018;104:695–700.

29. Benthien JP, Behrens P. Autologous matrix-induced chondrogenesis (AMIC): combining microfracturing and a collagen I/III matrix for articular cartilage resurfacing. Cartilage. 2010;1:65–8.

30. Lee YHD, Suzer F, Thermann H. Autologous matrix-induced chondrogenesis in the knee. Cartilage. 2014;5:145–53.

31. Benthien J, Behrens P. The treatment of chondral and osteochondral defects of the knee with autologous matrix-induced chondrogenesis (AMIC): method description and recent developments. Knee Surg Sports Traumatol Arthrosc. 2011;19:1316–9.

32. Kusano T, et al. Treatment of isolated chondral and osteochondral defects in the knee by autologous matrix-induced chondrogenesis (AMIC). Knee Surg Sports Traumatol Arthrosc. 2011;20:2109–15.

33. Gille J, et al. Outcome of autologous matrix induced chondrogenesis (AMIC) in cartilage knee surgery: data of the AMIC registry. Arch Orthop Trauma Surg. 2012;133:87–93.

34. Gille J, et al. Mid-term results of autologous matrix-induced chondrogenesis for treatment of focal cartilage defects in the knee. Knee Surg Sports Traumatol Arthrosc. 2010;18:1456–64.

35. Volz M, Schaumburger J, Frick H, Grifka J, Anders S. A randomized controlled trial demonstrating sustained benefit of autologous matrix-induced chondrogenesis over microfracture at five years. Int Orthop. 2017;41:797–804.

36. Anders S, Volz M, Frick H, Gellissen J. A randomized, controlled trial comparing autologous matrix-induced chondrogenesis (AMIC®) to microfracture: analysis of 1- and 2-year follow-up data of 2 centers. Open Orthop J. 2013;7:133–43.

37. Fossum V, Hansen AK, Wilsgaard T, Knutsen G. Collagen-covered autologous chondrocyte implantation versus autologous matrix-induced chondrogenesis: a randomized trial comparing 2 methods for repair of cartilage defects of the knee. Orthop J Sports Med. 2019;7:232596711986821.

38. de Girolamo L, et al. Autologous matrix-induced chondrogenesis (AMIC) and AMIC enhanced by autologous concentrated bone marrow aspirate (BMAC) allow for stable clinical and functional improvements at up to 9 years follow-up: results from a randomized controlled study. J Clin Med. 2019;8:392.

39. Beck A, Murphy DJ, Carey-Smith R, Wood DJ, Zheng MH. Treatment of articular cartilage defects with microfracture and autologous matrix-induced chondrogenesis leads to extensive subchondral bone cyst formation in a sheep model. Am J Sports Med. 2016;44:2629–43.

40. Whyte GP, McGee A, Jazrawi L, Meislin R. Comparison of collagen graft fixation methods in the porcine knee: implications for matrix-assisted chondrocyte implantation and second-generation autologous chondrocyte implantation. Arthroscopy. 2016;32:820–7.

41. Cassar-Gheiti AJ, Byrne DP, Kavanagh E, Mulhall KJ. Comparison of four chondral repair techniques in the hip joint: a biomechanical study using a physiological human cadaveric model. Osteoarthr Cartil. 2015;23:1018–25.

42. Endres M, et al. Synovial fluid recruits human mesenchymal progenitors from subchondral spongious bone marrow. J Orthop Res. 2007;25:1299–307.

43. Jin R, et al. Enzymatically-crosslinked injectable hydrogels based on biomimetic dextran–hyaluronic acid conjugates for cartilage tissue engineering. Biomaterials. 2010;31:3103–13.

44. Menzies DJ, et al. Tailorable cell culture platforms from enzymatically cross-linked multifunctional poly(ethylene glycol)-based hydrogels. Biomacromolecules. 2013;14:413–23.

45. Sharma B, et al. Human cartilage repair with a photoreactive adhesive-hydrogel composite. Sci Transl Med. 2013;5:167ra6.

46. Wang D-A, et al. Multifunctional chondroitin sulphate for cartilage tissue–biomaterial integration. Nat Mater. 2007;6:385–92.

47. Wolf MT, et al. Two-year follow-up and remodeling kinetics of ChonDux hydrogel for full-thickness cartilage defect repair in the knee. Cartilage. 2018:194760351880054. https://doi.org/10.1177/1947603518800547.

48. Erggelet C, et al. Regeneration of ovine articular cartilage defects by cell-free polymer-based implants. Biomaterials. 2007;28:5570–80.
49. Siclari A, Mascaro G, Kaps C, Boux E. A 5-year follow-up after cartilage repair in the knee using a platelet-rich plasma-immersed polymer-based implant. Open Orthop J. 2014;8:346–54.
50. Enea D, et al. Single-stage cartilage repair in the knee with microfracture covered with a resorbable polymer-based matrix and autologous bone marrow concentrate. Knee. 2013;20:562–9.
51. Hoemann CD, et al. Chitosan–glycerol phosphate/blood implants elicit hyaline cartilage repair integrated with porous subchondral bone in microdrilled rabbit defects. Osteoarthr Cartil. 2007;15:78–89.
52. Méthot S, et al. Osteochondral biopsy analysis demonstrates that BST-CarGel treatment improves structural and cellular characteristics of cartilage repair tissue compared with microfracture. Cartilage. 2016;7:16–28.
53. Stanish WD, et al. Novel scaffold-based BST-CarGel treatment results in superior cartilage repair compared with microfracture in a randomized controlled trial. J Bone Joint Surg. 2013;95:1640–50.
54. Shive MS, et al. BST-CarGel® treatment maintains cartilage repair superiority over microfracture at 5 years in a multicenter randomized controlled trial. Cartilage. 2015;6:62–72.
55. Choi K-H, Choi BH, Park SR, Kim BJ, Min B-H. The chondrogenic differentiation of mesenchymal stem cells on an extracellular matrix scaffold derived from porcine chondrocytes. Biomaterials. 2010;31:5355–65.
56. Jin CZ, Park SR, Choi BH, Park K, Min B-H. In vivo cartilage tissue engineering using a cell-derived extracellular matrix scaffold. Artif Organs. 2007;31:183–92.
57. Li TZ, et al. Using cartilage extracellular matrix (CECM) membrane to enhance the reparability of the bone marrow stimulation technique for articular cartilage defect in canine model. Adv Funct Mater. 2012;22:4292–300.
58. Chung J, et al. Cartilage extra-cellular matrix biomembrane for the enhancement of microfractured defects. Knee Surg Sports Traumatol Arthrosc. 2014;22:1249–59.
59. Commins J, et al. Biological mechanisms for cartilage repair using a biocartilage scaffold: cellular adhesion/migration and bioactive proteins. Cartilage. 2020:1947603519900803. https://doi.org/10.1177/1947603519900803.
60. Shieh AK, et al. Effects of micronized cartilage matrix on cartilage repair in osteochondral lesions of the talus. Cartilage. 2018:1947603518796125. https://doi.org/10.1177/1947603518796125.
61. Abrams GD, Mall NA, Fortier LA, Roller BL, Cole BJ. BioCartilage: background and operative technique. Oper Tech Sport Med. 2013;21:116–24.
62. Wang KC, Frank RM, Cotter EJ, Christian DR, Cole BJ. Arthroscopic management of isolated tibial plateau defect with microfracture and micronized allogeneic cartilage–platelet-rich plasma adjunct. Arthrosc Tech. 2017;6:e1613–8.
63. Solheim E, et al. Results at 10–14 years after microfracture treatment of articular cartilage defects in the knee. Knee Surg Sports Traumatol Arthrosc. 2014;24:1587–93.
64. Bae DK, Song SJ, Yoon KH, Heo DB, Kim TJ. Survival analysis of microfracture in the osteoarthritic knee-minimum 10-year follow-up. Arthroscopy. 2013;29:244–50.
65. Cassano JM, et al. Bone marrow concentrate and platelet-rich plasma differ in cell distribution and interleukin 1 receptor antagonist protein concentration. Knee Surg Sports Traumatol Arthrosc. 2016;26:333–42.
66. Holton J, Imam M, Ward J, Snow M. The basic science of bone marrow aspirate concentrate in chondral injuries. Orthop Rev. 2016;8:6659.
67. Murphy EP, McGoldrick NP, Curtin M, Kearns SR. A prospective evaluation of bone marrow aspirate concentrate and microfracture in the treatment of osteochondral lesions of the talus. Foot Ankle Surg. 2018;25:441–8.
68. Gigante A, Cecconi S, Calcagno S, Busilacchi A, Enea D. Arthroscopic knee cartilage repair with covered microfracture and bone marrow concentrate. Arthrosc Tech. 2012;1:e175–80.
69. Gobbi A, Whyte GP. One-stage cartilage repair using a hyaluronic acid-based scaffold with activated bone marrow-derived mesenchymal stem cells compared with microfracture: five-year follow-up. Am J Sports Med. 2016;44:2846–54.
70. Hussain N, Johal H, Bhandari M. An evidence-based evaluation on the use of platelet rich plasma in orthopedics—a review of the literature. Sicot J. 2017;3:57.
71. Re'em T, Kaminer-Israeli Y, Ruvinov E, Cohen S. Chondrogenesis of hMSC in affinity-bound TGF-beta scaffolds. Biomaterials. 2012;33:751–61.
72. Hapa O, et al. Does platelet-rich plasma enhance microfracture treatment for chronic focal chondral defects? An in-vivo study performed in a rat model. Acta Orthop Traumatol. 2013;47:201–7.
73. Milano G, et al. Repeated platelet concentrate injections enhance reparative response of microfractures in the treatment of chondral defects of the knee: an experimental study in an animal model. Arthroscopy. 2012;28:688–701.
74. Milano G, et al. The effect of platelet rich plasma combined with microfractures on the treatment of chondral defects: an experimental study in a sheep model. Osteoarthr Cartil. 2010;18:971–80.
75. Boffa A, et al. Platelet-rich plasma augmentation to microfracture provides a limited benefit for the treatment of cartilage lesions: a meta-analysis. Orthop J Sports Med. 2020;8:2325967120910504.

76. Zhu Y, et al. Adipose-derived stem cell: a better stem cell than BMSC. Cell Biochem Funct. 2008;26:664–75.

77. Nava S, et al. Long-lasting anti-inflammatory activity of human microfragmented adipose tissue. Stem Cells Int. 2019;2019:5901479.

78. Ceylan HH, et al. Can chondral healing be improved following microfracture? The effect of adipocyte tissue derived stem cell therapy. Knee. 2016;23:442–9.

79. Spakova T, et al. A preliminary study comparing microfracture and local adherent transplantation of autologous adipose-derived stem cells followed by intraarticular injection of platelet-rich plasma for the treatment of chondral defects in rabbits. Cartilage. 2017;9:410–6.

80. McQuilling JP, Vines JB, Kimmerling KA, Mowry KC. Proteomic comparison of amnion and chorion and evaluation of the effects of processing on placental membranes. Wounds Compend Clin Res Pract. 2017;29:E36–42.

81. Farr J, et al. A randomized controlled single-blind study demonstrating superiority of amniotic suspension allograft injection over hyaluronic acid and saline control for modification of knee osteoarthritis symptoms. J Knee Surg. 2019; https://doi.org/10.1055/s-0039-1696672.

82. Hao Y, Ma DH-K, Hwang DG, Kim W-S, Zhang F. Identification of antiangiogenic and anti-inflammatory proteins in human amniotic membrane. Cornea. 2000;19:348–52.

83. Raines AL, et al. Efficacy of particulate amniotic membrane and umbilical cord tissues in attenuating cartilage destruction in an osteoarthritis model. Tissue Eng A. 2017;23:12–9.

84. Willett NJ, et al. Intra-articular injection of micronized dehydrated human amnion/chorion membrane attenuates osteoarthritis development. Arthritis Res Ther. 2014;16:R47.

85. Morisset S, Frisbie DD, Robbins PD, Nixon AJ, McIlwraith CW. IL-1ra/IGF-1 gene therapy modulates repair of microfractured chondral defects. Clin Orthop Relat Res. 2007;462:221–8.

86. Akmal M, et al. The effects of hyaluronic acid on articular chondrocytes. J Bone Joint Surg Br. 2005;87-B:1143–9.

87. Patti AM, Gabriele A, Vulcano A, Ramieri MT, Rocca CD. Effect of hyaluronic acid on human chondrocyte cell lines from articular cartilage. Tissue Cell. 2001;33:294–300.

88. Doral MN, et al. Treatment of osteochondral lesions of the talus with microfracture technique and postoperative hyaluronan injection. Knee Surg Sports Traumatol Arthrosc. 2011;20:1398–403.

89. Sofu H, et al. Results of hyaluronic acid–based cell-free scaffold application in combination with microfracture for the treatment of osteochondral lesions of the knee: 2-year comparative study. Arthroscopy. 2017;33:209–16.

90. Legović D, et al. Microfracture technique in combination with intraarticular hyaluronic acid injection in articular cartilage defect regeneration in rabbit model. Coll Antropol. 2009;33:619–23.

91. Strauss E, Schachter A, Frenkel S, Rosen J. The efficacy of intra-articular hyaluronan injection after the microfracture technique for the treatment of articular cartilage lesions. Am J Sports Med. 2009;37:720–6.

Mats Brittberg

19.1 Introduction

All tissues consist of living cells and a damaged tissue needs a supply of active cells to be restored. Cartilage being a tissue having a very low number of cells is lacking blood vessels. Cell recruitment via the blood supply seen in intrinsic repair of other tissues is not possible in the cartilage matrix. Cells must be recruited directly from the joint, the bone marrow or synovium, or from cells introduced from sources external to the joint [1].

The cells of interest could be divided into four subgroups:

1. True committed autologous chondrocytes
2. True committed allograft chondrocytes
3. Chondrogeneic autologous progenitor cells
4. Chondrogeneic allograft progenitor cells

Cells can either be free in suspension or grown on scaffolds to become immature grafts. Cells already existing in mature chondral or osteochondral grafts can be used, where the graft acts as a carrier.

Acellular approaches aim to induce and facilitate the repair activity of native cell populations. One may make use of just an empty matrix, or of a matrix containing biological signalling agents that will recruit and trigger the differentiation of local stem cell populations resulting in the formation of a functionally repair tissue. Cellular technologies include direct cell isolation or laboratory isolation and in vitro expansion of the cells.

Cellular approaches include use of crushed/fragmented/particulated cartilage pieces in gels used either alone or in conjunction with matrices. Randomized studies have shown efficiencies of the use of internal recruitment of cells without any external manipulation.

Bone marrow mesenchymal stem cells (MSCs) are of interest as those cells can produce both the osseous part and the chondral part in repair of osteochondral defects. However, it has been shown that chondrocytes and MSCs differentiate and form different subtypes of cartilage, the hyaline and a mixed cartilage phenotype, respectively [2]. Subsequently, to be successful in tissue engineering of cartilage injuries, one has to pay attention to both the osseous and cartilaginous part; use of chondrocytes or chondrogeneic cells for the cartilage layers and bone marrow stem cells for the bony part. At the same time, increased knowledge is needed of which type of matrices that permits the cells used to differentiate the way that the different layers of cartilage

M. Brittberg (✉)
Cartilage Research Unit, University of Gothenburg, Gothenburg, Sweden

Region Halland Orthopaedics (RHO), Kungsbacka Hospital, Kungsbacka, Sweden
e-mail: mats.brittberg@regionhalland.se, mats.brittberg@telia.com

© ISAKOS 2021
A. J. Krych et al. (eds.), *Cartilage Injury of the Knee*,
https://doi.org/10.1007/978-3-030-78051-7_19

can be produced including the important calcified layer in between the chondrocyte repaired area and the subchondral bone. The aim is to direct the cells to the right position in a gradient repair, improve cell-to-cell interaction to be able to coordinate a tissue repair as near to complete regeneration as possible.

19.2 Intrinsic Repairs

19.2.1 Bone Marrow-Derived Repair Cells

Bone marrow stimulation is performed to recruit cells from the bone marrow and induce them into the area of cartilage damage. Subchondral drilling, abrasion arthroplasty, and microfractures are the classical methods to activate such a cell migration. However, the numbers of enough potent cells that are available for migration are few, and recent research has shown that it is best to go deep down in the bone to reach the larger vessels. Pericytes are cells surrounding blood vessels, and those cells are the ones to attract for cell migration and lesion repair tissue formation as they are most effective in repair [3].

Human mesenchymal stem cell numbers decline with age; a new-born has approximately one MSC in every 10,000 marrow cells, while someone at the age of 80 has one MSC in every 2,000,000 marrow cells [4]. Park et al. [5] highlight the importance of the correct definition of a stem cell. It is important to know that in stem cell therapy, the cells have been isolated from cells concentrated in a pellet and in vitro culture expanded. Finally, those cells have been characterized to have self-renewal capacity and could express specific cell surface markers. Park et al. [5] also suggest that stem cells derived from cell concentrates should be presented as cell-source aspirate concentrates. The expanded cells are more or less homogenous, while the concentrates are heterogeneous with fewer stem cells. This is important when comparing one-stage procedures with two-stage cell expansion procedures. For many years, pericytes were regarded as simple regulators of angiogenesis. They are now recog-

nized to have MSC (mesenchymal stem cell) characteristics, including multipotentiality, self-renewal, immunoregulation effects, and other important roles in tissue repair. However, Kurth et al. [6] have reported that MSCs isolated from the synovium in vivo are distinct from pericytes phenotypically and functionally. A local osteochondral cartilage defect can be repaired from the bone marrow by ingrowth of pericytes into the formed blood clot but some repair contribution may also appear from neighbouring synovia.

For small defects, deep bone marrow stimulation may be used to introduce such repair cells into the defect area. Defects less than 10 mm in diameter seem the best choice for such treatments while larger defects may be treated with a concomitant porous scaffold to trap the cells in the defect zone [7].

There are three ways to reach vascularity and induce bleeding with subsequent cell migration.

- Subchondral drilling
- Abrasion arthroplasty
- Microfracture

Recently, animal experimental studies have shown that, in the so-called deep drilling, one will reach larger subchondral blood vessels inducing a better repair performance compared to basic drilling and microfracturing [8]. These studies have induced a renaissance for subchondral drilling as treatment alternative to the popular microfracture technology. With this so-called nano-drilling a stronger repair tissue may be induced [9] and it seems that

- Deep drilling is better than shallow drilling and microfracture
- Small diameter drill holes are better than large

Different bone marrow stimulation procedures are still employed because they are easy to perform and cheap. It may be difficult to get a smooth filling of a cartilage defect following the various described bone marrow stimulation methods [10]. In recent years, researchers have developed techniques to augment cell ingrowth by implanting different porous materials into the debrided cartilage injury. With such augmentation, it is possible to induce a stronger and more even growth of cells into the cartilage defect [11–14].

The number of existing MSCs for repair is low, and the number of cells that can invade the lesion area after mechanical perforation varies considerably from patient to patient, and from young age to old. A concentrate of bone marrow aspirate (BMAC) is one way to increase number of cells to induce chondrogenesis [15]. BMAC is obtained through density gradient centrifugation of bone marrow aspirate (BMA), most often aspirated from the iliac crest [16]. A subcomponent of BMAC, bone marrow-derived mesenchymal stem cells (MSCs) seem to possess the ability to differentiate into cells important for osteogenesis and chondrogenesis. Cotter et al. in their review of BMAC [15] found that a modulation of the paracrine signalling may be the most important function of BM-MSCs.

Allogeneic bone marrow MSCs have not been used in isolation for local cartilage repairs in patients, but in a recent study combined the use of allogeneic MSCs with autologous chondrons. The expected trophic effects from the MSCs may stimulate recycled chondrons to improve the resulting repair cartilage [17].

19.3 Synovial and Adipose Cells

19.3.1 Synovial Derived MSCs

Chondrogeneic cells can also be retrieved from synovial tissue. Several in vitro and animal in vivo studies of cartilage repair using synovial stem cells have shown encouraging results [18]. The only one published human RCT study with 14 patients revealed good results concerning postoperative outcome, MRI, and histologic features after a two-stage implantation of synovial stem cells into an isolated cartilage defect of the femoral condyle. No graft failures were observed on MRI at the 2 years follow-up. Both synovial derived MSCs and the control chondrocytes demonstrated very good-to-excellent and good-to-very good infill, respectively, with no adverse

effects from the implant, regardless of the treatment [19].

19.3.2 Adipose Tissue-Derived MSCs

It is important to differ between adipose-derived MSCs and adipose stromal vascular fractions [5]. The number of MSCs from fat tissue is much greater than the amount obtained from a similar bone marrow aspirate but the in vitro chondrogeneic capacity is less than from culture expanded bone marrow MSCs [20]. In a human trial, human adipose MSCs were used as intra-articular injection in combination with microfracture and hyaluronic acid (HA) to improve joint function in patients with knee cartilage defects [21].

19.3.3 Adipose Tissue-Derived Stromal Vascular Fraction Cells

If one takes a piece of fat tissue or a lipoaspirate and centrifuge it, the portion of the resulting cell pellet is a mononuclear cell fraction of the fat [22]. Adipose MSCs have been used in rabbit experiments to induce articular cartilage repairs [23]. However, still there exist no human trials with this technique used for focal cartilage repairs but such cell fractions have instead been tried to treat osteoarthritis (OA) [24].

19.3.4 Umbilical Cord Blood-Derived MSCs

Human umbilical cord blood-derived MSCs have a high rate of cell proliferation and anti-inflammatory effects, suggesting that these cells could be used for cartilage tissue engineering [25–27]. The cells low immunogenicity make them an attractive prospect as an allogeneic cell source for cartilage repair [28]. The clinical use today has been focused on umbilical cord blood-derived MSCs for OA injection therapies [29] while there is lack of studies with those cells for focal cartilage repair. However, there is one centre using umbilical cord Wharton's jelly-derived MSCs embedded into collagen scaffolds. The group has not published any results but a technical note is published of how to use such cells in a scaffold via a trans-arthroscopic technique [30].

19.3.5 Menstrual Blood-Derived MSCs

In 2007, Meng et al. demonstrated that it was possible to isolate MSCs from menstrual blood [31]. Those isolated cells have greater proliferative and differentiation capacity than bone marrow-derived MSCs. However, further research is needed to determine those cell's chondrogeneic capacity [32].

19.3.6 Muscle-Derived Stem Cells

Among muscle stem cells, satellite stem cells are the most researched progenitor cells. Those cells can differentiate into osteoblasts, adipocytes, chondrocytes, and myocytes [33]. No human clinical study with such cells has so far been done.

19.3.7 Peripheral Blood Progenitor Cells

There is an increased interest of using peripheral blood as a source for chondrogeneic progenitor cells. Peripheral blood mononuclear cells have been shown to support cartilage healing. A method of drug administration containing granulocyte colony stimulating factor (G-CSF) has been used to mobilize those cells from the bone marrow [34]. In a rabbit experiment, bone marrow MSCs exhibited a more osteogenic potential and higher proliferation capacity than peripheral blood progenitor MSCs, whereas peripheral blood progenitor MSCs possessed a stronger adipogenic and chondrogeneic differentiation potential than bone marrow MSCs in vitro [35].

In a small RCT, cartilage lesions treated by an arthroscopic subchondral drilling plus postoperative intra-articular injections of autologous peripheral blood progenitor cells in combination with hyaluronic acid (HA) resulted in significant improvement of the repair tissue quality over the control treatment without PB-MSCs, verified by histologic and MRI evaluation. Clinically, however, no differences were found between the two treatment alternatives [36].

19.4 Autologous Chondrocytes

19.4.1 Autologous Chondrocytes (In Vitro Expanded)

The chondrocytes are few in number in the matrix, and their migration potential in the matrix is low. For this reason, the use of single chondrocytes for cartilage repair was initially not attractive. However with the knowledge of how to isolate chondrocytes from their matrix [37] and expand the cells in vitro [11, 38–42], the possibility to use the true cartilage repair cells increased. After extensive research of chondrocyte behaviours in vitro and an in vivo animal experiments [11, 38], the first autologous chondrocyte implantation (ACI) in humans was performed in October, 1987 [43]. Since that first operation, the technique has been developed and there are now four generations of ACI, with generation 3 being the most used.

- First-generation ACI with chondrocytes injected as a suspension under a periosteal sutured living membrane.
- Second-generation ACI with chondrocytes injected as a suspension under a sutured collagen inert non-living membrane.
- Third-generation ACI with chondrocytes grown in a porous scaffold and implanted as an immature graft or chondrocytes seeded on a cell carrier (see Figs. 19.1a–c and 19.2a–c).
- Fourth-generation ACI is mainly one-stage procedures with direct isolation of chondrocytes and implantation. Included into that

group of ACI also belongs cartilage fragment implantation (CAIS, CAFRIMA).

In vitro cell expansion and scaffold seeding are expensive procedures and subsequently, ACI has been mainly used for failed other cartilage procedures, the so-called second-line, or salvage surgeries. However, evidence of the efficacy and economics of getting it right first time means that the main indications today are:

1. Large chondral defects >2 cm
2. Large osteochondral defects >2 + bone grafting if defect depth >8 mm
3. All types of chondral and osteochondral defects with failed other types of cartilage repair

There is no age limit, but the surrounding cartilage should be of good quality.

It might then be important to differ between:

- Healthy cartilage.
- Degenerative cartilage (e.g., this type of cartilage could be seen after ACL and meniscal injuries and after repeated patella dislocation with local degeneration of cartilage structure but not a generalized joint disease).
- OA cartilage (Pre-OA, Early OA, Late OA).

ACI treatments can be used with surrounding healthy and also with surrounding degenerative cartilage sometimes on its way to pre-OA/early localized OA. A generalized early OA and further on to established full OA are not indications for an ACI.

As with other cartilage repairs, concomitant malalignment should be treated by unloading osteotomies in combination with the ACI procedure.

Very large cartilage defects may also benefit for an ACI in conjunction with an unloading osteotomy.

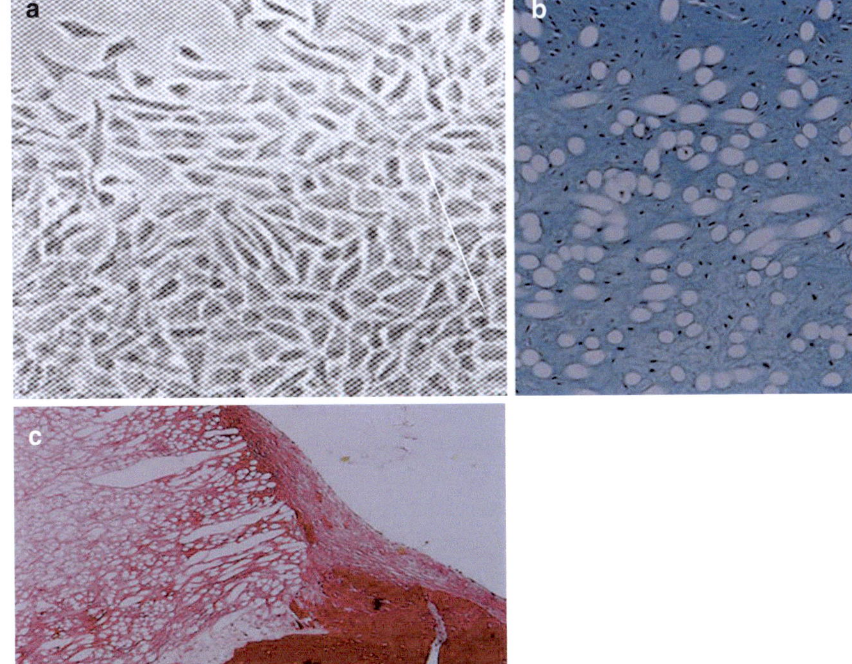

Fig. 19.1 (a) Chondrocytes in monolayer culture. (b) Chondrocytes grown in a Hyaff-11 matrice. (Image courtesy by Josefin Ekholm). (c) Chondrocytes in a Hyaff-11 matrice grown in an in vitro cartilage lesion model. (Image courtesy by Josefin Ekholm)

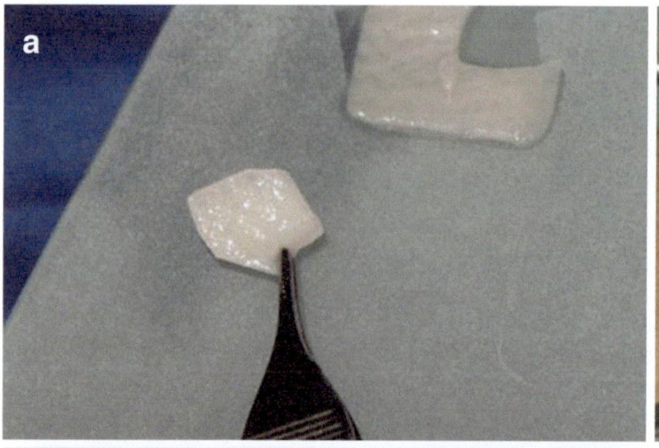
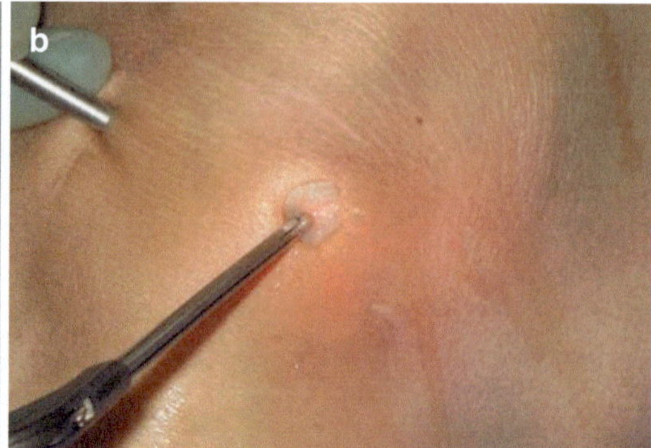
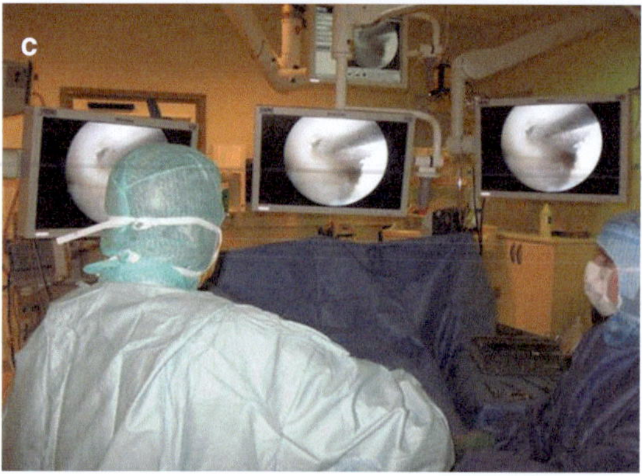

Fig. 19.2 (**a**) Chondrocyte graft (Hyaff-11 matrice with in vitro expanded chondrocytes) is prepared in size to be implanted trans-arthroscopic into a cartilage lesion. (**b**) The chondrocyte graft is hold by a grasper with plain sur- faces and is inserted via a small portal into the joint area. (**c**) The surgeon is delivering the chondrocyte graft into the debrided cartilage lesion with an arthroscopic plunger

19.4.2 Directly Isolated Autologous Chondrocytes

It is also possible to use chondrocytes, directly isolated without a time consuming in vitro expansion. It is then possible to use a combination of primary chondrocytes mixed with bone marrow MSCs to support cartilage tissue repair, without the need for cell culture [44]. The patient's cartilage biopsy and bone marrow aspirate are inserted into a semi-automated machine, termed the INSTRUCT cell processor, that isolates the chondrocytes, mixes them with marrow cells, adds fibronectin, and seeds the cell mixture to the scaffolds. The cell processor is able to produce a cell-scaffold implant within 1 h [45]. A prospective follow-up at 2 years with 40 patients operated on with this method was presented in 2020. Hyaline-like cartilage was observed on biopsies in at least 22 of the 40 patients [45].

19.4.3 Autologous Chondrons

Chondrocytes are embedded within an extracellular matrix (ECM). The chondrocyte with its immediate surrounding pericellular matrix (PCM) is a unit called a chondron [46]. The re-establishment of the PCM by isolated chondrocytes when implanted for cartilage repair is important. However, it is possible to isolate chondrons instead of bare chondrocytes. The chondrons have been used in a combination mix with allogeneic bone marrow MSCs to repair cartilage lesions [17]. From that study no treatment-related adverse events up to one year postoperatively was noted. At 12 months, all patients showed statistically significant improvement in clinical outcome compared to baseline. Of interest is the finding that Type VI collagen, a major component of the pericellular matrix, stabilizes the chondrocytes phenotypes and is critical for chondrocyte survival. The expression of type VI collagen is diminished after chondrocyte de-differentiation and restored during chondrocyte re-differentiation [47]. In tissue cultures, a complete pericellular matrix (PCM) is built in 6 weeks [47] but the time for implanted re-differentiated chondrocytes in scaffold to in vivo reconstruct a PCM is not known.

19.4.4 Allogeneic Chondrocytes (In Vitro Expanded)

Chondrocytes have major histocompatibility complex (MHC) class I and class II molecules but the cells are protected from contact with immunocompetent cells by the extracellular matrix. Furthermore, transplanted allogeneic cartilage is not rejected but in osteochondral allografted patients antibodies are found. The chondrocytes can also exert immunosuppressive and immunomodulatory effects on immunocompetent cells [48]. Clinically, in vitro expanded allogeneic chondrocytes have been transplanted in biodegradable, alginate-based, biocompatible scaffolds for the treatment of chondral and osteochondral lesions in the knee. Both short- and mid-term results up to 6 years showed satisfactory results and a good safety profile [49, 50]. Furthermore Olivos-Meza et al. have shown that it is possible to isolate viable chondrocytes from cadaveric human donors in samples processed in the first 48 hours post- mortem. There is no significant difference between the numbers of chondrocytes isolated from live or cadaveric donors. They also found that cryopreservation of cadaveric primary chondrocytes will not alter their chondrogeneic capacity [51].

19.4.5 Nasal, Auricular, and Costal Chondrocytes

Nasal chondrocytes are found in the hyaline cartilage of the nasal septum. From nasal septum biopsies, chondrocytes can be isolated, expanded, and cultured onto different types of scaffolds. Chondrocytes expanded from debrided joint carti-lage have in one study been compared with nasal chondrocytes. The chondrocytes derived from debrided joint cartilage exhibited an inferior proliferation rate than the nasal chondrocytes and a lower capacity to chondro-differentiate [52]. In a small safety study, nasal chondrocytes were isolated, expanded, and cultured onto collagen membranes to engineer cartilage grafts (30 × 40 × 2 mm) [53]. The engineered tissues were implanted into the femoral defects via mini-arthrotomy and assessed up to 2 years post-surgery. No adverse reactions were found and self-assessed patient reported outcomes were improved significantly. Radiological evaluations showed variable degrees of defect filling and repair tissue with similarities to surrounding native cartilage [53]. Furthermore, in an in vitro study, nasal, auricular, and costal chondrocytes were compared. Nasoseptal chondrocytes presented the strongest proliferation rate, whereas auricular chondrocytes obtained the highest total cell numbers using comparable cartilage sample weights [54].

Yoon et al. [55] recently presented a small safety study on seven patients treated by a costal chondrocyte-derived pellet-type autologous chondrocyte implantation. Implantation of the pellets was performed via minimal arthrotomy and secured with a fibrin sealant. Significant improvements were seen in all clinical scores from preoperative baseline to the 5-year follow-up and also significant improved MRI MOCART score [55].

19.4.6 Xenogeneic Chondrocytes

Recent research in animal transgenesis may facilitate the use of xenogeneic chondrocytes in tissue-engineering applications for clinical cartilage repair. However, the Covid-19 pandemic and other concerns may diminish the interest to use xenogeneic cells for tissue engineering. Sommaggio et al. [56, 57] have shown that complement activation contributes to rejection of xenogeneic cartilage and the authors also suggest a genetic-engineering approaches to prevent humoral rejection of xenogeneic chondrocytes for use in cartilage repair [56, 57].

19.4.7 Autologous Cartilage Fragments

The use of particulated or fragmented cartilage as a source for chondrocytes is regarded as a fourth generation ACI. From crushed cartilage, the most active chondrocytes may migrate out into a surrounding supportive scaffold, gel, or similar [58]. The procedure may then be used as a one-stage operation. A study has shown hand-minced cartilage performs as well as device-minced or un-minced cartilage regarding in vitro cell outgrowth but neither promoted matrix deposition after in vitro culture [59]. The first clinical study with minced or particulated cartilage was a randomized study studying the so-called CAIS (cartilage autograft implantation system) where the fragmented cartilage was compared with microfracture (MFX) treatment. Significant improvements in IKDC and KOOS with CAIS versus MFX were maintained at 24 months [60]. The CAIS technology uses a PDS scaffold for the minced cartilage. There are several other options for the support of minced cartilage. The Hyaff-11 scaffold (Hyalofast, Anika, Boston) is a promising scaffold for hand-minced cartilage in fibrin glue (CAFRIMA, Cartilage Fragment Implantation Membrane Augmented) [7].

19.4.8 Allogeneic Cartilage Fragments

The introduction of CAIS stimulated researchers and industry to develop a similar model using allogeneic cartilage fragments, mainly from juvenile cartilage. Most reports are from use in talar osteochondral lesions. There are no long follow-up studies present, but a recent publication was done in 45 patients followed for 24 months following patella cartilage lesions treated by juvenile cartilage fragments [61]. Particulated juvenile allograft tissue was found to be an acceptable cartilage restoration option for full-thickness cartilage lesions of the patella, offering satisfactory tissue defect fill at 6, 12, and 24 months after surgery. MRI of the repaired cartilage demonstrates progressive graft maturation over time [61]. In another patellofemoral lesion study, postoperative MRI revealed majority lesion fill in more than 69% of patients, but that persistent morphologic differences between graft site and normal adjacent cartilage remained [62].

19.4.9 IPS-Cells and Embryonic Cells

It is difficult to obtain functional chondrocytes from human embryonic stem cells (ESCs) even though new technologies are improving how to use such cells for cartilage tissue engineering [63]. Furthermore, the ethical issues associated with human ESCs are an important disadvantage of using such cells. Instead, induced pluripotential stem cells (iPSCs) may be more acceptable since large numbers of autologous cells can be derived from small starting populations [64, 65] (see Fig. 19.3a–c).

19.5 Summary

Although MSCs isolated from different tissues show similar phenotypic characteristics, it is not clear whether those cells are the same types of MSCs. Cells exhibit differing potential for proliferation and differentiation in response to stimulation with various growth factors. In a rabbit study with 6 groups treated by autogeneic MSCs from bone marrow, periosteum, synovium, adipose tissue, and muscle, the bone marrow-MSCs produced much more cartilage matrix than that of other groups. Furthermore, concern exists about the stability of mesenchymal stem cells to exhibit and maintain a chondrocyte phenotype since common in vitro protocols of chondrogenesis induce a program related to endochondral ossification which may finally yield only transient cartilage [66]. However, Sakaguchi et al. [67] looked instead at human MSCS from bone marrow, periosteum, synovium, skeletal muscle, and adipose tissue. They found that synovium-derived MSCs exhibited the highest capacity for chondrogenesis, followed by bone marrow-derived and periosteum-derived MSCs [67]. Today, clinically, MSCs from bone marrow are most commonly

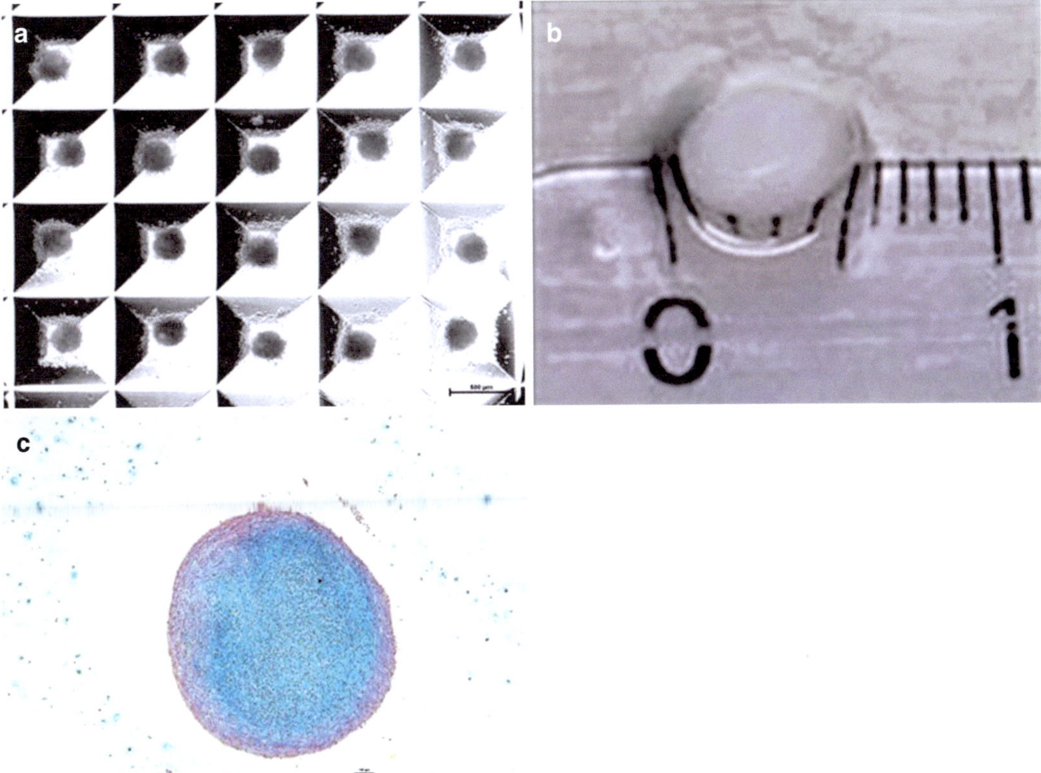

Fig. 19.3 (**a**) IPS-cells (induced pluripotent stem cells) have started to be differentiated in micro wells. (**b**) A small cartilage piece that has been produced by 3D printing with IPS-cells (induced pluripotent stem cells) and subsequent culture. (**c**) A small piece of cartilage, developed by 3D printed IPS-cells (induced pluripotent stem cells), cultured and sectioned. (Image courtesy by Stina Simonsson)

used due to ease of harvest (via the iliac crest) and that they have good chondrogenic potential. However, when comparing MSCs with chondrocytes, in contrast with MSCs, chondrocytes form cartilage only (and not bone) in an in vivo osteochondrogenic assay [68]. In another study, articular chondrocytes and iliac crest-derived MSCs were allowed to differentiate in pellet mass cultures. Significantly decreased expression of collagen type I was accompanied by increased expression of collagen types IIA and IIB during differentiation of chondrocytes, indicating differentiation towards a hyaline phenotype. Chondrogenesis in MSCs resulted in upregulation of collagen types I, IIA, IIB, and X, demonstrating differentiation towards cartilage of a mixed phenotype [2]. The authors suggest that chondrocytes and MSCs differentiate and form different subtypes of cartilage, a hyaline and a mixed cartilage phenotype. These findings may indicate that MSCs from other tissues may be confer a cartilage repair with characteristics that are different from repairs formed from chondrocytes, whose main purpose is producing cartilage [2]. DNA methylation is a process by which methyl groups are added to DNA. Methylation modifies the function of the DNA, and such a process is essential for normal tissue development [69]. In vitro engineered neo-cartilage tissue from primary chondrocytes, hPAC has been shown to exhibit a DNA methylation landscape that is almost identical (99% similarity) to autologous cartilage [69]. That finding was in contrast to neo-cartilage engineered from bone marrow-derived mesenchymal stem cells (MSCs) [69]. However, MSCs are interesting cells to use in combination with chondrocytes. Culturing human MSCs with human articular chondrocytes in HA-hydrogels enhances the mechanical properties and cartilage-specific ECM content of tissue-engineered cartilage. Furthermore, cocultures decreased the expression of collagen type X by MSCs and the risk of bone formation in the cartilage defect will be reduced [70].

There is a population of chondroprogenitor cells from the surface zone of articular cartilage and this population of cells can form large numbers of colonies from a low seeding density and is capable of extended culture without losing the chondrogenic phenotype. Those cells are of interest to use for cartilage repair. The embryonic development of articular cartilage progresses through appositional growth driven by that progenitor/stem cell subpopulation that resides in the articular surface [63, 71].

Based on findings related to different chondrogeneic cells and chondrocytes, one may stipulate that for chondrogeneic repair induction:

- Committed chondrocytes outperform mesenchymal stem cells [2].
- Young chondrocytes outperform old chondrocytes [72].
- Cartilage tissue progenitor cells outperform committed chondrocytes [73].

An allogeneic source of surface layer chondrocytes may be of future interest in combination with bone marrow cells in the bone area of an osteochondral repair. It might be important to turn a chondral defect into an osteochondral defect in order to induce a gradient repair. A gradient repair with chondrogeneic cells on top and osteogenic cells in the deep area could reproduce the important border zone between cartilage and bone tissues.

References

1. Yan H, Yu C. Repair of full-thickness cartilage defects with cells of different origin in a rabbit model. Arthroscopy. 2007;23(2):178–87.
2. Karlsson C, Brantsing C, Svensson T, Brisby H, Asp J, Tallheden T, Lindahl A. Differentiation of human mesenchymal stem cells and articular chondrocytes: analysis of chondrogenic potential and expression pattern of differentiation-related transcription factors. J Orthop Res. 2007;25(2):152–63.
3. Caplan AI. All MSCs are pericytes? Cell Stem Cell. 2008;3(3):229–30.
4. Goldberg VM. Stem cells in osteoarthritis. HSS J. 2012;8(1):59–61.
5. Park YB, Ha CW, Rhim JH, Lee HJ. Stem cell therapy for articular cartilage repair: review of the entity of cell populations used and the result of the clinical application of each entity. Am J Sports Med. 2018;46(10):2540–52.
6. Kurth TB, Dell'accio F, Crouch V, Augello A, Sharpe PT, De Bari C. Functional mesenchymal stem cell niches in adult mouse knee joint synovium in vivo. Arthritis Rheum. 2011;63(5):1289–300.
7. Brittberg M. Clinical articular cartilage repair—an up to date review. Ann Joint. 2018;3:1–8.
8. Chen H, Hoemann CD, Sun J, Chevrier A, McKee MD, Shive MS, Hurtig M, Buschmann MD. Depth of subchondral perforation influences the outcome of bone marrow stimulation cartilage repair. J Orthop Res. 2011;29(8):1178–84.
9. Eldracher M, Orth P, Cucchiarini M, Pape D, Madry H. Small subchondral drill holes improve marrow stimulation of articular cartilage defects. Am J Sports Med. 2014;42(11):2741–50.
10. Guo T, Noshin M, Baker HB, Taskoy E, Meredith SJ, Tang Q, Ringel JP, Lerman MJ, Chen Y, Packer JD, Fisher JP. 3D printed biofunctionalized scaffolds for microfracture repair of cartilage defects. Biomaterials. 2018;185:219–31.
11. Bentley G, Greer RB 3rd. Homotransplantation of isolated epiphyseal and articular cartilage chondrocytes into joint surfaces of rabbits. Nature. 1971;230(5293):385–8.
12. Cavallo C, Desando G, Columbaro M, Ferrari A, Zini N, Facchini A, Grigolo B. Chondrogenic differentiation of bone marrow concentrate grown onto a hyaluronan scaffold: rationale for its use in the treatment of cartilage lesions. J Biomed Mater Res A. 2013;101(6):1559–70.
13. Gao J, Dennis JE, Solchaga LA, Awadallah AS, Goldberg VM, Caplan AI. Tissue-engineered fabrication of an osteochondral composite graft using rat bone marrow-derived mesenchymal stem cells. Tissue Eng. 2001;7(4):363–71.
14. Gille J, Behrens P, Schulz AP, Oheim R, Kienast B. Matrix-associated autologous chondrocyte implantation: a clinical follow-up at 15 years. Cartilage. 2016;7(4):309–15.
15. Cotter EJ, Wang KC, Yanke AB, Chubinskaya S. Bone marrow aspirate concentrate for cartilage defects of the knee: from bench to bedside evidence. Cartilage. 2018;9(2):161–70.
16. Gobbi A, Karnatzikos G, Scotti C, Mahajan V, Mazzucco L, Grigolo B. One-step cartilage repair with bone marrow aspirate concentrated cells and collagen matrix in full-thickness knee cartilage lesions: results at 2-year follow-up. Cartilage. 2011;2(3):286–99.

17. de Windt TS, Vonk LA, Slaper-Cortenbach IC, van den Broek MP, Nizak R, van Rijen MH, de Weger RA, Dhert WJ, Saris DB. Allogeneic mesenchymal stem cells stimulate cartilage regeneration and are safe for single-stage cartilage repair in humans upon mixture with recycled autologous chondrons. Stem Cells. 2017;35(1):256–64.

18. To K, Zhang B, Romain K, Mak C, Khan W. Synovium-derived mesenchymal stem cell transplantation in cartilage regeneration: a PRISMA review of in vivo studies. Front Bioeng Biotechnol. 2019;7:314.

19. Akgun I, Unlu MC, Erdal OA, Ogut T, Erturk M, Ovali E, Kantarci F, Caliskan G, Akgun Y. Matrix-induced autologous mesenchymal stem cell implantation versus matrix-induced autologous chondrocyte implantation in the treatment of chondral defects of the knee: a 2-year randomized study. Arch Orthop Trauma Surg. 2015;135(2):251–63.

20. Parker AM, Katz AJ. Adipose-derived stem cells for the regeneration of damaged tissues. Expert Opin Biol Ther. 2006;6(6):1580–6.

21. Qiao Z, Tang J, Yue B, Wang J, Zhang J, Xuan L, Dai C, Li S, Li M, Xu C, Dai K, Wang Y. Human adipose-derived mesenchymal progenitor cells plus microfracture and hyaluronic acid for cartilage repair: a phase IIa trial. Regen Med. 2020; https://doi.org/10.2217/rme-2019-0068.

22. Zhang J, Du C, Guo W, Li P, Liu S, Yuan Z, Yang J, Sun X, Yin H, Guo Q, Zhou C. Adipose tissue-derived pericytes for cartilage tissue engineering. Curr Stem Cell Res Ther. 2017;12(6):513–21.

23. Oh SJ, Choi KU, Choi SW, Kim SD, Kong SK, Lee S, Cho KS. Comparative analysis of adipose-derived stromal cells and their secretome for auricular cartilage regeneration. Stem Cells Int. 2020;2020:8595940.

24. Hong Z, Chen J, Zhang S, Zhao C, Bi M, Chen X, Bi Q. Intra-articular injection of autologous adipose-derived stromal vascular fractions for knee osteoarthritis: a double-blind randomized self-controlled trial. Int Orthop. 2019;43(5):1123–34.

25. Ha CW, Park YB, Chung JY, Park YG. Cartilage repair using composites of human umbilical cord blood-derived mesenchymal stem cells and hyaluronic acid hydrogel in a Minipig model. Stem Cells Transl Med. 2015;4(9):1044–51.

26. Jin HJ, Bae YK, Kim M, Kwon SJ, Jeon HB, Choi SJ, et al. Comparative analysis of human mesenchymal stem cells from bone marrow, adipose tissue, and umbilical cord blood as sources of cell therapy. Int J Mol Sci. 2013;14(9):17986–8001.

27. Park YB, Ha CW, Kim JA, Han WJ, Rhim JH, Lee HJ, Kim KJ, Park YG, Chung JY. Single-stage cell-based cartilage repair in a rabbit model: cell tracking and in vivo chondrogenesis of human umbilical cord blood-derived mesenchymal stem cells and hyaluronic acid hydrogel composite. Osteoarthr Cartil. 2017;25(4):570–80.

28. Marmotti A, Mattia S, Castoldi F, Barbero A, Mangiavini L, Bonasia DE, Bruzzone M, Dettoni F, Scurati R, Peretti GM. Allogeneic umbilical cord-derived mesenchymal stem cells as a potential source for cartilage and bone regeneration: an in vitro study. Stem Cells Int. 2017;2017:1732094.

29. Song JS, Hong KT, Kim NM, Jung JY, Park HS, Lee SH, Cho YJ, Kim SJ. Implantation of allogenic umbilical cord blood-derived mesenchymal stem cells improves knee osteoarthritis outcomes: two-year follow-up. Regen Ther. 2020;14:32–9.

30. Sadlik B, Jaroslawski G, Puszkarz M, Blasiak A, Oldak T, Gladysz D, Whyte GP. Cartilage repair in the knee using umbilical cord Wharton's Jelly-derived mesenchymal stem cells embedded onto collagen scaffolding and implanted under dry arthroscopy. Arthrosc Tech. 2017;7(1):e57–63.

31. Meng X, Ichim TE, Zhong J, Rogers A, Yin Z, Jackson J, Wang H, Ge W, Bogin V, Chan KW, Thébaud B, Riordan NH. Endometrial regenerative cells: a novel stem cell population. J Transl Med. 2007;5:57.

32. Uzieliene I, Urbonaite G, Tachtamisevaite Z, Mobasheri A, Bernotiene E. The potential of menstrual blood-derived mesenchymal stem cells for cartilage repair and regeneration: novel aspects. Stem Cells Int. 2018;2018:5748126.

33. Biz C, Crimi A, Fantoni I, Pozzuoli A, Ruggieri P. Muscle stem cells: what's new in orthopedics? Acta Biomed. 2019;90(1-S):8–13.

34. Saw KY, Anz A, Merican S, Tay YG, Ragavanaidu K, Jee CS, McGuire DA. Articular cartilage regeneration with autologous peripheral blood progenitor cells and hyaluronic acid after arthroscopic subchondral drilling: a report of 5 cases with histology. Arthroscopy. 2011;27(4):493–506.

35. Fu WL, Zhou CY, Yu JK. A new source of mesenchymal stem cells for articular cartilage repair: MSCs derived from mobilized peripheral blood share similar biological characteristics in vitro and chondrogenesis in vivo as MSCs from bone marrow in a rabbit model. Am J Sports Med. 2014;42(3):592–601.

36. Saw KY, Anz A, Siew-Yoke Jee C, Merican S, Ching-Soong Ng R, Roohi SA, Ragavanaidu K. Articular cartilage regeneration with autologous peripheral blood stem cells versus hyaluronic acid: a randomized controlled trial. Arthroscopy. 2013;29(4):684–94.

37. Smith AU. Survival of frozen chondrocytes isolated from cartilage of adult mammals. Nature. 1965;205:782–4.

38. Brittberg M, Nilsson A, Lindahl A, Ohlsson C, Peterson L. Rabbit articular cartilage defects treated with autologous cultured chondrocytes. Clin Orthop Relat Res. 1996;326:270–83.

39. Chesterman PJ, Smith AU. Homotransplantation of articular cartilage and isolated chondrocytes. An experimental study in rabbits. J Bone Joint Surg Br. 1968;50(1):184–9.

40. Grande DA, Pitman MI, Peterson L, Menche D, Klein M. The repair of experimentally produced defects in rabbit articular cartilage by autologous chondrocyte transplantation. J Orthop Res. 1989;7(2):208–18.

41. Green WT. Articular cartilage repair, behaviour of rabbit chondrocytes during tissue culture and subsequent allografting. Clin Orthop. 1977;124:237–50.
42. Peterson L, Menche D, Grande D, Pitman M. Chondrocyte transplantation; an experimental model in the rabbit. In: Transaction from the 30th annual meeting Orthopaedic Research Society, Atlanta, 7–9 Feb 1984. p. 218.
43. Brittberg M, Lindahl A, Nilsson A, Ohlsson C, Isaksson O, Peterson L. Treatment of deep cartilage defects in the knee with autologous chondrocyte transplantation. N Engl J Med. 1994;331(14):889–95.
44. Hendriks J, Riesle J, van Blitterswijk CA. Co-culture in cartilage tissue engineering. J Tissue Eng Regen Med. 2007;1(3):170–8. Review.
45. Słynarski K, de Jong WC, Snow M, Hendriks JAA, Wilson CE, Verdonk P. Single-stage autologous chondrocyte-based treatment for the repair of knee cartilage lesions: two-year follow-up of a prospective single-arm multicenter study. Am J Sports Med. 2020;8:363546520912444.
46. Poole CA. Review. Articular cartilage chondrons: form, function and failure. J Anat. 1997;191(Pt 1):1–13.
47. Zhang Z. Chondrons and the pericellular matrix of chondrocytes. Tissue Eng B Rev. 2015;21(3):267–77.
48. Osiecka-Iwan A, Hyc A, Radomska-Lesniewska DM, Rymarczyk A, Skopinski P. Antigenic and immunogenic properties of chondrocytes. Implications for chondrocyte therapeutic transplantation and pathogenesis of inflammatory and degenerative joint diseases. Cent Eur J Immunol. 2018;43(2):209–19.
49. Almqvist KF, Dhollander AA, Verdonk PC, Forsyth R, Verdonk R, Verbruggen G. Treatment of cartilage defects in the knee using alginate beads containing human mature allogenic chondrocytes. Am J Sports Med. 2009;37(10):1920–9.
50. Dhollander AA, Verdonk PC, Lambrecht S, Verdonk R, Elewaut D, Verbruggen G, Almqvist KF. Midterm results of the treatment of cartilage defects in the knee using alginate beads containing human mature allogenic chondrocytes. Am J Sports Med. 2012;40(1):75–82.
51. Olivos-Meza A, Velasquillo Martínez C, Olivos Díaz B, Landa-Solís C, Brittberg M, Pichardo Bahena R, Ortega Sanchez C, Martínez V, Alvarez Lara E, Ibarra-Ponce de León JC. Co-culture of dedifferentiated and primary human chondrocytes obtained from cadaveric donor enhance the histological quality of repair tissue: an in vivo animal study. Cell Tissue Bank. 2017;18(3):369–81.
52. Lehoczky G, Wolf F, Mumme M, Gehmert S, Miot S, Haug M, Jakob M, Martin I, Barbero A. Intra-individual comparison of human nasal chondrocytes and debrided knee chondrocytes: relevance for engineering autologous cartilage grafts. Clin Hemorheol Microcirc. 2020;74(1):67–78.
53. Mumme M, Barbero A, Miot S, Wixmerten A, Feliciano S, Wolf F, Asnaghi AM, Baumhoer D, Bieri O, Kretzschmar M, Pagenstert G, Haug M, Schaefer DJ, Martin I, Jakob M. Nasal chondrocyte-based engineered autologous cartilage tissue for repair of articular cartilage defects: an observational first-in-human trial. Lancet. 2016;388(10055):1985–94.
54. He A, Xia H, Xiao K, Wang T, Liu Y, Xue J, Li D, Tang S, Liu F, Wang X, Zhang W, Liu W, Cao Y, Zhou G. Cell yield, chondrogenic potential, and regenerated cartilage type of chondrocytes derived from ear, nasoseptal, and costal cartilage. J Tissue Eng Regen Med. 2018;12(4):1123–32.
55. Yoon KH, Park JY, Lee JY, Lee E, Lee J, Kim SG. Costal chondrocyte-derived pellet-type autologous chondrocyte implantation for treatment of articular cartilage defect. Am J Sports Med. 2020;3:363546520905565. [Epub ahead of print]. https://doi.org/10.1177/0363546520905565.
56. Sommaggio R, Pérez-Cruz M, Brokaw JL, Máñez R, Costa C. Inhibition of complement component C5 protects porcine chondrocytes from xenogeneic rejection. Osteoarthr Cartil. 2013;21(12):1958–67.
57. Sommaggio R, Bello-Gil D, Pérez-Cruz M, Brokaw JL, Máñez R, Costa C. Genetic engineering strategies to prevent the effects of antibody and complement on xenogeneic chondrocytes. Eur Cell Mater. 2015;30:258–70.
58. Williams R, Khan IM, Richardson K, Nelson L, McCarthy HE, Analbelsi T, Singhrao SK, Dowthwaite GP, Jones RE, Baird DM, Lewis H, Roberts S, Shaw HM, Dudhia J, Fairclough J, Briggs T, Archer CW. Identification and clonal characterisation of a progenitor cell sub-population in normal human articular cartilage. PLoS One. 2010;5(10):e13246.
59. Levinson C, Cavalli E, Sindi DM, Kessel B, Zenobi-Wong M, Preiss S, Salzmann G, Neidenbach P. Chondrocytes from device-minced articular cartilage show potent outgrowth into fibrin and collagen hydrogels. Orthop J Sports Med. 2019;7(9):2325967119867618.
60. Cole BJ, Farr J, Winalski CS, Hosea T, Richmond J, Mandelbaum B, De Deyne PG. Outcomes after a single-stage procedure for cell-based cartilage repair: a prospective clinical safety trial with 2-year follow-up. Am J Sports Med. 2011;39(6):1170–9.
61. Grawe B, Burge A, Nguyen J, Strickland S, Warren R, Rodeo S, Shubin SB. Cartilage regeneration in full-thickness patellar chondral defects treated with particulated juvenile articular allograft cartilage: an MRI analysis. Cartilage. 2017;8(4):374–83.
62. Wang T, Belkin NS, Burge AJ, Chang B, Pais M, Mahony G, Williams RJ. Patellofemoral cartilage lesions treated with particulated juvenile allograft cartilage: a prospective study with minimum 2-year clinical and magnetic resonance imaging outcomes. Arthroscopy. 2018;34(5):1498–505.
63. Suchorska WM, Augustyniak E, Richter M, Łukjanow M, Filas V, Kaczmarczyk J, Trzeciak T. Modified methods for efficiently differentiating human embryonic stem cells into chondrocyte-like cells. Postepy Hig Med Dosw (Online). 2017;71:500–9.
64. Castro-Viñuelas R, Sanjurjo-Rodríguez C, Piñeiro-Ramil M, Hermida-Gómez T, Fuentes-Boquete IM,

de Toro-Santos FJ, Blanco-García FJ, Díaz-Prado SM. Induced pluripotent stem cells for cartilage repair: current status and future perspectives. Eur Cell Mater. 2018;36:96–109.

65. Yamashita A, Tamamura Y, Morioka M, Karagiannis P, Shima N, Tsumaki N. Considerations in hiPSC-derived cartilage for articular cartilage repair. Inflamm Regen. 2018;38:17.

66. Li Q, Tang J, Wang R, Bei C, Xin L, Zeng Y, Tang X. Comparing the chondrogenic potential in vivo of autogeneic mesenchymal stem cells derived from different tissues. Artif Cells Blood Substit Immobil Biotechnol. 2011;39(1):31–8.

67. Sakaguchi Y, Sekiya I, Yagishita K, Muneta T. Comparison of human stem cells derived from various mesenchymal tissues: superiority of synovium as a cell source. Arthritis Rheum. 2005;52:2521–9.

68. Tallheden T, Dennis JE, Lennon DP, Sjögren-Jansson E, Caplan AI, Lindahl A. Phenotypic plasticity of human articular chondrocytes. J Bone Joint Surg Am. 2003;85-A(Suppl 2):93–100.

69. Bomer N, den Hollander W, Suchiman H, Houtman E, Slieker RC, Heijmans BT, Slagboom PE, Nelissen RG, Ramos YF, Meulenbelt I. Neo-cartilage engineered from primary chondrocytes is epigenetically similar to autologous cartilage, in contrast to using mesenchymal stem cells. Ostcoarthr Cartil. 2016;24(8):1423–30.

70. Bian L, Zhai DY, Mauck RL, Burdick JA. Coculture of human mesenchymal stem cells and articular chondrocytes reduces hypertrophy and enhances functional properties of engineered cartilage. Tissue Eng A. 2011;17(7-8):1137–45.

71. Archer CW, Dowthwaite GP, Francis-West P. Development of synovial joints. Birth Defects Res C Embryo Today. 2003;69(2):144–55. Review.

72. Smeriglio P, Lai JH, Dhulipala L, Behn AW, Goodman SB, Smith RL, Maloney WJ, Yang F, Bhutani N. Comparative potential of juvenile and adult human articular chondrocytes for cartilage tissue formation in three-dimensional biomimetic hydrogels. Tissue Eng A. 2015;21(1-2):147–55.

73. Chang HX, Yang L, Li Z, Chen G, Dai G. Age-related biological characterization of mesenchymal progenitor cells in human articular cartilage. Orthopedics. 2011;34(8):e382–8.

Role of MSCs in Symptomatic Cartilage Defects

G. Jacob, K. Shimomura, and N. Nakamura

20.1 Introduction

It is difficult to determine the exact burden of chondral knee injuries in today's population since a great majority of lesions remain asymptomatic [1]. However, symptomatic lesions have posed a large clinical problem especially in athletes [2], and due to their hypocellularity and hypovascularity, cartilage displays poor natural healing [3]. We know that chondral injury predisposes to joint osteoarthritis (OA), and this is directly proportional to the grade of injury [4]. Various treatments have been employed for treating focal chondral lesions such as microfracture, autologous chondrocyte implantation (ACI), and osteochondral graft transfers. More recently, tissue-engineered options and stem cell therapies have been studied. The efficacy and indications for cell therapies in chondral defects are still under study with numerous pre-clinical, but only few clinical studies.

Mesenchymal stem cells (MSCs) have been the major focus of stem cell therapy due to their ease of procurement, rapid proliferation potential, and most importantly ability to differentiate into adipocyte, osteoblast, and chondrocyte cells [5, 6]. More recently, the paracrine functions of MSCs have been a topic of interest, and literature has suggested that exosomes secreted by MSCs potentially hold the key to superior tissue regeneration [7]. Tissue injury does stimulate endogenous MSC production in the joint but not in sufficient number for chondral repair [8–10]. In this chapter, we aim to describe the functions of MSCs and the roles they currently have in the treating chondral injuries.

20.2 Mesenchymal Stem Cells

20.2.1 Sources

MSCs have been isolated from various tissue sources and have demonstrated dissimilar differentiation capacities when their sources have been compared [11–14]. Popular sources include bone marrow [15], adipose [16], peripheral blood [17], and synovium [18]. Research has indicated synovium as a superior source when compared to bone marrow and adipose given differentiation capacity [11, 19]. Another important consideration has been the abundance and availability of MSCS where bone marrow, when compared to

G. Jacob · K. Shimomura
Department of Orthopaedic Surgery, Osaka University Graduate School of Medicine, Osaka, Japan
e-mail: kazunori-shimomura@umin.net

N. Nakamura (✉)
Institute for Medical Science in Sports, Osaka Health Science University, Osaka, Japan

Global Centre for Medical Engineering and Informatics, Osaka University, Osaka, Japan
e-mail: norimasa.nakamura@ohsu.ac.jp

© ISAKOS 2021
A. J. Krych et al. (eds.), *Cartilage Injury of the Knee*,
https://doi.org/10.1007/978-3-030-78051-7_20

adipose, is inferior [20, 21]. Synovial tissue also requires two-staged surgery and expansion due to limited tissue available from a biopsy. Theoretically, MSCs can be obtained from almost any human tissue and the major interest has been centered on the lack of immune response allowing for allogeneic administration [22]. Recently, sources have included periosteum, amnion, umbilical cord, and the induced pluripotent stem cell (iPS) [23]. Studies are still sparse in which these sources are used, and adipose and bone marrow remain the well-liked sources especially with concerns that iPS cells could lead to teratoma formation as they can differentiate into all three germ lines [23]. De-differentiated chondrocytes have also demonstrated stem cell-like characteristics and may also be a viable option in the future [24].

It has been noted that the body does have a natural intrinsic stem cell response to ACL and meniscal injury [25, 26]. It is thought that the local intra-articular bleeding brings MSCs and factors otherwise absent in the joint to the local joint environment. The reason for the MSCs marginal healing effect is postulated due to the upregulation of inflammatory markers which inhibit the regenerative actions of the cells. On introducing these synovial derived MSCs into rat knees post-ACL injury, it was found that the cells adhered to the injured ligament as opposed to the group with no ACL injury [27]. They postulated that the injured tissues expressed cytokines and chemokines which allowed for homing of the injected MSCs [28]. This means the body does have the ability to heal; however, it is somewhat hampered by the associated inflammatory processes and in the case of an isolated avascular chondral injury there is no presence of potential inflammatory or growth factors due to no intra-articular bleed [29].

20.2.2 Mechanisms of Action

The exact mechanism of action by MSCs remains unclear and earlier research hypothesized MSCs to function entirely by differentiation allowing them to repair and replace mesenchymal tissues. However, this is not a simple task and many studies have reported a lack of specific tissue differentiation in MSC therapies [30]. In vitro and in vivo studies have indicated that MSCs can be encouraged to differentiate toward chondrogenic lineage with the addition of certain growth factors and inductive agents, e.g., transforming growth factor-beta 1 (TGF-β1) [31], dexamethasone, bone morphogenic proteins, and insulin-like growth factors [32–34]. Due to the lack of differentiation of the MSCs themselves, it is now believed that MSCs could function primarily through paracrine signaling [7, 35]. This allows them to secrete anti-inflammatory, pro-regenerative, and immunomodulatory factors to enhance tissue repair [36–38]. The anti-inflammatory effects include downregulation of cytokines secreted by damaged cells such as interleukins and metalloproteinases [39]. In addition, molecules to promote cell proliferation and tissue healing are also secreted, namely transforming growth factor, vascular endothelial growth factor, and epithelial growth factor among others [40, 41].

Recently, extracellular vesicles (EVs) derived from MSCs have shown clinical promise in that they too express many of the advantages of stem cells among a few additional ones. Still, in early experimental phases, EVs derived from MSCs are much smaller and possess lower immunogenicity than MSCs [42]. They contain biologically active molecules that have anti-inflammatory and trophic properties similar to MSCs and can, therefore, affect cell proliferation, viability, and angiogenesis in a positive manner [43, 44]. Another major advantage is the long-term effectiveness of EVs in that they do not age and undergo senescence as with MSCs during expansion—therefore, they may have a longer lifespan of functionality [42]. In this way, MSC-derived EVs can aid in chondral regeneration and repair [45]. The use of EVs has remained in experimental studies only but data from these show potential for their use in chondral injury treatment. Table 20.1 highlights the advantages of using MSCs for cartilage repair. Figure 20.1

summarizes the various mechanisms of action of MSCs.

In contrast to previous belief, it seems as though MSCs are orchestrating the repair and regeneration of chondral tissue with their paracrine functions and secretion of EVs as opposed to regenerating and replacing the tissues.

20.2.3 Methods of Delivery

The delivery method of MSCs has now been extensively debated. MSCs can either be procured from the cell source such as bone marrow followed by centrifugation and then delivery as an injection or procured from the source, expanded in vitro and then delivered to the patient. Many researchers have advocated the expansion of cells before they are delivered to the chondral defect. The reasoning is to expand cell numbers as well as quality control and standardization of the treatment [46]. The obvious drawback is that the procedure becomes two-staged when compared to a single-stage harvest centrifuge and delivery. But another important concern has been the loss of cell phenotype and differentiation capacity during the expansion process [47, 48]. Various other techniques have been studied and many remain in pre-clinical phases. It is known that the addition of scaffolds and matrices provides a structural support to the delivered MSCs encouraging cell proliferation and differentiation [49]. These scaffolds have included materials such as collagen [50, 51], hyaluronic acid (HA) [52], and chitosan [53]. An ideal scaffold is required to be biocompatible, biodegradable, permeable, porous and possess some degree of mechanical strength. As mentioned earlier pre-clinical studies have also shown growing evidence that combining MSCs with growth factors can improve their chondrogenic differentiation capacity. These factors could be included in the matrix or scaffold intended for MSC delivery to a chondral defect and be a viable tool for MSC clinical therapies [54].

Table 20.1 The advantages of employing MSCs for chondral repair and regeneration are as follows

- Availability
- Low immunogenicity
- Multipotent
- Paracrine functions

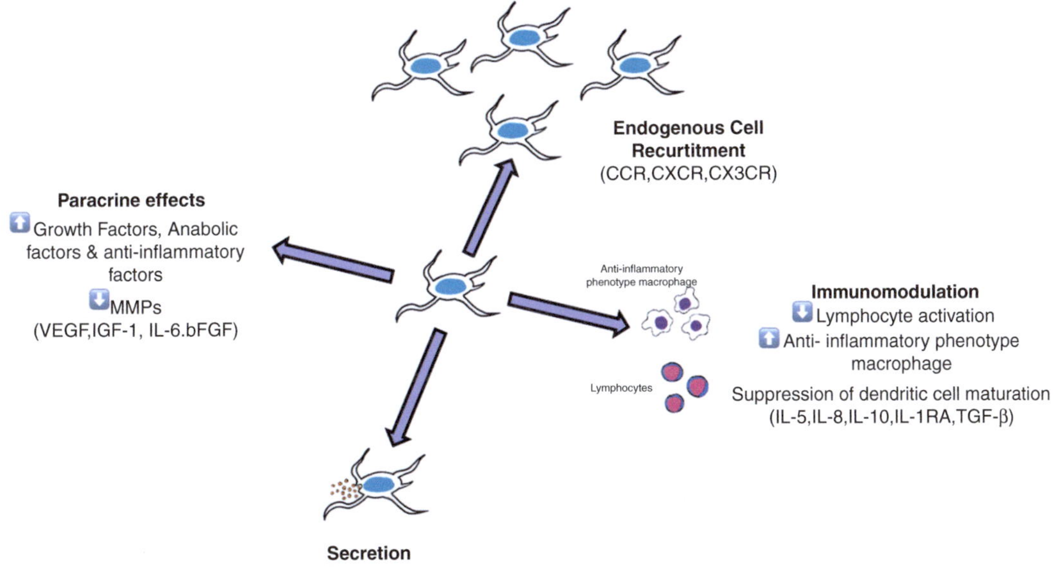

Fig. 20.1 Summarizing the various mechanisms of action of MSCs

20.3 Clinical Results of MSC Therapies

The use of MSCs in clinical settings has been viewed mainly as an investigational drug/agent in most healthcare systems. Regulations and lack of evidence mean the routine use of MSCs in chondral lesions is not recommended; however, some clinical trials have reported promising outcomes. In the past, bone marrow MSCs (BMMSC) were the most popular source but due to inadequacy in cell number more recent trials have been in favor of adipose-derived MSCs (AD-MSCs) and some synovium derived.

McIntyre et al. [55] performed a systematic review on MSC therapies and divided the studies into those assessing OA and those treating only focal chondral defects. They noted clinical benefit in at least one pain and one functional outcome measure in all included studies, but found the MRI (magnetic resonance imaging) results to be ambiguous. A more strict inclusion criterion was employed in a systematic review by Chahla et al. [56] where 6 studies could qualify, of which 3 addressed focal chondral defects. The total number of knees treated for chondral defects was 176 knees with a mean follow-up of 21 months. No adverse effects were reported in any of the included studies, but the outcome scores showed only modest improvement. Both reviews concluded the therapy was safe, but study design had a negative impact on the clarity of the results in MSC therapies making definite conclusions difficult. Most included studies were not controlled, not randomized and also employed adjuvant therapies such as platelet-rich plasma, fibrin glue, and scaffolds. For these types of studies, a placebo effect must be ruled out especially as patients do have a high level of expectation from such regenerative stem cell treatments.

Single-stage therapies are an attractive option for chondral injuries to reduce surgical time and treatment cost. de Windt et al. [57] performed a clinical trial in 35 patients where they recycled debrided chondral tissue using a rapid enzymatic isolation protocol and combined it with allogeneic MSCs in a ratio of 10:90 [58]. The mixture was then implanted into the defect site with the help of fibrin glue. During the 18 months follow-up, they reported significant improvement in clinical outcome scores and MRI scans at 12 months confirmed complete defect filling. A second-look arthroscopy showed stable grade I/II repair tissue and histology of the repair tissue showed tissue rich in proteoglycan content and collagen I and II content. Overall the repair tissue resembled that of hyaline-like tissue. They concluded that they were able to report similar results to autologous chondrocyte implantation while being more cost-effective. Another more recent stem cell therapy has been stromal vascular fraction (SVF) injections which are derived from lipoaspirates. SVF has demonstrated to be a rich source of stem cells [59]. The lipoaspirate is processed by first enzymatic digestion to remove adipocytes and then processed to contain a high percentage of stromal and vascular cells. These AD-MSCs, when injected into OA knee joints, have been proven to exhibit a large number of cells expressing CD34+ indicative of strong progenitor cell presence [60]. With regard to SVF being used in chondral defects, there is currently not much data. A case report by Salikhov et al. [61] added SVF to a microfracture repair of a chondral defect in a 36-year-old woman. They reported significant improvement in results however did not do a second-look arthroscopy. The postoperative MRI at 2 years showed good defect fill. Another report compared patients with chondral lesions who underwent microfracture alone versus in combination with SVF [62]. At 1 year follow-up, patients who underwent microfracture along with SVF injections had better outcome scores. This is not conclusive data but at present, the use of SVF has been used more in knee OA than in chondral defect treatment [63–65]. Yokota et al. [66] compared non-cultured SVF versus culture AD-MSCs in patients with knee OA and found that despite both treatments resulting in significant clinical improvement the results of AD-MSCs were superior. SVF has become a popular treatment in clinical settings as it is a one-stage therapeutic autologous option with no additional in vitro cell expansion, resulting in less cost and regulatory issues. However, two-staged cultured MSC treatments may remain

Table 20.2 Summarizing the clinical systematic reviews that reporting the use of MSCs for treatment of chondral defects

Author	Type of study	Number of studies included	Patient number	MSC source	Follow-up/ months	Results
McIntyre et al. [55]	Systematic review	14	451	Autologous BM, AD, IPFP	20.15	MSC therapies appear useful. Significant improvement in at least one PRO in each study. MRI outcome data is irregular. MSC therapies are safe with no adverse reactions reported.
Chahla et al. [56]	Systematic review	3	176	Autologous BM, PBPCs	21	All studies reported improvement in PROs. Improved MRI scores in all studies. A second-look arthroscopy and biopsy were done in one study and showed reported improvement. All studies reported MSC therapy as a safe treatment

Abbreviations: *BM* bone marrow, *AD* abdominal adipose, *IPFP* infra-patellar fat pad, *MSC* mesenchymal stem cell, *PRO* patient reported outcome, *MRI* magnetic resonance imaging, *PBPCs* peripheral blood progenitor cells

superior in that they have better quality control and a greater number of cells (Table 20.2).

20.4 Scaffold-Based Stem Cell Delivery Methods

Scaffold-based MSC treatments have been recently studied by combining biomaterials with MSCs [50, 67–69]. There have been many case series and reports demonstrating superior MRI, arthroscopy, and biopsy outcomes after these treatments which report repair tissue to resemble that of normal hyaline cartilage with a large amount of type II collagen and intense proteoglycan staining. Buda et al. [67] employed a hyaluronic acid membrane along with bone marrow concentrate in 20 patients and reported good defect fill and significantly improved clinical outcomes. Another technique reported by Enea et al. [68] used microfracture along with a polyglycolic/hyaluronan matrix augmented with bone marrow concentrate. They too reported superior clinical results and a hyaline-like cartilage repair. Collagen has also been used a scaffold alongside bone marrow aspirate and again reported to produce hyaline-like reparative tissue [50, 69, 70]. Kon et al. [71] published a review to assess whether there is a need for cells in the presence of a scaffold-based repair. They noted that acellular scaffold therapies too showed clinical benefit

similar to that of cell-based therapies and ended with a similar statement to other mentioned studies, in that study design and product heterogenicity prevented any definite conclusions to be drawn. They did question the use of cells, as cell culture and expansion are tedious when compared to a cell-free scaffold repair option. However, there is literature opposing this and in support of cellular therapies [72]. Despite these results, it must be noted that these are small studies and case reports with a small number of subjects, and they do not provide compelling levels of evidence yet. As these scaffold-based cellular therapeutic methods remain in pre-clinical or early clinical phases, further research and randomized trials are required to determine their value as a therapeutic option.

20.5 Scaffold-Free Methods

A new scaffold-free based therapy being explored is called Tissue-Engineered Construct (TEC). This is a natural scaffold-free MSC therapy for chondral repair [73]. Here, synovium was identified as the most appropriate MSC cell source given its strong chondrogenic potential and availability [11]. Ando et al. [74] cultured synovial MSCs in high density which led to extra cellular matrix synthesis. This was then detached from the culture plate using a pipette resulting in the formation of a three-dimensional structure, which could act as a natural scaffold. On further investigation, it was noted that TEC was abundant in collagen I and III, and on chondrogenic culture demonstrated a high glycosaminoglycan content and collagen II production [73]. Also, in another pre-clinical study, TEC demonstrated excellent adhesion to chondral defect sites without the need for any fixative methods [75]. Further large animal model in vivo studies performed using TEC demonstrated excellent chondral defect fill at 6 months post-implantation. Defects treated with TEC had significantly better modified ICRS histological scores and performed equal to that of normal cartilage when mechanically tested [76]. With the excellent pre-clinical data a first-in-human trial was conducted at Osaka University where five patients underwent TEC implantation for symptomatic chondral knee defects [77]. At 24 months post-surgery, all patients had significant improvement in self-assessed clinical scores with no adverse reactions, MRI, and a second-look arthroscopy confirmed stable and complete defect fill. Finally, Biopsy of the repair tissue resembled that of hyaline cartilage [77]. At present, a randomized control trial is underway to further understand and study the role of TEC in chondral repair.

20.6 Conclusion

MSCs demonstrate several desirable properties which theoretically make them the ideal tool and cellular candidate for regeneration of a chondral defect. In vitro studies have clearly shown superior chondrogenic differentiation, and newer techniques have enabled researchers to maintain cell phenotype even post expansion. With the large volume of pre-clinical data available many clinical studies have been performed, yet don't all possess similar outcomes. There is a great deal of variation in results and therefore guidelines and indications remain elusive, and there is still no consensus on a superior cell source. Current literature has a great deal of variation and short-comings in methodology and small sample sizes. Low quality literature is creating confusion and in effect delaying the publication of well-defined guidelines and recommendations. From the existing literature, MSC therapies appear safe with no major reported adverse effects. Many new strategies have shown potential, and with high quality rigorous clinical trials we will be able determine their effects in chondral repair. Currently, the use of MSCs should be as an investigational agent in high quality randomized trials with the hope of providing clarity on their potential and limitations.

References

1. da Cunha Cavalcanti FMM, Doca D, Cohen M, Ferretti M. Updating on diagnosis and treatment of chondral lesion of the knee. Rev Bras Ortop (Engl Ed). 2012;47(1):12–20.
2. Flanigan DC, Harris JD, Trinh TQ, Siston RA, Brophy RH. Prevalence of chondral defects in athletes' knees: a systematic review. Med Sci Sports Exerc. 2010;42(10):1795–801.
3. Li Y, Wei X, Zhou J, Wei L. The age-related changes in cartilage and osteoarthritis. BioMed Res Int. 2013;2013:916530.
4. Prakash D, Learmonth D. Natural progression of osteo-chondral defect in the femoral condyle. Knee. 2002;9(1):7–10.
5. Pittenger MF, Mackay AM, Beck SC, Jaiswal RK, Douglas R, Mosca JD, et al. Multilineage potential of adult human mesenchymal stem cells. Science. 1999;284(5411):143–7.
6. De Bari C, Roelofs AJ. Stem cell-based therapeutic strategies for cartilage defects and osteoarthritis. Curr Opin Pharmacol. 2018;40:74–80.
7. Barry F, Murphy M. Mesenchymal stem cells in joint disease and repair. Nat Rev Rheumatol. 2013;9(10):584–94.
8. Jones EA, Crawford A, English A, Henshaw K, Mundy J, Corscadden D, et al. Synovial fluid mesenchymal stem cells in health and early osteoarthritis: detection and functional evaluation at the single-cell level. Arthritis Rheum. 2008;58(6):1731–40.
9. Sekiya I, Ojima M, Suzuki S, Yamaga M, Horie M, Koga H, et al. Human mesenchymal stem cells in synovial fluid increase in the knee with degenerated cartilage and osteoarthritis. J Orthop Res. 2012;30(6):943–9.
10. Gupta PK, Das AK, Chullikana A, Majumdar AS. Mesenchymal stem cells for cartilage repair in osteoarthritis. Stem Cell Res Ther. 2012;3(4):1–9.
11. Sakaguchi Y, Sekiya I, Yagishita K, Muneta T. Comparison of human stem cells derived from various mesenchymal tissues: superiority of synovium as a cell source. Arthritis Rheum. 2005;52(8):2521–9.

12. Kolf CM, Cho E, Tuan RS. Mesenchymal stromal cells. Biology of adult mesenchymal stem cells: regulation of niche, self-renewal and differentiation. Arthritis Res Ther. 2007;9(1):204.

13. Strioga M, Viswanathan S, Darinskas A, Slaby O, Michalek J. Same or not the same? comparison of adipose tissue-derived versus bone marrow-derived mesenchymal stem and stromal cells. Stem Cells Dev. 2012;21(14):2724–52.

14. Stockmann P, Park J, Von Wilmowsky C, Nkenke E, Felszeghy E, Dehner JF, et al. Guided bone regeneration in pig calvarial bone defects using autologous mesenchymal stem/progenitor cells—a comparison of different tissue sources. J Cranio-Maxillofacial Surg. 2012;40(4):310–20.

15. van Buul GM, Villafuertes E, Bos PK, Waarsing JH, Kops N, Narcisi R, et al. Mesenchymal stem cells secrete factors that inhibit inflammatory processes in short-term osteoarthritic synovium and cartilage explant culture. Osteoarthr Cartil. 2012;20(10):1186–96.

16. Manferdini C, Maumus M, Gabusi E, Piacentini A, Filardo G, Peyrafitte JA, et al. Adipose-derived mesenchymal stem cells exert antiinflammatory effects on chondrocytes and synoviocytes from osteoarthritis patients through prostaglandin E2. Arthritis Rheum. 2013;65(5):1271–81.

17. Chong PP, Selvaratnam L, Abbas AA, Kamarul T. Human peripheral blood derived mesenchymal stem cells demonstrate similar characteristics and chondrogenic differentiation potential to bone marrow derived mesenchymal stem cells. J Orthop Res. 2012;30(4):634–42.

18. Koizumi K, Ebina K, Hart DA, Hirao M, Noguchi T, Sugita N, et al. Synovial mesenchymal stem cells from osteo- or rheumatoid arthritis joints exhibit good potential for cartilage repair using a scaffold-free tissue engineering approach. Osteoarthr Cartil. 2016;24(8):1413–22.

19. Mochizuki T, Muneta T, Sakaguchi Y, Nimura A, Yokoyama A, Koga H, et al. Higher chondrogenic potential of fibrous synovium- and adipose synovium-derived cells compared with subcutaneous fat-derived cells: distinguishing properties of mesenchymal stem cells in humans. Arthritis Rheum. 2006;54(3):843–53.

20. Mizuno H. Adipose-derived stem cells for tissue repair and regeneration: ten years of research and a literature review. J Nippon Med Sch. 2009;76(2):56–66.

21. Aust L, Devlin B, Foster SJ, Halvorsen YDC, Hicok K, du Laney T, et al. Yield of human adipose-derived adult stem cells from liposuction aspirates. Cytotherapy. 2004;6(1):7–14.

22. Chamberlain G, Fox J, Ashton B, Middleton J. Concise review: mesenchymal stem cells: their phenotype, differentiation capacity, immunological features, and potential for homing. Stem Cells. 2007;25(11):2739–49.

23. Vonk LA, De Windt TS, Slaper-Cortenbach ICM, Saris DBF. Autologous, allogeneic, induced pluripotent stem cell or a combination stem cell therapy? Where are we headed in cartilage repair and why: a concise review. Stem Cell Res Ther. 2015;6(1):94.

24. Jiang Y, Cai Y, Zhang W, Yin Z, Hu C, Tong T, et al. Human cartilage-derived progenitor cells from committed chondrocytes for efficient cartilage repair and regeneration. Stem Cells Transl Med. 2016;5(6):733–44.

25. Morito T, Muneta T, Hara K, Ju YJ, Mochizuki T, Makino H, et al. Synovial fluid-derived mesenchymal stem cells increase after intra-articular ligament injury in humans. Rheumatology. 2008;47(8):1137–43.

26. Matsukura Y, Muneta T, Tsuji K, Koga H, Sekiya I. Mesenchymal stem cells in synovial fluid increase after meniscus injury. Clin Orthop Relat Res. 2014;472(5):1357–64.

27. Kanaya A, Deie M, Adachi N, Nishimori M, Yanada S, Ochi M. Intra-articular injection of mesenchymal stromal cells in partially torn anterior cruciate ligaments in a rat model. Arthroscopy. 2007;23(6):610–7.

28. Sordi V, Malosio ML, Marchesi F, Mercalli A, Melzi R, Giordano T, et al. Bone marrow mesenchymal stem cells express a restricted set of functionally active chemokine receptors capable of promoting migration to pancreatic islets. Blood. 2005;106(2):419–27.

29. Sophia Fox AJ, Bedi A, Rodeo SA. The basic science of articular cartilage: structure, composition, and function. Sports Health. 2009;1(6):461–8.

30. Wyles CC, Houdek MT, Behfar A, Sierra RJ. Mesenchymal stem cell therapy for osteoarthritis: current perspectives. Stem Cells Cloning Adv Appl. 2015;8:117.

31. Barry F, Boynton RE, Liu B, Murphy JM. Chondrogenic differentiation of mesenchymal stem cells from bone marrow: differentiation-dependent gene expression of matrix components. Exp Cell Res. 2001;268(2):189–200.

32. Sekiya I, Colter DC, Prockop DJ. BMP-6 enhances chondrogenesis in a subpopulation of human marrow stromal cells. Biochem Biophys Res Commun. 2001;284(2):411–8.

33. Johnstone B, Hering TM, Caplan AI, Goldberg VM, Yoo JU. In vitro chondrogenesis of bone marrow-derived mesenchymal progenitor cells. Exp Cell Res. 1998;238(1):265–72.

34. Freyria AM, Mallein-Gerin F. Chondrocytes or adult stem cells for cartilage repair: the indisputable role of growth factors. Injury. 2012;43(3):259–65.

35. Hocking AM, Gibran NS. Mesenchymal stem cells: paracrine signaling and differentiation during cutaneous wound repair. Exp Cell Res. 2010;316(14):2213–9.

36. Céleste C, Ionescu M, Robin Poole A, Laverty S. Repeated intraarticular injections of triamcinolone acetonide alter cartilage matrix metabolism measured by biomarkers in synovial fluid. J Orthop Res. 2005;23(3):602–10.

37. Uccelli A, Moretta L, Pistoia V. Mesenchymal stem cells in health and disease. Nat Rev Immunol. 2008;8(9):726–36.

38. Le Blanc K, Frassoni F, Ball L, Locatelli F, Roelofs H, Lewis I, et al. Mesenchymal stem cells for

treatment of steroid-resistant, severe, acute graft-versus-host disease: a phase II study. Lancet. 2008;371(9624):1579–86.

39. Ruiz M, Cosenza S, Maumus M, Jorgensen C, Noël D. Therapeutic application of mesenchymal stem cells in osteoarthritis. Expert Opin Biol Ther. 2016;16(1):33–42.

40. Hofer HR, Tuan RS. Secreted trophic factors of mesenchymal stem cells support neurovascular and musculoskeletal therapies. Stem Cell Res Ther. 2016;7(1):1–4.

41. Murphy MB, Moncivais K, Caplan AI. Mesenchymal stem cells: environmentally responsive therapeutics for regenerative medicine. Exp Mol Med. 2013;45(11):e54.

42. Li JJ, Hosseini-Beheshti E, Grau GE, Zreiqat H, Little CB. Stem cell-derived extracellular vesicles for treating joint injury and osteoarthritis. Nanomaterials. 2019;9(2):261.

43. Kanazawa H, Fujimoto Y, Teratani T, Iwasaki J, Kasahara N, Negishi K, et al. Bone marrow-derived mesenchymal stem cells ameliorate hepatic ischemia reperfusion injury in a rat model. PLoS One. 2011;6(4):e19195.

44. Zhang HC, Liu XB, Huang S, Bi XY, Wang HX, Xie LX, et al. Microvesicles derived from human umbilical cord mesenchymal stem cells stimulated by hypoxia promote angiogenesis both in vitro and in vivo. Stem Cells Dev. 2012;21(18):3289–97.

45. Zhang S, Chuah SJ, Lai RC, Hui JHP, Lim SK, Toh WS. MSC exosomes mediate cartilage repair by enhancing proliferation, attenuating apoptosis and modulating immune reactivity. Biomaterials. 2018;156:16–27.

46. Torre ML, Lucarelli E, Guidi S, Ferrari M, Alessandri G, De Girolamo L, et al. Ex vivo expanded mesenchymal stromal cell minimal quality requirements for clinical application. Stem Cells Dev. 2015;24(6):677–85.

47. Yang YHK, Ogando CR, Wang See C, Chang TY, Barabino GA. Changes in phenotype and differentiation potential of human mesenchymal stem cells aging in vitro. Stem Cell Res Ther. 2018;9(1):1–4.

48. Bentivegna A, Miloso M, Riva G, Foudah D, Butta V, Dalprà L, et al. DNA methylation changes during in vitro propagation of human mesenchymal stem cells: implications for their genomic stability? Stem Cells Int. 2013;2013:192425.

49. Yamagata K, Nakayamada S, Tanaka Y. Use of mesenchymal stem cells seeded on the scaffold in articular cartilage repair. Inflamm Regen. 2018;38(1):4.

50. Kuroda R, Ishida K, Matsumoto T, Akisue T, Fujioka H, Mizuno K, et al. Treatment of a full-thickness articular cartilage defect in the femoral condyle of an athlete with autologous bone-marrow stromal cells. Osteoarthr Cartil. 2007;15(2):226–31.

51. Lubiatowski P, Kruczynski J, Gradys A, Trzeciak T, Jaroszewski J. Articular cartilage repair by means of biodegradable scaffolds. Transplant Proc. 2006;38(1):320–2.

52. Li L, Duan X, Fan Z, Chen L, Xing F, Xu Z, et al. Mesenchymal stem cells in combination with hyaluronic acid for articular cartilage defects. Sci Rep. 2018;8(1):1–1.

53. Mrugala D, Bony C, Neves N, Caillot L, Fabre S, Moukoko D, et al. Phenotypic and functional characterisation of ovine mesenchymal stem cells: application to a cartilage defect model. Ann Rheum Dis. 2008;67(3):288–95.

54. Bian L, Zhai DY, Tous E, Rai R, Mauck RL, Burdick JA. Enhanced MSC chondrogenesis following delivery of TGF-β3 from alginate microspheres within hyaluronic acid hydrogels in vitro and in vivo. Biomaterials. 2011;32(27):6425–34.

55. McIntyre JA, Jones IA, Han B, Vangsness CT. Intra-articular mesenchymal stem cell therapy for the human joint: a systematic review. Am J Sports Med. 2018;46(14):3550–63.

56. Chahla J, Piuzzi NS, Mitchell JJ, Dean CS, Pascual-Garrido C, LaPrade RF, et al. Intra-articular cellular therapy for osteoarthritis and focal cartilage defects of the knee: a systematic review of the literature and study quality analysis. J Bone Joint Surg Am. 2016;98(18):1511–21.

57. de Windt TS, Vonk LA, Slaper-Cortenbach ICM, Nizak R, van Rijen MHP, Saris DBF. Allogeneic MSCs and recycled autologous chondrons mixed in a one-stage cartilage cell transplantion: a first-in-man trial in 35 patients. Stem Cells. 2017;35(8):1984–93.

58. de Windt TS, Vonk LA, Slaper-Cortenbach ICM, van den Broek MPH, Nizak R, van Rijen MHP, et al. Allogeneic mesenchymal stem cells stimulate cartilage regeneration and are safe for single-stage cartilage repair in humans upon mixture with recycled autologous chondrons. Stem Cells. 2017;35(1):256–64.

59. Zuk PA, Zhu M, Mizuno H, Huang J, Futrell JW, Katz AJ, et al. Multilineage cells from human adipose tissue: implications for cell-based therapies. Tissue Eng. 2001;7(2):211–28.

60. Bunnell BA, Flaat M, Gagliardi C, Patel B, Ripoll C. Adipose-derived stem cells: isolation, expansion and differentiation. Methods. 2008;45(2):115–20.

61. Salikhov RZ, Masgutov RF, Chekunov MA, Tazetdinova LG, Masgutova G, Teplov OV, et al. The stromal vascular fraction from fat tissue in the treatment of osteochondral knee defect: case report. Front Med. 2018;5:154.

62. Bisicchia S, Bernardi G, Pagnotta SM, Tudisco C. Micro-fragmented stromal-vascular fraction plus microfractures provides better clinical results than microfractures alone in symptomatic focal chondral lesions of the knee. Knee Surg Sport Traumatol Arthrosc. 2019;11:1–9.

63. Fodor PB, Paulseth SG. Adipose derived stromal cell (ADSC) injections for pain management of osteoarthritis in the human knee joint. Aesthetic Surg J. 2016;36(2):229–36.

64. Yokota N, Yamakawa M, Shirata T, Kimura T, Kaneshima H. Clinical results following intra-articular injection of adipose-derived stromal vascu-

lar fraction cells in patients with osteoarthritis of the knee. Regen Ther. 2017;6:108–12.

65. Lapuente JP, Dos-Anjos S, Blázquez-Martínez A. Intra-articular infiltration of adipose-derived stromal vascular fraction cells slows the clinical progression of moderate-severe knee osteoarthritis: hypothesis on the regulatory role of intra-articular adipose tissue. J Orthop Surg Res. 2020;15:1–9.

66. Yokota N, Hattori M, Ohtsuru T, Otsuji M, Lyman S, Shimomura K, et al. Comparative clinical outcomes after intra-articular injection with adipose-derived cultured stem cells or noncultured stromal vascular fraction for the treatment of knee osteoarthritis. Am J Sports Med. 2019;47(11):2577–83.

67. Buda R, Vannini F, Cavallo M, Grigolo B, Cenacchi A, Giannini S. Osteochondral lesions of the knee: a new one-step repair technique with bone-marrow-derived cells. J Bone Joint Surg A. 2010;92(Suppl. 2):2–11.

68. Enea D, Cecconi S, Calcagno S, Busilacchi A, Manzotti S, Kaps C, et al. Single-stage cartilage repair in the knee with microfracture covered with a resorbable polymer-based matrix and autologous bone marrow concentrate. Knee. 2013;20(6):562–9.

69. Gobbi A, Karnatzikos G, Scotti C, Mahajan V, Mazzucco L, Grigolo B. One-step cartilage repair with bone marrow aspirate concentrated cells and collagen matrix in full-thickness knee cartilage lesions: results at 2-year follow-up. Cartilage. 2011;2(3):286–99.

70. Shetty AA, Kim SJ, Bilagi P, Stelzeneder D. Autologous collagen-induced chondrogenesis: single-stage arthroscopic cartilage repair technique. Orthopedics. 2013;36(5):e648–52.

71. Kon E, Roffi A, Filardo G, Tesei G, Marcacci M. Scaffold-based cartilage treatments: with or without cells? A systematic review of preclinical and clinical evidence. Arthroscopy. 2015;31(4):767–75.

72. Deng Z, Jin J, Zhao J, Xu H. Cartilage defect treatments: with or without cells? Mesenchymal stem cells or chondrocytes? Traditional or matrix-assisted? A systematic review and meta-analyses. Stem Cells Int. 2016;2016:9201492.

73. Ando W, Tateishi K, Katakai D, Hart DA, Higuchi C, Nakata K, et al. In vitro generation of a scaffold-free tissue-engineered construct (TEC) derived from human synovial mesenchymal stem cells: biological and mechanical properties and further chondrogenic potential. Tissue Eng A. 2008;14(12):2041–9.

74. Ando W, Tateishi K, Hart DA, Katakai D, Tanaka Y, Nakata K, et al. Cartilage repair using an in vitro generated scaffold-free tissue-engineered construct derived from porcine synovial mesenchymal stem cells. Biomaterials. 2007;28(36):5462–70.

75. Shimomura K, Ando W, Moriguchi Y, Sugita N, Yasui Y, Koizumi K, et al. Next generation mesenchymal stem cell (MSC)-based cartilage repair using scaffold-free tissue engineered constructs generated with synovial mesenchymal stem cells. Cartilage. 2015;6(2_Suppl):13S–29S.

76. Shimomura K, Ando W, Tateishi K, Nansai R, Fujie H, Hart DA, et al. The influence of skeletal maturity on allogenic synovial mesenchymal stem cell-based repair of cartilage in a large animal model. Biomaterials. 2010;31(31):8004–1177.

77. Shimomura K, Yasui Y, Koizumi K, Chijimatsu R, Hart DA, Yonetani Y, et al. First-in-human pilot study of implantation of a scaffold-free tissue-engineered construct generated from autologous synovial mesenchymal stem cells for repair of knee chondral lesions. Am J Sports Med. 2018;46(10):2384–93.

Scaffolds for Cartilage Repair

21

Elizaveta Kon, Daniele Altomare, Andrea Dorotei,
Berardo Di Matteo, and Maurilio Marcacci

21.1 Introduction

Biomimetic scaffolds are micro- or nanostructured biodegradable and biocompatible biomaterials implantable in the joint that can stimulate the generation of cartilage and the subchondral bone tissue. Biomimetic scaffolds may represent a step forward in the field of surgical cartilage repair, being a generally safe, one-step surgical strategy to repair cartilage and osteochondral defects. The scaffold has the goal to stimulate the potential of healing of native cells and tissues around the lesion. Recently, multilayer scaffolds mimicking the osteochondral unit have been developed. The goal of any of these scaffolds is to allow the healthy cartilage around the lesion to replicate the three-dimensional tissue structure, in order to fill the lesion. Ideally, chondrocytes are stimulated to migrate in the context of the scaffold and to produce extracellular matrix, restoring cartilage.

A multitude of scaffolds have been introduced to the market over the course of the past decade. In trying to classify these scaffolds, a crucial distinction has to be made between scaffolds that contain cells, and those that do not.

21.1.1 Cellulated Scaffold

The first generation of bioscaffolds was developed as an adjunct to optimize Autologous Chondrocyte Implantation (ACI), having the goal to provide the implanted chondrocytes a way to proliferate effectively in the context of the lesion, but also to recreate a three-dimensional and physiologic multilayered tissue. Therefore, the implant of a cellulated scaffold is a two-stage surgical procedure, requiring a first step, in which chondrocytes are harvested from a healthy portion of hyaline cartilage, and expanded in the laboratory with cultivation on the scaffold. The second step follows, in which the cellulated scaffold is implanted in the joint. The main drawbacks of this procedure are high costs, and necessity of two surgical interventions [1, 2].

E. Kon (✉)
Humanitas Clinical and Research Center, IRCCS,
Milan, Italy

First Moscow State Medical University, Sechenov
University, Moscow, Russia
e-mail: elizaveta.kon@humanitas.it

D. Altomare · A. Dorotei · B. Di Matteo
M. Marcacci
Humanitas Clinical and Research Center, IRCCS,
Milan, Italy

Department of Biomedical Sciences, Humanitas
University, Milan, Italy
e-mail: daniele.altomare@humanitas.it;
andrea.dorotei@humanitas.it;
berardo.dimatteo@humanitas.it;
maurilio.marcacci@humanitas.it

© ISAKOS 2021
A. J. Krych et al. (eds.), *Cartilage Injury of the Knee*,
https://doi.org/10.1007/978-3-030-78051-7_21

21.1.2 Cell-Free Scaffold

The most recent generation biomimetic scaffolds are implanted without cells. This implies that they do not have the goal to directly deliver chondrocytes in the location of the lesion. Rather, they focus on delivering a regenerative compartment in which autologous cells originating from the healthy borders of the lesion and from the subchondral bone can safely proliferate under the stimulation of load [3–5].

Further classification of the actual scaffolds available in clinical practice can be made according to the structure: first-generation scaffolds were single-layered, focused only on cartilage regeneration, not taking into account the different aspects of stimulation needed for the subchondral bone regeneration. The latest generation of scaffolds is multilayered, and every layer is made of a particular bioengineered tissue, with different materials to simulate the osseous surface versus the articular surface, in order to better mimic their particular structure and function [4].

21.2 Physical Properties of Scaffolds

In discussion of the characteristics of an ideal scaffold, the biophysical aspects of a scaffold to be considered should include the following:

1. Elastic strength resistance: 1–20 MPa. This allows both protection to cells, and also a certain mechanical stress in order to stimulate their proliferation.
2. Structure: a scaffold should be porous for the 80–90% of its entire volume, allowing for cells to grow in a three-dimensional structure. First-generation scaffolds were flat; therefore, the strength acting on the scaffold in this case led the chondrocyte to differentiate into fibroblasts, with consequentially a poor quality of the matrix produced.

In addition, biochemical aspects should include:

1. Biocompatibility: a perfect biocompatibility is needed in order to prevent any kind of foreign body reaction to biomaterial, which would mean a complete long-term failure of the scaffold.
2. Biodegradable: modern scaffolds are made of materials like agarose, aragonite, alginate, collagen, hyaluronic acid, and polymers (polylactic acid or PLA, and polyglycolic acid or PGA). These kinds of materials are practical to the activity of macrophagic cells. An ideal scaffold should provide a guide to the progressive restoration of healthy cartilage and bone. Once achieved, the scaffold should be completely resorbed, in order to allow a biologic replacement of the extracellular matrix.
3. Bioactivity: an ideal scaffold should provide a biochemical stimulation to cell replication. In order to do this, scaffolds can contain growth factors like BMP, TGF-ß, or IGF.

Overall, biomimetic scaffolds are growing in popularity as a potential therapeutic option for isolated cartilage lesion repair. Advantages of scaffold-based surgical approaches include:

1. Single-stage, standardized procedure: reducing both the burden for the patients and the surgeon.
2. Cost reduction: Cell-based procedures can be very expensive due to chondrocyte culture cost and its requirement for two-stage surgery. Scaffold utilization could represent a less expensive solution.
3. Future perspective: 3D printing could lead to complete customization of the procedure to address a specific defect. In the near future, a customized scaffold, based on a CT study of the lesion, will be available [6].

21.3 Surgical Indication

Biomimetic scaffolds are indicated for patients who sustained a symptomatic chondral or osteochondral lesion of various etiology: traumatic, post-traumatic, degenerative, or osteochondritis dissecans. In addition, new scaffold indications are extended to the include more diffuse chondral and osteochondral lesions associated with early osteoarthritis [3]. However, the classic indication for utilization of a scaffold is for a relatively young patient that is physically active, and not responding to conservative therapy. *Contraindications would include* older, obese patients, especially if they have diffuse OA in their knee. Further contraindication is a maligned limb or an unstable knee that is not addressed at the time of surgery.

21.4 Rehabilitation Protocol

Discharge of the patient is usually scheduled 1 or 2 days after the procedure. An early rehabilitation protocol is advocated after implantation of a scaffold. Weight-bearing is delayed by 3–5 weeks postoperatively, with the use of two crutches and progressive increase of weight-bearing after this period. Isometric and isotonic exercises are encouraged from the very early postoperative, in addition to neuromuscular electrical stimulation (NMES). Swimming pool exercises are recommended from the fourth week postoperatively [7].

21.5 Cell-Free Scaffolds Available in Clinical Practice

Scaffolding is an emergent surgical technique, quickly rising in popularity due to new nanotechnologies available and 3D printing devices. Several cell-free scaffolds have been introduced over the last decade and, by the time this chapter has been written, other scaffolds may have been designed and their release dates have been scheduled for the very near future.

A general overview of the main cell-free scaffolds currently available on the market is presented. A distinction must be made between chondral and osteochondral scaffolds, in particular:

- Osteochondral scaffolds: such as MaioRegen®, Agili-C™, Trufit®, aim to replicate the osteochondral unit in its entirety.
- Chondral scaffolds: such as autologous matric-induced chondrogenesis (AMIC®) with Chondro-Gide®, are designed as membranous cell-free scaffolds, aiming to provide support to the migration of chondrocytes from the periphery of the lesion, and to replace only the chondral portion of the osteochondral unit.

21.5.1 MaioRegen® (Fin-Ceramica S.p.A., Faenza, Italy)

MaioRegen is an osteochondral, nanostructured, biomimetic scaffold with a porous three-dimensional (3D) tri-layer composite structure, mimicking the entire osteochondral anatomy. The cartilaginous layer is made of type I collagen, the intermediate layer consists in a combination of type I collagen (60%) and hydroxyapatite (HA) (40%), and the lower layer is a mineralized blend of type I collagen (30%) and HA (70%), reproducing the subchondral bone layer.

The surgical procedure is performed with pneumatic tourniquet and a medial or lateral parapatellar approach is used to expose the lesion.

- Step 1: The defect is prepared as follows: the sclerotic subchondral bone is removed until 8 mm deep site with stable shoulder is created for implant. The defect is then templated with an aluminum foil obtaining the exact size and shape that are needed. The lesion implantation site must be smooth and regular (Figs. 21.1 and 21.2).
- Step 2: The scaffold is then accurately measured and cut for the corresponding implant site. Fibrin glue is added to ensure stability once implanted (Figs. 21.3–21.5).
- Step 3: The scaffold is finally implanted by press-fit and the addition of fibrin glue for stability is recommended. Flexion/extension maneuvers to check the stability of the scaffold are performed (Fig. 21.6) [8].

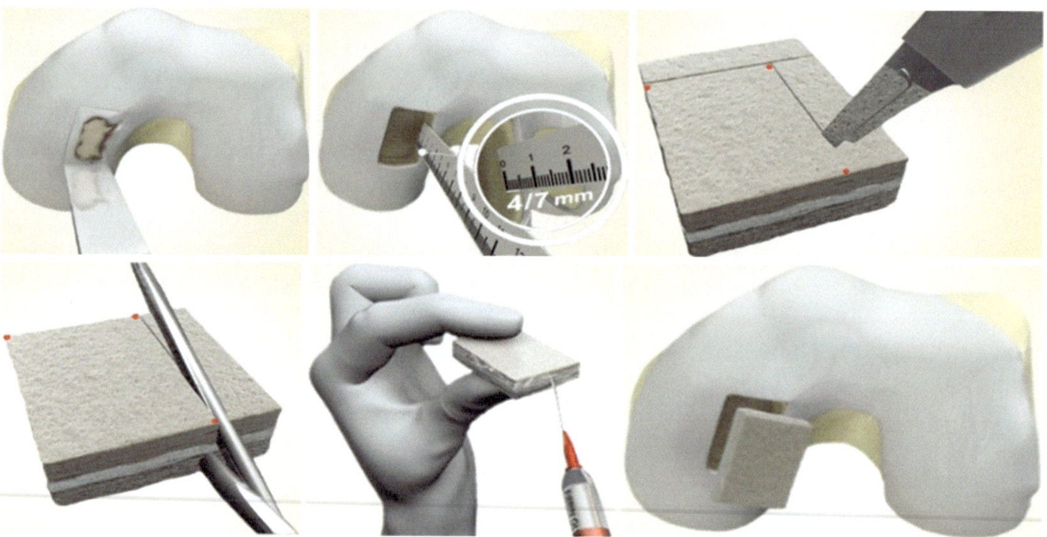

Figs. 21.1–21.6 MaioRegen® surgical procedure

21.5.2 Agili-C™ (Cartiheal (2009) Ltd., Israel)

Agili-C™ is an aragonite-based osteochondral scaffold. It is a rigid cell-free implant designed in two layers: the bone phase (calcium carbonate in the aragonite crystalline form) and the superficial cartilage phase (modified aragonite). This biphasic structure aims to reproduce the anatomic subchondral bone layer. The scaffold is implanted by press-fit, with the superficial layer being 1–2 mm deeper than the surrounding cartilage [1].

Surgical procedure: A classic arthroscopic or parapatellar arthrotomy (medial or lateral) approach can be used to expose the lesion.

- Step 1: Perform exposure of the lesion and preparation of the implant site to stable vertical borders. A cartilage cutter can be used to ensure smooth and regular edges to avoid invagination of the tissues during implant insertion (Figs. 21.7–21.9).
- Step 2: Scaffold implant after careful measurement. Press-fit technique is used until the desired position is reached, 2 mm below the surface of the articular cartilage. In case of

multiple implants, a 5 mm bone bridge must be present as a divider (Figs. 21.10–21.12). Postoperative stability tests are performed.

21.5.3 AMIC® Chondro-Gide® (Geistlich)

Chondro-Gide®, a bio-derived porcine collagen membrane, can be used with cells for ACI of combined with microfracture in the Autologous Matrix-Induced Chondrogenesis (AMIC) technique. AMIC is a one-step treatment for repairing cartilage lesions [9–13].

AMIC Surgical procedure: mini-open surgery.

- Step 1: Prepare the surgical site. Using a standard, minimally invasive anterior approach, open the knee joint. Remove damaged and unstable cartilage with a scalpel and curette until a stable, perpendicular shoulder surrounds the defect (Figs. 21.13 and 21.14).
- Step 2: Measure the defect. Place the sterile aluminum template included with the Chondro-Gide® in the defect to obtain an exact impression of the defect. Cut out the

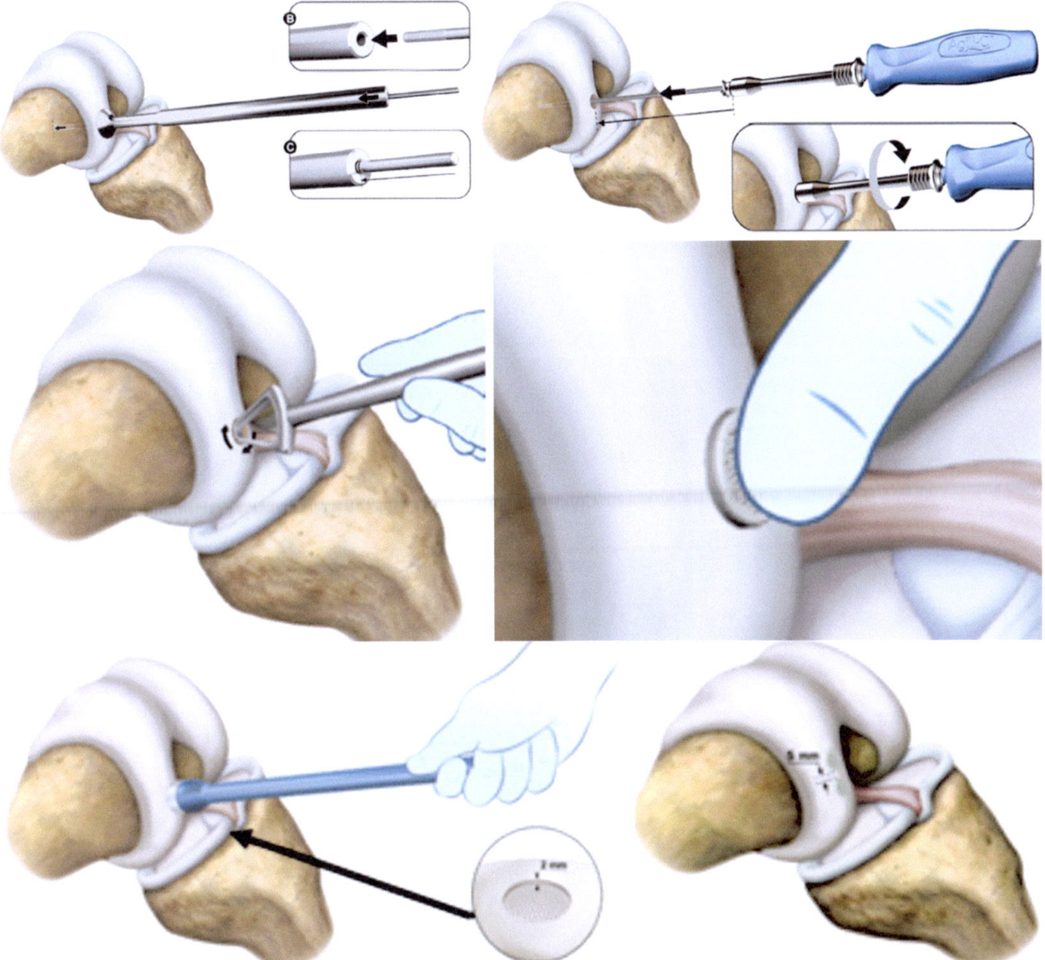

Figs. 21.7–21.12 Agili-C™ surgical procedure

imprint and transfer it onto the membrane (Figs. 21.15 and 21.16).

- Step 3: Perforate the Bone. Use a sharp awl or drill to perforate the subchondral bone at the base of the lesion. Start at the periphery of the lesion and then move towards the center at intervals of 3–4 mm (Figs. 21.17 and 21.18).
- Step 4: Position and suture or glue the Chondro-Gide® membrane. Place the Chondro-Gide into the defect and then fix it with suture (Vicryl or PDS 6/0) or fibrin glue (Figs. 21.19–21.22).

AMIC Surgical procedure: For arthroscopic application.

- Step 1: Prepare the surgical site. Use a sharp curette to remove cartilage fragments and create smooth vertical defect walls (Fig. 21.23).
- Step 2: Measure the defect size. Using a probe, measure the defect size. Turn the probe in different directions to determine the diameter and shape of the defect (Fig. 21.24).
- Step 3: Prepare the Chondro-Gide. When trimming the Chondro-Gide, remember to cut it 10–15% smaller than the defect itself, as the area of the Chondro-Gide will expand once moistened (Fig. 21.25).
- Step 4: Microfracture using a 1.2 mm K-wire, perforate the subchondral bone at the base of the lesion. Working from the periphery of the

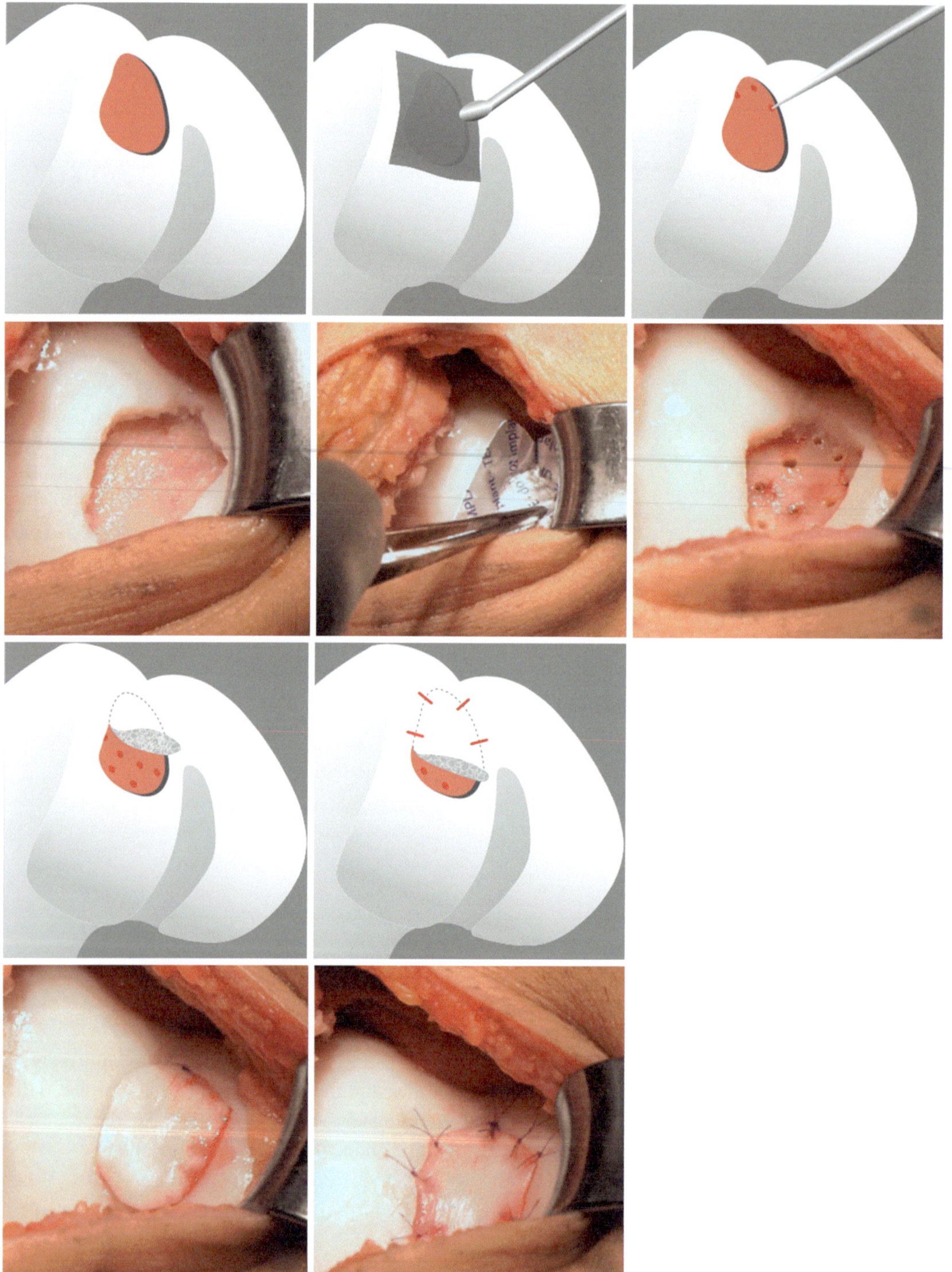

Figs. 21.13–21.22 AMIC® Chondro-Gide® mini-open surgical procedure

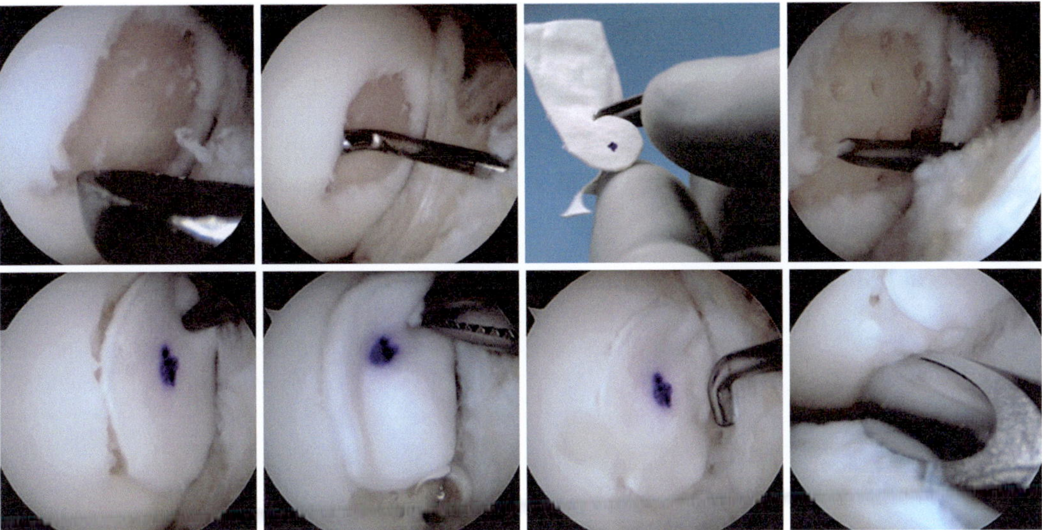

Figs. 21.23–21.30 AMIC® Chondro-Gide® arthroscopic surgical procedure

lesion towards the center, insert holes at intervals of 3–4 mm (Fig. 21.26).
- Step 5: Position the Chondro-Gide®. Use forceps or a clamp to place the membrane in the defect. To prevent delamination of the membrane, make sure the Chondro-Gide is sitting flush inside the defect (Fig. 21.27).
- Step 6: Apply the glue. Inject fibrin glue into the space between the Chondro-Gide and the defect. With a probe or a shaver, remove the excess fibrin glue (Figs. 21.28–21.30).

21.6   Clinical Results

Literature about the results of scaffolds in humans is still scarce. There is a general lack of evidence, which highlights the low numbers of scaffolds implanted over the last several decades.

A systematic review by Andriolo et al. [4], in 2019 synthetized the best studies available among the literature, especially about cell-free scaffold. Gille et al. [14] in 2010 reported a good mid-term outcome in 27 patients treated with Autologous Matrix-Induced Chondrogenesis (AMIC technique), with a significant increase in every functional score both at 12 and 24 months. Kusano et al. [11] in 2012 for the first time implemented in their study an MRI evaluation, showing an incomplete or homogeneous tissue filling at 36 months of follow-up, despite a significant improvement in clinical outcome scores. Schuttler et al. [15] in 2014 delved into the topic of tissue filling, evaluating MRI integration at 4-years follow-up, showing a good MRI result in all the 15 patients included in their study. Anders et al. were the very first, in 2013, to compare AMIC to Mfx, showing a better result at 12–24 months for patients treated with Mfx + AMIC, despite a good result was obtained even with Mfx alone.

Roessler et al. [16] in 2015 reported on the use of cell-free collagen type I matrix for the treatment of large, symptomatic, cartilage defects in a cohort of 28 patients, obtaining a complete defect filling after 24 months in 24 out of 28 patients. This demonstrates the reliability of this procedure even for challenging, larger cartilage lesions at early follow-up. Sofu et al. [17] in 2017 once again demonstrated the superiority of a Hyaluronic Acid-Based Cell-Free scaffold in combination with microfracture, versus microfracture alone. Randomizing 43 patients in two subgroups, they obtained better clinical outcome scores in the subgroup treated with Scaffolding + Mfx, compared to the subgroup treated with Mfx alone. They also reported a relatively short time from surgery to return to non-impact sports activities with 7.8 months in the scaffold subgroup compared to 9.2 months in the Mfx alone subgroup. Despite those good results, complete filling of the lesion was achieved only in 36.8% of the patients treated with scaffold implantation, and in the 16.6% of the patients treated with Mfx alone.

Sadlik et al. [10] in 2017 firstly described clinical results of AMIC implanted with an all-inside arthroscopic technique, in particular treating patellar cartilage defects. Reporting on the arthroscopic technique, Schagemann et al. in 2018 compared AMIC performed with mini-arthrotomy vs arthroscopic technique, reporting no significant difference in the two subgroups.

Hoburg et al. [18] in 2018 focused on the osteochondral unit, analyzing results of AMIC combined with bone grafting for the treatment of large osteochondral defects with a bone-bed deficiency. They obtained good clinical results, with a complete filling of the lesions in about two patients out of 3 at 4 years postoperatively. Finally, Schuttler et al. [3] 2019 reported an increased failure rate for scaffolds at follow-up longer than 5 years, especially in larger defects. This study was the first to highlight the possibility of long-term failure of this procedure, and the lack of evidence in the current literature about the long-term follow-up of this procedure. Further studies are needed to better estimate the real impact that this procedure can achieve in treating symptomatic cartilage lesion in younger and active patients.

21.6.1 MaioRegen® Clinical Results

According to in vivo and in vitro studies, this scaffold is able to guide differentiation of the host cells towards cartilage on the surface and towards bone underneath so that the entire osteochondral layer is regenerated. The authors report good results at 12 months postoperatively in 27 patients with symptomatic OCD of the femoral condyles, with further increase at 24 months and no correlation between size and outcome [19]. Delcogliano et al. [7] show good clinical results at 24 months follow-up in 19 patients with large articular defects. Berruto et al. [20] confirmed good clinical results after 2 years of follow-up in a multicenter study of 49 patients with large osteochondral lesions. Guérin et al. (2020) [8] evaluated clinical and imaging outcomes to assess any existing correlation between short-term (2 years) clinical outcome and MRI features. They found that MaioRegen® is a valid option at short-term follow-up for treating large focal osteochondral defects in knees of young patients, but no correlation was found between knee functional scores and MRI appearance.

21.6.2 AMIC® Chondro-Gide® (Geistlich) Clinical Results

A 10-year follow-up study by Kaiser et al. [21] investigated the use of AMIC® in the treatment of chondral and osteochondral defects in the knee of 33 patients. Average Lysholm Scores and Visual Analog Scores (VAS) for pain improved significantly when the pre-operative values were compared to the results at 2- and 10-year postoperative. Importantly, the improvement of these key scores was maintained over the 2–10-year follow-up. This study demonstrated that AMIC offers significant improvement over the pre-operative status, as well as long-term durability of results.

In a multicenter, randomized, controlled 3-arm study by Volz et al. [9] in 2017 compared Mfx vs AMIC, focusing on long-term result, especially at 2 and 5 years of follow-up. They noticed a degradation of good outcome results for Mfx after 2 years of follow-up, while AMIC was able to maintain a good outcome even at 5 years of follow-up. Most recently, in a 2019 systematic review [22] and meta-analysis of AMIC outcomes, significantly reduced pain and improved function was reported from baseline to early follow-up. A retrospective analysis by Schiavoni Panni et al. [23] noted that AMIC® was effective when treating full-thickness knee cartilage defects larger than 2 cm² in 21 patients after 7-year follow-up. Most recently, Fossum et al. [24] conducted a prospective, randomized, controlled study to assess the outcomes of ACI-C and AMIC in chondral and osteochondral defects of the distal femur and patella. They found that the mean function and pain baseline scores showed significant improvement at 1 and 2 years postoperatively.

21.6.3 Agili-C™ (Cartiheal (2009) Ltd., Israel) Clinical Results

Preclinical analysis [25] reveals the safety and the potential of this scaffold, demonstrating the ability to recruit cell from the surrounding tissues allowing a good regeneration of the entire osteochondral unit. Most recently, (2019) Chubinskaya et al. [1] investigated the ex vivo Agili-C potential of repairing full-thickness cartilage defects, focusing on the potential in stimulating cartilage in-growth through chondrocytes migration into the 3D interconnected porous structure of the scaffold. The analysis supports the potential of Agili-C™ scaffold to stimulate cartilage regeneration and repair. At the moment, a European multicenter clinical trial is currently being performed, and results should be available shortly.

In summary, scaffolds have been designed to treat a variety of clinical cartilage injuries and have been shown to be a good option for surgical treatment of chondral and osteochondral defects in early follow-up studies. There are currently both cell-based scaffolds, and non-cell-based options available with advantages and disadvantages to each approach. Long-term results are needed to further assess the durability of these scaffolds.

References

1. Chubinskaya S, Di Matteo B, Lovato L, Iacono F, Robinson D, Kon E. Agili-C implant promotes the regenerative capacity of articular cartilage defects in an ex vivo model. Knee Surg Sport Traumatol Arthrosc. 2019;27(6):1953–64.
2. Pascarella A, Ciatti R, Pascarella F, Latte C, Di Salvatore MG, Liguori L, et al. Treatment of articular cartilage lesions of the knee joint using a modified AMIC technique. Knee Surg Sport Traumatol Arthrosc. 2010;18(4):509–13.
3. Schüttler K-F, Götschenberg A, Klasan A, Stein T, Pehl A, Roessler PP, et al. Cell-free cartilage repair in large defects of the knee: increased failure rate 5 years after implantation of a collagen type I scaffold. Arch Orthop Trauma Surg. 2019;139(1):99–106.
4. Andriolo L, Reale D, Di Martino A, Boffa A, Zaffagnini S, Filardo G. Cell-free scaffolds in cartilage knee surgery: a systematic review and meta-analysis of clinical evidence. Cartilage. 2019; https://doi.org/10.1177/1947603519852406.
5. Efe T, Theisen C, Fuchs-Winkelmann S, Stein T, Getgood A, Rominger MB, et al. Cell-free collagen type I matrix for repair of cartilage defects-clinical and magnetic resonance imaging results. Knee Surg Sports Traumatol Arthrosc. 2012;20(10):1915–22.
6. Shetty AA, Kim SJ, Shetty V, Jang JD, Huh SW, Lee DH. Autologous collagen induced chondrogenesis (ACIC: Shetty–Kim technique)—a matrix based acellular single stage arthroscopic cartilage repair technique. J Clin Orthop Trauma. 2016;7:164–9.
7. Delcogliano M, de Caro F, Scaravella E, Ziveri G, De Biase CF, Marotta D, et al. Use of innovative biomimetic scaffold in the treatment for large osteochondral lesions of the knee. Knee Surg Sport Traumatol Arthrosc. 2014;2:1260–9.
8. Guérin G, Pujol N. Repair of large condylar osteochondral defects of the knee by collagen scaffold. Minimum two-year outcomes. Orthop Traumatol Surg Res. 2020;106:475–9.
9. Volz M, Schaumburger J, Frick H, Grifka J, Anders S. A randomized controlled trial demonstrating sustained benefit of autologous matrix-induced chondrogenesis over microfracture at five years. Int Orthop. 2017;41(4):797–804.
10. Sadlik B, Puszkarz M, Kosmalska L, Wiewiorski M. All-arthroscopic autologous matrix-induced chondrogenesis-aided repair of a patellar cartilage defect using dry arthroscopy and a retraction system. J Knee Surg. 2017;30(9):925–9.
11. Kusano T, Jakob RP, Gautier E, Magnussen RA, Hoogewoud H, Jacobi M. Treatment of isolated chondral and osteochondral defects in the knee by autologous matrix-induced chondrogenesis (AMIC). Knee Surg Sport Traumatol Arthrosc. 2012;20(10):2109–15.
12. Anders S, Volz M, Frick H, Gellissen J. A randomized, controlled trial comparing autologous matrix-induced chondrogenesis (AMIC®) to microfracture: analysis of 1- and 2-year follow-up data of 2 centers. Open Orthop J. 2013;7(1):133–43.
13. Dhollander A, Moens K, Van Der Maas J, Verdonk P, Almqvist KF, Victor J. Treatment of patello-femoral cartilage defects in the knee by autologous matrix-induced chondrogenesis (AMIC). Acta Orthop Belg. 2014;80(2):251–9.
14. Gille J, Behrens P, Volpi P, De Girolamo L, Reiss E, Zoch W, et al. Outcome of autologous matrix induced chondrogenesis (AMIC) in cartilage knee surgery: data of the AMIC Registry. Arch Orthop Trauma Surg. 2013;133(1):87–93.
15. Schüttler KF, Schenker H, Theisen C, Schofer MD, Getgood A, Roessler PP, et al. Use of cell-free collagen type I matrix implants for the treatment of small cartilage defects in the knee: clinical and mag-

netic resonance imaging evaluation. Knee Surg Sport Traumatol Arthrosc. 2014;22(6):1270–6.

16. Roessler PP, Pfister B, Gesslein M, Figiel J, Heyse TJ, Colcuc C, et al. Short-term follow up after implantation of a cell-free collagen type I matrix for the treatment of large cartilage defects of the knee. Int Orthop. 2015;39(12):2473–9.

17. Sofu H, Kockara N, Oner A, Camurcu Y, Issın A, Sahin V. Results of hyaluronic acid-based cell-free scaffold application in combination with microfracture for the treatment of osteochondral lesions of the knee: 2-year comparative study. Arthroscopy. 2017;33(1):209–16.

18. Hoburg A, Leitsch JM, Diederichs G, Lehnigk R, Perka C, Becker R, et al. Treatment of osteochondral defects with a combination of bone grafting and AMIC technique. Arch Orthop Trauma Surg. 2018;138(8):1117–26.

19. Filardo G, Kon E, Di Martino A, Busacca M, Altadonna G, Marcacci M. Treatment of knee osteochondritis dissecans with a cell-free biomimetic osteochondral scaffold: clinical and imaging evaluation at 2-year follow-up. Am J Sports Med. 2013;41(8):1786–93.

20. Berruto M, Delcogliano M, De Caro F, Carimati G, Uboldi F, Ferrua P, et al. Treatment of large knee osteochondral lesions with a biomimetic scaffold: results of a multicenter study of 49 patients at 2-year follow-up. Am J Sports Med. 2014;42(7):1607–17.

21. Kaiser N, Jakob RP, Pagenstert G, Tannast M, Petek D. Stable clinical long term results after AMIC in the aligned knee. Arch Orthop Trauma Surg. 2020; https://doi.org/10.1007/s00402-020-03564-7.

22. Steinwachs MR, Gille J, Volz M, Anders S, Jakob R, De Giromlamo L, et al. Systematic review and meta-analysis of the clinical evidence on the use of autologous matrix-induced chondrogenesis in the knee. Cartilage. 2019; https://doi.org/10.1177/1947603519870846.

23. Schiavone Panni A, Del Regno C, Mazzitelli G, D'Apolito R, Corona K, Vasso M. Good clinical results with autologous matrix-induced chondrogenesis (Amic) technique in large knee chondral defects. Knee Surg Sports Traumatol Arthrosc. 2018;26(4):1130–6.

24. Fossum V, Hansen AK, Wilsgaard T, Knutsen G. Collagen-covered autologous chondrocyte implantation versus autologous matrix-induced chondrogenesis: a randomized trial comparing 2 methods for repair of cartilage defects of the knee. Orthop J Sport Med. 2019;7(9) https://doi.org/10.1177/2325967119868212.

25. Kon E, Filardo G, Robinson D, Eisman JA, Levy A, Zaslav K, et al. Osteochondral regeneration using a novel aragonite-hyaluronate bi-phasic scaffold in a goat model. Knee Surg Sport Traumatol Arthrosc. 2014;22(6):1452–64.

Osteochondral Autograft for Treatment of Small Cartilage Injuries

Christopher M. LaPrade, Clayton W. Nuelle, Taylor Ray, and Seth L. Sherman

22.1 Introduction

Articular cartilage injury of the knee remains a challenging problem for orthopedic surgeons and their patients. Focal chondral or osteochondral lesions have been reported in 19% of patients undergoing arthroscopic surgery in a prospective study with other retrospective studies reporting numbers as high as 40% [1, 2]. Symptomatic focal cartilage defects cause dysfunction as measured by patient reported outcome (PROs) similar to arthroplasty patients and worse than patients undergoing ACL reconstruction [3].

Given this high level of disability, multiple treatment methods have evolved to address these injuries including microfracture, osteochondral autologous transplantation (OAT), osteochondral allograft transplantation (OCA), and autologous chondrocyte implantation (ACI). Historically, microfracture was the first-line treatment for smaller lesions. However, an increasing body of evidence has demonstrated poor long-term outcomes of microfracture, variable return-to-play, and the need for subsequent salvage cartilage res-

toration [4–8]. As such, the incidence of micro fracture has significantly decreased while evolving techniques such as OAT has become a more viable option for symptomatic smaller focal defects in the active population [9, 10]. The purpose of this chapter is to review the indications and surgical technique for OAT in the knee joint, as well as the clinical outcomes and basic science supporting this technique.

22.2 Surgical Technique

The OAT surgical technique typically involves one of two procedures: the single plug or mosaicplasty [11]. As the name entails, single plug technique involves the transplantation of a single 6–10 mm osteochondral graft that fills the entirety of the cartilage defect. The mosaicplasty technique involves multiple small osteochondral grafts producing a "mosaic" structure (Fig. 22.1). Both can both be performed arthroscopically or with a mini or larger arthrotomy. Typically, an arthrotomy may be required for larger or more posterior lesions due to the difficulty achieving a proper insertion angle at these locations [11, 12].

For both techniques, a donor site is identified from one of three typical low weightbearing locations that have been identified as having ideal curvature for recipient sites (Fig. 22.2): the superior medial trochlea, superior lateral trochlea, and/or the lateral aspect of intercondylar notch

C. M. LaPrade · T. Ray · S. L. Sherman (✉)
Department of Orthopedic Surgery, Stanford University, Stanford, CA, USA
e-mail: shermans@stanford.edu

C. W. Nuelle
Orthopaedic Surgery Sports Medicine, Missouri Orthopaedic Institute, Columbia, MO, USA

© ISAKOS 2021
A. J. Krych et al. (eds.), *Cartilage Injury of the Knee*,
https://doi.org/10.1007/978-3-030-78051-7_22

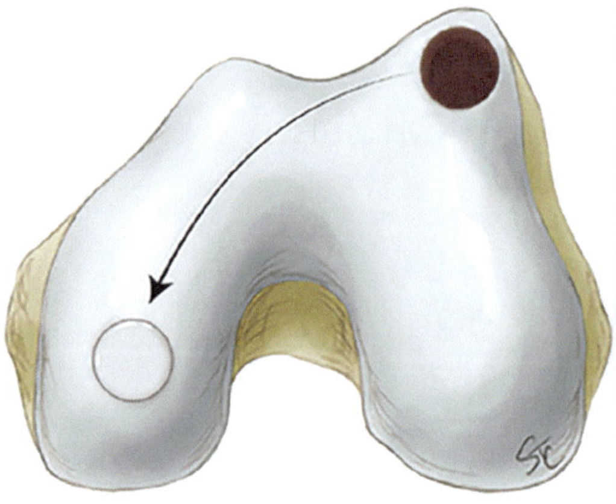
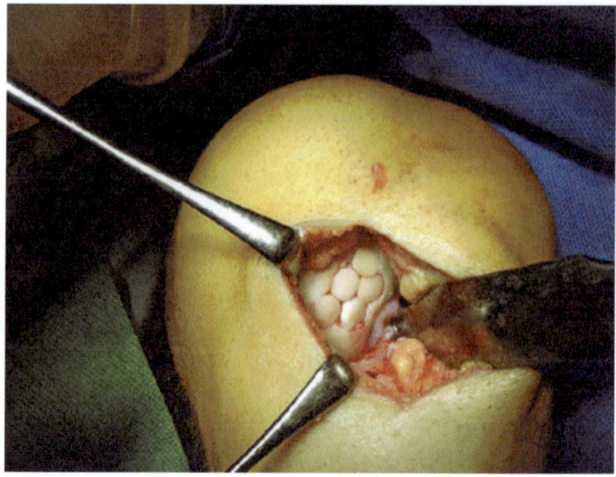

Fig. 22.1 (**a**) Illustration demonstrating the single plug technique, which involves the transplantation of a single 6–10 mm osteochondral graft to fill the cartilage defect. (Used with permission from Sherman et al (2017), Reprinted from Sports Medicine Clinics, Vol 36/Issue 3, Seth L. Sherman, Emil Thyssen, Clayton W. Nuelle, Osteochondral Autologous Transplantation, 489–500, Copyright (2017), with permission from Elsevier [or Applicable Society Copyright Owner]). (**b**) The mosaic-plasty technique involves multiple small osteochondral grafts producing a "mosaic" structure as seen in this clinical photo. (Used with permission from Hangody et al (2008), Reprinted from Injury, Vol 39/Issue 3, László Hangody, Gábor Vásárhelyi, László Rudolf Hangody, Zita Sükösd, György Tibay, Lajos Bartha, Gábor Bodó, Autologous osteochondral grafting—Technique and long-term results, 32–39, Copyright (2008), with permission from Elsevier [or Applicable Society Copyright Owner])

[11]. The lateral trochlear flare superior to the sulcus terminalis provides the largest surface area with minimal contact pressures. After selecting a graft site for harvesting, a donor harvester is placed perpendicular and flush with articular cartilage (Fig. 22.3). The harvester is then gently impacted with a mallet to 12–15 mm to ensure there is adequate subchondral bone. The harvester is then turned 180° to disengage the graft. If multiple grafts are harvested, separation of at least 2–3 mm is recommended so that each site remains perpendicular with the cartilage surface and ensure that the condyles are not weakened. These donor sites can be left in situ allowing for fibrocartilaginous fill or preferentially grafted with recipient bone plugs, allograft bone chips, or other bone void filler [11, 12].

At the site of cartilage defect, a harvester is used to remove the bone and to create a socket for the donor graft. The harvester should be positioned perpendicular and impacted 2 mm less than the donor graft. The recipient site is then debrided with the goal of having perpendicular walls around the defect to ensure bone-to-bone healing. A graft delivery tube is then inserted around the graft harvester, followed by a graft pusher that is inserted ensuring that the graft is flush with the edges of the delivery tube. The delivery tube is then placed perpendicular to the recipient site, and the graft is slowly advanced into the defect until it is flush with the surrounding cartilage. A tamp can be used to gently compress the graft, without causing graft fracture or chondrocyte injury [5, 11] (Fig. 22.4). Additional steps specific to a mosaicplasty procedure include using multiple grafts in the same fashion as above. Care should be provided to place larger grafts in the center of the defect, as well as positioning the deepest part of each graft to touch the base of the defect and be directed towards the center. This will ensure the proper convex orientation of the donor site, instead of a flat surface if all placed parallel [11].

There are advantages and disadvantages for each technique. The single plug technique has the potential to restore the entire defect with congruent hyaline cartilage; however, this technique is limited by the size of the lesion and limited donor-site availability. The mosaicplasty technique allows for harvesting of donor grafts from multiple sites and a technically easier matching of the articular cartilage surface; nevertheless,

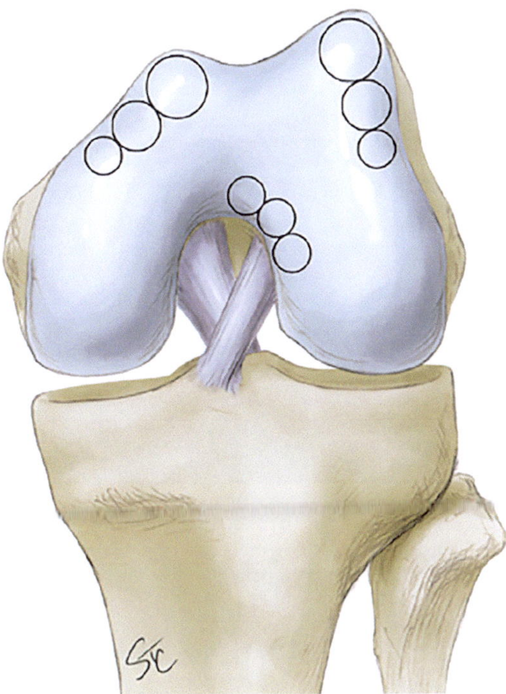

Fig. 22.2 Illustration demonstrating harvest sites for osteochondral autograft transplantation. Typically, the superior medial trochlea, superior lateral trochlea, and/or the lateral aspect of intercondylar notch are chosen given their low weightbearing demands and curvature that is most conducive for the common recipient sites. (Used with permission from Sherman et al (2017), Reprinted from Sports Medicine Clinics, Vol 36/Issue 3, Seth L. Sherman, Emil Thyssen, Clayton W. Nuelle, Osteochondral Autologous Transplantation, 489–500, Copyright (2017), with permission from Elsevier [or Applicable Society Copyright Owner])

the mosaicplasty technique results in increased space between donor grafts and leads to the increased possibility of fibrocartilage ingrowth and decreased hyaline cartilage [11].

22.3 Surgical Indications

Strict indications for OAT are imperative to increase the chance of achieving a successful outcome. In the knee, OAT is typically indicated for lesions in the femoral condyle, patella, or trochlea. Of note, with regard to the patella, there is a mismatch between the thickness of the cartilage surface of donor and recipient sites that can lead to an uneven subchondral bone plate even with a flush articular cartilage surface [11]. For this and other reasons (such as donor-site morbidity within the patellofemoral joint), it may be warranted to consider other cartilage restoration alternatives such as cell-based repair (such as MACI) or osteochondral allograft for larger defects of the patella.

Typically, most studies have advocated proceeding with OAT for lesions between 1 and 2 cm in diameter (1–4 cm^2) given that defects less than 1 cm are typically less symptomatic, while lesions larger than 2 cm^2 require multiple grafts and are limited by donor harvest site availability (Figs. 22.4 and 22.5). Typically, larger lesions are treated with OCA or MACI. In addition, OAT is typically indicated for symptomatic International Cartilage Repair Society (ICRS) grade III or IV defects in an active patient. While microfracture may be chosen as a therapy with an intact subchondral bone plate, athletes should be informed of clinical outcome differences, timeframes, and expectations for return-to-play, and possible need for further surgery if choosing microfracture over OAT [11, 13–15].

With regard to patient-specific indications, OAT is typically reserved for patients who remain symptomatic after failure of conservative treatment. Some relative contraindications include Body Mass Index (BMI) greater than 40, age greater than 50, knee osteoarthritis with greater than grade 2 on the Kellgren-Lawrence scale, and previous infections, tumors, or inflammatory arthritis of the knee joint [11, 14].

In addition, if there are concurrent injuries or malalignment of the knee joint, these should also be addressed at the time of surgery or prior to surgery. This includes planning for possible ligamentous repair or reconstruction (i.e., ACL reconstruction) or meniscal repair at the time of surgery. In addition, if an osteotomy is required for varus, valgus, or patellofemoral malalignment, this should also be addressed as a staged or combined procedure [7, 11].

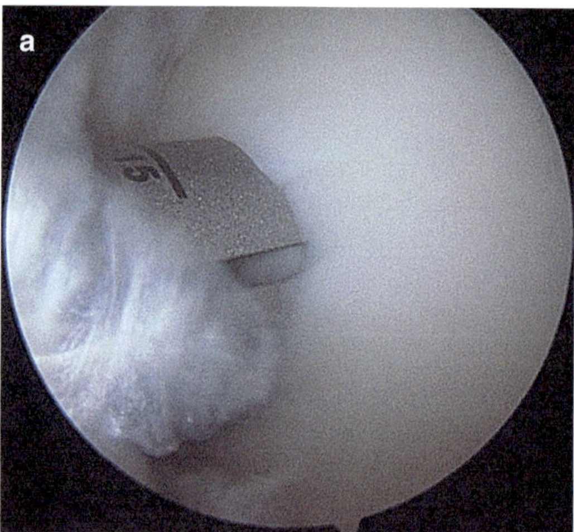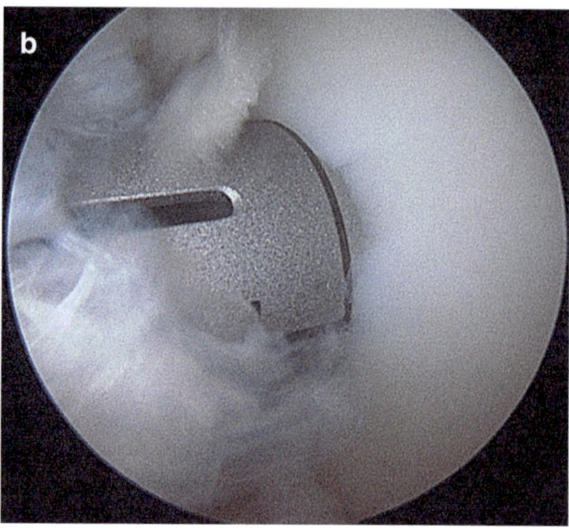

Fig. 22.3 (**a**) Intraoperative photograph showing the harvesting of an osteochondral autologous transplantation (OAT) graft from the lateral aspect of intercondylar notch. The donor harvester is placed perpendicular and flush with articular cartilage. (**b**) Photograph showing the donor site being impacted with a mallet to 12–15 mm to ensure there is adequate subchondral bone

22.4 Clinical Outcomes

22.4.1 Randomized Controlled Trials

While there remains a need for further investigation of the efficacy of treatment for focal cartilage defects, increasing numbers of clinical studies have been recently published evaluating the short- and long-term clinical outcomes of OAT versus alternative treatments. However, there is a paucity of level 1 studies investigating different cartilage treatments. Gudas et al. reported that in a 10-year follow-up of OAT versus microfracture in lesions less than 4 cm^2, both groups resulted in significantly higher clinical outcome scores on the ICRS scale [4]. Nevertheless, OAT resulted in significantly higher scores based on ICRS and Tegner scores versus microfracture and also had a significantly decreased rate of failure in comparison to microfracture, 14% versus 38%, respectively. In addition, there were no signs of osseous loosening in OAT patients based on magnetic resonance imaging (MRI) at either 1-year or 10-year follow-up [4]. Solheim et al. (2018) performed a level 1 study evaluating microfracture versus mosaicplasty OAT at minimum of 15-year follow-up.

The mean Lysholm scores were significantly higher, and clinically significant, for the OAT group versus the pre-operative scores at all time points, as well as compared to the microfracture group at all time points at 12 months, 5 years, 10 years, and 15 years [5]. In a level 2 comparative study, Jungmann et al. also followed patients with nonoperatively treated cartilage injuries against those treated with OAT and reported decreased progression of degenerative MRI changes at a mean of 6 years [14] (Table 22.1).

22.4.2 Cost-Effectiveness

Everhart et al. investigated the cost-effectiveness of each of the cartilage treatments over a 10-year follow-up [6]. In their systematic review, they reported that in their baseline model all treatments (microfracture, OAT, OCA, ACI) were cost-effective; however, when incorporating a minimal clinical difference, microfracture as the initial treatment for lesions over 3 cm^2 was found to be the least cost-effective, while microfracture for lesions under 3 cm^2 and OAT (evaluated separately as 1 or 2 plugs and 3 or 4 plugs) were the most cost-effective treatments [6]. In a similar

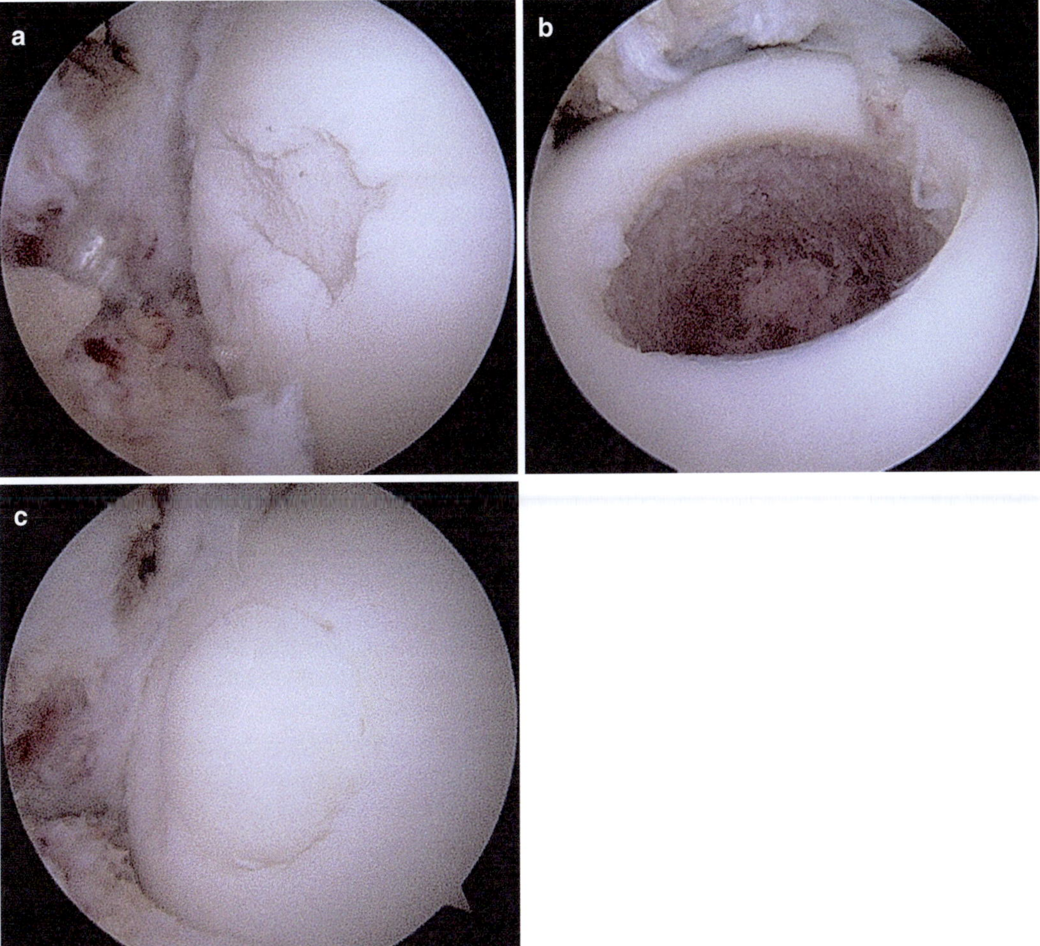

Fig. 22.4 (**a**) Intraoperative arthroscopy photograph of an osteochondral defect. (**b**) Photograph demonstrating the recipient site that has been debrided to create perpen- dicular walls around the defect to ensure bone-to-bone healing. (**c**) Photograph showing the final construct after osteochondral autologous transplantation (OAT)

study evaluating the different procedures (microfracture, OAT, OCA, ACI), Jones et al. demonstrated that OAT and ACI met the minimal clinical important difference (MCID) values at short-, medium-, and long-term follow-up in terms of International Knee Documentation Committee (IKDC), Lysholm, and Visual Analog Scale (VAS) pain for all available data, while microfracture did not meet the VAS pain levels at medium-term follow-up (and lacked any available long-term data for any of the above clinical outcome scales) [8].

22.4.3 Return-to-Sport

Given that many patients undergoing OAT are active athletes, two recent reviews have investigated the return-to-sport following different treatments [7, 16]. These studies found similar outcomes with OAT having a significantly improved return-to-sport in comparison to microfracture [7], with both studies reporting the highest rate of return-to-sport with OAT (89–93%) in comparison to OCA (88% for both), ACI (82–84%), and microfracture (58–75%) [7, 16]. In

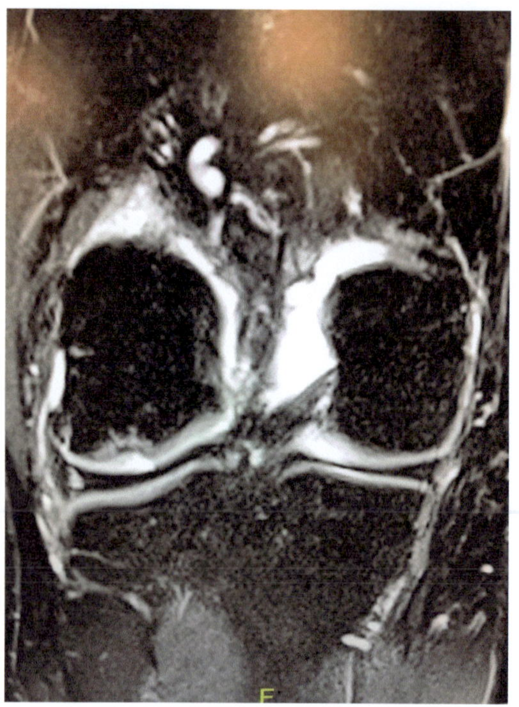

Fig. 22.5 T2 weighted coronal magnetic resonance imaging (MRI) demonstrating a lateral femoral condyle osteochondral defect prior to surgical intervention. Typical indications recommend lesions between 1 and 2 cm in diameter (1–4 cm²) as being optimal candidates for osteochondral autologous transplantation (OAT)

addition, Krych et al. reported OAT was resulted in a significantly shorter in time to return-to-sport (at an average of 5 months) than OCA, ACI, and microfracture [16].

22.4.4 Contrasting Findings

It should be noted that not all clinical studies have demonstrated improved clinical outcomes or significantly better outcomes than alternative therapies. Pareek et al. (2016) reported on a systematic review of outcomes after OAT at a 10-year follow-up and found that while IKDC and Lysholm clinical outcome scores significantly increased, the Tegner scores did not significantly change [17].

Lim et al. had a level 2 study comparing microfracture to ACI and OAT and did not find a significant difference in Lysholm, Tegner, or HSS scores at minimum 3-year follow-up [15]. In addition, Ulstein et al. reported on a level 2 study, at a median follow-up of 10 years comparing microfracture or OAT mosaicplasty [18]. They did not report significant differences between Lysholm, KOOS, isokinetic muscle strength, and radiographic osteoarthritis based on the Kellgren-Lawrence scale [18]. It should be noted that the total patient populations in both level 2 studies were low (25 and 30 patients, respectively), while one was limited to an average of 5-year follow-up [15], while the other included lesions up to 6 cm², which is above the recommended surgical indications for OAT [18].

22.4.5 Complications

Recent studies have investigated the complication rates of cartilage procedures. Gowd et al. reported that both open and arthroscopic OAT procedures resulted in less than 2% complication rates at 30-day follow-up, with no significant difference between different cartilage procedures [10]. In a systematic review with a 10-year follow-up, it was reported that the reoperation rate after OAT was 19% with a clinical failure of 29% [17].

A systematic review evaluated the donor-site morbidity that occurs after OAT mosaicplasty and reported approximately 5.9% in 1473 knee-to-knee transfers and 16.9% in 268 knee-to-talus transfers. There was no correlation between size of the defect and the number and size of the plugs [19]. Other studies have reported on donor-site morbidity after transfer from the knee to the talus (6.7% to 10.8% in a meta-analysis) [20] and capitellum (12.8%) [21].

22.5 Basic Science Studies

There are very few biomechanical studies in the literature; however, there are few studies investigating the effect of graft orientation in the knee joint. Walter et al. (2020) measured friction using dissipated energy (DE) and found that leaving

Table 22.1 Table summarizing the clinical outcome studies for osteochondral autograft transplantation (OAT)

Study	Level of evidence	Number of patients	Follow-up (mean years)	Results
Campbell et al. (2016) [7]	Level IV, Systematic review	1117	3.6	OAT with significantly higher return-to-sport than MF (89% vs 75%)
Everhart et al. (2020) [6]	Level IV, Systematic review	1145	8.6	Systematic review of 22 studies demonstrated OAT and MF for lesions <3 cm^2 were most cost-effective, MF >3 cm^2 were not cost-effective when including MCID
Gudas et al. (2012) [4]	Level I, RCT	57	10.4	OAT with significantly lower rate of failure and higher ICRS and Tegner scores vs OAT at minimum 9-year follow-up
Jones et al. (2019) [8]	Level IV, Systematic review and meta-analysis	3894	Varying	OAT met MCID for all available clinical outcome scores, MF did not meet MCID for VAS pain in the mid-term (long-term was not available for MF)
Jungmann et al. (2019) [14]	Level II, Retrospective cohort	32	5.7	OAT with decreased progression of degenerative changes on MRI vs nonoperatively treated cartilage lesions
Krych et al. (2016) [16]	Level IV, Systematic review	2549	3.9	OAT with significantly higher return-to-sport (93% vs 58%) and faster return-to-sport vs MF
Lim et al. (2012) [15]	Level II, Prospective cohort	30	5	At mid-term follow-up, there was no significant difference between OAT and MF for Lysholm, HSS, or Tegner scales
Pareek et al. (2016) [17]	Level IV, Systematic review	610	10.2	At 10-year follow-up, OAT resulted in significantly higher IKDC and Lysholm scores, while Tegner scores were not significantly different
Solheim et al. (2018) [5]	Level I, RCT	40	16	Lysholm scores were significantly higher for the OAT group vs MF at all time points in a minimum 15-year follow-up
Ulstein et al. (2014) [18]	Level II, Prospective cohort	25	9.8	OAT and MF without significant differences in Lysholm, KOOS, isokinetic muscle strength, or radiographic changes

RCT randomized controlled trial, *MF* microfracture, *OAT* osteochondral autologous transplantation, *MRI* magnetic resonance imaging, *MCID* minimal clinically significant difference, *VAS* visual analog scale, *IKDC* international knee documentation committee, *HSS* hospital for special surgery, *KOOS* knee injury and osteoarthritis outcome score

grafts 1 mm proud led to significantly increased DE versus the native knee. This effect was not found for grafts 1 mm deep [22]. In a similar study using peak contact pressures using a swine model, Koh et al. found that grafts elevated and sunk both 0.5 and 1 mm all resulted in increased pressures versus native knees [23]. Lastly, Bauer et al. evaluated the alignment of graft alignment and found no difference between aligned and 90° rotated grafts [24].

In an in vivo canine model, McCarthy et al. investigated OAT vs OCA at a 1-year follow-up [25]. This study found that there were no significant differences between the groups in terms of histologic evidence of hyaline cartilage, biome-chanical testing through use of indentation testing, radiographic evaluation of joint space narrowing, ICRS scores, or MRI evaluation of bony incorporation [25].

22.6 Conclusion

Osteochondral autograft transplantation (OAT) is becoming increasing utilized as a treatment option for focal small cartilage and osteochondral defects. This article reviews the surgical technique and surgical indications for this procedure. Clinical outcome studies have demonstrated promising initial results for OAT, with the need for further randomized controlled trials to evaluate the long-term effectiveness of OAT versus other available techniques.

References

1. Hjelle K, Solheim E, Strand T, Muri R, Brittberg M. Articular cartilage defects in 1,000 knee arthroscopies. Arthroscopy. 2002;18(7):730–4.
2. Widuchowski W, Widuchowski J, Trzaska T. Articular cartilage defects: study of 25,124 knee arthroscopies. Knee. 2007;14(3):177–82.
3. Heir S, Nerhus TK, Røtterud JH, et al. Focal cartilage defects in the knee impair quality of life as much as severe osteoarthritis: a comparison of knee injury and osteoarthritis outcome score in 4 patient categories scheduled for knee surgery. Am J Sports Med. 2010;38(2):231–7.
4. Gudas R, Gudaite A, Pocius A, et al. Ten-year follow-up of a prospective, randomized clinical study of mosaic osteochondral autologous transplantation versus microfracture for the treatment of osteochondral defects in the knee joint of athletes. Am J Sports Med. 2012;40(11):2499–508.
5. Solheim E, Hegna J, Strand T, Harlem T, Inderhaug E. Randomized study of long-term (15-17 years) outcome after microfracture versus mosaicplasty in knee articular cartilage defects. Am J Sports Med. 2018;46(4):826–31.
6. Everhart JS, Campbell AB, Abouljoud MM, Kirven JC, Flanigan DC. Cost-efficacy of knee cartilage defect treatments in the United States. Am J Sports Med. 2020;48(1):242–51.
7. Campbell AB, Pineda M, Harris JD, Flanigan DC. Return to sport after articular cartilage repair in athletes' knees: a systematic review. Arthroscopy. 2016;32(4):651–668.e1.
8. Jones KJ, Kelley BV, Arshi A, McAllister DR, Fabricant PD. Comparative effectiveness of cartilage repair with respect to the minimal clinically important difference. Am J Sports Med. 2019;47(13):3284–93.
9. Frank RM, Cotter EJ, Hannon CP, Harrast JJ, Cole BJ. Cartilage restoration surgery: incidence rates, complications, and trends as reported by the American Board of Orthopaedic Surgery part II candidates. Arthroscopy. 2019;35(1):171–8.
10. Gowd AK, Cvetanovich GL, Liu JN, et al. Management of chondral lesions of the knee: analysis of trends and short-term complications using the national surgical quality improvement program database. Arthroscopy. 2019;35(1):138–46.
11. Sherman SL, Thyssen E, Nuelle CW. Osteochondral autologous transplantation. Clin Sports Med. 2017;36(3):489–500.
12. Inderhaug E, Solheim E. Osteochondral autograft transplant (mosaicplasty) for knee articular cartilage defects. JBJS Essent Surg Tech. 2019;9(4):e34.1–2.
13. Chahla J, Stone J, Mandelbaum BR. How to manage cartilage injuries? Arthroscopy. 2019;35(10):2771–3.
14. Jungmann PM, Gersing AS, Baumann F, et al. Cartilage repair surgery prevents progression of knee degeneration. Knee Surg Sports Traumatol Arthrosc. 2019;27(9):3001–13.
15. Lim HC, Bae JH, Song SH, Park YE, Kim SJ. Current treatments of isolated articular cartilage lesions of the knee achieve similar outcomes. Clin Orthop Relat Res. 2012;470(8):2261–7.
16. Krych AJ, Pareek A, King AH, Johnson NR, Stuart MJ, Williams RJ 3rd. Return to sport after the surgical management of articular cartilage lesions in the knee: a meta-analysis. Knee Surg Sports Traumatol Arthrosc. 2017;25(10):3186–96.
17. Pareek A, Reardon PJ, Maak TG, Levy BA, Stuart MJ, Krych AJ. Long-term outcomes after osteochondral autograft transfer: a systematic review at mean follow-up of 10.2 years. Arthroscopy. 2016;32(6):1174–84.
18. Ulstein S, Årøen A, Røtterud JH, Løken S, Engebretsen L, Heir S. Microfracture technique versus osteochondral autologous transplantation mosaicplasty in patients with articular chondral lesions of the knee: a prospective randomized trial with long-term follow-up. Knee Surg Sports Traumatol Arthrosc. 2014;22(6):1207–15.
19. Andrade R, Vasta S, Pereira R, et al. Knee donor-site morbidity after mosaicplasty—a systematic review. J Exp Orthop. 2016;3(1):31.
20. Shimozono Y, Seow D, Yasui Y, Fields K, Kennedy JG. Knee-to-talus donor-site morbidity following autologous osteochondral transplantation: a meta-analysis with best-case and worst-case analysis. Clin Orthop Relat Res. 2019;477(8):1915–31.
21. Matsuura T, Hashimoto Y, Kinoshita T, et al. Donor site evaluation after osteochondral autograft transplantation for capitellar osteochondritis dissecans. Am J Sports Med. 2019;47(12):2836–43.
22. Walter C, Trappe D, Beck A, Jacob C, Hofmann UK. Effect of graft positioning on dissipated energy in knee osteochondral autologous transplantation-A biomechanical study. J Orthop Res. 2020;38(8):1727–34.
23. Koh JL, Wirsing K, Lautenschlager E, Zhang LO. The effect of graft height mismatch on contact pressure following osteochondral grafting: a biomechanical study. Am J Sports Med. 2004;32(2):317–20.
24. Bauer C, Göçerler H, Niculescu-Morzsa E, et al. Effect of osteochondral graft orientation in a biotribological test system. J Orthop Res. 2019;37(3):583–92.
25. McCarthy EC, Fader RR, Mitchell JJ, Glenn RE Jr, Potter HG, Spindler KP. Fresh osteochondral allograft versus autograft: twelve-month results in isolated canine knee defects. Am J Sports Med. 2016;44(9):2354–65.

Osteochondral Allograft Transplantation

23

Luís Eduardo Tírico, Marco Kawamura Demange, and William Bugbee

23.1 Introduction

Fresh osteochondral allograft transplantation is a procedure that utilizes mature hyaline cartilage with living chondrocytes that are capable of supporting the cartilage matrix [1]. Hyaline cartilage possesses characteristics that make it attractive for transplantation. It is an avascular tissue, and therefore does not require a blood supply, meeting its metabolic needs through diffusion from synovial fluid. It is an aneural structure and does not require innervation for function. It is relatively immunoprivileged, as the chondrocytes are imbedded within a matrix

L. E. Tírico · M. K. Demange (✉)
Orthopedic Surgery, Hospital das Clinicas HCMFUSP, Faculdade de Medicina, University of São Paulo, São Paulo, São Paulo, Brazil
e-mail: luis.tirico@hc.fm.usp.br; demange@usp.br; marco.demange@hc.fm.usp.br

W. Bugbee
Department of Orthopaedic Surgery, Scripps Clinic, La Jolla, CA, USA

Joint Reconstruction and Replacement, Scripps Clinic, La Jolla, CA, USA

Cartilage Restoration Service, Scripps Clinic, La Jolla, CA, USA

Lower Extremity Joint Reconstruction, Scripps Clinic, La Jolla, CA, USA

Shiley Center for Orthopaedic Research and Education, Scripps Clinic, La Jolla, CA, USA
e-mail: bugbee.william@scrippshealth.org

and are relatively protected from host immune surveillance. It has been shown that chondrocytes remain viable for up to 6 weeks during hypothermal storage in nutritive culture medium which gives the surgeon an acceptable therapeutic window [2–4].

The other component of the osteochondral allograft (OCA) is the osseous portion. This functions generally as a support for the articular cartilage, as well as a vehicle to allow attachment and fixation of the graft to the host. The osseous portion of the graft is quite different from the hyaline portion, as it is a vascularized tissue, and cells are not thought to survive transplantation; rather, the osseous structure functions as a scaffold for healing to the host by creeping substitution. Generally, the osseous portion of the graft is limited to a few millimeters. It is helpful to consider a fresh osteochondral allograft as a composite graft of both bone and cartilage, with a living mature hyaline cartilage portion and a non-living subchondral bone portion. It is also important to understand that allografting procedure is a tissue or organ transplantation, as the graft essentially is transplanted as an intact structural and functional unit replacing a diseased or absent component in the recipient joint. The transplantation of mature hyaline cartilage obviates the need to rely on techniques that induce cells to form cartilage tissue, which are central to other restorative procedures.

© ISAKOS 2021
A. J. Krych et al. (eds.), *Cartilage Injury of the Knee*,
https://doi.org/10.1007/978-3-030-78051-7_23

23.2 History

The concept of treating articular cartilage diseases with bone and cartilage substitution in the knee has now a history of more than a century since the first joint transplantation was described by Lexer in 1908 [5]. Lexer published his early experience with "joint allotransplantation" by three different methods; half joint replacement, both articular surfaces replacement and total joint transplantation, including joint capsule. All transplants were obtained by fresh amputated legs at the same day of surgery. However, he acknowledged that joint transplantation is not an easy procedure and that he was not able to promise successful and permanent results. By 1925, Lexer had documented 34 hemi or whole knee allogenic implants in humans and reported a 50% success rate. Animal and clinical studies concerning transplantation and immunology were carried out in the 1970s, demonstrating that transplanted fresh cadaver cartilage is viable [6–8]. Gross and colleagues began reporting on their experience with small fragment and partial joint osteochondral allografts for post-traumatic and peri-articular tumor reconstruction [9, 10]. In the 1980s, Meyers and Convery first applied this technique to specific chondral and osteochondral diseases such as chondromalacia, osteoarthritis, and osteonecrosis, developing the shell-shaped graft [11, 12]. Later in the 1990s, Garrett first reported on the use of allograft plugs for the treatment of osteochondritis dissecans of the knee [13]. In the last 20 years, a large number of basic scientific and clinical studies have been performed. These studies and the expansion of availability of fresh allografts have led to an increasing popularity of fresh allografts and the inclusion of this procedure as part of the cartilage repair paradigm for the treatment of chondral or osteochondral lesions in the knee [14–18].

Historically, the obstacles presented have led to the development of fresh allograft programs only at specialized centers that have a close association with an experienced tissue bank and have put significant investment of resources into setting up protocols specific for safe and effective transplantation of fresh osteochondral tissue.

Recently, fresh osteochondral grafts have become commercially available in North America, and thus more accessible to the orthopedic surgical community. The age criterion for the donor pool for fresh grafts is generally between 15 and 40 years of age. The joint surface must also pass a visual inspection for cartilage quality. These criteria ensure, but do not guarantee, acceptable tissue for transplantation. It is extremely important to acknowledge that fresh human tissue is unique, and no two donors have the same characteristics. Adherence to tissue-banking standards and to protocols and processes in quality control are critical for both safety and efficacy of fresh allografts. Storage of fresh osteochondral allografts prior to transplantation is an important consideration. Historically, fresh grafts were transplanted within 7 days of donor death, obviating the need for prolonged tissue storage. Current tissue bank protocols call for prolonged storage of fresh osteochondral allografts (for up to 60 days) while processing and donor testing is completed. Recent studies on allograft storage have shown significant deterioration in cell viability, cell density, and metabolic activity with prolonged storage of fresh osteochondral allografts. Small but statistically significant changes are first detected after storage for 7 days; these changes are pronounced after storage for 28 days [19]. A recent study analyzed the clinical consequences of these storage-induced graft changes and demonstrated that storage up to 28 days prior to allograft implantation does not appear to significantly affect the clinical outcome of osteochondral allografting compared to a short-term storage and implantation within 7 days, despite the fact that chondrocyte viability decreases over storage time [20].

23.3 Immunology

The cornerstone of an allografting procedure is the availability of fresh osteochondral tissue. The rationale for fresh tissue is predicated on the concept of maximizing the quality of the articular cartilage in the graft. It has been demonstrated, primarily through retrieval studies, that viable chondrocytes and relatively preserved cartilage matrix are present many years after transplantation. These experiences have generally supported the use of fresh versus frozen tissue for small osteochondral allografts in the setting of reconstruction of chondral and osteochondral defects. Currently, small-fragment osteochondral allografts are not HLA or blood type-matched, and are utilized fresh, rather than frozen or processed. In addition, post-allograft patients received no immunosuppressive medication regimen to prevent an immune-mediated response. Despite current practices, the success rate of osteochondral allografts has been high enough to support its continued implementation [21–25]. However, the immunologic ramifications of this procedure remain an important consideration and might allow its use to further improve this treatment and prevent graft failures secondary to host rejection. While graft failure is often identified by radiographic evidence of bony nonunion, late fragmentation, graft collapse or fracture, and/or cartilage deterioration [26], few studies investigate cellular and/or structural causes for such failures. Research to date has revealed several important factors in graft survival, including cartilage cell viability after storage and effective osseous support [27, 28]. Despite no clear demonstration in prior studies, the host's immunologic response might also play a key role in the success of osteochondral allografts [29].

Historically, osteochondral allograft immunology has been studied for use in tumor reconstruction. It is well understood that allograft immunogenicity is reduced by freezing or freeze-drying techniques [8, 30, 31]; however, these methods of preserving allografts are known to cause a significant decrease in viable chondrocytes available to sustain the hyaline cartilage allograft tissue [32]. Studies have clearly revealed that isolated articular chondrocytes and matrix components are immunogenic but the intact hyaline cartilage matrix is relatively immunoprivileged [30, 33]. Observations suggest that the intact articular matrix protects the chondrocytes because of its structure, therefore making it difficult for cell-surface antigens to be recognized by the body's immune system.

The role of the host immune system with potential graft rejection has not been clearly determined. Two retrieval studies of human failed fresh osteochondral allografts showed little or no histologic evidence of immune-mediated response and no evidence of frank transplant rejection [26, 34]. Conversely, studies by Stevenson [35] in canines and Sirlin et al. [36] in humans have shown sensitization to fresh osteochondral allograft transplants with the development of anti-HLA class I antibodies in a significant number of allograft recipients. These studies demonstrate activating the recipient's humoral immune system and validating the potential interplay between the host body's immune system and fresh osteochondral graft rejection.

A study performed by Hunt et al. [29] evaluated the relationship between total graft area and development of antibodies and the effect of post-allograft antibody formation on clinical outcomes. Patients that had negative preoperative anti-HLA class I cytotoxic antibody screen that converted to a positive antibody response postoperatively were matched to a similar group who were negative pre- and postoperatively for anti-HLA class I cytotoxic antibodies. There were no significant differences in failure type, failure rate, time to failure, graft type, graft area, or graft location between antibody-positive and antibody-negative groups. At last follow-up, no significant difference was found on clinical scores for the surviving anti-HLA antibody-positive and antibody-negative groups ($P = 0.482$). However, the authors found that the development of anti-HLA cytotoxic antibodies after fresh, non-matched osteochondral allograft transplantation of the knee appears to be related to graft size. A large osteochondral graft (>10 cm^2) was 36 times more likely to elicit an antibody response than a small graft (<5 cm^2) ($P < 0.05$). Although in this study the authors evaluated the incidence of antibody formation and the effect on graft performance and clinical outcome, it should be noted that little is known about the potential systemic effects of development of anti-HLA antibodies. Studies designed to investigate the relationship between graft size and levels of circulating antibodies, in comparison to types of allograft failure, would be useful to elucidate some of the subtle details associated with the immunogenic response due to the implanted allografts.

The HLA matching of all allograft patients with the allograft donor is logistically difficult and expensive. If future studies confirm the effect of HLA antigens on the clinical outcome of osteochondral allografting, HLA typing may be a necessary. The obstacles incurred while putting this into practice would be considerable. Not only the expense of the immunologic testing but also the vast size of the donor pool required to support histocompatibility and graft size requirements would have to be considered. Presently, a shortage of allograft tissue available for transplanting exists and the inclusion of HLA typing would adversely affect this already limited resource. Until definitive evidence is available, matching will likely remain optional.

23.4 Allograft Recovery, Processing, and Storage

Understanding the process of tissue procurement, testing, and storage is critically important in the allografting procedure.

Prior to 1998, the use of fresh OCA in North America was restricted to a few institutions which maintained their own systems for retrieving, processing, and storing tissues for their own clinical use. These allografts were stored in lactated Ringer's solution, which could maintain the biochemical and biomechanical properties of the graft for 7 days, with transplantation within 1 week of donor death [37, 38]. Around 1999, OCAs became commercially available from tissue banks whose guidelines for procurement and processing were established by the American Association of Tissue Banks under oversight from the Food and Drug Administration (FDA) [39, 40]. Allograft tissue is harvested within 24 h of donor death, ideally from donors between the ages of 13 and 35 years old with grossly healthy articular cartilage.

Chondrocyte viability is critically important for maintenance of the material properties of the graft, which correlates directly with the clinical success of OCA transplantation [4, 19]. Chondrocytes maintain the extracellular matrix, thereby maintaining the material properties of the graft if they are kept viable in storage. Gross et al. demonstrated that long-term survival of OCAs in vivo depended on the presence of viable chondrocytes, intact extracellular matrix, and incorporation of host bone [1]. Furthermore, chondrocyte viability at the articular surface (superficial zone) is important for long-term graft survival. Following transplantation, several studies have demonstrated preservation of chondrocyte viability over time. Retrieval studies of OCAs after revision have shown high donor chondrocyte viability many years after transplantation [3]. The processing and storage of OCAs (frozen, cryopreserved, or fresh) has different effects on chondrocyte viability. Biomechanical and biochemical composition of cartilage deteriorates over storage time, correlating with decreasing chondrocyte viability [41]. Freezing grafts at −80 °C maintains less than 5% chondrocyte viability, and the extracellular matrix deteriorates due to a lack of viable chondrocytes to maintain the matrix [42, 43].

Currently, fresh OCAs maintain the highest chondrocyte viability among the available storage options [2, 44]. Chondrocyte viability begins to decrease, and biomechanical properties deteriorate in fresh OCAs stored hypothermically at 4 °C for greater than 7 days [2]. A 2009 study by Pallante et al. demonstrated increased chondrocyte viability throughout all zones when fresh grafts were stored at 37 °C as compared to 4 °C, with acceptable percentage (80%) of viable chondrocytes after 28 days of storage [45]. This study increased the effective length of time a graft could be stored prior to transplantation. This increased timeframe is critically important, as tissue banks currently hold OCA tissue until the completion of microbiologic and serologic testing is completed, generally a minimum of 14 days [46]. Other recent studies have also indicated that a transition of storage to physiologic (37 °C) or room temperature (25 °C) improves the viability of

OCAs during storage [44, 45]. Improved allograft processing that may safely allow for earlier graft implantation (as was practiced prior to commercialization) and storage technology that may increase chondrocyte viability and preserve extracellular matrix properties to allow longer storage to continue to be active areas of research.

There is tremendous interest outside the USA in fresh allograft technology. However numerous regulatory, logistic and cultural issues have historically been difficult to overcome. Setting up an allograft program outside the USA is facilitated by an association with an existing University affiliated tissue bank. In addition, every country has unique regulations that need to be considered, depending on whether the health care system is public or private, and if a current frozen transplantation program is already a routine.

23.5 Indications

Major indications for an OCA transplantation as a primary treatment for cartilage repair are symptomatic full-thickness chondral and subchondral defects greater than 2–3 cm^2 in diameter or focal lesions of ICRS grade III–IV with subchondral damage greater than 6–10 mm (i.e., OCD, focal avascular osteonecrosis, post-traumatic defects). Furthermore, it is indicated as a salvage procedure after primary failed cartilage restoration techniques, such as microfracture, osteochondral autograft transplantation (OAT), autologous chondrocyte implantation (ACI), or primary failed OCA transplantation (Complex Reconstruction).

Most commonly, OCA transplantation is used to treat femoral defects but in selected cases it is also possible to address tibial chondral defects (entire tibial and meniscal surface may be transplanted) or bipolar ("kissing") lesions of the femur, tibia, and patella. Osteochondral allografts are versatile when addressing even very large, complex, or multiple lesions in topographically challenging environments, especially if they involve an osseous component.

Table with indications?

Cartilage Repair
- Chondral or osteochondral defects larger than 2 cm^2
- Osteochondritis dissecans
- Revision of previous failed cartilage repair surgery
- Subchondral bone lesions without full-thickness cartilage defect

Complex Reconstruction
- Post-traumatic peri-articular fracture malunion
- Single compartment arthritis or multifocal degenerative lesions
- Massive type III or IV osteochondritis dissecans
- Osteonecrosis of the femoral condyle

23.6 Contraindications

Absolute Contraindications [47]
- Advanced multicompartmental OA
- Inflammatory arthropathies

Relative Contraindications
- Smoking
- Alcohol abuse
- Chronic steroid use
- Ligamentous instability
- Uncorrected joint malalignment
- Obesity (BMI >30 kg/m^2)
- Absence of >50% of the ipsilateral meniscus

Typically, there are no absolute age limitations but inferior outcomes have been reported in patients older than 40 years [47–50].

23.7 Preoperative Planning

When considering using OCA for cartilage repair the surgeon needs to understand that a compatible donor must be found in order to match the recipient defect characteristics with donor morphology and a scheduled surgical procedure with a specific date and time is not always possible. Many times, the patient receives notice that a donor is available 7–10 days before the surgical procedure, in order to perform transplantation of graft with high cell viability.

One of the main steps in an OCA procedure is matching the donor with the recipient. Currently, this is done by size alone. Small-fragment fresh osteochondral allografts are not human leukocyte antigen-(HLA-) or blood type-matched between donor and recipient and no immunosuppression is used. For exact perioperative planning, anteroposterior radiographs of the knee joint in full extension (weight bearing) are routinely used. The mediolateral dimension of the tibia, just below the joint surface is measured, correcting for magnification (Fig. 23.1). The donor graft is measured at the tissue bank performing a direct measurement on the donor tibial plateau using a caliper. In order to address additional pathologies, a series of standard radiographs needs to be done (including weight-bearing AP view with 45° knee flexion, lateral view, patellar view, and standing bilateral long-leg alignment view). Additionally, CT and MRI scans can be helpful

to assess the cartilage integrity, the extent of bone involvement as well as concomitant ligamentous and/or meniscal pathologies. CT and MRI can also be used to measure the width of the proximal tibia for matching donor and recipient (Fig. 23.2). Matching donor with the recipient is usually considered acceptable if the difference is between ±2 mm [51]. When performing a press-fit plug (dowel) technique, size of the donor tibial width should be equal or larger than the recipient, in order to have the convexity of the donor femoral condyle similar or flatter in shape comparing with the recipient. The true size of the articular lesion is often underestimated (up to 60%) within imaging diagnostics [52, 53]. Therefore, if applicable it is always helpful to examine images recorded during previous surgical procedures (i.e., arthroscopy). However, it should be noted that there is a significant variability in anatomy, which is not reflected in any preoperative imaging. In particular where the affected condyle is larger, flatter, and wider. In these cases, a larger donor should be used. It is the responsibility of the surgeon to inspect the graft and to confirm the adequacy of the size match and quality of the allograft tissue prior to surgery.

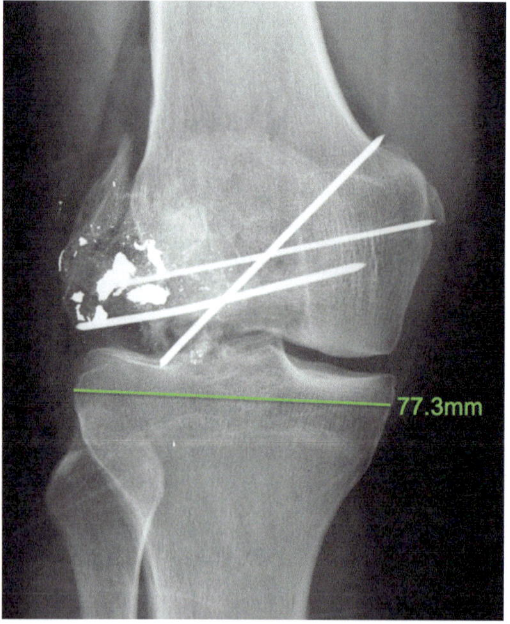

Fig. 23.1 Anteroposterior right knee radiograph with mediolateral proximal tibial plateau size measurement. Correction for magnification is imperative when using radiograph for matching. (All figures are from author's personal database)

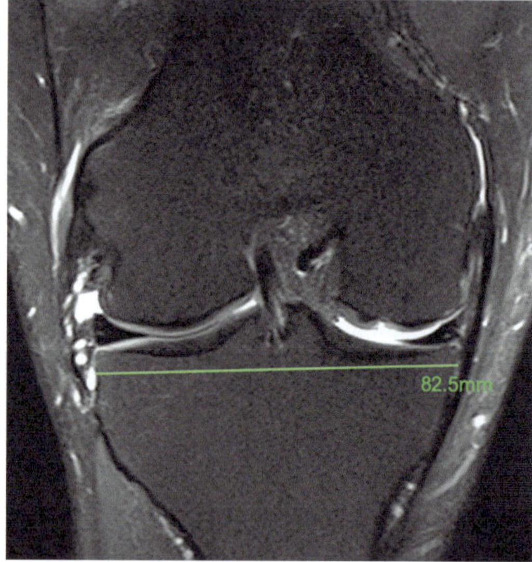

Fig. 23.2 MRI used to measure the width of the proximal tibia for matching donor and recipient. There is no need to correct for magnification when using MRI or CT scans. (All figures are from author's personal database)

23.8 Surgical Techniques

The two commonly used techniques for the preparation and implantation of osteochondral allografts include the press-fit plug technique and the shell graft technique. Each technique has advantages and disadvantages. The press-fit plug technique is a similar in principle to autologous osteochondral transfer (OAT). A number of commercially available instruments can be used to perform this type of procedure. This technique is optimal for contained condylar lesions between 15 and 35 mm in diameter. Fixation is generally not required due to the stability achieved with the press-fit. Disadvantages include the fact that very posterior femoral condyle and tibial plateau lesions are not conducive to the use of a circular coring system and may be more amenable to shell allografts. Additionally, the more ovoid or elongated a lesion is in shape, the more normal cartilage needs to be sacrificed at the recipient site in order to accommodate the circular donor plug. Shell grafts are technically more difficult to perform and typically require fixation. However, depending on the technique employed, less normal cartilage may need to be sacrificed.

23.8.1 Press-Fit Plug Technique

The surgical procedure is performed with the patient in a supine position. An anteromedial or anterolateral 5 cm arthrotomy is executed, depending where the lesion is located. The size of the lesion is recorded. When performing the dowel osteochondral allograft technique, a 2.5 mm Kirschner guide wire is drilled in the center of the lesion and 15–30 mm cylindrical templates is used to measure the appropriate size of the repair. The recipient site is debrided and prepared with circular reamers. Depth of the debridement is determined when healthy bleeding subchondral bone is encountered and is usually no more than 3–7 mm of subchondral bone, yielding a total prepared recipient site depth of 5–10 mm (Fig. 23.3a–d). Donor grafts are typically cored out at the exact same (orthotopic) location as the lesion on the recipient, and then

trimmed to the same thickness. Pulsatile lavage (1–2 L) is used on the donor graft, in order to wash out potentially immunogenic marrow elements from the osseous portion of the graft and to reduce overall allograft bioburden. The graft is then inserted by hand in the appropriate rotation, and then it is gently pressed into place manually and with manually cycling the joint. Finally, very gentle tamping is performed to fully seat the graft when needed (Fig. 23.4a–f). Fixation is achieved by a press-fit technique in the majority of cases with supplemental fixation using absorbable internal fixation devices in a minority of cases.

23.8.2 Press-Fit Plug Technique Postoperative Management

Initial postoperative management includes attention to control of pain, swelling, and restoration of limb control and range of motion. Patients generally are maintained on touch-down weight bearing for 4–6 weeks, depending on the size of the graft and stability of fixation. Patients with patellofemoral grafts are allowed weight bearing as tolerated in extension, and generally are limited to 45° of flexion for the first 4 weeks, utilizing an immobilizer or range-of-motion brace. Closed chain exercise such as cycling is introduced between weeks 2 and 4. Weight bearing is progressed slowly between the second and fourth month, with full weight bearing utilizing a cane or crutch. Full weight bearing and normal gait pattern are generally tolerated between the third and fourth month. Recreation and sports are not reintroduced until joint rehabilitation is complete and radiographic healing has been demonstrated, which generally occurs no earlier than 4–6 months postoperatively.

23.8.3 Shell Technique

Although the press-fit plug technique is generally preferred for most lesions, the surgeon should be prepared to perform a shell graft if the lesion size or location do not allow for proper placement of the dowel graft instru-

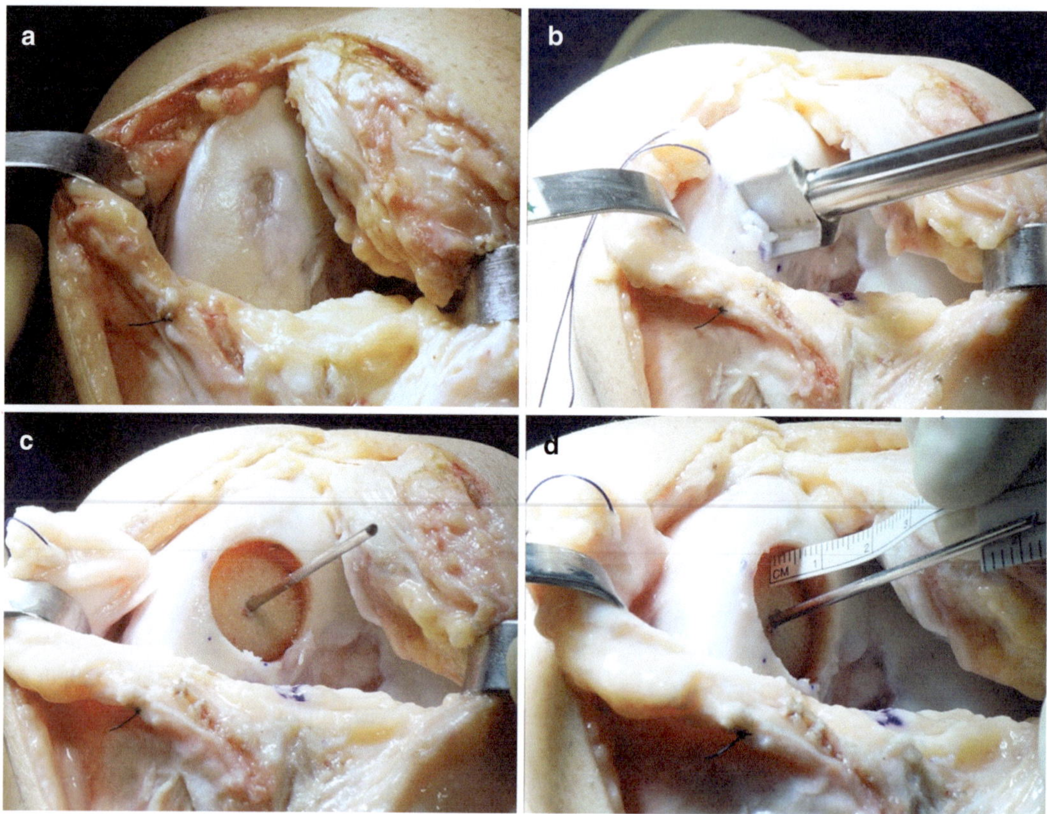

Fig. 23.3 (a) Image of osteochondritis dissecans on the medial femoral condyle. (b) Recipient site debridement and preparation with circular reamer. (c) Depth of the debridement is determined when healthy bleeding subchondral bone is encountered. (d) Depth measurement in four quadrants, usually the total prepared recipient site depth is no more than 5–11 mm. (All figures are from author's personal database)

ments. For the shell graft technique, the defect is identified through the previously described arthrotomy, and the dimensions of the lesion are marked with a surgical pen. Commonly, a more extended surgical approach is needed when performing a shell technique, once allografts are usually larger in size or lesions are located in areas of difficult access through small incisions. Using motorized burrs, sharp curettes, and osteotomes, the subchondral bone is removed down to a depth of 4–5 mm. The shape is transferred to the graft, using length, width and depth measurements or a foil template. Anatomical parameters of the recipient defect can be used to match size and location in the donor graft. A saw is used to cut the basic graft shape from the donor condyle, initially slightly over sizing the graft by a few millimeters. Excess bone and cartilage are removed as necessary through multiple trial fittings until a perfect fit is achieved. The graft and host bed are then copiously irrigated, and the graft is placed flush with the articular surface. The need for fixation is based on the degree of inherent stability. Compression screws can be used for fixation (Fig. 23.5a–h). After cycling the knee through a full range of motion to ensure graft stability, standard closure is performed. Initial postoperative management includes attention to control of pain, swelling, and restoration of limb control and range of motion. Patients generally are main-

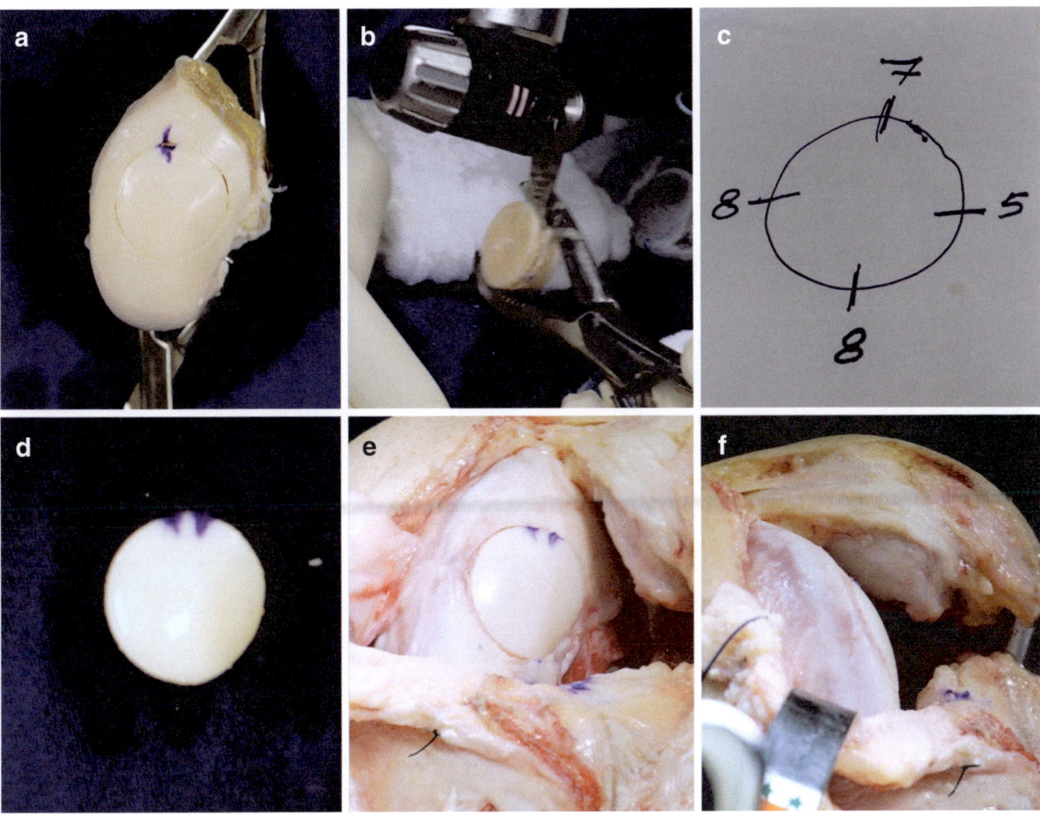

Fig. 23.4 (**a**) Donor grafts are cored out at the exact same (orthotopic) location as the lesion on the recipient. (**b**) Trimming of the graft to the same thickness as the recipient socket. (**c**) Recipient socket depth template in four quadrants. (**d**) Final plug before implantation. (**e**) The graft inserted in the appropriate rotation. (**f**) Lateral view of the graft, matching host condylar curvature. A flush position to the articular surface should be aimed. (All figures are from author's personal database)

tained on touch-down weight bearing for 4–6 weeks, depending on the size of the graft and stability of fixation. Patients with patellofemoral grafts are allowed weight bearing as tolerated in extension, and generally are limited to 45° of flexion for the first 4 weeks, utilizing an immobilizer or range-of-motion brace. Closed chain exercise such as cycling is introduced between weeks 2 and 4. Full weight bearing is progressed slowly between the second and fourth month utilizing a cane or crutch. Full weight bearing and normal gait pattern are generally tolerated between the third and fourth month. Recreation and sports are not reintroduced until joint rehabilitation is complete and radiographic healing has been demonstrated, which generally occurs no earlier than 6 months postoperatively.

23.8.4 Shell Technique Postoperative Management

Initial postoperative management includes attention to control of pain, swelling, and restoration of limb control and range of motion. Patients generally are maintained on touch-down weight bearing for 4–6 weeks, depending on the size of the graft and stability of fixation. Patients with patellofemoral grafts are allowed weight bearing as tolerated in extension, and generally are limited to 45° of flexion for the first 4 weeks, utilizing an immobilizer or range-of-motion brace. Closed chain exercise such as cycling is introduced between weeks 2 and 4. Weight bearing is progressed slowly between the second and fourth month, with full weight bearing utilizing a cane or crutch. Full weight bearing and normal gait pattern are gener-

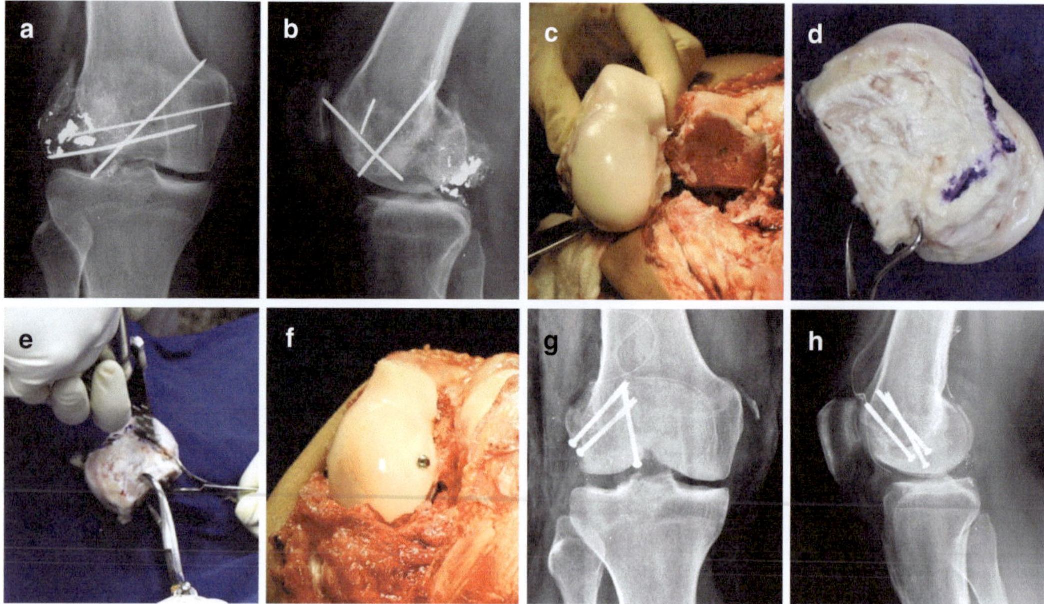

Fig. 23.5 (**a**) Right knee anteroposterior radiographic view showing a complex comminuted fracture of the lateral femoral condyle, with previous failed fixation. (**b**) Lateral view showing a large fragment of the posterior portion of the lateral femoral condyle displaced and fragmented from the distal femur. (**c**) Large anterolateral parapatellar incision. A saw blade was used to cut the recipient condyle in its distal and posterior parts, with a 90° angle to increase stability following fixation. Donor's lateral femoral condyle that will be prepared for transplantation. (**d**) Photograph of the donor femoral condyle. A marking pen was used to match recipient's defect and donor's condyle measurements, to obtain a perfect match. (**e**) A free-hand technique using a saw blade is utilized to prepare the donor femoral condyle. (**f**) Transplantation of the lateral femoral condyle and fixation with metal screws avoiding the weight-bearing part of the condyle. (**g**) Postoperative right knee anteroposterior radiographic view showing restoration of the anatomy and shape of the lateral femoral condyle. (**h**) Lateral radiographic view showing the contour of the transplanted lateral femoral condyle, matching the native anatomy. Matching size of donor and recipient is extremely important when performing a shell allograft technique. (All figures are from author's personal database)

ally tolerated between the third and fourth month. Recreation and sports are not reintroduced until joint rehabilitation is complete and radiographic healing has been demonstrated, which generally occurs no earlier than 6 months postoperatively.

23.9 Outcomes of Fresh Osteochondral Allograft Transplantation

23.9.1 Factors Affecting Outcome

23.9.1.1 Age

There are an abundance of studies that have described age-related decline in chondrocyte function, such as reductions in proliferative potential, sulfated glycosaminoglycan production, collagen deposition, and responsiveness to growth factors [54, 55]. In this way, it is logical that younger patients have better clinical outcome scores and better repair cartilage fill on magnetic resonance imaging (MRI) in different cartilage repair strategies [56–59].

A study performed by Murphy et al. [25] analyzed outcomes of osteochondral allograft transplantation of the knee in the pediatric and adolescent population in patients younger than 18 years with a focus on subjective outcome measures and allograft survivorship. A total of 39 patients (43 knees), with a mean age of 16.4 years (range, 11.0–17.9 years), underwent OCA transplantation for treatment of chondral and osteochondral lesions. The most common underlying causes of the lesions were osteochondritis dissecans (61%), avascular necrosis (16%), and traumatic chondral injury (14%) and the mean allograft size was 8.4 cm². Five knees experienced clinical failure at a median of 2.7 years (range, 1.0–14.7 years). The authors reported four failures that were successfully revised with another allograft and one patient underwent prosthetic arthroplasty 8.6 years after revision allograft. Graft survivorship was 90% at 10 years. The mean International Knee Documentation Committee (IKDC) scores improved from 42 preoperatively to 75 postoperatively, and the Knee Society function (KS-f) score improved from 69 to 89 (both $P < 0.05$). The authors concluded that OCA transplantation is a useful treatment option in pediatric and adolescent patients with 88% good/excellent results and 80% salvage rate of clinical failures with an additional allograft.

The effect of patient age on outcomes after OCA was also studied by Frank et al. [60] comparing patients aged ≥40 years compared with a group of patients aged <40 years of age. In an analysis of a prospective collective data of patients with minimum follow-up of 2 years, reoperation rate, failure rate, and patient-reported outcome scores were reviewed. Failure was defined as revision OCA, conversion to knee arthroplasty, or gross appearance of graft failure at second-look arthroscopic surgery. A total of 170 patients who underwent OCA with a mean follow-up of 5.0 ± 2.7 years (range, 2.0–15.1 years) were included, with 115 patients aged <40 years (mean age, 27.6 ± 7.3 years) and 55 patients aged ≥40 years (mean age, 44.9 ± 4.0 years). The authors found no differences in the number of previous procedures between the groups ($P = 0.085$) and no differences in the reoperation rate (<40 years: 38%; ≥40 years: 36%; $P = 0.867$), time to reoperation (<40 years: 2.12 ± 1.90 years; ≥40 years: 3.43 ± 3.43 years; $P = 0.126$), or failure rate (<40 years: 13%; ≥40 years: 16%; $P = 0.639$) between the older and younger groups. Patients in both groups demonstrated significant improvement in Lysholm, IKDC, and Knee Injury and Osteoarthritis Outcome Score (KOOS), Western

Ontario and McMaster Universities Osteoarthritis Index (WOMAC), and Short Form-12 (SF-12) physical (all: $P < 0.001$) scores compared with preoperative values. Interesting findings were that patients aged ≥40 years demonstrated significantly higher KOOS symptom ($P = 0.015$) subscores compared with patients aged <40 years and patients aged <40 years demonstrated lower KOOS symptom subscores postoperatively compared with older patients, potentially attributable to higher expectations of return to function postoperatively as compared with older patients. The same finding that age doesn't influence outcome following OCA was described by Nuelle et al. [60] comparing patients that were successfully treated with OCA (53 patients, 71%) and patients that were unsuccessful following OCA. Success was defined by analysis of Visual Analog Scale (VAS) pain score of 0 or improvement in score (decrease) of 2 or more at final follow-up. According to authors, patients with successful outcomes were younger on average (33.0 vs 37.2 years); however, this difference in age was not statistically significant ($P = 0.23$).

A recent study performed by Wang et al. [50] evaluated outcomes of OCA transplantation of the knee in patients aged 40 years and older characterized survivorship, predictors of failure, and clinical outcomes of osteochondral allograft transplantation (OCA) of the knee among this cohort. Failure was defined by any removal or revision of the allograft or conversion to arthroplasty. The authors reported that among 51 patients (mean age, 48 years; range, 40–63 years; 65% male), a total of 52 knees had symptomatic focal cartilage lesions (up to 2 affected areas) that were classified as Outerbridge grade 4 at the time of OCA and did not involve substantial bone loss requiring shell allografts or additional bone grafting. The mean duration of follow-up was 3.6 years (range, 2–11 years). After OCA, 21 knees (40%) underwent reoperation, including 14 failures (27%) consisting of revision OCA ($n = 1$), unicompartmental knee arthroplasty ($n = 5$), and total knee arthroplasty ($n = 8$). Mean time to failure was 33 months, and 2- and 4-year survivorship rates were 88% and 73%, respectively. Male sex (hazard ratio = 4.18, 95%

CI = 1.12–27.13) and a higher number of previous ipsilateral knee operations (hazard ratio = 1.70 per increase in 1 surgical procedure, 95% CI = 1.03–2.83) were predictors of failure in this cohort. A more advanced grade in the Kellgren-Lawrence osteoarthritis classification on preoperative radiographs was associated with higher failure rates in the Kaplan-Meier analysis but not the multivariate model. At final follow-up, clinically significant improvements were noted in the pain (mean score, 47.8–67.6) and physical functioning (56.8–79.1) subscales of the Short Form-36, as well as the IKDC subjective form (45.0–63.6), KOOS-Activities of Daily Living (64.5–80.1), and overall condition statement (4.5–6.8) ($P < 0.001$). A higher failure rate was found in this series of patients aged ≥40 years who were treated with OCA as compared with other studies of younger populations. However, the authors concluded that for select older patients, OCA can be a good midterm treatment option for cartilage defects of the knee.

23.9.1.2　Location

Anatomic location of the osteochondral lesion and thus the allograft may correlate with clinical results. It is important to understand that clinical outcomes seen in one particular location cannot be translated to other locations, once each site of the knee has its own characteristics and can behave differently following OCA transplantation.

Clinical outcomes and survival of OCA transplantation for femoral condyles defects were studied by Tirico et al. [21] reporting on 200 knees that underwent OCA transplantation for isolated osteochondral lesions on the femoral condyle utilizing a thin-plug technique with commercially available surgical instruments. In this cohort, all patients that were treated with shell grafts were excluded. The medial femoral condyle was affected in 69% of knees. A single thin-plug graft was used in 145 knees (72.5%), and 2 grafts were used in 55 knees (27.5%). Mean allograft area treated was 6.3 cm^2, and graft thickness was 6.5 mm, where all grafts were prepared with the minimum amount of bone necessary for fixation. At last follow-up, patients had

clinically meaningful improvement in pain, function, and quality of life on IKDC and KOOS scores. Satisfaction following OCA procedure was reported by 89% of patients and survivorship of the allograft was 95.6% at 5 years and 91.2% at 10 years. Reoperations were performed in 52 knees (26%), of which 16 (8% of entire cohort) were defined as allograft failures (4 OCA revisions, 1 arthrosurface, 6 unicompartmental knee arthroplasties, and 5 total knee arthroplasties). The median time to failure was 4.9 years. OCA transplantation for femoral condyle osteochondral lesions with a thin-plug graft technique resulted in significant improvement in clinical scores, high patient satisfaction, and low reoperation and clinical failure rates.

Results of OCA transplantation in the patellofemoral joint was evaluated in a Systematic Review performed by Chahla et al. [22]. Their systematic search identified 8 studies with a total of 129 patients that were treated with OCA transplantation for patella, trochlea, or bipolar defects in the patellofemoral joint. The methods of graft procurement and storage time included fresh (121 patients, 93.8%), and cryopreserved (8 patients, 6.2%) grafts. The mean survival rate was 87.9% at 5 years and 77.2% at 10 years. All studies reported significant improvement in at least one clinical score. All four studies that utilized IKDC scores reported a significant improvement from baseline to postoperative follow-up ($P < 0.001$), with an aggregate preoperative IKDC score of 41.8 and postoperative IKDC score of 68.1. The aggregate mean improvement in total IKDC score from preoperative to final follow-up was 26.3. Studies with the modified D'Aubigné-Postel scores reported significant postoperative improvement ($P < 0.001$), with mean preoperative 12.2, and mean postoperative of 15.9. The aggregate mean preoperative KSS-F score was 53.4 and postoperative was 80.2. OCA transplantation for the patellofemoral joint yielded improved postoperative outcomes with high patient satisfaction and survival rates at short- to medium- and long-term follow-up. Additionally, although the mean reoperation rate was 51.6%, the most common reoperation performed was hardware removal (31.8%), which is common in all patellar realignment series. Finally, while heterogeneous definitions for failure were used among the reviewed studies, the overall mean failure rate was 20.1%, which is similar to various other biologic cartilage restorative procedures at the tibiofemoral compartments.

The use of fresh osteochondral allograft (FOCA) for post-traumatic tibial osteochondral defects was studied by Abolghasemian et al. [61] evaluating long-term outcomes of this procedure and factors impacting graft survivorship in patients treated with OCA transplantation for tibial plateau defects, associated or not to a realignment osteotomy. The authors studied 113 knees (15 medial and 98 lateral tibial defects), a meniscal allograft, and a realignment osteotomy were used in 77 (68%) and 74 (65%) of the cases, respectively. At a mean follow-up of 13.8 years (range, 1.7–34 years), 46 knees either had been converted to total knee arthroplasty or had surgical indication for this surgery, and in two additional cases, the patient had undergone reoperation with revision OCA, and thus, a total of 48 knees (48 patients) experienced failure of OCA transplantation. The mean time to failure was 11.6 years (range, 1.7–34 years) after the transplantation procedure. The remaining 65 patients had a mean follow-up of 15.5 years (range, 4.3–31.7 years). The Kaplan-Meier survival function analysis showed a graft survivorship of 90% at 5 years (95% confidence interval [CI], 83–94%), 79% at 10 years (95% CI, 70–86%), 64% at 15 years (95% CI, 53–73%), and 47% at 20 years (95% CI, 34–59%) following transplantation. This study suggests that OCA transplantation for post-traumatic tibial osteochondral defects results in favorable outcomes for over a decade, and while the outcome may be inferior to that of OCA procedures involving the femoral condyle, it is a viable treatment option for those of young age with large, traumatic osteochondral lesions of the tibial plateau, once usually the other surgical option in these patients is either an arthrodesis or some type of knee replacement. Older age at the time of surgery, involvement of the medial tibial plateau, and a higher number of previous surgeries adversely affected graft survivorship with this procedure.

23.9.1.3 Diagnosis

Diagnosis can also affect outcomes following OCA transplantation. In general, a focal chondral defect, commonly seen following an acute traumatic event or in patients with osteochondritis dissecans have better clinical outcomes than chronic degenerative lesions or in cases of early osteoarthritis. Recently, there has been an effort of expanding indications of OCA transplantation to more severe and chronic pathologies. However, outcomes and survivorship may not be as good as compared to other pathologies that presents with focal cartilage defects.

One of the best indications to perform an OCA transplantation is osteochondritis dissecans (OCD) of the knee. OCD lesions are typically found in young patients with pristine meniscal, ligament, and cartilage status, despite the single lesion of OCD. Fresh osteochondral allograft (OCA) transplantation is theoretically an attractive option because it can restore both the osseous and chondral components caused by the OCD lesion. Sadr et al. [23] evaluated 135 patients (149 knees) who underwent OCA for OCD of the knee. The median age at the time of surgery was 21 years (range, 12–55 years and the majority of lesions involved the medial femoral condyle (62%). Other involved areas were the lateral femoral condyle (29%), with the remaining lesions on the trochlea (6%), patella (1%), or two anatomic locations (2%). The mean allograft size was 7.3 cm^2. A dowel technique was used for small- and medium-sized lesions, and a shell allograft technique or a multiple dowel technique was used for larger lesions (127 knees had a dowel, 19 knees had a shell, and 3 knees had both a dowel and shell). All clinical outcome measures improved significantly at latest follow-up ($P < 0.001$). Reoperations were performed in 34 (23%) knees; however, only 8% were classified as OCA failures that were treated with revision OCA or allograft removal. The median follow-up duration was 6.3 years and the mean time to failure was 6.1 years. OCA survivorship was 95% at 5 years and 93% at 10 years. Satisfaction with the OCA procedure was obtained in 95% of the patients.

Shasha et al. [14] presented a study that assessed survivorship and long-term functional outcome following OCA transplantation for unipolar post-traumatic tibial plateau defects in young, high-demand patients. In this study, 65 patients underwent OCA transplantation for tibial plateau fractures using a shell technique. A meniscal allograft was used in 39 knees (60%). The average age of the patients was 42.8 years, and allograft reconstruction was performed at an average of 4 years after trauma. Graft nonunion, fragmentation, collapse, resorption, and degenerative changes were recorded. Several patients with less than 5 years of follow-up had undergone early conversion to total knee replacement. Kaplan-Meier survivorship analysis was used to predict the length of time that the graft had remained intact and functioning. The end points that were used to defined survivorship (failure) were an HSS score of <70 points, a patient's decision to proceed with knee arthroplasty, or revision of the allograft for any reason. At the end of the study period, 44 (68%) of the 65 grafts were in situ and functioning at an average of 12.9 ± 5.1 years. Their analysis showed 95% survival at 5 years, 80% survival at 10 years; 65% survival at 15 years, and 46% survival at 20 years. Although some patients with severe degenerative changes had a good HSS score, on the average, the HSS score decreased among patients who were classified as having more severe degenerative changes ($P < 0.001$). Good to excellent results on the basis of the HSS score were found in 86% of the patients at an average of 12 years (range, 5–24 years). Only 39% of the knees had moderate to severe degenerative changes at the time of the final follow-up. The authors found an interesting correlation between severe degenerative changes and the HSS score. The HSS score did not degrade over time in the absence of degenerative changes. The authors conclude that OCA transplantation for tibial plateau fractures successfully provides an enduring stable and functional knee in young, high-demand patients. The presence of the tibial allograft did not make knee arthroplasty technically more difficult and their study showed that osteochondral allograft-

ing can delay total knee arthroplasty while enabling good knee function.

Similar results were found by Gracitelli et al. [62] evaluating patients that were treated with OCA transplantation as a salvage procedure for fractures of the knee, including tibial plateau (74%), femoral condyle (15%), and patella fractures (10%). Thirty-nine patients (39 knees) comprised their study population, including 24 males and 15 females with an average age of 34 years (range = 16–54 years). Scores on the modified Merle D'Aubigné-Postel, IKDC, and KS-F improved from the preoperative visit to latest follow-up. Following the OCA transplantation, 19 of 39 knees (49%) had further surgery, of these, 10 knees (26%) were considered OCA failures (3 OCA revisions, 6 total knee arthroplasties (TKA), and 1 patellectomy). Survivorship of the OCA was 82.6% at 5 years and 69.6% at 10 years.

Avascular necrosis of the knee can be seen in young patients following systemic high-dose corticosteroid therapy for autoimmune disease or primary malignancy. Steroid-induced lesions form in the subchondral bone, with eventual fracture and progression to overlying chondrosis, joint collapse, and arthritis. The femoral condyles are the second most common site to be affected, after the femoral head. Treatment of steroid-associated osteonecrosis remains controversial, with proposed therapeutic approaches including activity modification and surgical intervention, however regardless of the etiology, symptomatic, high-grade osteonecrotic lesions of the distal femur generally require TKA for definitive treatment. Young patients, however, are more likely to continue placing high demands on their replaced joints and are thus more likely to require future revisions of TKA procedures due to aseptic loosening and polyethylene wear, when biological repair strategies such as osteochondral allograft (OCA) transplantation of the femoral condyles could be used as a durable method to postpone the need for arthroplasty in young active patients. A long-term follow-up retrospective review performed by Early et al. [63]. Evaluated 25 patients (33 knees) with and average age of 25 years (range, 16–48 years) who were treated with OCA transplantation for osteonecrosis of the knee. Patient's underlying diagnoses were primarily related to an autoimmune disorder (44% of patients with underlying diagnosis of systemic lupus erythematosus, ulcerative colitis, Crohn's disease, or myositis) or malignancy (32% of patients with underlying diagnosis of leukemia or Hodgkin's lymphoma), with the remainder of underlying diagnoses being less common causes to receive high-dose corticosteroid therapy. Patients included in this series were initial candidates for arthroplasty but were referred to allografting as an alternative treatment option. Sixteen surgeries were bilateral. Twenty-five knees had unicondylar lesions (13 lateral, 12 medial), whereas 8 knees had bicondylar involvement (medial and lateral femoral condyles in the same knee) and received allografts to both condyles. Mean total allograft surface area was 10.6 cm^2 (range, 4.0–19.0 cm^2). Seventeen out of 33 (51.5%) knees had multiple grafts; these included cases of bicondylar involvement, large lesions using dowel technique, or additional non-structural particulate bone allografting of necrotic areas beneath the grafts. Overall, patients required an average of 1.7 osteochondral allografts per knee (range 1–4). Nine of 33 knees (27%) had further surgery following the OCA transplantation. Of these, eight knees (24% of entire cohort) underwent further surgery that involved graft removal and were classified as OCA failures (3 revision OCA transplantations and 5 conversions to TKA). Mean time to OCA failure (including OCA revisions and conversions to TKA) was 7.8 years (range 1.6–13.7 years). Graft survivorship was 90% at 5 years and 82% at 10 years. Among the 25 knees that had the allograft in situ, the mean follow-up duration was 11.0 years (range, 2.9–29 years). Pain and function scores decreased from early follow-up to long-term follow-up, but all scores were statistically better at latest follow-up than preoperatively.

The results of osteochondral allografting for OA conditions and kissing lesions of the knee are difficult to summarize. Gross et al. have reported 75% 10-year survivorship of tibial grafts in the management of post-traumatic OA [14, 16, 64]

and up to 75% good to excellent outcomes using allografts for patellofemoral disease. Gortz et al. [17] reported 90% graft survival rate at 6 years in steroid-induced osteonecrosis of the femoral condyles. The outcome of bipolar tibiofemoral disease, in patients attempting to defer arthroplasty, shows high patient satisfaction but a 60% reoperation rate and 30% rate of conversion to TKA at average of 6 years. In a longer follow-up analysis of this same cohort, Early et al. [63] noted an increase in the rate of new arthroplasties (15%) or other surgical intervention (27%) on affected knees compared with previous findings at mean 5.6 years' follow-up in 2010 (4% and 15%, respectively). Of the 8 knees requiring additional surgical intervention, 4 involved bicondylar lesions, 4 involved above-average necrotic area (range 11.6–19.0 vs. 10.6 cm^2), and 6 were performed using shell allograft technique, showing that large lesions requiring multiple grafts, or to require allografting in multiple areas in the knee, commonly found in more advanced stages of OA, may present worse outcomes than single and focal osteochondral defects in the knee. A reduced graft survivorship in OA population may reflect the higher level of lesion complexity in patients with OA, combined with underlying disease burden from patient's primary diagnoses. Recent studies have shown an increased failure rate of OCA transplantation for bipolar OCA transplantation for knee OA. Stannard et al. [65] presented short-term outcomes following unipolar, multisurface, and bipolar osteochondral allograft transplantations in the knee in 194 patients, where 88 patients were treated with bipolar grafts. Bipolar lesion was defined as any pathology involving two opposing articulating surfaces, including patellofemoral, femorotibial, and/or femoromeniscal compartment. In a mean follow-up of 3.5 years documented failures occurred in 26 patients (13%), with all undergoing TKA for treatment. Bipolar cases comprised 22 (85%) failures, making bipolar transplantation significantly ($P = 0.008$) and 3.8 times more likely than unipolar grafts to be associated with failure. While most studies document the majority of revisions and failures occurring in the first year after OCA transplantation for OA patients, results with this technique for OA must be interpreted with caution until long-term follow-up data are available.

23.9.1.4 Size

Fresh osteochondral allograft (OCA) transplantation is most commonly performed as a treatment for lesions larger than 2–4 cm^2.

The relationship between size of the lesion and prognosis was studied by Tirico et al. [66] evaluating 156 knees (143 patients) treated with OCA transplantation for distal femoral condyle osteochondral lesions of the knee. The total area of the allograft was used as a surrogate for the absolute size of the lesion and was categorized as small (<5 cm^2), medium (5–8 cm^2), or large (>8 cm^2). The mean allograft area was 6.4 cm^2 (range, 2.3–11.5 cm^2). Thirty-six of 156 allografts (23.1%) were categorized as small, 76 of 156 (48.7%) were categorized as medium, and 44 of 156 (28.2%) were categorized as large. The graft failure rate was similar for all absolute size groups, occurring in 2 of 36 (5.6%) small grafts, 3 of 76 (3.9%) medium grafts, and 4 of 44 (9.1%) large grafts ($P = 0.507$). Survivorship of the graft at 5 years for the small, medium, and large absolute size groups was 97.2%, 100.0%, and 92.5%, respectively ($P = 0.445$), showing that for femoral condyle defects, lesion size does not influence subjective outcomes of pain and function after OCA transplantation.

Giorgini et al. [67] found that improvement in IKDC scores was lower when lesions were larger than 8 cm^2. Similar results were found by Bugbee evaluating a cohort of 402 knees in a long-term follow-up series. Survivorship of all grafts in 12 years; including different location, diagnosis, and age; was 90% for grafts smaller than 8 cm^2 and 64% when larger than 8 cm^2. So, in general, smaller thin-plug grafts for OCD lesions might have higher survivorship than a large tibial plateau and meniscal graft for a salvage complex tibial post-traumatic arthritic lesion.

23.9.1.5 Storage Time

Tissue culture media allow a longer storage time but lead to chondrocyte death within the tissue [41]. Historically, the use of fresh OCAs was limited to specialized centers with tissue banks that could safely recover, process, and test tissue rapidly to allow transplantation within 7 days, thereby maximizing chondrocyte cell viability. The increasing popularity of OCA transplantation has led to a need for new protocols that would allow for prolonged viable storage of osteochondral grafts to permit greater availability and wider distribution of fresh OCAs to treat more patients outside of specialized centers. Several storage methods have been investigated to try to optimize chondrocyte viability with each showing noticeable declines in chondrocyte viability after Day 14, decreasing below acceptable levels (typically considered to be 70% viable cells) by 28 days after procurement. Storage media were shown to have an effect on chondrocyte viability, with tissue culture media allowing a longer storage time than Ringer's lactate solution [41]. Storage temperature was also studied, and currently, most storage protocols use 4 °C as a standard, which provides improved chondrocyte viability (over Ringer's lactate solution) up to 28 days. However, studies did show that, even in nutritive media, prolonged storage of fresh OCA tissue leads to variable but predictable chondrocyte death within the tissue. Although the effect of chondrocyte death from prolonged storage has been studied in animal models, the clinical consequence in humans has not been studied extensively.

A matched-pair study performed by Schmidt et al. [20] compared 75 patients who received "early release" grafts between September 1997 and September 2002 (mean storage time, 6.3 days [range, 1–14 days]) and 75 patients who received "late release" grafts between October 2002 and August 2008 (mean storage time, 20.0 days [range, 16–28 days]). Patients were matched 1:1 by age, diagnosis, and graft size and clinical outcome measures including reoperations and failures were recorded. Among patients with grafts remaining in situ, the mean follow-up was 11.9 years (range, 2.0–16.8 years) and 7.8 years (range, 2.3–11.1 years) for the early and late release groups, respectively. The total reoperation rate was 42.7% (32/75) of knees in the early release group and 30.7% (23/75) of knees in the late release group ($P = 0.127$). OCA failure occurred in 25.3% (19/75) of patients in the early release group and 12.0% (9/75) of patients in the late release group ($P = 0.036$) and the median time to failure was 3.5 years (range, 1.7–13.8 years) and 2.7 years (range, 0.3–11.1 years) for the early and late release groups, respectively. The 5-year survivorship of the OCA was 85% for the early release group and 90% for the late release group ($P = 0.321$). The results of this matched-pair study suggest that OCAs with prolonged storage up to 28 days do not adversely affect clinical outcomes. The late release group had a significantly lower clinical failure rate than the early release group (12.0% vs 25.3%, respectively; $P < 0.05$). The overall 5-year reoperation rate was similar between groups. This result was unexpected based on basic science and animal studies, that prolonged storage would lead to inferior clinical outcomes [41]. Other variables may be more important in affecting overall outcomes. Although the authors performed a matched-pair analysis to account for patient differences, the early release group had surgeries performed before 2002 and the late release group after 2002, resulting in different lengths of follow-up. Inherent improvements in surgical techniques, such as new instrumentation and surgeon experience, may have also played a role in outcomes.

In an animal model, Cook et al. [44] developed and examined the feasibility of storing osteochondral allografts for up to 60 days using the new media system in terms of chondrocyte viability and risk for bacterial contamination. In this study, their solution was able to maintain sufficient (>70%) chondrocyte viability for up to 60 days in 83% of stored allografts in 25 °C. This system was also studied in human tissue with good cell viability up to 56 days after procurement [68]. Other authors have also investigated different solutions and media in an effort to increase storage time of grafts with high cell viability [69, 70]. Increasing storage time of grafts would improve availability of grafts, provide grafts with high cell viability, allow for prescreening of donors for safety, and facilitate more convenient scheduling of surgery.

23.10 Return to Sport

Due to improved surgical technique and better donor graft availability during the last two decades, osteochondral allograft (OCA) transplantation has become an increasingly relevant and regarded surgical option in the cartilage repair paradigm in young and active patients who desire to return to athletic activity [71, 72]. In a recent systematic literature review with 1117 included patients, Campbell et al. reported a return-to-sport rate of also 88% after OCA transplantation (89% for OAT, 84% for ACI, and 75% for microfracture [72]. Furthermore, the authors could show that athletes who were younger had a shorter preoperative duration of symptoms, underwent no previous surgical interventions, participated in a more rigorous rehabilitation protocol, had a smaller cartilage defect, and had a significantly better prognosis after surgery.

In an effort to evaluate the rate of RTS, clinical outcome, and risk factors for not returning to physical activity following OCA transplantation, Krych et al. [73] reported an overall return to sport of 88% (38/43) of patients, with 79% (34/43) returning to the previous level of physical activity. The average time to RTS was 9.6 ± 3.0 months (range, 7–13). Activities of daily living and clinical outcome measures were significantly improved from baseline to last follow-up. Factors correlated to non-return to sport in this series were age older than 25 years and preoperative symptoms greater than 12 months.

Bugbee et al. identified 142 patients (149 knees) who underwent primary OCA transplantation in the knee and participated in sport or recreational activity prior to cartilage injury and did not have a major concomitant surgery (osteotomy, anterior cruciate ligament repair, or meniscal allograft) at the time of the OCA. Level of activity was classified as highly competitive athlete, well-trained and frequently sporting, sporting sometimes, or non-sporting to describe their activity level before injuring their knee. Patients included in this study were either highly competitive athlete (67/145, 45%) or well-trained and frequently sporting (82/149, 55%). At a mean follow-up of 6 years (range, 1.0–

15.8 years), 75.2% (112 of 149 knees) had returned to sport or recreational activity following the OCA. Among the entire cohort of 149 knees, regardless of return-to-sport status, 71% achieved "very good" to "excellent" knee function following the OCA, and 79% were able to participate in a high level of activity (moderate, strenuous, or very strenuous activities) as assessed on the IKDC subjective evaluation form. Among the 24.8% (37 of 149 knees) who did not return to sport or activity, reasons included both knee-related problems and lifestyle characteristics. Survivorship of allografts was 91% at 5 years and 89% at 10 years [74].

23.11 Complications

Early complications unique to the allografting procedure are few. There does not appear to be any increased risk of surgical site infection with the use of allografts as compared with other procedures. The use of a mini-arthrotomy in the knee decreases the risk of postoperative stiffness. Occasionally, one sees a persistent effusion, which is typically a sign of over-use, but which may indicate an immune-mediated synovitis. Delayed union or nonunion of the fresh allograft is the most common early finding. This is evidenced by persistent discomfort and/or visible graft-host interface on serial radiographic evaluation. Delayed union or nonunion is more common in larger grafts, such as those used in the tibial plateau, or in the setting of compromised bone, such as in the treatment of osteonecrosis. In this setting, patience is essential and complete healing or recovery may take an extended period. Decreasing activities, the institution of weight-bearing precautions or use of braces, may be helpful in the early management of a delayed healing. In this setting, careful evaluation of serial radiographs can provide insight into the healing process; and MRI scans are rarely diagnostic, particularly prior to 6 months postoperatively, as they typically show extensive signal abnormality that is difficult to interpret. The natural history of the graft that fails to achieve adequate osteointegration is unpredictable. Clinical symptoms may be minimal, or there may be progressive clinical deterioration and radiographic evidence of fragmentation, fracture, or collapse.

23.12 Summary

OCA is a well-established procedure and may achieve excellent long-term clinical results to treat symptomatic large cartilage lesions (chondral and osteochondral) defects with the correct indications and patient selection.

References

1. Czitrom AA, Keating S, Gross AE. The viability of articular cartilage in fresh osteochondral allografts after clinical transplantation. J Bone Joint Surg Am. 1990;72(4):574–81.
2. Williams RJ 3rd, Dreese JC, Chen CT. Chondrocyte survival and material properties of hypothermically stored cartilage: an evaluation of tissue used for osteochondral allograft transplantation. Am J Sports Med. 2004;32(1):132–9.
3. Williams SK, Amiel D, Ball ST, Allen RT, Tontz WL, Emmerson BC, et al. Analysis of cartilage tissue on a cellular level in fresh osteochondral allograft retrievals. Am J Sports Med. 2007;35(12):2022–32. https://doi.org/10.1177/0363546507305017.
4. Williams SK, Amiel D, Ball ST, Allen RT, Wong VW, Chen AC, et al. Prolonged storage effects on the articular cartilage of fresh human osteochondral allografts. J Bone Joint Surg Am. 2003;85-A(11):2111–20.
5. Lexer E. Substitution of whole or half joints from freshly amputated extremities by free plastic operations. Surg Gynecol Obstet. 1908;6:601–7.
6. Elves MW. Immunological studies of osteoarticular allografts. Proc R Soc Med. 1971;64(6):644.
7. Volkov M. Allotransplantation of joints. J Bone Joint Surg. 1970;52(1):49–53.
8. Elves MW, Ford CH. A study of the humoral immune response to osteoarticular allografts in the sheep. Clin Exp Immunol. 1974;17(3):497–508.
9. Gross AE, Silverstein EA, Falk J, Falk R, Langer F. The allotransplantation of partial joints in the treatment of osteoarthritis of the knee. Clin Orthop Relat Res. 1975;108:7–14.
10. Pritzker KP, Gross AE, Langer F, Luk SC, Houpt JB. Articular cartilage transplantation. Hum Pathol. 1977;8(6):635–51.
11. Meyers MH, Jones RE, Bucholz RW, Wenger DR. Fresh autogenous grafts and osteochondral allografts for the treatment of segmental collapse in osteonecrosis of the hip. Clin Orthop Relat Res. 1983;174:107–12.

12. Convery FR, Meyers MH, Akeson WH. Fresh osteochondral allografting of the femoral condyle. Clin Orthop Relat Res. 1991;273:139–45.
13. Garrett JC. Fresh osteochondral allografts for treatment of articular defects in osteochondritis dissecans of the lateral femoral condyle in adults. Clin Orthop Relat Res. 1994;303:33–7.
14. Shasha N, Krywulak S, Backstein D, Pressman A, Gross AE. Long-term follow-up of fresh tibial osteochondral allografts for failed tibial plateau fractures. J Bone Joint Surg Am. 2003;85-A(Suppl 2):33–9.
15. Williams RJ, Ranawat AS, Potter HG, Carter T, Warren RF. Fresh stored allografts for the treatment of osteochondral defects of the knee. J Bone Joint Surg. 2007;89(4):718–26. https://doi.org/10.2106/jbjs.f.00625.
16. Gross AE, Kim W, Las Heras F, Backstein D, Safir O, Pritzker KP. Fresh osteochondral allografts for posttraumatic knee defects: long-term followup. Clin Orthop Relat Res. 2008;466(8):1863–70. https://doi.org/10.1007/s11999-008-0282-8.
17. Gortz S, De Young AJ, Bugbee WD. Fresh osteochondral allografting for steroid-associated osteonecrosis of the femoral condyles. Clin Orthop Relat Res. 2010;468(5):1269–78. https://doi.org/10.1007/s11999-010-1250-7.
18. Bugbee WD, Khanna G, Cavallo M, McCauley JC, Gortz S, Brage ME. Bipolar fresh osteochondral allografting of the tibiotalar joint. J Bone Joint Surg Am. 2013;95(5):426–32. https://doi.org/10.2106/jbjs.l.00165.
19. Ball ST, Amiel D, Williams SK, Tontz W, Chen AC, Sah RL, et al. The effects of storage on fresh human osteochondral allografts. Clin Orthop Relat Res. 2004;418:246–52.
20. Schmidt KJ, Tirico LE, McCauley JC, Bugbee WD. Fresh osteochondral allograft transplantation: is graft storage time associated with clinical outcomes and graft survivorship? Am J Sports Med. 2017;45(10):2260–6. https://doi.org/10.1177/0363546517704846.
21. Tirico LEP, McCauley JC, Pulido PA, Bugbee WD. Osteochondral allograft transplantation of the femoral condyle utilizing a thin plug graft technique. Am J Sports Med. 2019;47(7):1613–20. https://doi.org/10.1177/0363546519844212.
22. Chahla J, Sweet MC, Okoroha KR, Nwachukwu BU, Hinckel B, Farr J, et al. Osteochondral allograft transplantation in the patellofemoral joint: a systematic review. Am J Sports Med. 2019;47(12):3009–18. https://doi.org/10.1177/0363546518814236.
23. Sadr KN, Pulido PA, McCauley JC, Bugbee WD. Osteochondral allograft transplantation in patients with osteochondritis dissecans of the knee. Am J Sports Med. 2016;44(11):2870–5. https://doi.org/10.1177/0363546516657526.
24. Cameron JI, Pulido PA, McCauley JC, Bugbee WD. Osteochondral allograft transplantation of the femoral trochlea. Am J Sports Med. 2016;44(3):633–8. https://doi.org/10.1177/0363546515620193.
25. Murphy RT, Pennock AT, Bugbee WD. Osteochondral allograft transplantation of the knee in the pediatric and adolescent population. Am J Sports Med. 2014;42(3):635–40. https://doi.org/10.1177/0363546513516747.
26. Oakeshott RD, Farine I, Pritzker KP, Langer F, Gross AE. A clinical and histologic analysis of failed fresh osteochondral allografts. Clin Orthop Relat Res. 1988;233:283–94.
27. Gross AE, Shasha N, Aubin P. Long-term followup of the use of fresh osteochondral allografts for posttraumatic knee defects. Clin Orthop Relat Res. 2005;435:79–87. https://doi.org/10.1097/01.blo.0000165845.21735.05.
28. Ghazavi MT, Pritzker KP, Davis AM, Gross AE. Fresh osteochondral allografts for post-traumatic osteochondral defects of the knee. J Bone Joint Surg. 1997;79(6):1008–13.
29. Hunt HE, Sadr K, Deyoung AJ, Gortz S, Bugbee WD. The role of immunologic response in fresh osteochondral allografting of the knee. Am J Sports Med. 2014;42(4):886–91. https://doi.org/10.1177/0363546513518733.
30. Friedlaender GE. Immune responses to osteochondral allografts. Current knowledge and future directions. Clin Orthop Relat Res. 1983;174:58–68.
31. Friedlaender GE, Horowitz MC. Immune responses to osteochondral allografts: nature and significance. Orthopedics. 1992;15(10):1171–5.
32. Pegg DE, Wusteman MC, Wang L. Cryopreservation of articular cartilage. Part 1: conventional cryopreservation methods. Cryobiology. 2006;52(3):335–46. https://doi.org/10.1016/j.cryobiol.2006.01.005.
33. Langer F, Gross AE, West M, Urovitz EP. The immunogenicity of allograft knee joint transplants. Clin Orthop Relat Res. 1978;132:155–62.
34. Kandel RA, Pritzker KP, Langer F, Gross AE. The pathologic features of massive osseous grafts. Hum Pathol. 1984;15(2):141–6.
35. Stevenson S. The immune response to osteochondral allografts in dogs. J Bone Joint Surg Am. 1987;69(4):573–82.
36. Sirlin CB, Brossmann J, Boutin RD, Pathria MN, Convery FR, Bugbee W, et al. Shell osteochondral allografts of the knee: comparison of mr imaging findings and immunologic responses. Radiology. 2001;219(1):35–43.
37. Meyers MH, Akeson W, Convery FR. Resurfacing of the knee with fresh osteochondral allograft. J Bone Joint Surg Am. 1989;71(5):704–13.
38. Beaver RJ, Mahomed M, Backstein D, Davis A, Zukor DJ, Gross AE. Fresh osteochondral allografts for post-traumatic defects in the knee. A survivorship analysis. J Bone Joint Surg. 1992;74(1):105–10.
39. Csonge L, Bravo D, Newman-Gage H, Rigley T, Conrad EU, Bakay A, et al. Banking of osteochondral allografts, part II. Preservation of chondrocyte viability during long-term storage. Cell Tissue Bank. 2002;3(3):161–8.

40. Csonge L, Bravo D, Newman-Gage H, Rigley T, Conrad EU, Bakay A, et al. Banking of osteochondral allografts. Part I. Viability assays adapted for osteochondrol and cartilage studies. Cell Tissue Bank. 2002;3(3):151–9. https://doi.org/10.102 3/A:1023665418244.

41. Pallante AL, Chen AC, Ball ST, Amiel D, Masuda K, Sah RL, et al. The in vivo performance of osteochondral allografts in the goat is diminished with extended storage and decreased cartilage cellularity. Am J Sports Med. 2012;40(8):1814–23. https://doi.org/10.1177/0363546512449321.

42. Enneking WF, Mindell ER. Observations on massive retrieved human allografts. J Bone Joint Surg Am. 1991;73(8):1123–42.

43. Judas F, Rosa S, Teixeira L, Lopes C, Ferreira MA. Chondrocyte viability in fresh and frozen large human osteochondral allografts: effect of cryoprotective agents. Transplant Proc. 2007;39(8):2531–4. https://doi.org/10.1016/j.transproceed.2007.07.028.

44. Cook JL, Stoker AM, Stannard JP, Kuroki K, Cook CR, Pfeiffer FM, et al. A novel system improves preservation of osteochondral allografts. Clin Orthop Relat Res. 2014;472(11):3404–14. https://doi.org/10.1007/s11999-014-3773-9.

45. Pallante AL, Bae WC, Chen AC, Gortz S, Bugbee WD, Sah RL. Chondrocyte viability is higher after prolonged storage at 37 C than at 4 C for osteochondral grafts. Am J Sports Med. 2009;37(1_Suppl):24S–32S. https://doi.org/10.1177/0363546509351496.

46. Tirico LE, Demange MK, Santos LA, de Rezende MU, Helito CP, Gobbi RG, et al. Development of a fresh osteochondral allograft program outside North America. Cartilage. 2016;7(3):222–8. https://doi.org/10.1177/1947603515618484.

47. Chui K, Jeys L, Snow M. Knee salvage procedures: the indications, techniques and outcomes of large osteochondral allografts. World J Orthop. 2015;6(3):340–50. https://doi.org/10.5312/wjo.v6.i3.340.

48. Capeci CM, Turchiano M, Strauss EJ, Youm T. Osteochondral allografts: applications in treating articular cartilage defects in the knee. Bull Hosp Joint Dis. 2013;71(1):60–7.

49. Behery O, Siston RA, Harris JD, Flanigan DC. Treatment of cartilage defects of the knee: expanding on the existing algorithm. Clin J Sport Med. 2014;24(1):21–30. https://doi.org/10.1097/jsm.0000000000000004.

50. Wang D, Kalia V, Eliasberg CD, Wang T, Coxe FR, Pais MD, et al. Osteochondral allograft transplantation of the knee in patients aged 40 years and older. Am J Sports Med. 2018;46(3):581–9. https://doi.org/10.1177/0363546517741465.

51. Gortz S, Bugbee WD. Allografts in articular cartilage repair. J Bone Joint Surg Am. 2006;88(6):1374–84.

52. Campbell AB, Knopp MV, Kolovich GP, Wei W, Jia G, Siston RA, et al. Preoperative MRI underestimates articular cartilage defect size compared with findings at arthroscopic knee surgery. Am J Sports Med. 2013;41(3):590–5. https://doi.org/10.1177/0363546512472044.

53. Gomoll AH, Yoshioka H, Watanabe A, Dunn JC, Minas T. Preoperative measurement of cartilage defects by MRI underestimates lesion size. Cartilage. 2011;2(4):389–93. https://doi.org/10.1177/1947603510397534.

54. Blaney Davidson EN, Scharstuhl A, Vitters EL, van der Kraan PM, van den Berg WB. Reduced transforming growth factor-beta signaling in cartilage of old mice: role in impaired repair capacity. Arthritis Res Ther. 2005;7(6):R1338–47. https://doi.org/10.1186/ar1833.

55. Barbero A, Grogan S, Schafer D, Heberer M, Mainil-Varlet P, Martin I. Age related changes in human articular chondrocyte yield, proliferation and post-expansion chondrogenic capacity. Osteoarthr Cartil. 2004;12(6):476–84. https://doi.org/10.1016/j.joca.2004.02.010.

56. Goyal D, Keyhani S, Goyal A, Lee EH, Hui JH, Vaziri AS. Evidence-based status of osteochondral cylinder transfer techniques: a systematic review of level I and II studies. Arthroscopy. 2014;30(4):497–505. https://doi.org/10.1016/j.arthro.2013.12.023.

57. Goyal D, Keyhani S, Lee EH, Hui JH. Evidence-based status of microfracture technique: a systematic review of level I and II studies. Arthroscopy. 2013;29(9):1579–88. https://doi.org/10.1016/j.arthro.2013.05.027.

58. Goyal D, Goyal A, Keyhani S, Lee EH, Hui JH. Evidence-based status of second- and third-generation autologous chondrocyte implantation over first generation: a systematic review of level I and II studies. Arthroscopy. 2013;29(11):1872–8. https://doi.org/10.1016/j.arthro.2013.07.271.

59. Mithoefer K, McAdams T, Williams RJ, Kreuz PC, Mandelbaum BR. Clinical efficacy of the microfracture technique for articular cartilage repair in the knee: an evidence-based systematic analysis. Am J Sports Med. 2009;37(10):2053–63. https://doi.org/10.1177/0363546508328414.

60. Nuelle CW, Nuelle JA, Cook JL, Stannard JP. Patient factors, donor age, and graft storage duration affect osteochondral allograft outcomes in knees with or without comorbidities. J Knee Surg. 2017;30(2):179–84. https://doi.org/10.1055/s-0036-1584183.

61. Abolghasemian M, Leon S, Lee PTH, Safir O, Backstein D, Gross AE, et al. Long-term results of treating large posttraumatic tibial plateau lesions with fresh osteochondral allograft transplantation. J Bone Joint Surg Am. 2019;101(12):1102–8. https://doi.org/10.2106/jbjs.18.00802.

62. Gracitelli GC, Tirico LE, McCauley JC, Pulido PA, Bugbee WD. Fresh osteochondral allograft transplantation for fractures of the knee. Cartilage. 2017;8(2):155–61. https://doi.org/10.1177/1947603516657640.

63. Early S, Tirico LEP, Pulido PA, McCauley JC, Bugbee WD. Long-term retrospective follow-up of fresh osteochondral allograft transplantation for

steroid-associated osteonecrosis of the femoral condyles. Cartilage. 2018:1947603518809399. https://doi.org/10.1177/1947603518809399.

64. Torga Spak R, Teitge RA. Fresh osteochondral allografts for patellofemoral arthritis: long-term followup. Clin Orthop Relat Res. 2006;444:193–200. https://doi.org/10.1097/01.blo.0000201152.98830.ed.

65. Stannard JP, Cook JL. Prospective assessment of outcomes after primary unipolar, multisurface, and bipolar osteochondral allograft transplantations in the knee: a comparison of 2 preservation methods. Am J Sports Med. 2020;48(6):1356–64. https://doi.org/10.1177/0363546520907101.

66. Tirico LEP, McCauley JC, Pulido PA, Bugbee WD. Lesion size does not predict outcomes in fresh osteochondral allograft transplantation. Am J Sports Med. 2018;46(4):900–7. https://doi.org/10.1177/0363546517746106.

67. Giorgini A, Donati D, Cevolani L, Frisoni T, Zambianchi F, Catani F. Fresh osteochondral allograft is a suitable alternative for wide cartilage defect in the knee. Injury. 2013;44(Suppl 1):S16–20. https://doi.org/10.1016/s0020-1383(13)70005-6.

68. Stoker AM, Stannard JP, Kuroki K, Bozynski CC, Pfeiffer FM, Cook JL. Validation of the Missouri osteochondral allograft preservation system for the maintenance of osteochondral allograft quality during prolonged storage. Am J Sports Med. 2018;46(1):58–65. https://doi.org/10.1177/0363546517727516.

69. Calvo R, Espinosa M, Figueroa D, Pozo LM, Conget P. Assessment of cell viability of fresh osteochondral allografts in N-acetylcysteine-enriched medium. Cartilage. 2020;11(1):117–21. https://doi.org/10.1177/1947603518786547.

70. Denbeigh JM, Hevesi M, Paggi CA, Resch ZT, Bagheri L, Mara K, et al. Modernizing storage conditions for fresh osteochondral allografts by optimizing viability at physiologic temperatures and conditions. Cartilage. 2019:1947603519888798. https://doi.org/10.1177/1947603519888798.

71. Krych AJ, Pareek A, King AH, Johnson NR, Stuart MJ, Williams RJ 3rd. Return to sport after the surgical management of articular cartilage lesions in the knee: a meta-analysis. Knee Surg Sports Traumatol Arthrosc. 2016; https://doi.org/10.1007/s00167-016-4262-3.

72. Campbell AB, Pineda M, Harris JD, Flanigan DC. Return to sport after articular cartilage repair in athletes' knees: a systematic review. Arthroscopy. 2016;32(4):651–68.e1. https://doi.org/10.1016/j.arthro.2015.08.028.

73. Krych AJ, Robertson CM, Williams RJ 3rd. Return to athletic activity after osteochondral allograft transplantation in the knee. Am J Sports Med. 2012;40(5):1053–9. https://doi.org/10.1177/0363546511435780.

74. Nielsen ES, McCauley JC, Pulido PA, Bugbee WD. Return to sport and recreational activity after osteochondral allograft transplantation in the knee. Am J Sports Med. 2017;45(7):1608–14. https://doi.org/10.1177/0363546517694857.

Emerging Cartilage Repair Options

24

Mario Hevesi, Bradley M. Kruckeberg,
Aaron J. Krych, and Daniel B. F. Saris

24.1 Introduction

Articular cartilage defects cause pain and progression to osteoarthritis (OA), and there exists a critical need for safe and cost-effective interventions. These defects have limited healing potential secondary to the poor regenerative capacity and the avascular nature of cartilage. As a result, chondral lesions can be a source of pain and mechanical symptoms as well as a risk factor for post-traumatic osteoarthritis. Focal cartilage defects impair quality of life in a similar fashion to severe osteoarthritis, causing long-term dysfunction and deterioration of the entire joint [1].

Historical treatment strategies for articular cartilage defects have been limited in success. Whereas palliative treatment options offer limited and short-term symptom relief, articular cartilage restoration has demonstrated effectiveness in reducing pain and functional disability. A variety of surgical options are available to treat cartilage lesions, and these include microfracture, osteochondral allograft transplantation (OCA), and autologous chondrocyte implantation (ACI). Microfracture is the most commonly performed method of cartilage restoration by marrow stimulation for small defects. This technique relies on the influx of marrow products (stem cells, growth factors, and platelets) to form a fibrin clot, which is slowly remodeled into a fibrocartilage scar. This technique has limited outcomes and usefulness due to poor performance in large defects and inferior long-term outcomes compared to more advanced treatment methods. Osteochondral allograft transplantation demonstrates clinically favorable long-term outcomes, with published revision-free survival of 66–69% at 20 years of follow-up [2]. However, the use of OCA remains limited by the fact that these grafts are obtained from young deceased donors, leading to logistical scheduling challenges and lack of scalability of this efficacious resource. While efforts are underway to optimize OCA and expand graft quality availability, autologous approaches remain attractive, given the potential to restore joint biology and repair native tissues [3, 4].

Successful cartilage repair requires an abundance of cells, growth factors, and intricate modulation of the cellular regenerative process. PRP has

M. Hevesi · B. M. Kruckeberg · A. J. Krych
Orthopedics and Sports Medicine, Mayo Clinic,
Rochester, MN, USA

Department of Orthopedic Surgery, Mayo Clinic,
Rochester, MN, USA
e-mail: Hevesi.mario@mayo.edu;
Kruckeberg.bradley@mauo.edu;
Krych.aaron@mayo.edu

D. B. F. Saris (✉)
Orthopedics and Sports Medicine, Mayo Clinic,
Rochester, MN, USA

Department of Orthopedic Surgery, Mayo Clinic,
Rochester, MN, USA

Department of Orthopedics, University Utrecht,
Utrecht, The Netherlands
e-mail: Saris.daniel@mayo.edu

© ISAKOS 2021
A. J. Krych et al. (eds.), *Cartilage Injury of the Knee*,
https://doi.org/10.1007/978-3-030-78051-7_24

demonstrated trophic and anti-inflammatory properties utilizing in vitro models [5]. Additionally, PRP has shown favorable outcomes in the treatment of knee osteoarthritis, with the potential to be used synergistically with other surgical products to enhance the healing environment.

Cell-based strategies such as autologous chondrocyte implantation (ACI) have demonstrated better durability over microfracture, due to formation of hyaline-like cartilage over fibrocartilage [6]. However, there are disadvantages of ACI, including costly and logistically challenging need for two-stage surgery with ex vivo expansion of the chondrocytes.

Human mesenchymal stem/stromal cells (MSCs) can also be used to improve cartilage regeneration models. The use of MSCs in cartilage repair is promising, with both small and large animal models as well as pilot studies in man demonstrating safety and efficacy in cartilage regeneration [7, 8].

Finally, the combination of chondrocytes with other cell types has gained recent attention given that cells respond to their environment and can be positively influenced by the presence of other cell types [9, 10]. The combination of cells opens the door to single-stage cartilage repair as both orchestrating [stromal] cells and chondrocyte building blocks can be provided simultaneously, without the need for ex vivo expansion.

24.2 Key Concepts

- Evolving use of Platelet-Rich Plasma for Cartilage Treatment
- Emergence and growth of cell-based therapies:
  - Autologous Chondrocyte Implantation
  - Stem/Stromal Cell-Based Therapeutics
  - Single-Stage Auto/Allo Cartilage Repair

24.2.1 Platelet-Rich Plasma for Cartilage Treatment

Platelet-rich plasma (PRP) has received significant attention in recent years as a potential treatment for knee osteochondral defects and osteoarthritis. PRP contains growth factors, modulating local inflammatory responses as well as cellular proliferation and differentiation involved in healing processes [5].

The literature has demonstrated that PRP studies are quite varied with regard to their processing, composition, timing, and indications. A recent systematic review showed that only 10%, or 11/105 studies, provided a comprehensive report with clear description of preparation in composition of the PRP investigated [11]. Furthermore, PRP varies significantly with regard to its platelet, growth factor, and leukocyte composition from patient to patient [11]. Recent efforts have shown that leukocyte composition may be a key factor in the treatment efficacy of knee osteoarthritis [12]. There does appear to be a delicate balance with leukocytes and platelets, as each has important catabolic properties, but, in excess have the ability to upregulate certain proteins such as matrix metalloproteinases, leading to detrimental changes to the surrounding tissues.

Favorable outcomes of intra-articular injections of PRP when compared to saline [13], corticosteroids [14], and hyaluronic acid (HA) [15] have been reported in several blinded, randomized controlled trials (RCT). Other RCTs have demonstrated significant improvement but similar results between PRP and HA [16, 17]. In vitro studies and early clinical observations have also shown a potential synergistic interaction between PRP and HA [18, 19].

The utilization of PRP as an augmentation in the treatment of chondral defects is currently evolving. PRP as an augmentation to microfracture in the treatment of small chondral lesions may provide additional benefit at short-term follow-up, even up to 12 months [20], but did not reach the minimally clinically important difference (MCID) in a recent meta-analysis [21]. While the use of PRP for the treatment of knee cartilage defects and osteoarthritis is becoming increasing popular, its implementation and outcomes remain under scientific debate, in particular due to its heterogeneous nature and preparation. Furthermore, PRP provides a one-time dose of factors which does not have the capacity to for long-term modulation and feedback regulation-inhibition. Given this, emerging treatment options for cartilage repair increasingly involve cell-based therapies that open the door for sustained, modulated healing and regeneration.

24.2.2 Autologous Chondrocyte Implantation

Cell-based strategies have demonstrated better durability over microfracture, due to the formation of hyaline-like cartilage over fibrocartilage [6]. Indeed, a growing body of evidence suggests that microfracture does no better than debridement alone [22, 23]. Given this, we increasingly recommend consideration of debridement for small chondral defects, to better preserve the subchondral plate, should future ACI or other biologic therapy be warranted. Furthermore, this approach has been postulated to limit the occurrence of intralesional osteophyte formation or subchondral plate fracture as well as allow for cell-based biologic intervention without having to treat the full-depth osteochondral unit, such as with OCA.

In several RCTs, we have demonstrated cell-based ACI has superior clinical outcomes and better structure repair compared to scar formation after microfracture [24–27]. Technically, ACI requires precise debridement to stable defect edges as well as close matching of defect geography to the implanted membrane. For this, we prefer to use a cookie cutter technique in order to provide efficient operative workflow, precisely cut defect edges, and a form-fitting ACI membrane [28].

It is important to note that there are several disadvantages of ACI, including the need for two-stage surgery with ex vivo expansion of the chondrocytes. This delays the final rehabilitation of the patients, and in some cases makes quadriceps atrophy and deconditioning of the affected extremity worse over time. In addition, this procedure is very costly, and is continuously challenged by payers.

24.2.3 Stem/Stromal Cell-Based Therapeutics

Stem/stromal cells represent a population of cells that demonstrate the ability for self-renewal, long-term viability, and multilinear culture [29]. Embryonically, mesenchymal stem/stromal cells (MSCs) are derived from the mesoderm and are distinguished by their capacity to divide into connective tissues including ligament, bone, and cartilage leading to evolving interest in their therapeutic use for orthopedic care [29, 30].

Stem/stromal cell preparations exist in varying formulations spanning from point-of-care aspirates to culture-expanded and characterized cell populations. Classic stem/stromal investigations in musculoskeletal repair were centered initially about bone marrow mesenchymal stem/stromal cells (BMSCs) [31]. While bone marrow is relatively enriched in MSCs as compared to other adult tissues, we caution efforts to employ bone marrow aspirate as a robust source of stem/stromal cells given that MSCs comprise only 0.01–0.001% of the harvested cell population [30, 32]. In contrast, the stromal vascular fraction (SVT) of adipose tissue contains approximately 500-fold the stem/stromal cell concentration of bone marrow [33, 34].

Adipose-derived mesenchymal stem/stromal cells (AMSCs) have also demonstrated growing interest and promise in regenerative therapeutics including cartilage repair. AMSCs differ from BMSCs in the relative ease of adipose isolation, both in clinic and in the OR, as well as the quantity of tissue that can be readily harvested in most patients depending on habitus. AMSCs have been demonstrated to differentiate into fibrocytes and tenocytes in addition to adipogenic, myogenic, and chondrogenic tissues and are therefore a natural target for tendon repair/regeneration studies [35–37]. In a recent RNA sequencing analysis of AMSCs and BMSCs obtained from the same human donors, Zhou et al. found that AMSCs demonstrated lower expression of Human Leukocyte Antigen I (HLA I) as well as higher immunosuppression capacity when compared with the BMSC population [38]. This is desirable given that limitations in HLA effect can enable allogeneic stem cell application, easing logical preparations, especially as they relate to culture-expanded formulations [39, 40]. Furthermore, the immunomodulatory effect of stem cells may also play a key role in ligament healing given that multiple groups have proposed and reported on the positive histologic effects and recreation of native-like tendon-bone interfaces with immuno-suppression and macrophage inhibition [41–43].

24.2.4 Single-Stage Auto/Allo Cartilage Repair

Finally, the combination of chondrocytes with other cell types has also gained attention as others showed that cells respond to their environment and can be positively influenced by the presence of other cell types [9, 10]. Indeed, direct contact between MSCs and dedifferentiated articular chondrocytes recently showed improvement of the cartilage phenotype of dedifferentiated articular chondrocytes [44, 45]. Therefore, combining articular chondrocytes with other cell types can help us overcome barriers and improve the traditional ACI-approach.

In their first-in-man trial, de Windt et al. demonstrated that one-stage application of allogeneic BMSCs mixed with 10–20% defect-derived autologous chondrons resulted in significant improvements in Knee Injury and Osteoarthritis Outcome Score (KOOS) as well as visual analog scale (VAS) which was durable at 18 months of follow-up [39, 46]. Furthermore, MRI demonstrated complete defect filling as well as integration with host tissue, while 32 s-look arthroscopies with tissue biopsy demonstrated that the regenerate contained only autologous DNA, supporting that MSCs provide a transient orchestrating effect whereas autologous cells are needed for defect healing.

Recently, our team has initiated an analogous trial under US Clinical trial NCT03672825. Preliminary results using allogeneic AMSCs mixed with defect-derived autologous chondrocytes demonstrate no significant adverse events and satisfactory outcomes at 3–18 months of follow-up. Formal results of this 25 patient Phase I Clinical Trial are forthcoming.

24.3 Conclusions

Cartilage defects substantially affect patient quality of life, and there remains a critical need for safe and cost-effective interventions. The recent technovolution of cartilage treatment has been rapid, with newly emerging options for repair. Methods of PRP preparation are increasingly nuanced and demonstrate promise in growth factor delivery and use as an adjuvant to advanced biologic therapies. Cell-based approaches represent the latest in emerging cartilage repair options. The latest in the evolutionary line of cell-based therapies is represented by single-stage combination autologous/allogeneic treatments which increasingly address and overcome the logistical challenges of two-stage treatments while providing the signal orchestration and autologous cells needed for defect repair.

References

1. Heir S, Nerhus TK, Rotterud JH, Loken S, Ekeland A, Engebretsen L, et al. Focal cartilage defects in the knee impair quality of life as much as severe osteoarthritis: a comparison of knee injury and osteoarthritis outcome score in 4 patient categories scheduled for knee surgery. Am J Sports Med. 2010;38(2):231–7.
2. Familiari F, Cinque ME, Chahla J, Godin JA, Olesen ML, Moatshe G, et al. Clinical outcomes and failure rates of osteochondral allograft transplantation in the knee: a systematic review. Am J Sports Med. 2017; https://doi.org/10.1177/0363546517732531.
3. Denbeigh JM, Hevesi M, Paggi CA, Resch ZT, Bagheri L, Mara K, et al. Modernizing storage conditions for fresh osteochondral allografts by optimizing viability at physiologic temperatures and conditions. Cartilage. 2019; https://doi.org/10.1177/1947603519888798.
4. Hevesi M, Denbeigh JM, Paggi CA, Galeano-Garces C, Bagheri L, Larson AN, et al. Fresh osteochondral allograft transplantation in the knee: a viability and histologic analysis for optimizing graft viability and expanding existing standard processed graft resources using a living donor cartilage program. Cartilage. 2019; https://doi.org/10.1177/1947603519880330.
5. Filardo G, Kon E, Roffi A, Di Matteo B, Merli ML, Marcacci M. Platelet-rich plasma: why intra-articular? A systematic review of preclinical studies and clinical

evidence on PRP for joint degeneration. Knee Surg Sports Traumatol Arthrosc. 2015;23(9):2459–74.

6. Pareek A, Carey JL, Reardon PJ, Peterson L, Stuart MJ, Krych AJ. Long-term outcomes after autologous chondrocyte implantation: a systematic review at mean follow-up of 11.4 years. Cartilage. 2016;7(4):298–308.

7. Mokbel A, El-Tookhy O, Shamaa AA, Sabry D, Rashed L, Mostafa A. Homing and efficacy of intra-articular injection of autologous mesenchymal stem cells in experimental chondral defects in dogs. Clin Exp Rheumatol. 2011;29(2):275–84.

8. Marquass B, Schulz R, Hepp P, Zscharnack M, Aigner T, Schmidt S, et al. Matrix-associated implantation of predifferentiated mesenchymal stem cells versus articular chondrocytes: in vivo results of cartilage repair after 1 year. Am J Sports Med. 2011;39(7):1401–12.

9. Fischer J, Dickhut A, Rickert M, Richter W. Human articular chondrocytes secrete parathyroid hormone-related protein and inhibit hypertrophy of mesenchymal stem cells in coculture during chondrogenesis. Arthritis Rheum. 2010;62(9):2696–706.

10. Hwang NS, Varghese S, Puleo C, Zhang Z, Elisseeff J. Morphogenetic signals from chondrocytes promote chondrogenic and osteogenic differentiation of mesenchymal stem cells. J Cell Physiol. 2007;212(2):281–4.

11. Chahla J, Cinque ME, Piuzzi NS, Mannava S, Geeslin AG, Murray IR, et al. A call for standardization in platelet-rich plasma preparation protocols and composition reporting: a systematic review of the clinical orthopaedic literature. J Bone Joint Surg Am. 2017;99(20):1769–79.

12. Riboh JC, Saltzman BM, Yanke AB, Fortier L, Cole BJ. Effect of leukocyte concentration on the efficacy of platelet-rich plasma in the treatment of knee osteoarthritis. Am J Sports Med. 2016;44(3):792–800.

13. Smith PA. Intra-articular autologous conditioned plasma injections provide safe and efficacious treatment for knee osteoarthritis: an FDA-sanctioned, randomized, double-blind, placebo-controlled clinical trial. Am J Sports Med. 2016;44(4):884–91.

14. Forogh B, Mianehsaz E, Shoaee S, Ahadi T, Raissi GR, Sajadi S. Effect of single injection of platelet-rich plasma in comparison with corticosteroid on knee osteoarthritis: a double-blind randomized clinical trial. J Sports Med Phys Fitness. 2016;56(7–8):901–8.

15. Dai WL, Zhou AG, Zhang H, Zhang J. Efficacy of platelet-rich plasma in the treatment of knee osteoarthritis: a meta-analysis of randomized controlled trials. Arthroscopy. 2017;33(3):659–70, e1.

16. Filardo G, Di Matteo B, Di Martino A, Merli ML, Cenacchi A, Fornasari P, et al. Platelet-rich plasma intra-articular knee injections show no superiority versus viscosupplementation: a randomized controlled trial. Am J Sports Med. 2015;43(7):1575–82.

17. Di Martino A, Di Matteo B, Papio T, Tentoni F, Selleri F, Cenacchi A, et al. Platelet-rich plasma versus hyaluronic acid injections for the treatment of knee osteoarthritis: results at 5 years of a double-blind, randomized controlled trial. Am J Sports Med. 2019;47(2):347–54.

18. Chen WH, Lo WC, Hsu WC, Wei HJ, Liu HY, Lee CH, et al. Synergistic anabolic actions of hyaluronic acid and platelet-rich plasma on cartilage regeneration in osteoarthritis therapy. Biomaterials. 2014;35(36):9599–607.

19. Saturveithan C, Premganesh G, Fakhrizzaki S, Mahathir M, Karuna K, Rauf K, et al. Intra-articular hyaluronic acid (HA) and platelet rich plasma (PRP) injection versus hyaluronic acid (HA) injection alone in patients with grade III and IV knee osteoarthritis (OA): a retrospective study on functional outcome. Malays Orthop J. 2016;10(2):35–40.

20. Manunta AF, Manconi A. The treatment of chondral lesions of the knee with the microfracture technique and platelet-rich plasma. Joints. 2013;1(4):167–70.

21. Boffa A, Previtali D, Altamura SA, Zaffagnini S, Candrian C, Filardo G. Platelet-rich plasma augmentation to microfracture provides a limited benefit for the treatment of cartilage lesions: a meta-analysis. Orthop J Sports Med. 2020;8(4):2325967120910504.

22. Hevesi M, Bernard C, Hartigan DE, Levy BA, Domb BG, Krych AJ. Is microfracture necessary? Acetabular chondrolabral debridement/abrasion demonstrates similar outcomes and survival to microfracture in hip arthroscopy: a multicenter analysis. Am J Sports Med. 2019;47(7):1670–8.

23. Gudas R, Gudaite A, Mickevicius T, Masiulis N, Simonaityte R, Cekanauskas E, et al. Comparison of osteochondral autologous transplantation, microfracture, or debridement techniques in articular cartilage lesions associated with anterior cruciate ligament injury: a prospective study with a 3-year follow-up. Arthroscopy. 2013;29(1):89–97.

24. Saris D, Price A, Widuchowski W, Bertrand-Marchand M, Caron J, Drogset JO, et al. Matrix-applied characterized autologous cultured chondrocytes versus microfracture: two-year follow-up of a prospective randomized trial. Am J Sports Med. 2014;42(6):1384–94.

25. Saris DB, Vanlauwe J, Victor J, Almqvist KF, Verdonk R, Bellemans J, et al. Treatment of symptomatic cartilage defects of the knee: characterized chondrocyte implantation results in better clinical outcome at 36 months in a randomized trial compared to microfracture. Am J Sports Med. 2009;37(Suppl 1):10s–9s.

26. Saris DB, Vanlauwe J, Victor J, Haspl M, Bohnsack M, Fortems Y, et al. Characterized chondrocyte implantation results in better structural repair when treating symptomatic cartilage defects of the knee in a randomized controlled trial versus microfracture. Am J Sports Med. 2008;36(2):235–46.

27. Brittberg M, Recker D, Ilgenfritz J, Saris DBF. Matrix-applied characterized autologous cultured chondrocytes versus microfracture: five-year follow-up of a prospective randomized trial. Am J Sports Med. 2018;46:1343–51.

28. Hevesi M, Krych AJ, Saris DBF. Treatment of cartilage defects with the matrix-induced autologous

chondrocyte implantation cookie cutter technique. Arthrosc Tech. 2019;8(6):e591–e6.

29. Zuk PA, Zhu M, Ashjian P, De Ugarte DA, Huang JI, Mizuno H, et al. Human adipose tissue is a source of multipotent stem cells. Mol Biol Cell. 2002;13(12):4279–95.

30. Sullivan MO, Gordon-Evans WJ, Fredericks LP, Kiefer K, Conzemius MG, Griffon DJ. Comparison of mesenchymal stem cell surface markers from bone marrow aspirates and adipose stromal vascular fraction sites. Front Vet Sci. 2016;2:82.

31. Bianco P. "Mesenchymal" stem cells. Annu Rev Cell Dev Biol. 2014;30:677–704.

32. Oedayrajsingh-Varma MJ, van Ham SM, Knippenberg M, Helder MN, Klein-Nulend J, Schouten TE, et al. Adipose tissue-derived mesenchymal stem cell yield and growth characteristics are affected by the tissue-harvesting procedure. Cytotherapy. 2006;8(2):166–77.

33. Fraser JK, Wulur I, Alfonso Z, Hedrick MH. Fat tissue: an underappreciated source of stem cells for biotechnology. Trends Biotechnol. 2006;24(4):150–4.

34. Tremolada C, Colombo V, Ventura C. Adipose tissue and mesenchymal stem cells: state of the art and Lipogems® technology development. Curr Stem Cell Rep. 2016;2(3):304–12.

35. Norelli JB, Plaza DP, Stal DN, Varghese AM, Liang H, Grande DA. Tenogenically differentiated adipose-derived stem cells are effective in Achilles tendon repair in vivo. J Tissue Eng. 2018;9:2041731418811183.

36. Torres-Torrillas M, Rubio M, Damia E, Cuervo B, Del Romero A, Peláez P, et al. Adipose-derived mesenchymal stem cells: a promising tool in the treatment of musculoskeletal diseases. Int J Mol Sci. 2019;20(12):3105.

37. Hevesi M, LaPrade M, Saris DBF, Krych AJ. Stem cell treatment for ligament repair and reconstruction. Curr Rev Musculoskelet Med. 2019;12(4):446–50.

38. Zhou W, Lin J, Zhao K, Jin K, He Q, Hu Y, et al. Single-cell profiles and clinically useful properties of human mesenchymal stem cells of adipose and bone marrow origin. Am J Sports Med. 2019;47(7):1722–33.

39. de Windt TS, Vonk LA, Slaper-Cortenbach IC, van den Broek MP, Nizak R, van Rijen MH, et al. Allogeneic mesenchymal stem cells stimulate cartilage regeneration and are safe for single-stage cartilage repair in humans upon mixture with recycled autologous chondrons. Stem Cells. 2017;35(1):256–64.

40. Dalle JH, Balduzzi A, Bader P, Lankester A, Yaniv I, Wachowiak J, et al. Allogeneic stem cell transplantation from HLA-mismatched donors for pediatric patients with acute lymphoblastic leukemia treated according to the 2003 BFM and 2007 International BFM studies: impact of disease risk on outcomes. Biol Blood Marrow Transplant. 2018;24(9):1848–55.

41. Hays PL, Kawamura S, Deng XH, Dagher E, Mithoefer K, Ying L, et al. The role of macrophages in early healing of a tendon graft in a bone tunnel. J Bone Joint Surg Am. 2008;90(3):565–79.

42. Hu J, Yao B, Yang X, Ma F. The immunosuppressive effect of Siglecs on tendon-bone healing after ACL reconstruction. Med Hypotheses. 2015;84(1):38–9.

43. Kawamura S, Ying L, Kim HJ, Dynybil C, Rodeo SA. Macrophages accumulate in the early phase of tendon-bone healing. J Orthop Res. 2005;23(6):1425–32.

44. Chen WH, Lai MT, Wu AT, Wu CC, Gelovani JG, Lin CT, et al. In vitro stage-specific chondrogenesis of mesenchymal stem cells committed to chondrocytes. Arthritis Rheum. 2009;60(2):450–9.

45. Tsuchiya K, Chen G, Ushida T, Matsuno T, Tateishi T. The effect of coculture of chondrocytes with mesenchymal stem cells on their cartilaginous phenotype in vitro. Mater Sci Eng C. 2004;24(3):391–6.

46. de Windt TS, Vonk LA, Slaper-Cortenbach ICM, Nizak R, van Rijen MHP, Saris DBF. Allogeneic MSCs and recycled autologous chondrons mixed in a one-stage cartilage cell transplantion: a first-in-man trial in 35 patients. Stem Cells. 2017;35(8):1984–93.

One-Step Chondral and Subchondral Lesion Treatment with MSCs

Alberto Gobbi, Ignacio Dallo, and Eleonora Irlandini

25.1 Introduction

Articular cartilage in the knee is a highly specialized tissue, not only responsible for load bearing, but also for providing a smooth gliding interface within any joint. Nonetheless, due to the avascular nature of the tissue and specialized cells with low mitotic potential, cartilage has limited healing capacity. As it is well-known that cartilage once damaged does not heal, surgical intervention may be needed to achieve repair of the chondral defects. Failure to obtain good functional outcome can lead to cartilage degeneration, which could subsequently result in the development of osteoarthritis (OA) [1, 2]. Almost 60% incidence of chondral lesions has been reported in all patients between 40 and 50 years of age [3, 4]. Chondral lesions are usually a result of an acute injury or repetitive microtrauma in high impact or cutting sports and are commonly seen along anterior cruciate ligament (ACL) tear [5, 6]. An overuse injury, due to limb malalignment or joint instability, may also lead to cartilage damage [7]. Due to the fact that OA treatment is very complex and expensive [8], it is crucial to treat such injuries early and effectively. Research is currently focusing on preventive interventions and therapeutic solutions that will enhance tissue regeneration and the reduction of degenerative mechanisms [9].

Over the years, a number of techniques in cartilage restoration have been developed aiming to prolong the durability of cartilage repair. Autologous chondrocyte implantation (ACI) has shown to stimulate the production of hyaline-like repair tissue, providing longer clinical improvement for the patient [10, 11]. Evolution of this technique led to the development and use of scaffolds that allowed cell ingrowth, but has not eliminated the need for chondrocyte harvest and cultivation. That is why, the idea of performing a one-step procedure, avoiding the need of a two-stage surgical procedures and reducing the costs of the operation by approximately five times. One-step procedures use of bone marrow aspirate concentrate (BMAC) that contains multipotent stem cells (MSCs) and growth factors, and that are placed within a hyaluronan-based scaffold for the treatment of chondral injuries. Treatment options that take into account the subchondral bone are still limited. Osteo-core-plasty is a new, minimally invasive procedure for treating subchondral lesions. During osteo-core-plasty, the surgeon injects bone marrow and small dowels of autologous bone into the affected area under fluoroscopic imaging control in order to fill the intertrabecular space, thereby inducing improved bone remodeling.

A. Gobbi (✉) · I. Dallo · E. Irlandini
O.A.S.I. Bioresearch Foundation, Gobbi N.P.O.,
Milan, Italy
e-mail: gobbi@cartilagedoctor.it

© ISAKOS 2021
A. J. Krych et al. (eds.), *Cartilage Injury of the Knee*,
https://doi.org/10.1007/978-3-030-78051-7_25

25.2 One Step Treatments for Chondral and Osteochondral Injuries

25.2.1 HA-BMAC

Bone marrow aspirate concentrate (BMAC) contains bone marrow stem cells (BMSCs) and growth factors that are a promising option for cartilage repair and regeneration [12–15]. The BMSCs interact with a non-woven hyaluronan-based scaffold, the HYAFF 11, that supports cellular adhesion, migration, and proliferation, promoting the synthesis of extracellular matrix components under static culture conditions [16–18]. Nejadnik et al. compared the clinical outcomes of patients treated with first-generation ACI and patients treated with autologous BMSCs. The authors concluded that BMSCs are as effective as ACI for articular cartilage repair [19]. At our institution, we compared patients treated with matrix-induced autologous chondrocyte implantation (MACI) to patients treated with BMSCs using the same scaffold. Both groups improved but we did not notice any significant statistical differences between the two groups at 3 years follow-up, concluding that both techniques were viable and effective [20]. Many clinical studies have demonstrated that the hyaluronic acid-based scaffold with activated bone marrow aspirate concentrate (HA-BMAC) technique is a valuable method for the treatment of full-thickness cartilage lesions of the knee [21]. Different sizes of osteochondral lesions can be treated, from small injuries to large defects (up to 22 cm^2) showing good clinical outcomes at long-term follow-up [22–25]. The HA-BMAC technique has proven to be effective in treatment for patients over 45 years of age [26].

25.2.2 Indications

The HA-BMAC technique is not a "one-size fits all" for damaged joints, but may be extremely effective when applied for a carefully selected group of patients. This procedure is a good solution for cartilage repair in all compartments in patients with less than 60 years of age and a body mass index (BMI) less than 30. It is also crucial that all concomitant injuries are addressed during the surgery. Malalignment if present, should be corrected at the time of the repair, as well as any kind of ligament instability or meniscal injury. This treatment is not indicated in older (>60 years), obese (BMI > 30) with severe tricompartmental OA. Patients with untreated malalignment (varus /valgus >5°) or knee instability and those who have had multiple intra-articular injections with steroids in the 3 months preceding the procedure, as well as hip disorders leading to abnormal gait, general systemic illnesses, such as rheumatic diseases, Bechterew's syndrome, chondrocalcinosis, gout, and neurovascular diseases are also contraindications.

25.2.3 The Procedure

The entire procedure is performed under general anesthesia. The patient is positioned supine for standard knee arthroscopy. The ipsilateral iliac crest is prepared and exposed for bone marrow aspiration. Examination of the knee under anesthesia is done to recognize the concomitant pathologies that will be addressed during the surgery. All cartilage lesions are then identified during diagnostic arthroscopy. At the time of the procedure, it is necessary to choose whether the procedure will be performed arthroscopically or via arthrotomy. Arthroscopic intervention is only possible if the lesion can be fully visualized with the arthroscope and reached with instruments. If not, the procedure should be continued through an arthrotomy. Thorough debridement of the loose chondral tissue is necessary, ensuring that the border of the lesion is vertical to the subchondral plane. The calcified cartilage layer overlying the subchondral bone is removed. Care must be taken to not violate the subchondral plate. BMAC preparation is started after the lesion is prepared. Approximately 60 mL of bone marrow from the ipsilateral iliac crest is harvested, using a dedicated aspiration kit. The aspirate is centrifuged with a commercially available system to obtain the concentrated bone marrow (Angel, Arthrex, Cytomedix, Gaithersburg, MD). The dimensions of the lesion have to be measured to prepare the matching implant using a three-dimensional hyaluronic acid-based scaffold (Hyalofast, Anika Therapeutics, Bedford MA USA Srl, Abano Terme, Italy). It is also possible to prepare an aluminum foil template of the lesion, and then cut the scaffold to correspond to the contour of the aluminum foil model. When the scaffold is ready, BMAC is activated with batroxobin enzyme (Plateltex Act, Plateltex SRO, Bratislava, Slovakia). The activation process is necessary for BMAC to form a clot, which is then applied onto the prepared scaffold forming a sticky implant that is easy to apply to the lesion (Fig. 25.1).

According to the chosen approach, previously prepared HA-BMAC is then implanted into the lesion. If an open technique is selected, the surgeon should apply HA-BMAC directly onto the defect. If needed, fibrin glue is added to secure the graft

further. The knee is then flexed and extended to check graft stability. If the surgeon chooses an arthroscopic approach, fluid needs to be completely drained, and the lesion should be inspected arthroscopically after fluid drainage to ensure that the circumferential border is stable. The scaffold is introduced into the joint via the working portal through a valveless cannula using a grasper. The implant is placed gently filling the cartilage defect. A hook can be used to press-fit the scaffold into the lesion. The crucial part of the procedure is to check the implant stability. The joint is moved through a range of motion several times while the scaffold is observed with the arthroscope. If needed, fibrin glue is applied to improve implant stability. The working portals are sutured, but a drain should not be inserted into the joint [24–26].

A recently described technique by Sadlik et al. [27] to repair osteochondral injury using mor-

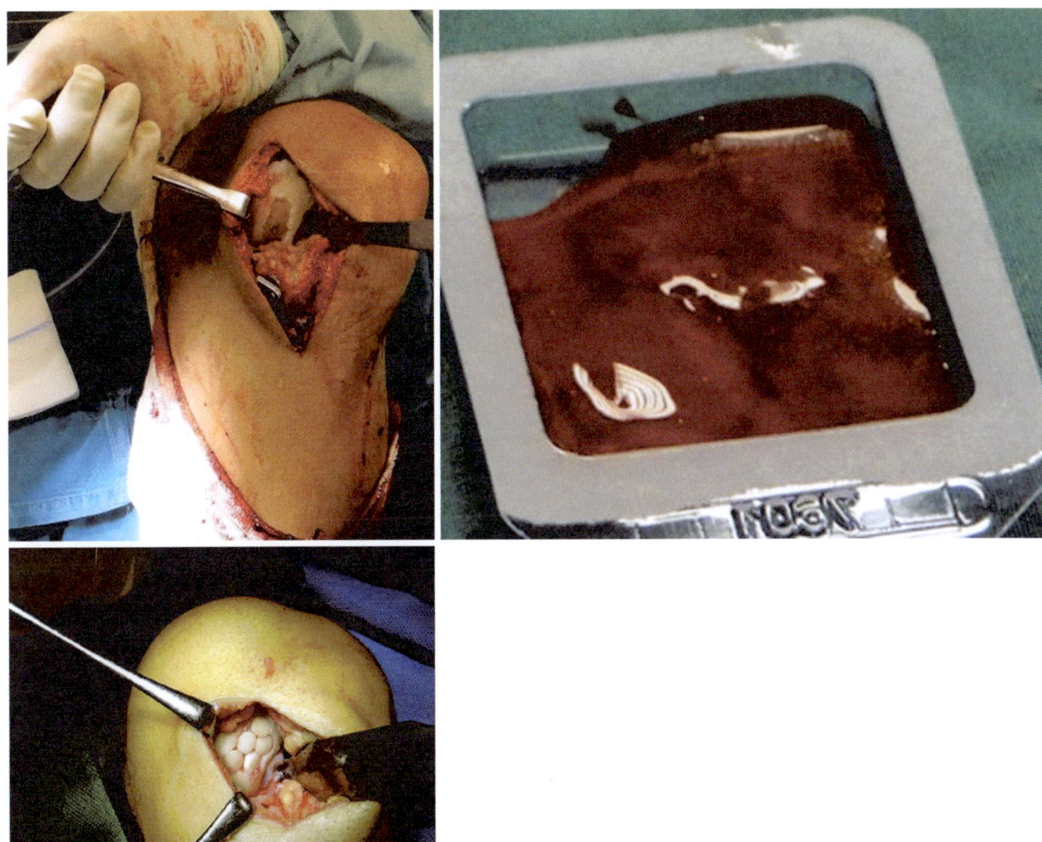

Fig. 25.1 Intraoperative images of HA-BMAC technique

selized bone grafting and mesenchymal stem cells sourced from bone marrow aspirate has been termed Biologic Inlay Osteochondral Reconstruction (BIOR). This technique uses a hyaluronic acid-based scaffold embedded with BMAC in association with a malleable bone graft inlay. Although only preliminary clinical outcome data is currently available for osteochondral pathology treated with BIOR, [27] this type of cell-based, single-stage reconstruction procedure is expected to become a preferred method of surgical treatment, given the cost-effective nature and technical versatility of the technique.

Box 25.1 Pearls and Pitfalls of HA-BMAC Cartilage Repair

Pearls
- Complete exposure of the cartilage lesion is essential and may be problematic in the patellofemoral compartment. Use traction methods as needed to provide a comfortable working space
- If dimensions of the prepared cartilage defect are difficult to measure, use an aluminum foil template or similar material to assist with accurate scaffold size matching
- The hyaluronic acid-based scaffold composition is symmetrical; after creation of the HA-BMAC graft, implantation may proceed with either side placed against the subchondral bone

Pitfalls
- Arthroscopic cartilage repair should proceed only in cases where the entirety of the defect can be appreciated and treated in a minimally invasive manner; repair should be performed in an open manner otherwise
- Confirm secure graft seating within the cartilage defect by cycling the knee under arthroscopic visualization; failure to do so may increase the risk of graft delamination in the postoperative period

25.3 One-Step Treatment for Subchondral Bone Lesions

25.3.1 Osteo-Core-Plasty

Osteo-Core-Plasty (Marrow Cellution™) is a minimally invasive subchondral bone augmentation procedure that provides both biologic and structural components to provide optimized environment for regeneration. It is a fluoroscopic guided, minimally invasive, autologous, biologic procedure that allows necrotic bone segment resection and transplant living, live, intact bone segments that have the capabilities to reincorporate naturally without foreign body implantation [28]. It is an approach that could potentially overcome the issue of centrifugation techniques wherein there is an increase level of peripheral blood nucleated cells which contain very few stem or progenitor cells. It uses multiple small volume draws (1 mL) from a single puncture that utilizes lateral flow from multiple sites near the inner cortical bone space in bone marrow (SSLM method). It is identified that this anatomical location contains a high number of bone marrow stem or progenitor cells [29].

Osteo-Core-Plasty starts with bone marrow aspiration process. All the materials and instruments are prepared. Aseptic technique is applied over the iliac crest and operative site. First is to heparinize all kit components using 2.000 units/mL heparin. Then, the introducer needle with sharp stylet is inserted just past cortex into the medullary space. Sharp stylet is then removed. Syringe is attached and 1 mL marrow is aspirated to ensure proper positioning of needle tip. The syringe is after removed. Blunt Stylet is inserted and locked. Introducer Needle may now be advanced to desired depth. Guide Grip is now rotated to skin level. Blunt Stylet is then removed. The Aspiration Cannula is then inserted and secured. The syringe is attached and 1 mL marrow is aspirated. A Guide Grip is held at handle and rotated 360° counterclockwise then another 1 mL is aspirated. Guide Grip could be rotated as needed and could be reassembled for additional puncture sites [28] (Fig. 25.2).

Application could be done arthroscopically or open access method. Arthroscopic method is done with fluoroscopic guidance. Necrotic Tissue Zone is identified. K-wire is then inserted to target zone and cannulated drill is inserted over the K-Wire. K-Wire and necrotic bone core are then removed. Extraction/Delivery Tool containing Marrow Cellution Bone Core Graft. The probe is inserted to push bone core graft to target zone position. Lastly, Marrow Cellution™ is injected as liquid bone graft [28] (Fig. 25.3).

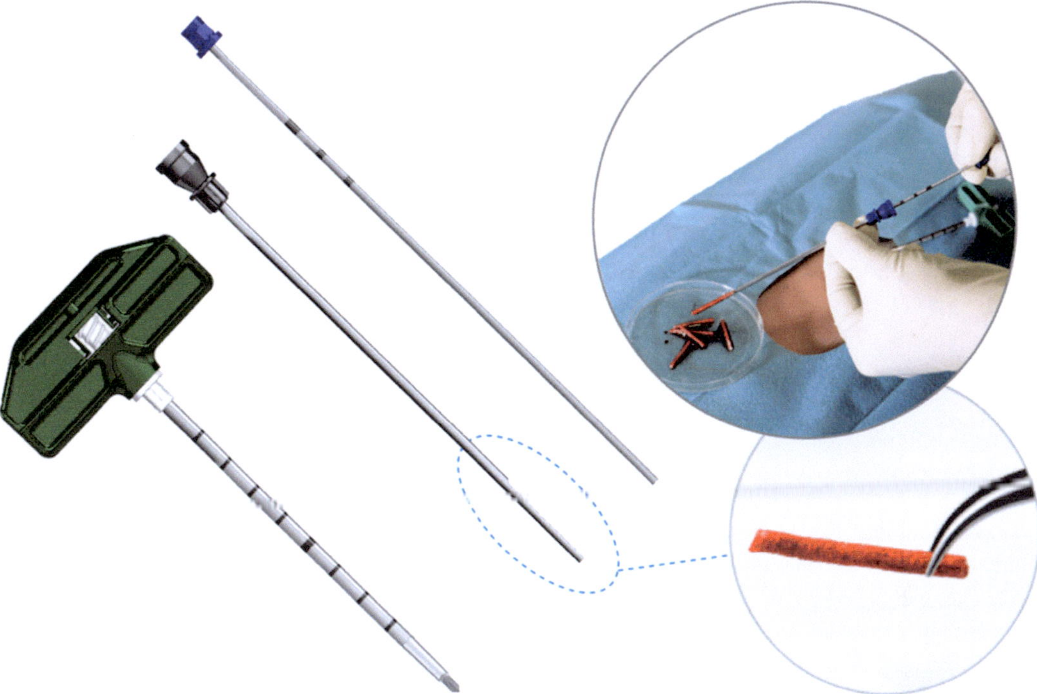

Fig. 25.2 Osteo-Core-Plasty (Marrow Cellution™). Instruments required (Reproduced with permission)

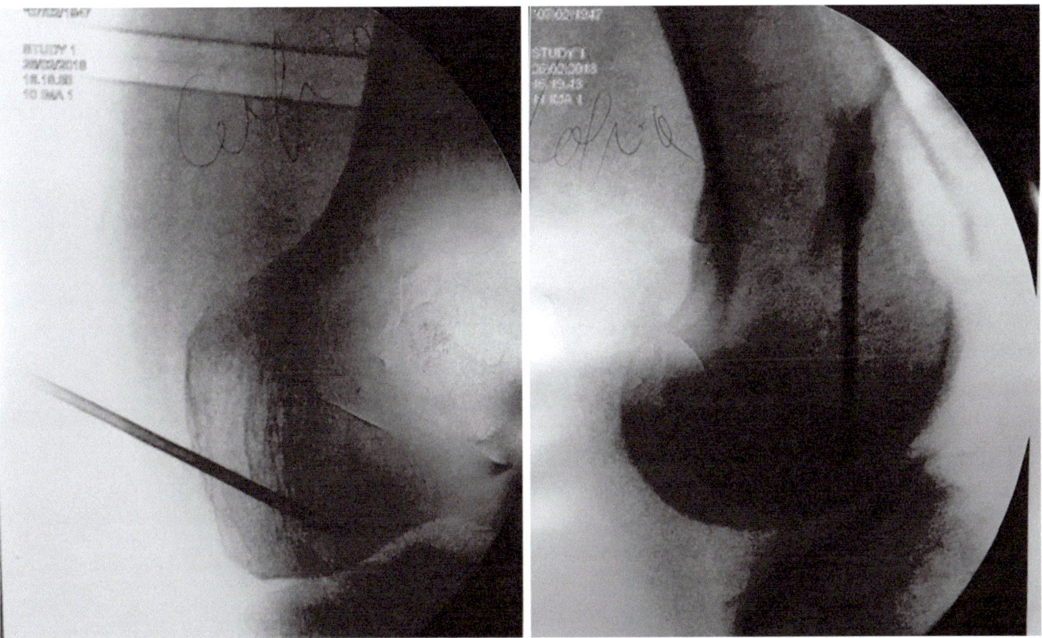

Fig. 25.3 Osteo-Core-Plasty. The procedure under radioscopic guidance

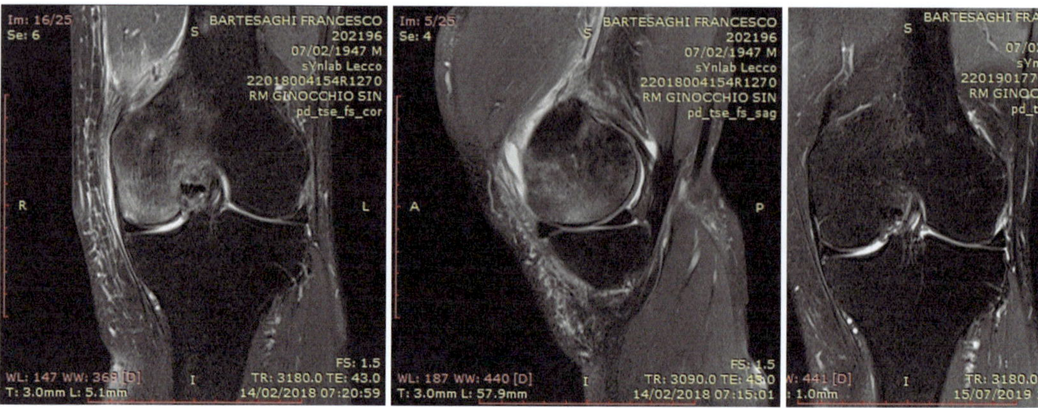

Fig. 25.4 MRI pre-op and 12 months post-op. of a case example with a BML in the medial femoral condyle treated with osteo-core-plasty

Open technique is also done with fluoroscopic guidance wherein the necrotic tissue zone is identified. The cartilage bed is now debrided. After debridement, cannulated drill is inserted to required depth. Necrotic core is removed. Extraction/Delivery Tool containing Marrow Cellution™ Bone Core Graft is then inserted. Then Probe is used to push Bone Core Graft to Distal Position. Then, Marrow Cellution™ Liquid Bone Graft is injected. Then the Marrow Cellution™ Saturated Matrix Scaffold Membrane is applied. Finally, Fibrin Glue is applied to seal the membrane [28].

Studies show that bone marrow samples containing a relatively high CFU-fs/mL and CD34+/mL can be attained without the need for centrifugation using the Marrow Cellution™ system. The level of CFU-fs/mL was significantly higher in the Osteo-Core-Plasty compared to BMACs in side by side comparison from the same patients using the contralateral iliac crest [29]. Another study showed that the Osteo-Core-Plasty had over twice as many fibroblast-like colony forming units (CFU-f) and only half as many nucleated cells compared to centrifugation techniques. Moreover, the Osteo-Core-Plasty showed same numbers of CD34+ and CD117+ cells compared to centrifugation techniques [29].

There are several benefits of Osteo-Core-Plasty. It allows the clinician to retain the product entirely on the sterile area rather than necessitating the product to leave the sterile area for centrifugation and re-enter the sterile area for administration to the patient, decreases procedural expenses, and maintains all the cells and growth factors obtained during aspiration. Users of this technique reported that another advantage is the ability to advance into and retreat from the marrow area in both precise and controlled manner [30] (Fig. 25.4).

Box 25.2 Pearls and Pitfalls of Osteo-Core-Plasty

Pearls
- During bone marrow aspiration change the trocar direction to obtain BMA from different places
- Assess the lesion both with MRI and radiography
- Use AP and lateral fluoroscopic images to determine the application site precisely
- Decompress the lesion with a cannula
- Keep the trocar inserted in the cannula for 5–7 min to allow BMA to clot
- Perform arthroscopy to confirm lack of intra-articular leakage

Pitfalls
- Breach of the cortex during decompression
- Imprecise BMA application and intra-articular leakage
- Premature removal of the trocar and cannula
- Leaving other intra-articular pathologies untreated

25.4 Postoperative Rehabilitation

25.4.1 Immediate Postoperative Protocol at the Hospital

First day after the surgery the patient is taught static exercises to prevent vascular complications and muscle hypotrophy. The limb is placed on a continuous passive motion (CPM) machine on a continuous or intermittent basis for the next few days or weeks, the range of motion is set according to the site and size of the lesion. The patient stays in the hospital for approximately 3 days, where the physiotherapist trains the patient on non-weight bearing crutch assisted walking with a straight leg brace. The brace is to be worn day and night and removed only when doing rehabilitation exercises and during showering.

25.4.2 Postoperative Rehabilitation Protocol

All patients follow a standard rehabilitation protocol after HA-BMAC implantation. However, this program should be modified according to the patient's progress and capabilities. The program is divided into four phases, each phase lasting from 6 to 12 weeks.

25.4.2.1 Proliferative/ Protective Phase (0–6 Weeks)

This phase aims to protect the implanted scaffold from excessive loads and shearing forces. The goal for the patient is to gain full extension with gradual recovery of knee flexion by the end of this phase. The patient can start toe touch ambulation by the end of third week and partial weight bearing at sixth week. The brace should be locked at 0° of extension during ambulation and at nights for at least 4 weeks. Mobilization may begin at the third week with the aim to achieve flexion of 120° by the end of 6 weeks. Strengthening exercises should start immediately with static exercises progressing to pool exercises by 3 weeks and cycling by the end of 4 weeks. Pain and swelling are controlled with cryotherapy, stockings, and anti-inflammatory drugs. Next phase

can begin when the patient regains complete passive extension and flexion of approximately 120° with minimum pain, swelling, and adequate quadriceps recruitment.

25.4.2.2 Transition Phase (6–12 Weeks)

After 6 weeks, gait retraining begins to increase the muscle strength and to gradually increase functional activities. The brace should be maintained until there is sufficient quadriceps strength for ambulation. Full weight bearing without crutches is started 8–12 weeks post-implantation as tolerated. It is important to start multidirectional patella mobilization exercises along with active and passive range of motion (ROM) exercises. Next phase of rehabilitation can begin after achieving pain-free full range of motion, about 70% quadriceps and flexor strength compared to contralateral limb and normal gait pattern.

25.4.2.3 Maturation Phase (12–24 Weeks)

At this period of time, focus is on increasing the quadriceps and flexors muscle strength and resistance, as well as an increase in functional activities. Patient can progress to next phase of rehabilitation if side-to-side quadriceps and flexor strength of 90% is achieved.

25.4.2.4 Functional Recovery Phase (24–52 Weeks)

During this phase, patients gradually return to functional activity without limitations. It involves both closed and open chain exercises with progressive weight bearing and plyometric exercises. The goal of these exercises is to improve patient's proprioception, agility, and coordination, so that patient can safely go back to sporting activities.

25.5 Conclusions

Single-step cartilage repair eliminates the need for a two-step procedure, thereby reducing the cost and morbidity to the patient.

Associated comorbidities such as malalignment, meniscus deficiency, or ligament laxity

Table 25.1 Summary of the growth factors and cytokines in bone marrow aspirate concentrate

Growth factor/ cytokine	Principle action	Signaling pathway	Reference
TGF β1, TGF β2, TGF β3	Chondrocyte proliferation + differentiation	SMAD-2 and SMAD-3	
BMP-2	Chondrocyte proliferation, matrix synthesis and hypertrophy	SMAD-1, SMAD-5, SMAD-8, TAK-1	
BMP-7	Increase ECM production		
IL-I/IL-1β	Inflammatory response-cell migration/recruitment to site of injury	Mitogen activated kinases (JNK, P38, ERK1/2)	
IL-8	Inflammatory response; MSC homing to site to injury; Increased VEGF production; chondrocyte hypertrophy	Mitogen activated kinase; P38	[15, 24]
VEGF	Promotes angiogenesis to sub-chondral bone and supports cartilage growth	HIF-1, Runx2	[28, 29]
PDGF	Wound healing, collagen synthesis, angiogenesis, suppression of IL-1β, enhanced BMP signaling	ERK 1/2, down-regulation of NF-kB signaling	
IGF-1	Increased synthetic and metabolic activity- increased collagen and proteoglycan synthesis, chondrogenic differentiation	PI-3K, ERK 1/2	
FGF-2	Chondrogenic differentiation, MSC homing	ERK 1/2, STATI/P21	
FGF-18	Chondrogenic differentiation, enhanced BMP signaling		

JNK C-Jun N-terminal kinase, *ERK* extracellular signal-related kinases, *TAK-1* TGF-β activating kinase 1 (TAK-1), *STAT1* signal transducer and activator of transcription-1, *PI-3K* phosphoinositide 3-kinase, *Runx2* Runt-domain transcription factor family-2, *HIF-1* hypoxia inducible factor-1, *NK-kB* nuclear factor kappa beta

must be addressed to provide an optimal environment for cartilage repair.

HA-BMAC is a safe and accessible procedure that provides good to excellent clinical outcomes at long-term follow-up in small or large lesions, single or multiple injuries, and various compartments.

Osteo-core-plasty is a new minimally invasive procedure with reported efficacy in the treatment of painful subchondral bone lesions. It may be particularly important for younger, active patients who wish to reduce pain.

There is still a need for high-powered randomized controlled studies comparing different treatment options for chondral and subchondral lesions before definitive recommendations can be made (Tables 25.1 and 25.2).

Table 25.2 Cellular characterization

	n	Median (Range)
Pre-spin measures		
Viability, %	24	97.8 (75.2–99.4)
MNCs, %	25	38.5 (26.0–57.5)
Total MNCs/µL	25	6100 (1950–27,000)
HSCs, %	25	3.2 (0.04–21.0)
MSCs, %	25	0.03 (0.00–0.60)
Total MNCs × MSCs, %	25	198 (0–2673)
WBCs, 1000/µL	25	13.0 (3.9–62.8)
RBCs, Mil/µL	25	3.33 (0.17–4.44)
HCTs, %	25	32.0 (1.6–38.2)
Platelets, 1000/µL	25	95 (7–399)
Post-spin measures		
Viability, %	22	97.0 (85.4–99.6)
MNCs, %	23	56.2 (25.8–87.9)
Total MNCs/µL	23	16,000 (2900–210.000)
HSCs, %	23	4.4 (1.2–14.0)
MSCs, %	23	0.05 (0.0–0.9)
Total MNCs × MSCs, %	23	688 (8.7–28,980)
WBCs, 1000/µL	23	31.4 (5.6–97.2)
RBCs, Mil/µL	23	0.96 (0.63–3.65)
HCTs, %	23	8.5 (3.5–34.0)
Platelets, 1000/µL	22	422 (52–1515)
Total HSCs injected	23	4,620,000 (174,000–130,200,000)
Total MSCs injected	23	34,400 (435–1,449,000)

HCT hematocrit, *HSC* hematopoietic stem cell, *Mil* million, *MNC* mononuclear cell, *MSC* mesenchymal stem cell, *n* number of patient samples analyzed, *RBC* red blood cell, *WBC* white blood cell

References

1. Hunter W. On the structure and diseases of articulating cartilage. Philos Trans R Soc Lond B Biol Sci. 1743;9:277.
2. Mankin HJ. The response of articular cartilage to mechanical injury. J Bone Joint Surg Am. 1982;64(3):460–6.
3. Widuchowski W, Widuchowski J, Trzaska T. Articular cartilage defects: study of 25,124 knee arthroscopies. Knee. 2007;14:177–82.
4. Flanigan DC, Harris JD, Trinh TQ, Siston RA, Brophy RH. Prevalence of chondral defects in athletes' knees: a systematic review. Med Sci Sports Exerc. 2010;42:1795–801.
5. Johnson DL, Urban WP Jr, Caborn DN, et al. Articular cartilage changes seen with magnetic resonance imaging-detected bone bruises associated with acute anterior cruciate ligament rupture. Am J Sports Med. 1998;26:409–14.
6. Lohmander LS, Roos H, Dahlberg L, et al. Temporal patterns of stromelysin-1, tissue inhibitor, and proteoglycan fragments in human knee joint fluid after injury to the cruciate ligament or meniscus. J Orthop Res. 1994;12:21–8.
7. Mandelbaum BR, Browne JE, Fu F, et al. Articular cartilage lesions of the knee. Am J Sports Med. 1998;26:853–61.
8. Kotlarz H, Gunnarsson CL, Fang H, Rizzo JA. Insurer and out-of-pocket costs of osteoarthritis in the US: evidence from national survey data. Arthritis Rheum. 2009;60(12):3546–53.
9. Takeda H, Nakagawa T, Nakamura K, Engebretsen L. Prevention and management of knee osteoarthritis and knee cartilage injury in sports. Br J Sports Med. 2011;45(4):304–9. Epub 2011 Feb 25
10. Marcacci M, Berruto M, Brocchetta D, et al. Articular cartilage engineering with Hyalograft(R) C: 3-year clinical results. Clin Orthop Relat Res. 2005;435:96–105.
11. Gobbi A, Kon E, Berruto M, et al. Patellofemoral full-thickness chondral defects treated with second-generation autologous chondrocyte implantation: results at 5 years' follow-up. Am J Sports Med. 2009;37:1083–92.
12. Caplan AI. Mesenchymal stem cells: cell-based reconstructive therapy in orthopedics. Tissue Eng. 2005;11(7–8):1198–211.
13. Caplan AI. Mesenchymal stem cells: the past, the present, the future. Cartilage. 2010;1(1):6–9.
14. Dimarino AM, Caplan AI, Bonfield TL. Mesenchymal stem cells in tissue repair. Front Immunol. 2013;4:201.
15. Huselstein C, Li Y, He X. Mesenchymal stem cells for cartilage engineering. Biomed Mater Eng. 2012;22:69–80.
16. Pasquinelli G, Orrico C, Foroni L, Bonafè F, Carboni M, Guarnieri C, et al. Mesenchymal stem cell interaction with a non-woven hyaluronan-based scaffold suitable for tissue repair. J Anat. 2008;213(5):520–30.
17. Lisignoli G, Cristino S, Piacentini A, Zini N, Noël D, Jorgensen C, et al. Chondrogenic differentiation of murine and human mesenchymal stromal cells in a hyaluronic acid scaffold: differences in gene expression and cell morphology. J Biomed Mater Res A. 2006;77(3):497–506.
18. Facchini A, Lisignoli G, Cristino S, Roseti L, De Franceschi L, Marconi E, et al. Human chondrocytes and mesenchymal stem cells grown onto engineered scaffold. Biorheology. 2006;43(3–4):471–80.
19. Nejadnik H, Hui JH, Feng Choong EP, Tai BC, Lee EH. Autologous bone marrow-derived mesenchymal stem cells versus autologous chondrocyte implantation: an observational cohort study. Am J Sports Med. 2010;38(6):1110–6.
20. Gobbi A, Chaurasia S, Karnatzikos G, Nakamura N. Matrix-induced autologous chondrocyte implantation versus multipotent stem cells for the treatment of large patellofemoral chondral lesions: a nonrandomized prospective trial. Cartilage. 2015;6(2):82–97.

21. Gobbi A, Karnatzikos G, Sankineani SR. One-step surgery with multipotent stem cells for the treatment of large full-thickness chondral defects of the knee. Am J Sports Med. 2014;42(3):64857.

22. Gobbi A, et al. Biologic arthroplasty for full-thickness cartilage lesions of the knee: results at three years follow-up (SS-56). Arthroscopy. 2013;29(6):e27.

23. Gobbi A, Karnatzikos G, Scotti C, Mahajan V, Mazzucco L, Grigolo B. One-step cartilage repair with bone marrow aspirate concentrated cells and collagen matrix in full-thickness knee cartilage lesions: results at 2-year follow-up. Cartilage. 2011;2(3):286–99.

24. Gobbi A, Whyte GP. Long-term clinical outcomes of one-stage cartilage repair in the knee with hyaluronic acid-based scaffold embedded with mesenchymal stem cells sourced from bone marrow aspirate concentrate. Am J Sports Med. 2019;47(7):1621–8.

25. Whyte GP, Gobbi A, Sadlik B. Dry arthroscopic single-stage cartilage repair of the knee using a hyaluronic acid-based scaffold with activated bone marrow-derived mesenchymal stem cells. Arthrosc Tech. 2016;5(4):e913–8.

26. Gobbi A, Scotti C, Karnatzikos G, Mudhigere A, Castro M, Peretti GM. One-step surgery with multi-potent stem cells and Hyaluronan-based scaffold for the treatment of full-thickness chondral defects of the knee in patients older than 45 years. Knee Surg Sports Traumatol Arthrosc. 2017;25(8):2494–501.

27. Sadlik B, et al. Biologic inlay osteochondral reconstruction: arthroscopic one-step osteochondral lesion repair in the knee using morselized bone grafting and hyaluronic acid-based scaffold embedded with bone marrow aspirate concentrate. Arthrosc Tech. 2017;6(2):e383–9.

28. Osteo-Core-Plasty™ with Marrow Cellution™|Aspire Medical Innovation [Internet]. [cited 2020 Mar 3]. https://aspire-medical.eu/marrowcellution/osteo-core-plasty-with-marrow-cellution/.

29. Scarpone M, Kuebler D, Chambers A, De Filippo CM, Amatuzio M, Ichim TE, et al. Isolation of clinically relevant concentrations of bone marrow mesenchymal stem cells without centrifugation. J Transl Med [Internet]. 2019 [cited 2020 Mar 9];17:10. https://doi.org/10.1186/s12967-018-1750-x.

30. Swedowski D, Gobbi A, Irlandini E. Osteo-core plasty: a minimally invasive approach for subchondral bone marrow lesions of the knee. Arthrosc Tech. 2020;9(11):e1773–7.

Cartilage Restoration and Stabilization Strategies for the Patellofemoral Joint

Joseph D. Lamplot, Andreas H. Gomoll, and Sabrina M. Strickland

26.1 Introduction

Cartilage defects within the patellofemoral joint (PFJ) are common and can cause pain and dysfunction. Chondral lesions may result from macrotrauma, including a direct impact injury or patellar instability event, or microtrauma, such as abnormal joint loading due to chronic patellar subluxation or repetitive high loading [1]. Patellofemoral (PF) cartilage disease often occurs in the setting of other pathologies including patellar maltracking and instability. Nonetheless, focal chondral lesions still do frequently occur even in the absence of these other pathologies [2, 3]. Multiple studies have demonstrated that high-grade focal chondral or osteochondral lesions occur in up to 61–66% of patients undergoing knee arthroscopy, with one third of these lesions occurring in the PFJ [4, 5]. Among patients with high-grade articular cartilage lesions within the knee, the patella is the second most common location after the medial femoral condyle [1, 4, 5]. However, the true prevalence of these defects is difficult to determine since a large percentage are asymptomatic due to, in part, the aneural nature of articular cartilage.

It is imperative to understand that chondrosis does not necessarily equal pain and should be considered a diagnosis of exclusion after considering all other identifiable factors including malalignment and instability. Many patients with anterior knee pain do not have cartilage defects, while many patients with chondrosis have no pain [1]. Nonetheless, if left untreated, PF cartilage defects may lead to osteoarthritis [6, 7]. Risk factors for focal chondral lesions within the PFJ include trochlear dysplasia, patella alta, and abnormal patellar tilt [8]. Trochlear lesions occur more commonly in males and tend to present at an older age than patellar lesions [8]. Patellar lesions occur more commonly in females and at a younger age, and they have a closer association with anatomic risk factors including trochlear dysplasia and patella alta [8]. The natural history of a subset of patients with PFJ chondral lesions is progression to OA, which occurs at a younger age than tibiofemoral OA [8]. It is likely that the anatomic risk factors of trochlear dysplasia and patellar malalignment lead to premature chondral degeneration and eventual PFJ OA [8, 9].

Several factors contribute to the challenges of performing cartilage restoration procedures

J. D. Lamplot (✉) · A. H. Gomoll · S. M. Strickland
Orthopedics, Sports Medicine—Hospital for Special Surgery, New York, NY, USA
e-mail: joseph.daniel.lamplot@emory.edu;
gomolla@hss.edu; stricklands@hss.edu

© ISAKOS 2021
A. J. Krych et al. (eds.), *Cartilage Injury of the Knee*,
https://doi.org/10.1007/978-3-030-78051-7_26

within the PFJ compared to other areas of the knee [10]. These include the high shear and compressive stresses within the joint, which are further increased in the setting of chondral injuries [11]. Furthermore, the complex topography of the PFJ and heterogeneity of anatomy between patients can complicate efforts to restore anatomic congruity [10]. Additionally, the patella contains the thickest cartilage in the body with different structural characteristics than femoral cartilage [10], and as such, auto- or allografts from femoral donor sites may not adapt to the stresses encountered within the PFJ [12–14]. In most cases, treatment is initially non-operative, with the exception of acute injuries resulting in loose bodies. The goal of cartilage repair and restoration surgery within the PFJ is to alleviate pain and restore function. Surgical options can be categorized as palliative, reparative, restorative, and reconstructive. It currently remains unknown whether these treatments slow or halt the progression to PFJ OA due to the challenges of long-term studies of 20 years or more. Historically, outcomes following cartilage restoration within the PFJ have been inferior to those within the tibiofemoral joint due to the complex biomechanics of the former; however, more recent studies have demonstrated almost equivalent outcomes [12, 13, 15–20].

26.2 History and Physical Exam

Although history and physical exam are neither sensitive nor specific for cartilage injury, it remains an important component of clinical decision-making. Possible etiologies of cartilage lesions within the PFJ include patellar instability/dislocation, acute direct trauma, repetitive mictrotrauma, maltracking, and idiopathic causes. Chondral defects of the patella can be seen in up to 95% of patients after a patellar dislocation, and most do not necessitate cartilage restoration or repair surgery [21]. One study of pediatric patients with surgically treated patellar instability demonstrated that PF articular cartilage damage was present in 63% of knees, with the patella involved in 61% and the trochlea in 20% of cases [22]. Repetitive activities that may put the PFJ at risk include jumping, squatting, and crawling (firefighters). While patients frequently complain of anterior knee pain, it is important to determine the specific location of pain (margin of patella, deep to the patella), the position of the knee at which pain occurs, and activities that exacerbate pain. The presence or absence of swelling and mechanical symptoms should be noted. Focal pain without mechanical symptoms is likely secondary to subchondral bone overload [1].

Diagnostic components of the physical exam related to PFJ pathology include gait analysis and examination of tibiofemoral and patellar alignment. Specifically, static valgus malalignment, dynamic valgus during a single-leg squat, and rotational malalignment with increased tibial torsion or femoral anteversion should be assessed and may be seen in patients with patellar chondral lesions [1]. The location of tenderness to palpation (medial, lateral, distal, retropatellar) and its concordance with the location of the cartilage lesion(s) should be determined. Patellar tracking should be carefully evaluated and is best evaluated in a sitting position. Specific items to assess include J-sign and subluxation during quadriceps contraction in extension. Anatomic risk factors for maltracking include trochlear dysplasia, patella alta, increased tibial tubercle to trochlear-groove distance (TT-TG) and lateral soft tissue contracture. A J-sign in terminal extension suggests trochlear dysplasia and/or significant patella alta [1]. Other structures to evaluate include ligamentous and soft tissue contracture and laxity with patellar apprehension, patellar glide, patellar tilt, effusion, and crepitus.

26.3 Imaging

Beyond characterizing cartilage lesions, imaging studies can allow identification of malalignment and other associated pathology. Initial imaging includes standard anteroposterior (AP), 45-degree posteroanterior (PA), lateral and Merchant radiographs. Merchant views can demonstrate PFJ congruence, tilt, subluxation, and joint space narrowing. The true lateral view can be used to assess for trochlear dysplasia [23].

PFJ alignment is evaluated by patellar height, tilt, and TT-TG distance [24]. MRI is routinely obtained to assess chondral lesions as well as subchondral bone involvement. While helpful in estimating the grade and size of lesions, MRI has been reported to underestimate lesion size by up to 60% [25]. Anatomic indices that should be measured in patients with PF pathology include measures of patellar height such as (1) the Caton-Deschamps patellar height ratio, (2) the Blackburn-Peele index, and (3) the patellar trochlear overlap index, and the TT-TG distance [24, 26].

26.4 Treatment Indications

Indications for cartilage repair or restoration surgery in the PFJ include persistent pain and dysfunction secondary to focal, full-thickness chondral defects despite non-operative management. Bipolar lesions are not an absolute contraindication, while significant joint space narrowing is. Distal lateral chondral defects of the patella in symptomatic patients undergoing tibial tubercle osteotomy (TTO) for instability may be debrided or left alone, as these lesions will be offloaded by the osteotomy [27]. Inferomedial patellar chondral defects from patellar dislocation that do not cross the median patellar ridge may also generally be debrided or left alone. Loose bodies with or without a history of acute injury or instability event can be treated with either removal or, if tissue quality is sufficient, repair of the chondral or osteochondral fragment [28, 29]. In the setting of acute loose bodies, surgical treatment is warranted.

26.5 Non-operative Management

With few exceptions, the initial management of articular cartilage lesions includes relative rest, activity modification, and physical therapy, with or without non-steroidal anti-inflammatories (NSAIDs). Physical therapy should first focus on restoration of range of motion and flexibility followed by progressive strengthening including the core, hip, and quadriceps muscles, emphasizing a "Core to Floor" approach [30]. In general, non-operative measures are typically attempted prior to proceeding with cartilage restoration surgery. Traumatic lesions, especially in younger patients and in those with a symptomatic loose body resulting from an acute injury, may be treated more expediently. Injections may be considered in patients with degenerative lesions. While there is a lack of evidence to support their use specifically for focal PF chondral lesions, corticosteroid or viscosupplementation may alleviate pain by decreasing inflammation [31]. Bracing or taping is a noninvasive and generally inexpensive measure that may also be attempted to unload PF chondral lesions, albeit with limited evidence to support their use [32–34]. After failing an extensive course of non-operative management, a minority of patients will warrant consideration for surgical management.

26.6 Surgical Management of Cartilage Defects

Cartilage surgery within the PFJ aims to relieve pain, restore function, improve quality of life, and potentially delay the onset of OA and need for knee arthroplasty. Cartilage procedures generally include debridement (chondroplasty), microfracture (Mfx) with or without adjuvant treatment, osteochondral autograft transfer (OAT), osteochondral allograft (OCA), particular juvenile allograft cartilage (PJAC), perforated allograft cartilage, and matrix-assisted chondrocyte implantation (MACI). While there is increasing evidence that these procedures result in improved pain and function in patients with PFJ cartilage defects, it remains unclear whether or not these procedures slow or prevent the progression of OA [35, 36]. Cartilage procedures can be divided into four categories: palliative, reparative, restorative, and reconstructive [1]. Palliative options include loose body removal and chondroplasty, which solely aim to relieve painful mechanical symptoms. Reparative techniques fix the chondral or osteochondral fragment that is injured and are generally only performed in the acute or subacute setting. Restorative techniques are cell-based and include marrow stimulation, including Mfx, MACI, and PJAC. Reconstructive methods, such as OAT and OCA, utilize transplantation of autograft or allograft tissue to the injury site to reconstruct the injured osteochondral unit.

Adequate exposure is critical to facilitate defect preparation and implantation or fixation. An open approach is often recommended, and a parapatellar arthrotomy may be made either medial or lateral on the same side as the lesion. If patellar eversion is required to reach the defect, the arthrotomy is typically extended into the quadriceps tendon. Alternatively, a subvastus or midvastus approach may be performed. For patellar lesions, the patella usually requires eversion, which may not be necessary for trochlear lesions. For central lesions, a medial parapatellar approach may be preferred, as the patella is more easily subluxed laterally. If multiple concomitant procedures are performed, an approach that allows good access for all procedures should be selected.

26.7 Patellar Dislocation: Osteochondral Fracture and Chondral Shear Injuries

Acute patellar dislocations typically result from a contact or noncontact flexion-rotation injury, direct blow to the patella, or forced knee hyperextension and may result in osteochondral fragment fractures or chondral shear injuries of the patella, trochlea, or femoral condyle [37, 38]. These injuries commonly occur in active pediatric and adolescent patients who often have many years of future impact activities, and as such, may benefit from preservation of their native cartilage [37]. Skeletally immature patients are particularly susceptible to these injuries because the calcified cartilage layer is incompletely formed, resulting in a weak interface between the articular cartilage and underlying subchondral bone [38, 39]. Multiple studies have reported that greater than one third of patients with a first-time acute patellar dislocation have an osteochondral fracture identified on MRI [40], most commonly occurring on the medial facet of the patella [21, 41, 42]. Osteochondral injury resulting in loose bodies has been reported in 5–50% of acute patellar instability cases [29]. In most cases, fragment excision or surgical repair may be considered acutely due to mechanical symptoms as well as the potential for loose body migration and damage to surrounding uninjured cartilage [40]. Furthermore, the loose fragment tends to swell over time resulting in chondral degeneration [38]. The threshold size of a loose osteochondral or chondral fragment warranting operative intervention remains unclear, with some studies suggesting that fragments less than 10 mm [42] and others suggesting that fragments less than 15 mm can benefit from a trial of non-operative management [43]. However, if visualized on preoperative imaging, the authors recommend removal of loose bodies with repair on a case-by-case basis depending on fragment size, quality lesion location.

When possible, attempts should be made to preserve the native articular cartilage, which has superior histological and long-term wear characteristics compared to other cartilage restoration techniques [38]. However, the decision of whether to excise or fix the fragment can be difficult. Fixation of osteochondral fractures is recommended if the fragment is of an adequate size (i.e., greater than approximately 10 mm in diameter) [42] and has adequate bony tissue to facilitate stable fixation and bone-to-bone healing [38, 44]. In general, if the resulting defect is relatively small (less than 10 mm in diameter), then fragment excision may be performed alone or in combination with a cartilage restoration procedure [42, 43]. Isolated fragment excision has improved clinical outcomes when the donor site is the patella compared to the femoral condyle [42, 45]. Repair is recommended for relatively large osteochondral fractures when the fragment's cartilage is in good condition [40]. Patellar osteochondral fragment fixation requires an arthrotomy. Fixation methods include metallic headless compression screws, trans-patellar suture fixation, and bioabsorbable implants, including screws and pins [40]. Bioabsorbable implants typically do not require removal unless they migrate or become symptomatic [46]. Metallic headless compression screws are typi-

cally removed at approximately 12 weeks postoperative or when radiographic healing has occurred. Skeletally immature patients treated with bioabsorbable implants have been reported to have higher rates of healing and lower complication rates than those with closed physes [47].

There is a growing body of evidence to support the fixation of isolated chondral shear injuries of the knee in pediatric and adolescent patients. Historically, chondral-only fragments were removed rather than fixed, as it was believed that repair would fail due to poor healing potential [48, 49]. Recent case reports have contradicted this dogma, suggesting that healing and good clinical outcomes can occur following chondral fragment to bone fixation (Fig. 26.1) [37, 50, 51]. In a case series of 15 patients undergoing fixation of chondral-only fragments within the knee, Fabricant et al. [37] reported successful short-term healing

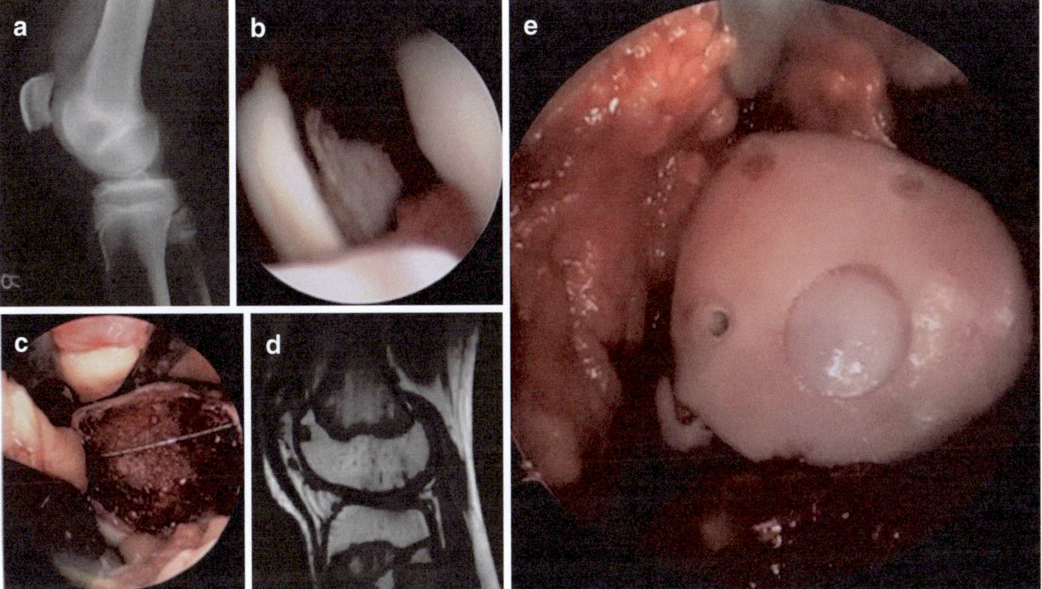

Fig. 26.1 A 16-year-old male with first-time patellar dislocation with associated chondral shear injury to lateral femoral condyle. (**a**) Preoperative lateral radiograph indicates skeletally immaturity. (**b**) Arthroscopic image demonstrating large loose chondral-only fragment. (**c**) Intraoperative photo demonstrates defect size of 20 mm × 22 mm. (**d**) Postoperative MRI demonstrates OAT plug. (**e**) Chondral fragment fixed with four absorbable tacks peripherally and a single 6 mm OAT plug. OAT plug serves as fragment fixation and support for the large chondral fragment

in the majority of pediatric and adolescent patients with chondral-only fragments originating from the patella, trochlea, or lateral femoral condyle with median surface area of 492.0 mm^2 fixed with bioabsorbable implants. One patient in this series failed to heal, with no implant-related complications in any of the other patients.

26.8 Debridement/Chondroplasty

Cartilage lesions that are not causing pain most often do not need to be treated. Unless a patient presents with patellofemoral pain or anterior-based mechanical symptoms, patellofemoral chondral lesions should be ignored during a knee arthroscopy performed for meniscectomy or reasons other than anterior knee pain. There is limited evidence in the literature to support the use of chondroplasty in the PFJ [52, 53]. However, a large number of surgeons continue to perform this procedure [54]. We reserve chondroplasty for patients with frank anteriorly based mechanical symptoms, in cases in which a cartilage biopsy is being performed, and for irreparable chondral or osteochondral lesions who are not candidates for cartilage restoration surgery. This includes patients with relatively small lesions (<1 cm^2), relatively older patients who have failed an extensive course of non-operative treatment, and some high-level athletes with a desire to return to play sooner than the rehabilitation following a cartilage restoration surgery would allow.

26.9 Microfracture

Mfx remains one of the most commonly performed cartilage restoration surgeries within the PFJ, second only to autologous chondrocyte implantation (MACI) (29.6% vs. 45.5%). Results of Mfx appear to be inferior within the PFJ compared to the femoral condyles [55, 56]. Results do seem to be improved in younger patient populations who likely have a more metabolically active marrow milieu [55–57]. A recent systematic review investigated clinical outcomes after Mfx within the PFJ, reporting improvements in clinical outcomes in all included studies following Mfx, with greater improvements in younger patients [58]. No recommendations were made regarding treatment guidelines as they relate to lesion size or grade. Studies have suggested that Mfx could be considered for PFJ chondral lesions 2 cm^2 and less [10, 59, 60]. We do not utilize Mfx within the PFJ for several reasons, including concerns about the durability and longevity of the resulting fibrocartilage repair tissue [55, 56, 59–61]. Additionally, patellar lesions are often not completely shouldered, and circumferential shouldering is essential for adequate fibrocartilage fill. Achieving a perpendicular trajectory to the patellar subchondral bone with the Mfx awl or drill is technically difficult and may warrant an open approach although there are angled drill shaver attachments that make an arthroscopic approach feasible. There are also fewer mesenchymal stem cells within the patellar bone marrow than the distal femoral marrow. Finally, shear forces are relatively high within the PFJ compared to the femoral condyles [10]. Because the fibrocartilage resulting from Mfx has inferior biomechanical properties compared to hyaline cartilage, these shear forces are not as well tolerated [10].

Two randomized controlled trials (RCTs) have demonstrated superior clinical outcomes following MACI and OAT compared to Mfx for chondral lesions within the knee [62, 63]. Unfortunately, results in these two studies were not reported according to knee compartment. Solheim et al. [62] reported clinically significant improvements in Lysholm scores at short-, medium-, and long-term (15-year) follow-up after mosaicplasty compared to Mfx. Saris et al. [63] reported a significant improvement in multiple KOOS subscales and fewer treatment failures (12.5% vs 31.9%, $p = 0.016$) following MACI compared to Mfx. While Kreuz et al. [55, 56] reported acceptable results after Mfx of the femoral condyles in young patients, there were diminishing results following Mfx within the PFJ between 18 and 36 months postoperative [64]. Recently, there has been an increased interest in Mfx "plus" in which marrow stimulation is augmented with a scaffold or paste in an attempt to mechanically stabilize the clot formed at the repair site, thereby providing a more favorable environment for cell differentiation [65]. One such treatment option is autologous matrix-induced chondrogenesis (AMIC), in which a collagen membrane is placed within the chondral defect following MFx in order to provide an environment in which MSCs can adhere to and proliferate, thereby improving fibrocartilage formation. In an RCT of patients undergoing either Mfx or AMIC for chondral lesions within any knee compartment, Volz et al. [66] reported a deterioration at 2 years postoperative following patellar Mfx, whereas results were sustained at 5 years following AMIC. Dhollander et al. [67] reported good clinical outcomes at mean 2 year follow-up for the treatment of isolated patellar or trochlear defects although there was a 30% rate of intralesional osteophyte formation and slight MRI deterioration between 1 and 2 years postoperative. Gobbi et al. [68] reported improved results following treatment of grade IV chondral injuries of the femoral condyles or patella treated with a hyaluronic acid-based scaffold with activated bone marrow aspirate concentrate (HA-BMAC) compared to Mfx [68]. Results were not reported according to knee compartment. Altogether, while Mfx is an inexpensive and relatively simple procedure, clinical outcomes within the PFJ seem to favor other cartilage restoration strategies.

26.10 Osteochondral Autograft Transfer (OAT)

Osteochondral autograft transfer (OAT) may be considered for relatively small defects within the PFJ measuring 1–3 cm². The size of the lesion relative to the patient's harvest site should be considered, as donor site morbidity can result when using multiple large plugs. Plugs are typically harvested from the lesser-weightbearing periphery of the trochlea, and less commonly from the intercondylar notch using an all-arthroscopic approach [10, 11, 13, 14]. Peripheral trochlear lesions can often be managed with an all-arthroscopic technique, while patellar lesions require an arthrotomy in order to position instrumentation perpendicular to the articular surface. One particular challenge of OAT for PFJ lesions is difficult in matching the complex topography and varying cartilage thickness of donor and recipient sites [1, 10]. Patellar subchondral bone is also generally harder than femoral condylar bone. As such, a drill rather than the typically used hand-powered trephine should be considered for recipient site preparation in this setting.

Improved outcomes following OAT throughout the knee joint have been reported for lesions <2 cm² [69]. Specifically within the patella, improved outcomes have been reported in patients treated with a single OAT plug compared to multiple plugs [11], among patients who did not require concomitant realignment osteotomy [14], and among patients with isolated traumatic chondral lesions [14]. Inferior outcomes have been reported following PFJ OAT among patients older than 50 [13], larger lesion surface area [11, 13, 14, 69], and in cases with both medial and lateral patellar facet lesions [14]. Astur et al. [11] reported significant improvements in functional and patient-reported outcomes at minimum 2-year follow-up and 100% osseous integration at 1 year following isolated patella OAT. Figueroa et al. [70] reported 100% good or excellent clinical outcomes and 100% ICRS grade IA scores on MRI at minimum 2 years following patellar OAT. Hangody et al. [13] reported 79% good to excellent outcomes following patellar OAT using a mosaicplasty technique at minimum 10-year follow-up. More recently, Emre et al. reported significant clinical improvement without any complications or repeat surgeries following patellofemoral mosaicplasty [71]. Nho et al. [14] reported significant improvements in IKDC scores and good cartilage fill (67–100%) in all patients at minimum 18-month follow-up after patellar OAT. We consider utilizing OAT for relatively small patellar lesions (<2 cm^2) with subchondral bone involvement which precludes the use of cell-based options such as MACI or PJAC.

26.11 Osteochondral Allograft

Osteochondral allograft (OCA) historically has been considered a salvage procedure used to treat large osteochondral defects in patients who have failed a prior surgery who are poor candidates for arthroplasty procedures [10]. Concerns related to OCA include long-term chondrocyte viability and graft resorption, and as with most cartilage restoration procedures, outcomes within the PFJ have generally been inferior to those in the tibiofemoral joint [10]. OCA may be considered for relatively large defects (>2 cm^2) and for lesions in which the subchondral bone is compromised, precluding the use of cell-based options. OCA is among the most technically challenging cartilage restoration techniques, particularly within the PFJ. Recent results following OCA within the PFJ have been acceptable and improved results have been seen within the trochlea compared to the patella [72, 73]. Cameron et al. [72] reported a 91.7% graft survivorship rate at 10-year follow-up, a 21% revision rate, and 89% patient satisfaction following trochlear OCA. Gracitelli et al. [73] reported 78% survival at 10 years and 55.8% survival at 15-year follow-up with a 61% revision rate and 89% patient satisfaction for isolated patellar OCA. In a study of OCA for both isolated and bipolar lesions, Jamali et al. [74] reported 75% good or excellent results. Meric et al. [75] reported inferior survivorship in bipolar lesions compared to focal lesions. The authors utilize

OCA in salvage situations for larger lesions (>2 cm^2) in which subchondral bone injury precludes the use of cell-based options.

26.12 Autologous Chondrocyte Implantation

Autologous chondrocyte implantation (MACI) techniques have evolved over the past two decades. First-generation techniques involved the use of a periosteal patch (pACI), second-generation techniques (cACI) used a type I/III collagen membrane; and the current third-generation technique seeds and cultivates a collagen membrane with chondrocytes prior to implantation (matrix-induced autologous chondrocyte implantation or MACI) [76]. Overall, MACI is the most commonly performed advanced cartilage restoration procedure in the PFJ [77, 78]. MACI has been FDA approved for over 20 years. Due to the complex topography of the PFJ that makes OAT and OCA technically difficult, focal contained chondral lesions of the patella and trochlea may be more amenable to cell-based techniques [10]. MACI is typically indicated for the treatment of medium to large full-thickness cartilage defects and considered second-line for lesions smaller than 2 cm^2 [10] (Fig. 26.2). Relative contraindications include uncontained and bipolar lesions. As with other cartilage procedures, careful assessment of lower extremity alignment, patellar stability, and tracking must be performed preoperatively, and associated pathology should be treated in a concomitant fashion.

While results of earlier generations of MACI were disappointing within the PFJ, currently reported results are nearly as good as within the femoral condyles, with good to excellent results reported across multiple studies in 71–93% of cases [15, 79–82]. It is likely that several variables impact clinical outcomes. One study reported better outcomes following MACI for patellar compared to trochlear lesions [83].

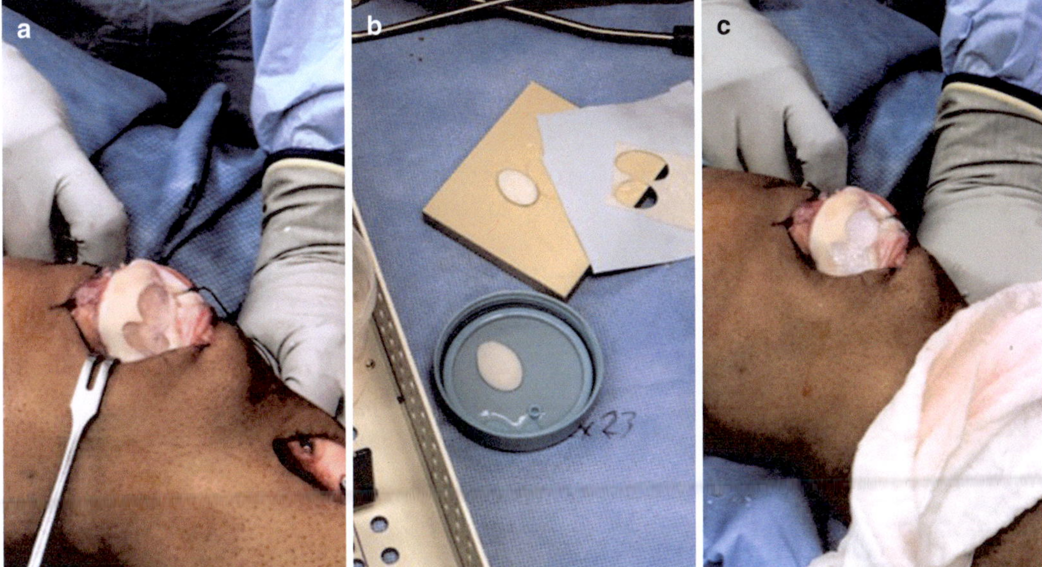

Fig. 26.2 Multifocal patellar lesions treated with MACI. (**a**) Large multifocal patellar chondral lesions without subchondral bone involvement. Lesions involve the medial and lateral facets of the patella. Post-debridement, the lesions coalesce along the median patellar ridge. (**b**) The post-debridement lesion size is templated, and the MACI implant is prepared using a custom cutter, yielding two implants for the defects. (**c**) The MACI implants completely fill the defects and are secured in place using fibrin glue, obviating the need for suture fixation

Another study reported inferior outcomes for degenerative compared to acute lesions [83]. However, it remains unclear how lesion location (medial, lateral, or central) impacts outcomes [3, 6, 84]. It also remains unclear whether bipolar lesions result in inferior outcomes compared to unipolar lesion [3, 15, 18, 85] and whether lesion size or containment impacts outcomes [3, 83]. Multiple studies have reported similar clinical outcomes when comparing the PFJ to the femoral condyles [86, 87], while one study reported improved outcomes following MACI in the femoral condyles [88]. Minas et al. [89] reported similar long-term survivorship between tibiofemoral and patellofemoral grafts but earlier failure among those that did fail in the PFJ group. MRI studies have demonstrated improved defect fill over time [90], with complete fill in 30–40% of patients [15, 68, 91–94]. Farr et al. [95] reported only three failures out of 39 defects at mean 3.1-year follow-up. Gomoll et al. [3] reported nine failures among 110 patients at min-

imum 4-year follow-up, with a 92% satisfaction rate and no significant difference between unipolar and bipolar lesions. Zarkadis et al. [96] reported three failures among 72 army personnel at mean 4.5-year follow-up, with 78% return to occupational specialties.

Multiple studies have demonstrated that outcomes of MACI in the setting of prior marrow stimulation are inferior to MACI without prior marrow stimulation [36, 87, 97]. This is likely due in part to alteration of subchondral bony architecture which can result in the formation of intralesional osteophytes [98] and subchondral cysts [99, 100]. The presence of intralesional osteophytes or cysts should be considered a contraindication to cell-based therapies, and osteochondral replacement should be considered in these situations. Alternatively, an MACI sandwich technique can be utilized in which diseased subchondral bone is removed and grafted with autologous bone followed by MACI [101]. MACI is our preferred method of cartilage restoration within the PFJ. Subchondral edema alone does not preclude the use of cell-based options such as MACI, but if cystic changes or intralesional osteophytes are identified on preoperative imaging or encountered intraoperatively, then an osteochondral-replacing option must be considered.

26.13 Particulated Juvenile Allograft Cartilage

PJAC, a relatively newer cartilage restoration option with an evolving role, is minced cartilage allograft cut into approximately 1 mm cubes from juvenile donors younger than 13 years old [102]. Juvenile chondrocytes may be more metabolically active and are utilized due to their superior production of extracellular matrix and likely improved cartilage quality [103, 104]. Chondrocytes from particulated cartilage migrate to form new hyaline-like repair tissue that integrates with surrounding tissue. Unlike MACI, it is a single-stage procedure that does not require a separate biopsy (Fig. 26.3). It is typically used for small to medium well-contained defects, with most experts agreeing on post-debridement lesion size between 1 and 6 cm^2 [105, 106]. Relative contraindications include bipolar lesions and subchondral bone loss although concomitant

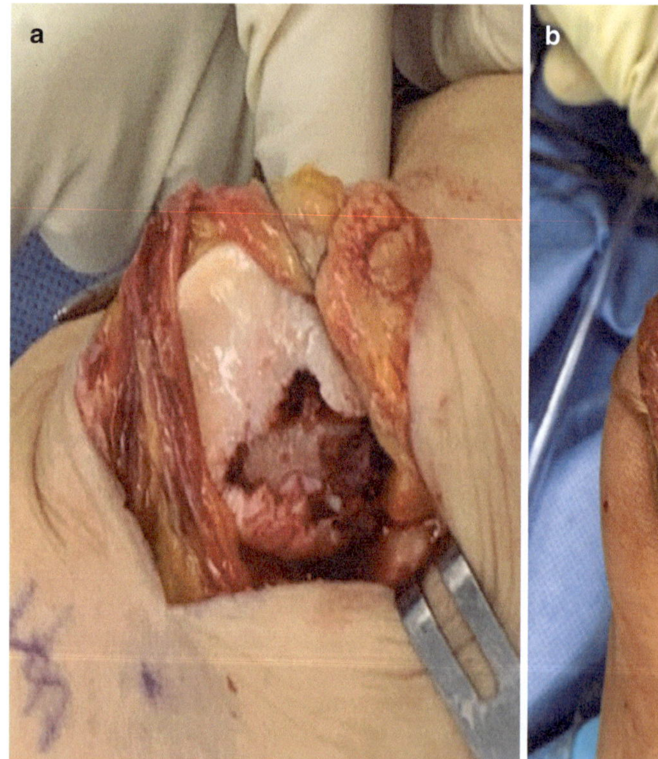

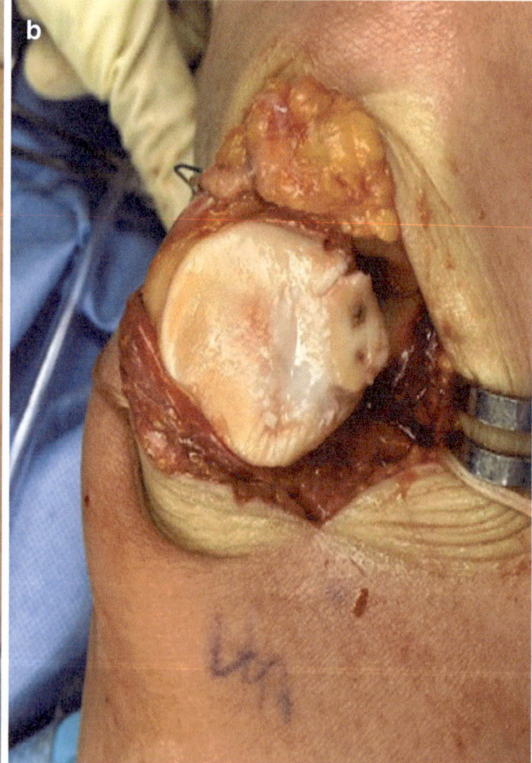

Fig. 26.3 A 27-year-old female with 16 mm × 16 mm osteochondral fragment from medial facet of patella extending to median patellar ridge following lateral patellar dislocation. (a) Intraoperative photo demonstrates post-debridement lesion size. (b) Partial osteochondral fragment fixation was performed with two bioabsorbable bone fixation nails to the medial aspect of medial facet and PJAC to fill the remainder of the defect

bone grafting has been described [106]. Defect preparation is similar to MACI and MACI. The area of the lesion should be determined, and depending on manufacturer, one packet of PJAC typically covers approximately 2.0–2.5 cm². During preparation, the excess of the liquid media is discarded and the pieces are arranged in one layer touching or nearly touching each other. One recommended technique for PJAC preparation is replicating the defect size and shape by pressing a piece of aluminum foil into the post-debridement defect and then filling base of the foil mold with a layer of fibrin glue followed by the PJAC. After approximately 5–10 min, the preparation can be implanted directly into the prepared defect. It can be helpful to use a freer elevator or other small instrument to facilitate precise placement of the preparation within the defect in an anatomic orientation. The preparation is relatively malleable and typically conforms well to the lesion. It is important that the preparation be recessed below or at the level of the surrounding shoulders of the defect in order to decrease the compressive and shear forces encountered by the preparation. Once the preparation is placed in an appropriate orientation within the defect, it is sealed into place with another layer of fibrin glue. We recommend against any irrigation after PJAC implantation and also against the use of intra-articular drains, when possible.

While data following PJAC is relatively limited, outcomes have generally been favorable [104, 107]. Magnetic resonance imaging and clinical evaluation of chondral lesions treated with allografts juvenile cells. Farr et al. [108] reported significant improvements in multiple KOOS subscales and IKDC scores, with T2-weighted MRI scores approximating normal articular cartilage by 2 years postoperative following PJAC for femoral and trochlear defects. Tompkins et al. [109] reported 89% mean defect fill and at mean 28-month follow-up of PJAC for grade IV chondral defects of the patella. Of 15 knees, there were three cases of mild graft hypertrophy and two with gross graft hypertrophy requiring arthroscopic debridement. Grawe et al. [110] reported that 85% of patients had good cartilage defect fill on MRI at 12 months postoperative following PJAC of the patella. Wang et al. [111] reported significant improvements in IKDC and KOS-ADL scores among patients undergoing PJAC for patellar or trochlear lesions, with lesion fill exceeding 67% in 69% of lesions at mean 3.8-year follow-up. Outcomes were not affected by lesion location or concomitant TTO. Additional studies are needed to better determine indications and clinical outcomes following PJAC.

26.14 Perforated Allograft Cartilage

Perforated allograft cartilage, which are cryopreserved osteochondral equivalent implants, attempts to combine the benefits of OCA with cell-based treatments [112]. The product is malleable and easily conforms to the complex anatomy of the PFJ. Furthermore, the cryopreserved nature allows for a longer shelf life than other cartilage restoration options. The product is perforated to allow chondrocyte egress and vertical integration with the underlying subchondral plate. There is limited data to support the use of perforated allograft cartilage at this time.

26.15 Choosing an Appropriate Cartilage Repair Therapy

There are multiple factors to consider when deciding on the appropriate cartilage restoration method for defects within the PFJ. The status of the subchondral bone is an important consideration. For lesions with intact subchondral bone without intralesional osteophytes or cysts, surface cell-based options including MACI or PJAC can be considered. As discussed earlier, of all cartilage treatment options within the PFJ, the largest amount of data is available for MACI. If the subchondral bone is compromised, then options that replace the subchondral bone including OAT and OCA should be considered. Small lesions (approximately <2 cm²) may be appropriate for OAT and PJAC, while medium-sized defects (approximately 2–4 cm²) may be appropriate for MACI and PJAC. Large lesions (approximately >4–6 cm²) may be considered for MACI or OCA. Due to the amount of supportive data in favor of MACI, we generally favor MACI over other cell-based options. If the subchondral bone is compromised, we favor OCA, unless the lesion size is small, in which case OAT is considered.

26.16 Associated Procedures and Patellofemoral Cartilage Restoration

Concurrent procedures should be selected according to the pathology present. Abnormal pathology should be corrected to restore PF biomechanics and protect the cartilage repair [8]. Factors initially responsible for chondral damage should be addressed at the time of surgery or possibly in a staged fashion, with cartilage restoration surgery occurring last [36]. Commonly required associated procedures include tibial tubercle osteotomy (TTO), lateral retinacular lengthening, and MPFL reconstruction (Fig. 26.4).

26.16.1 Tibial Tubercle Osteotomy

TTO is the most common procedure performed concomitantly with PF cartilage restoration surgery and has reported as being performed in 30–75% of cases [3, 15, 81, 82, 94, 113]. A more detailed discussion of TTO can be found in Chap. 8. Selective osteotomy should be performed when warranted in the setting of malalignment or recurrent patellar instability and also may be performed to offload cartilage lesions depending on defect location [3, 15]. Concomitant procedures to address trochlear dysplasia and patella alta are less commonly performed, unless indicated for severe dysplasia or Caton-Deschamps Index >1.3 [8]. TTO is often performed for recurrent patellar instability or for symptomatic focal chondral lesions, most commonly affecting the inferior

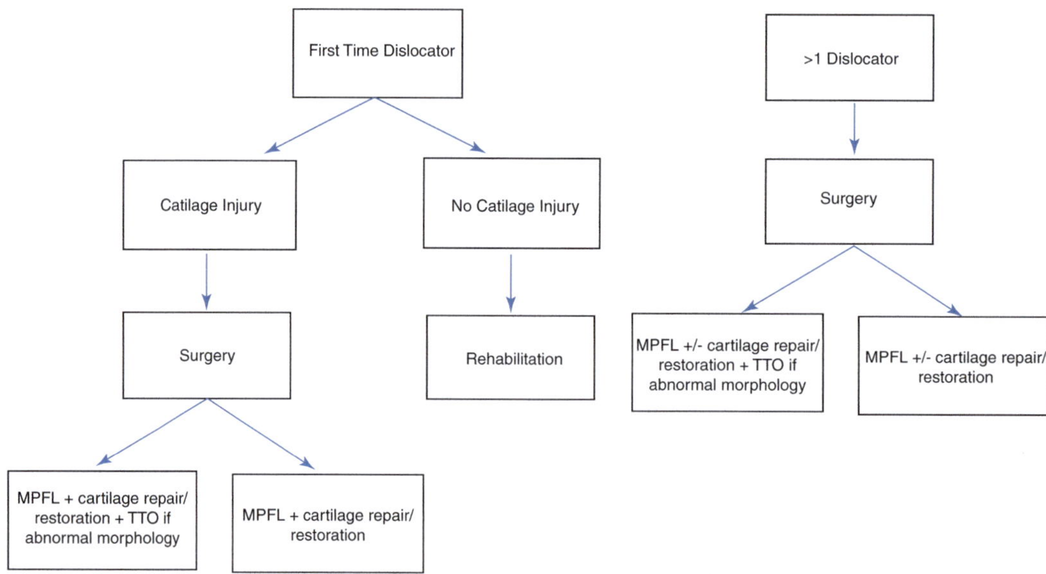

Fig. 26.4 Treatment algorithm for patients with first-time and recurrent patellar dislocations

and lateral aspect of the patella when used as a load shifting operating [114]. A Maquet, or purely anteriorization osteotomy, and an Elmslie-Trillat, or purely medializing osteotomy, allow correction in only one plane. The anteromedialization (AMZ) TTO allows correction in both the coronal and sagittal planes: Medialization results in offloading of the lateral facet, while anteriorization leads to offloading of the distal pole and a decrease in overall PF stresses [114]. Contraindications of isolated AMZ TTO include proximal pole, medial and panpatellar chondrosis. Pain should be concordant with the biomechanical abnormality that will be corrected by the osteotomy [27, 114–116]. If the TTO will lead to increased load over the areas of chondrosis, it is not advisable.

Originally described by Fulkerson, the AMZ TTO is the most commonly performed TTO [8]. Care should be taken to prevent over-medialization during TTO [117]. In the setting of an elevated TT-TG distance, the goal is to normalize TT-TG in the range of 5–10 mm. While anteriorization of 2 cm can reduce compressive forces across the PFJ by 50%, excessive elevation can result in wound healing complications, and while the maximum anteriorization recommended is patient-dependent, it should not exceed 17 mm and is more typically between 10 and 15 mm [118]. Depending on the indication for surgery (instability, offloading of chondral lesion, or both), the slope of an AMZ TTO is titrated accordingly. The steepest slope typically attempted is 60° and results in more chondral offloading and decreases in patellofemoral forces, while a shallower AMZ TTO is typically used in the setting of recurrent instability. A straight anteriorization (Maquet) is a rarely performed and largely historical procedure but may be considered when TT-TG is within normal limits and the goal of surgery is to decrease patellofemoral forces.

Outcomes following AMZ depend on the location of chondral lesion(s). Pidoriano and Fulkerson [27] demonstrated that patients undergoing AMZ TTO without cartilage restoration had 87% good or excellent outcomes when the cartilage lesions were located on the inferior pole and lateral facet of the patella. Conversely, all patients with central trochlear involvement had poor outcomes, and only 55% and 20% of those with medial facet or proximal pole/diffuse patellar lesions, respectively, had good or excellent outcomes. Clinical outcomes following TTO alone have been reported as poorer when patellar chondral lesions are grade III or IV [114]. Lateral lesions within the trochlea and bipolar lesions warrant consideration of a TTO [3, 15, 81, 82]. Ogura et al. [36] reported a 79% graft survival rate following MACI of bipolar PF chondral lesions at 10 years postoperative, with the best survival rates observed among patients who underwent concomitant TTO (91% survival at 5 and 10 years). The worst survival rates were seen in patients with prior marrow stimulation (43% at 5 and 10 years). The results of this study are comparable with previous studies of unipolar lesions within the PFJ [80, 119]. Consistent with these findings, several other studies have reported no difference between outcomes for unipolar and bipolar lesions [3, 15].

While some studies have reported improved results following cartilage restoration surgery with concomitant TTO [17, 82, 120], others have reported similar results with and without TTO when selective osteotomy was performed according to lesion location and patellofemoral alignment [8, 15, 81, 121]. A multicenter study of 110 patients treated with MACI in which 69% of patients underwent concomitant AMZ TTO reported good to excellent results in 86% of patients at 7.5-year follow-up [3]. Gillogly et al. [80] similarly reported good to excellent results in 83% of patients who underwent MACI with concomitant AMZ TTO. Altogether, current data suggests that appropriately tracking knees perform well following cartilage repair surgery, regardless of whether a TTO is needed to achieve normal tracking.

26.16.2 Soft Tissue Procedures

Concomitant lateral retinacular release has been reported as being performed in 20–60% of cases of PF cartilage restoration, often along with TTO [3, 18, 82, 89]. Although MPFL reconstruction is less frequently performed than TTO, it should be considered in the setting of recurrent instability in the absence of bony malalignment. Siebold et al. [122] reported outcomes following concomitant MPFL reconstruction and MACI among patients with recurrent patellar dislocation and grade IV chondral lesions with a mean defect size of 7.2 cm^2, reporting no episodes of recurrent instability, improved subjective and objective outcomes scores and complete defect fill in 80% of lesions. In the setting of patellar dislocation resulting in chondral or osteochondral injury, we routinely perform an MPFL reconstruction with or without TTO, as there is increasing evidence to support superior outcomes following MPFL reconstruction compared to repair, even in the acute setting [123]. In the setting of patellar instability, we will also perform TTO (typically AMZ) if there is significant lateralization of the tibial tubercle relative to the trochlear groove, generally above 15–20 mm on a case-by-case basis.

26.17 Rehabilitation

We recommend immediate protected motion with a continuous passive motion (CPM) machine used 6–8 h daily for 6 weeks and a goal of 90° reached by 2–3 weeks postoperative. Unless contraindicated due to another concomitant procedure such as a TTO, the patient is allowed weightbearing as tolerated with the knee locked in full extension in a brace. Flexed knee loading, such as stairs or squatting, is not permitted for a minimum of 3 months postoperatively. Although there is currently evidence to support accelerated weightbearing protocol following MACI [124], we typically do not allow a return to running and plyometric activities for 12 months and strenuous cutting activities for 18 months when the graft has fully matured.

26.18 Complications

In addition to complications common to most knee procedures including infection and postoperative stiffness, there are several issues related to the various cartilage restoration treatment options. Postoperative concerns with Mfx include persistent knee pain, recurrent knee effusions, incomplete defect filling, poor integration with surrounding articular cartilage, and deterioration of functional outcomes necessitating alternative restoration or arthroplasty procedures [10]. Complication and failure rates with OAT are relatively low in comparison to other cartilage restoration techniques and include stiffness requiring manipulation under anesthesia (3–9%) and graft failure (zero to 8%) [10]. Complications specific to cell-based therapies include a biologic failure to form appropriate repair tissue and delamination of a well-formed graft, typically due to trauma [18, 119]. Graft hypertrophy was common following first-generation MACI but less of an issue with second-generation MACI and MACI [87, 90, 91, 93, 108]. Graft hypertrophy has been reported after PJAC [108]. Complications related to TTO include nonunion of the tubercle, tibia fracture, shingle fracture, over-medialization with resulting medial instability, patella baja, delayed wound healing, skin necrosis, and symptomatic hardware [118]. It is imperative to begin early range of motion following TTO to minimize the risk of patella baja. We recommend touch-down weightbearing for a period of four or more weeks, with a minimum of 6 weeks if distalization is performed, as the likelihood of nonunion is higher when the distal fragment is fully detached. Home exercises during the first 4 weeks include dangling, heel slides, and quad sets until formal physical therapy begins at 4 weeks postoperative.

26.19 Conclusion

While several methods of cartilage restoration within the PFJ have been described, there is a lack of comparative studies between the various treatment options and often wide variability among patient characteristics both within and across studies. As such, there is currently a lack of consensus regarding the "best" treatment option(s) for symptomatic, focal PFJ cartilage lesions. Native articular cartilage should be preserved when possible and if the osteochondral fragment has a sufficient amount of bone and healthy cartilage. There is a growing body of evidence to support repair of chondral-only shear injuries which typically occur during acute patellar dislocations in skeletally immature patients. Cell-based therapies including MACI and PJAC may be considered when the injury does not extend deep into the subchondral bone. Subchondral bony involvement beyond marrow edema, such as intralesional osteophytes or subchondral cysts, warrants consideration of osteochondral reconstruction such as OAT or OCA. In general, concomitant pathology such as patellar malalignment or ligamentous instability should be corrected concurrently or in a staged fashion. Further research, including RCTs evaluating various cell-based therapies with one another and/or against osteochondral reconstruction techniques, are desirable (but challenging) to better delineate proper indications for these treatment options. Long-term outcomes studies will determine whether these treatments slow or halt the progression of OA, thereby altering the natural history of focal chondral or osteochondral injuries.

References

1. Pinkowsky GJ, Farr J. Considerations in evaluating treatment options for patellofemoral cartilage pathology. Sports Med Arthrosc Rev. 2016;24(2):92–7.
2. Frank RM, Lee S, Levy D, Poland S, Smith M, Scalise N, et al. Osteochondral allograft transplantation of the knee: analysis of failures at 5 years. Am J Sports Med. 2017;45(4):864–74.
3. Gomoll AH, Gillogly SD, Cole BJ, Farr J, Arnold R, Hussey K, et al. Autologous chondrocyte implantation in the patella: a multicenter experience. Am J Sports Med. 2014;42(5):1074–81.
4. Aroen A, Loken S, Heir S, Alvik E, Ekeland A, Granlund OG, et al. Articular cartilage lesions in 993 consecutive knee arthroscopies. Am J Sports Med. 2004;32(1):211–5.
5. Curl WW, Krome J, Gordon ES, Rushing J, Smith BP, Poehling GG. Cartilage injuries: a review of 31,516 knee arthroscopies. Arthroscopy. 1997;13(4):456–60.
6. Niemeyer P, Steinwachs M, Erggelet C, Kreuz PC, Kraft N, Kostler W, et al. Autologous chondrocyte implantation for the treatment of retropatellar cartilage defects: clinical results referred to defect localisation. Arch Orthop Trauma Surg. 2008;128(11):1223–31.
7. Rosenberger RE, Gomoll AH, Bryant T, Minas T. Repair of large chondral defects of the knee with autologous chondrocyte implantation in patients 45 years or older. Am J Sports Med. 2008;36(12):2336–44.
8. Ambra LF, Hinckel BB, Arendt EA, Farr J, Gomoll AH. Anatomic risk factors for focal cartilage lesions in the patella and trochlea: a case-control study. Am J Sports Med. 2019;47(10):2444–53.
9. Mehl J, Otto A, Willinger L, Hapfelmeier A, Imhoff AB, Niemeyer P, et al. Degenerative isolated cartilage defects of the patellofemoral joint are associated with more severe symptoms compared to trauma-related defects: results of the German Cartilage Registry (KnorpelRegister DGOU). Knee Surg Sports Traumatol Arthrosc. 2019;27(2):580–9.
10. Brophy RH, Wojahn RD, Lamplot JD. Cartilage restoration techniques for the patellofemoral joint. J Am Acad Orthop Surg. 2017;25(5):321–9.
11. Astur DC, Arliani GG, Binz M, Astur N, Kaleka CC, Amaro JT, et al. Autologous osteochondral transplantation for treating patellar chondral injuries: evaluation, treatment, and outcomes of a two-year follow-up study. J Bone Joint Surg Am. 2014;96(10):816–23.
12. Filardo G, Kon E, Andriolo L, Di Martino A, Zaffagnini S, Marcacci M. Treatment of "patellofemoral" cartilage lesions with matrix-assisted autologous chondrocyte transplantation: a comparison of patellar and trochlear lesions. Am J Sports Med. 2014;42(3):626–34.
13. Hangody L, Fules P. Autologous osteochondral mosaicplasty for the treatment of full-thickness defects of weight-bearing joints: ten years of experimental and clinical experience. J Bone Joint Surg Am. 2003;85-A(Suppl 2):25–32.
14. Nho SJ, Foo LF, Green DM, Shindle MK, Warren RF, Wickiewicz TL, et al. Magnetic resonance imaging and clinical evaluation of patellar resurfacing with press-fit osteochondral autograft plugs. Am J Sports Med. 2008;36(6):1101–9.
15. Farr J. Autologous chondrocyte implantation improves patellofemoral cartilage treatment outcomes. Clin Orthop Relat Res. 2007;463:187–94.
16. Nawaz SZ, Bentley G, Briggs TW, Carrington RW, Skinner JA, Gallagher KR, et al. Autologous chondrocyte implantation in the knee: mid-term to long-term results. J Bone Joint Surg Am. 2014;96(10):824–30.
17. Trinh TQ, Harris JD, Siston RA, Flanigan DC. Improved outcomes with combined autologous chondrocyte implantation and patellofemoral osteotomy versus isolated autologous chondrocyte implantation. Arthroscopy. 2013;29(3):566–74.

18. Vasiliadis HS, Lindahl A, Georgoulis AD, Peterson L. Malalignment and cartilage lesions in the patellofemoral joint treated with autologous chondrocyte implantation. Knee Surg Sports Traumatol Arthrosc. 2011;19(3):452–7.

19. Andrade R, Nunes J, Hinckel BB, Gruskay J, Vasta S, Bastos R, et al. Cartilage restoration of patellofemoral lesions: a systematic review. Cartilage. 2019;1947603519893076

20. Hinckel BB, Pratte EL, Baumann CA, Gowd AK, Farr J, Liu JN, et al. Patellofemoral cartilage restoration: a systematic review and meta-analysis of clinical outcomes. Am J Sports Med. 2020;363546519886853

21. Nomura E, Inoue M, Kurimura M. Chondral and osteochondral injuries associated with acute patellar dislocation. Arthroscopy. 2003;19(7):717–21.

22. Luhmann SJ, Smith JC, Schootman M, Prasad N. Recurrent patellar instability: implications of preoperative patellar crepitation on the status of the patellofemoral articular cartilage. J Pediatr Orthop. 2019;39(1):33–7.

23. Gomoll AH, Minas T, Farr J, Cole BJ. Treatment of chondral defects in the patellofemoral joint. J Knee Surg. 2006;19(4):285–95.

24. Camp CL, Stuart MJ, Krych AJ, Levy BA, Bond JR, Collins MS, et al. CT and MRI measurements of tibial tubercle-trochlear groove distances are not equivalent in patients with patellar instability. Am J Sports Med. 2013;41(8):1835–40.

25. Gomoll AH, Yoshioka H, Watanabe A, Dunn JC, Minas T. Preoperative measurement of cartilage defects by mri underestimates lesion size. Cartilage. 2011;2(4):389–93.

26. Dejour H, Walch G, Nove-Josserand L, Guier C. Factors of patellar instability: an anatomic radiographic study. Knee Surg Sports Traumatol Arthrosc. 1994;2(1):19–26.

27. Fulkerson JP, Becker GJ, Meaney JA, Miranda M, Folcik MA. Anteromedial tibial tubercle transfer without bone graft. Am J Sports Med. 1990;18(5):490–6. discussion 6-7

28. Colvin AC, West RV. Patellar instability. J Bone Joint Surg Am. 2008;90(12):2751–62.

29. Pedowitz JM, Edmonds EW, Chambers HG, Dennis MM, Bastrom T, Pennock AT. Recurrence of patellar instability in adolescents undergoing surgery for osteochondral defects without concomitant ligament reconstruction. Am J Sports Med. 2019;47(1):66–70.

30. Chiu JK, Wong YM, Yung PS, Ng GY. The effects of quadriceps strengthening on pain, function, and patellofemoral joint contact area in persons with patellofemoral pain. Am J Phys Med Rehabil. 2012;91(2):98–106.

31. Campbell KA, Erickson BJ, Saltzman BM, Mascarenhas R, Bach BR Jr, Cole BJ, et al. Is local viscosupplementation injection clinically superior to other therapies in the treatment of osteoarthritis of the knee: a systematic review of overlapping meta-analyses. Arthroscopy. 2015;31(10):2036–45. e14

32. Hunter DJ, Harvey W, Gross KD, Felson D, McCree P, Li L, et al. A randomized trial of patellofemoral bracing for treatment of patellofemoral osteoarthritis. Osteoarthritis Cartilage. 2011;19(7):792–800.

33. McWalter EJ, Hunter DJ, Harvey WF, McCree P, Hirko KA, Felson DT, et al. The effect of a patellar brace on three-dimensional patellar kinematics in patients with lateral patellofemoral osteoarthritis. Osteoarthritis Cartilage. 2011;19(7):801–8.

34. Yanke AB, Wuerz T, Saltzman BM, Butty D, Cole BJ. Management of patellofemoral chondral injuries. Clin Sports Med. 2014;33(3):477–500.

35. Knutsen G, Drogset JO, Engebretsen L, Grontvedt T, Ludvigsen TC, Loken S, et al. A randomized multicenter trial comparing autologous chondrocyte implantation with microfracture: long-term follow-up at 14 to 15 years. J Bone Joint Surg Am. 2016;98(16):1332–9.

36. Ogura T, Bryant T, Minas T. Long-term outcomes of autologous chondrocyte implantation in adolescent patients. Am J Sports Med. 2017;45(5):1066–74.

37. Fabricant PD, Yen YM, Kramer DE, Kocher MS, Micheli LJ, Lawrence JTR, et al. Fixation of traumatic chondral-only fragments of the knee in pediatric and adolescent athletes: a retrospective multicenter report. Orthop J Sports Med. 2018;6(2):2325967117753140.

38. Kramer DE, Pace JL. Acute traumatic and sports-related osteochondral injury of the pediatric knee. Orthop Clin North Am. 2012;43(2):227–36. vi

39. Flachsmann R, Broom ND, Hardy AE, Moltschaniwskyj G. Why is the adolescent joint particularly susceptible to osteochondral shear fracture? Clin Orthop Relat Res. 2000;381:212–21.

40. Bauer KL. Osteochondral injuries of the knee in pediatric patients. J Knee Surg. 2018;31(5):382–91.

41. Nietosvaara Y, Aalto K, Kallio PE. Acute patellar dislocation in children: incidence and associated osteochondral fractures. J Pediatr Orthop. 1994;14(4):513–5.

42. Seeley MA, Knesek M, Vanderhave KL. Osteochondral injury after acute patellar dislocation in children and adolescents. J Pediatr Orthop. 2013;33(5):511–8.

43. Palmu S, Kallio PE, Donell ST, Helenius I, Nietosvaara Y. Acute patellar dislocation in children and adolescents: a randomized clinical trial. J Bone Joint Surg Am. 2008;90(3):463–70.

44. Chotel F, Knorr G, Simian E, Dubrana F, Versier G, French AS. Knee osteochondral fractures in skeletally immature patients: French multicenter study. Orthop Traumatol Surg Res. 2011;97(8 Suppl):S154–9.

45. Mashoof AA, Scholl MD, Lahav A, Greis PE, Burks RT. Osteochondral injury to the mid-lateral weight-bearing portion of the lateral femoral condyle associated with patella dislocation. Arthroscopy. 2005;21(2):228–32.

46. Tabaddor RR, Banffy MB, Andersen JS, McFeely E, Ogunwole O, Micheli LJ, et al. Fixation of juve-

nile osteochondritis dissecans lesions of the knee using poly 96L/4D-lactide copolymer bioabsorbable implants. J Pediatr Orthop. 2010;30(1):14–20.

47. Millington KL, Shah JP, Dahm DL, Levy BA, Stuart MJ. Bioabsorbable fixation of unstable osteochondritis dissecans lesions. Am J Sports Med. 2010;38(10):2065–70.

48. Buckwalter JA. Articular cartilage: injuries and potential for healing. J Orthop Sports Phys Ther. 1998;28(4):192–202.

49. Tew S, Redman S, Kwan A, Walker E, Khan I, Dowthwaite G, et al. Differences in repair responses between immature and mature cartilage. Clin Orthop Relat Res. 2001;(391 Suppl):S142–52.

50. Nakamura N, Horibe S, Iwahashi T, Kawano K, Shino K, Yoshikawa H. Healing of a chondral fragment of the knee in an adolescent after internal fixation. A case report. J Bone Joint Surg Am. 2004;86(12):2741–6.

51. Siparsky PN, Bailey JR, Dale KM, Klement MR, Taylor DC. Open reduction internal fixation of isolated chondral fragments without osseous attachment in the knee: a case series. Orthop J Sports Med. 2017;5(3):2325967117696281.

52. Galloway MT, Noyes FR. Cystic degeneration of the patella after arthroscopic chondroplasty and subchondral bone perforation. Arthroscopy. 1992;8(3):366–9.

53. Schonholtz GJ, Ling B. Arthroscopic chondroplasty of the patella. Arthroscopy. 1985;1(2):92–6.

54. Arshi A, Cohen JR, Wang JC, Hame SL, McAllister DR, Jones KJ. Operative management of patellar instability in the united states: an evaluation of national practice patterns, surgical trends, and complications. Orthop J Sports Med. 2016;4(8):2325967116662873.

55. Kreuz PC, Erggelet C, Steinwachs MR, Krause SJ, Lahm A, Niemeyer P, et al. Is microfracture of chondral defects in the knee associated with different results in patients aged 40 years or younger? Arthroscopy. 2006a;22(11):1180–6.

56. Kreuz PC, Steinwachs MR, Erggelet C, Krause SJ, Konrad G, Uhl M, et al. Results after microfracture of full-thickness chondral defects in different compartments in the knee. Osteoarthritis Cartilage. 2006b;14(11):1119–25.

57. Blevins FT, Steadman JR, Rodrigo JJ, Silliman J. Treatment of articular cartilage defects in athletes: an analysis of functional outcome and lesion appearance. Orthopedics. 1998;21(7):761–7. discussion 7-8

58. Smoak JB, Kluczynski MA, Bisson LJ, Marzo JM. Systematic review of patient outcomes and associated predictors after microfracture in the patellofemoral joint. J Am Acad Orthop Surg Glob Res Rev. 2019;3(11)

59. Mestriner AB, Ackermann J, Gomoll AH. Patellofemoral cartilage repair. Curr Rev Musculoskelet Med. 2018;11(2):188–200.

60. Oussedik S, Tsitskaris K, Parker D. Treatment of articular cartilage lesions of the knee by microfracture or autologous chondrocyte implantation: a systematic review. Arthroscopy. 2015;31(4):732–44.

61. Behery O, Siston RA, Harris JD, Flanigan DC. Treatment of cartilage defects of the knee: expanding on the existing algorithm. Clin J Sport Med. 2014;24(1):21–30.

62. Solheim E, Hegna J, Strand T, Harlem T, Inderhaug E. Randomized study of long-term (15-17 years) outcome after microfracture versus mosaicplasty in knee articular cartilage defects. Am J Sports Med. 2018;46(4):826–31.

63. Saris D, Price A, Widuchowski W, Bertrand-Marchand M, Caron J, Drogset JO, et al. Matrix-applied characterized autologous cultured chondrocytes versus microfracture: two-year follow-up of a prospective randomized trial. Am J Sports Med. 2014;42(6):1384–94.

64. Petri M, Broese M, Simon A, Liodakis E, Ettinger M, Guenther D, et al. CaReS (MACT) versus microfracture in treating symptomatic patellofemoral cartilage defects: a retrospective matched-pair analysis. J Orthop Sci. 2013;18(1):38–44.

65. Albright JC, Daoud AK. Microfracture and microfracture plus. Clin Sports Med. 2017;36(3):501–7.

66. Volz M, Schaumburger J, Frick H, Grifka J, Anders S. A randomized controlled trial demonstrating sustained benefit of Autologous Matrix-Induced Chondrogenesis over microfracture at five years. Int Orthop. 2017;41(4):797–804.

67. Dhollander A, Moens K, Van der Maas J, Verdonk P, Almqvist KF, Victor J. Treatment of patellofemoral cartilage defects in the knee by autologous matrixinduced chondrogenesis (AMIC). Acta Orthop Belg. 2014;80(2):251–9.

68. Gobbi A, Whyte GP. One-stage cartilage repair using a hyaluronic acid-based scaffold with activated bone marrow-derived mesenchymal stem cells compared with microfracture: five-year follow-up. Am J Sports Med. 2016;44(11):2846–54.

69. Pareek A, Reardon PJ, Macalena JA, Levy BA, Stuart MJ, Williams RJ 3rd, et al. Osteochondral autograft transfer versus microfracture in the knee: a meta-analysis of prospective comparative studies at midterm. Arthroscopy. 2016;32(10):2118–30.

70. Figueroa D, Melean P, Calvo R, Gili F, Zilleruelo N, Vaisman A. Osteochondral autografts in full thickness patella cartilage lesions. Knee. 2011;18(4):220–3.

71. Emre TY, Atbasi Z, Demircioglu DT, Uzun M, Kose O. Autologous osteochondral transplantation (mosaicplasty) in articular cartilage defects of the patellofemoral joint: retrospective analysis of 33 cases. Musculoskelet Surg. 2017;101(2):133–8.

72. Cameron JI, Pulido PA, McCauley JC, Bugbee WD. Osteochondral allograft transplantation of the femoral trochlea. Am J Sports Med. 2016;44(3):633–8.

73. Gracitelli GC, Meric G, Briggs DT, Pulido PA, McCauley JC, Belloti JC, et al. Fresh osteochondral allografts in the knee: comparison of primary transplantation versus transplantation after failure of previous subchondral marrow stimulation. Am J Sports Med. 2015;43(4):885–91.

74. Jamali AA, Emmerson BC, Chung C, Convery FR, Bugbee WD. Fresh osteochondral allografts: results in the patellofemoral joint. Clin Orthop Relat Res. 2005;437:176–85.

75. Meric G, Gracitelli GC, Gortz S, De Young AJ, Bugbee WD. Fresh osteochondral allograft transplantation for bipolar reciprocal osteochondral lesions of the knee. Am J Sports Med. 2015;43(3):709–14.

76. Basad E, Wissing FR, Fehrenbach P, Rickert M, Steinmeyer J, Ishaque B. Matrix-induced autologous chondrocyte implantation (MACI) in the knee: clinical outcomes and challenges. Knee Surg Sports Traumatol Arthrosc. 2015;23(12):3729–35.

77. Edwards PK, Ebert JR, Janes GC, Wood D, Fallon M, Ackland T. Arthroscopic versus open matrix-induced autologous chondrocyte implantation: results and implications for rehabilitation. J Sport Rehabil. 2014;23(3):203–15.

78. Ferruzzi A, Buda R, Faldini C, Vannini F, Di Caprio F, Luciani D, et al. Autologous chondrocyte implantation in the knee joint: open compared with arthroscopic technique. Comparison at a minimum follow-up of five years. J Bone Joint Surg Am. 2008;90(Suppl 4):90–101.

79. Gigante A, Enea D, Greco F, Bait C, Denti M, Schonhuber H, et al. Distal realignment and patellar autologous chondrocyte implantation: mid-term results in a selected population. Knee Surg Sports Traumatol Arthrosc. 2009;17(1):2–10.

80. Gillogly SD, Arnold RM. Autologous chondrocyte implantation and anteromedialization for isolated patellar articular cartilage lesions: 5- to 11-year follow-up. Am J Sports Med. 2014;42(4):912–20.

81. Minas T, Bryant T. The role of autologous chondrocyte implantation in the patellofemoral joint. Clin Orthop Relat Res. 2005;436:30–9.

82. Pascual-Garrido C, Slabaugh MA, L'Heureux DR, Friel NA, Cole BJ. Recommendations and treatment outcomes for patellofemoral articular cartilage defects with autologous chondrocyte implantation: prospective evaluation at average 4-year follow-up. Am J Sports Med. 2009;37(Suppl 1):33S–41S.

83. Gobbi A, Kon E, Berruto M, Francisco R, Filardo G, Marcacci M. Patellofemoral full-thickness chondral defects treated with Hyalograft-C: a clinical, arthroscopic, and histologic review. Am J Sports Med. 2006;34(11):1763–73.

84. Macmull S, Jaiswal PK, Bentley G, Skinner JA, Carrington RW, Briggs TW. The role of autologous chondrocyte implantation in the treatment of symptomatic chondromalacia patellae. Int Orthop. 2012;36(7):1371–7.

85. Peterson L, Vasiliadis HS, Brittberg M, Lindahl A. Autologous chondrocyte implantation: a long-term follow-up. Am J Sports Med. 2010;38(6):1117–24.

86. Cvetanovich GL, Riboh JC, Tilton AK, Cole BJ. Autologous chondrocyte implantation improves knee-specific functional outcomes and health-related quality of life in adolescent patients. Am J Sports Med. 2017;45(1):70–6.

87. Pestka JM, Bode G, Salzmann G, Sudkamp NP, Niemeyer P. Clinical outcome of autologous chondrocyte implantation for failed microfracture treatment of fullthickness cartilage defects of the knee joint. Am J Sports Med. 2012;40(2):325–31.

88. Behrens P, Bitter T, Kurz B, Russlies M. Matrix-associated autologous chondrocyte transplantation/implantation (MACT/MACI)–5-year follow-up. Knee. 2006;13(3):194–202.

89. Minas T, Von Keudell A, Bryant T, Gomoll AH. The John Insall Award: a minimum 10-year outcome study of autologous chondrocyte implantation. Clin Orthop Relat Res. 2014;472(1):41–51.

90. Ebert JR, Robertson WB, Woodhouse J, Fallon M, Zheng MH, Ackland T, et al. Clinical and magnetic resonance imaging-based outcomes to 5 years after matrix-induced autologous chondrocyte implantation to address articular cartilage defects in the knee. Am J Sports Med. 2011;39(4):753–63.

91. Bartlett W, Skinner JA, Gooding CR, Carrington RW, Flanagan AM, Briggs TW, et al. Autologous chondrocyte implantation versus matrix-induced autologous chondrocyte implantation for osteochondral defects of the knee: a prospective, randomised study. J Bone Joint Surg Br. 2005;87(5):640–5.

92. Bentley G, Biant LC, Carrington RW, Akmal M, Goldberg A, Williams AM, et al. A prospective, randomised comparison of autologous chondrocyte implantation versus mosaicplasty for osteochondral defects in the knee. J Bone Joint Surg Br. 2003;85(2):223–30.

93. Ebert JR, Fallon M, Smith A, Janes GC, Wood DJ. Prospective clinical and radiologic evaluation of patellofemoral matrix-induced autologous chondrocyte implantation. Am J Sports Med. 2015;43(6):1362–72.

94. Meyerkort D, Ebert JR, Ackland TR, Robertson WB, Fallon M, Zheng MH, et al. Matrix-induced autologous chondrocyte implantation (MACI) for chondral defects in the patellofemoral joint. Knee Surg Sports Traumatol Arthrosc. 2014;22(10):2522–30.

95. Farr J 2nd. Autologous chondrocyte implantation and anteromedialization in the treatment of patellofemoral chondrosis. Orthop Clin North Am. 2008;39(3):329–35. vi

96. Zarkadis NJ, Belmont PJ Jr, Zachilli MA, Holland CA, Kinsler AR, Todd MS, et al. Autologous chondrocyte implantation and tibial tubercle osteotomy for patellofemoral chondral defects: improved pain relief and occupational outcomes Among

US Army Servicemembers. Am J Sports Med. 2018;46(13):3198–208.

97. Minas T, Gomoll AH, Rosenberger R, Royce RO, Bryant T. Increased failure rate of autologous chondrocyte implantation after previous treatment with marrow stimulation techniques. Am J Sports Med. 2009;37(5):902–8.

98. Mithoefer K, McAdams T, Williams RJ, Kreuz PC, Mandelbaum BR. Clinical efficacy of the microfracture technique for articular cartilage repair in the knee: an evidence-based systematic analysis. Am J Sports Med. 2009;37(10):2053–63.

99. Chen H, Chevrier A, Hoemann CD, Sun J, Ouyang W, Buschmann MD. Characterization of subchondral bone repair for marrow-stimulated chondral defects and its relationship to articular cartilage resurfacing. Am J Sports Med. 2011;39(8):1731–40.

100. Orth P, Goebel L, Wolfram U, Ong MF, Graber S, Kohn D, et al. Effect of subchondral drilling on the microarchitecture of subchondral bone: analysis in a large animal model at 6 months. Am J Sports Med. 2012;40(4):828–36.

101. Minas T, Ogura T, Headrick J, Bryant T. Autologous chondrocyte implantation "sandwich" technique compared with autologous bone grafting for deep osteochondral lesions in the knee. Am J Sports Med. 2018;46(2):322–32.

102. Farr J, Yao JQ. Chondral defect repair with particulated juvenile cartilage allograft. Cartilage. 2011;2(4):346–53.

103. Bonasia DE, Martin JA, Marmotti A, Amendola RL, Buckwalter JA, Rossi R, et al. Cocultures of adult and juvenile chondrocytes compared with adult and juvenile chondral fragments: in vitro matrix production. Am J Sports Med. 2011;39(11):2355–61.

104. Buckwalter JA, Bowman GN, Albright JP, Wolf BR, Bollier M. Clinical outcomes of patellar chondral lesions treated with juvenile particulated cartilage allografts. Iowa Orthop J. 2014;34:44–9.

105. Farr J, Cole BJ, Sherman S, Karas V. Particulated articular cartilage: CAIS and DeNovo NT. J Knee Surg. 2012;25(1):23–9.

106. Riboh JC, Cole BJ, Farr J. Particulated articular cartilage for symptomatic chondral defects of the knee. Curr Rev Musculoskelet Med. 2015;8(4):429–35.

107. Pascual-Garrido C, Gold SL, Snikeris J, Burge A, Nguyen J, Potter HG, et al. Magnetic resonance imaging and clinical evaluation of chondral lesions treated with allografts juvenile cells. Orthopaed J Sports Med. 2013;1(4_suppl):2325967113S00030.

108. Farr J, Tabet SK, Margerrison E, Cole BJ. Clinical, radiographic, and histological outcomes after cartilage repair with particulated juvenile articular cartilage: a 2-year prospective study. Am J Sports Med. 2014;42(6):1417–25.

109. Tompkins M, Hamann JC, Diduch DR, Bonner KF, Hart JM, Gwathmey FW, et al. Preliminary results of a novel single-stage cartilage restoration technique: particulated juvenile articular cartilage allograft for chondral defects of the patella. Arthroscopy. 2013;29(10):1661–70.

110. Grawe B, Burge A, Nguyen J, Strickland S, Warren R, Rodeo S, et al. Cartilage regeneration in full-thickness patellar chondral defects treated with particulated juvenile articular allograft cartilage: an MRI analysis. Cartilage. 2017;8(4):374–83.

111. Wang T, Belkin NS, Burge AJ, Chang B, Pais M, Mahony G, et al. Patellofemoral cartilage lesions treated with particulated juvenile allograft cartilage: a prospective study with minimum 2-year clinical and magnetic resonance imaging outcomes. Arthroscopy. 2018;34(5):1498–505.

112. Redondo ML, Naveen NB, Liu JN, Tauro TM, Southworth TM, Cole BJ. Preservation of knee articular cartilage. Sports Med Arthrosc Rev. 2018;26(4):e23–30.

113. Vanlauwe JJ, Claes T, Van Assche D, Bellemans J, Luyten FP. Characterized chondrocyte implantation in the patellofemoral joint: an up to 4-year follow-up of a prospective cohort of 38 patients. Am J Sports Med. 2012;40(8):1799–807.

114. Pidoriano AJ, Weinstein RN, Buuck DA, Fulkerson JP. Correlation of patellar articular lesions with results from anteromedial tibial tubercle transfer. Am J Sports Med. 1997;25(4):533–7.

115. Bellemans J, Cauwenberghs F, Witvrouw E, Brys P, Victor J. Anteromedial tibial tubercle transfer in patients with chronic anterior knee pain and a sub-luxation-type patellar malalignment. Am J Sports Med. 1997;25(3):375–81.

116. Naranja RJ Jr, Reilly PJ, Kuhlman JR, Haut E, Torg JS. Long-term evaluation of the Elmslie-Trillat-Maquet procedure for patellofemoral dysfunction. Am J Sports Med. 1996;24(6):779–84.

117. Kuroda S, Sugawara Y, Yamashita K, Mano T, Takano-Yamamoto T. Skeletal Class III oligodontia patient treated with titanium screw anchorage and orthognathic surgery. Am J Orthod Dentofacial Orthop. 2005;127(6):730–8.

118. Middleton KK, Gruber S, Shubin Stein BE. Why and where to move the tibial tubercle: indications and techniques for tibial tubercle osteotomy. Sports Med Arthrosc Rev. 2019;27(4):154–60.

119. Mandelbaum B, Browne JE, Fu F, Micheli LJ, Moseley JB Jr, Erggelet C, et al. Treatment outcomes of autologous chondrocyte implantation for fullthickness articular cartilage defects of the trochlea. Am J Sports Med. 2007;35(6):915–21.

120. Henderson IJ, Lavigne P. Periosteal autologous chondrocyte implantation for patellar chondral defect in patients with normal and abnormal patellar tracking. Knee. 2006;13(4):274–9.

121. Brittberg M, Lindahl A, Nilsson A, Ohlsson C, Isaksson O, Peterson L. Treatment of deep cartilage

defects in the knee with autologous chondrocyte transplantation. N Engl J Med. 1994;331(14):889–95.

122. Siebold R, Karidakis G, Fernandez F. Clinical outcome after medial patellofemoral ligament reconstruction and autologous chondrocyte implantation following recurrent patella dislocation. Knee Surg Sports Traumatol Arthrosc. 2014;22(10):2477–83.

123. Camanho GL, Viegas Ade C, Bitar AC, Demange MK, Hernandez AJ. Conservative versus surgical treatment for repair of the medial patellofemoral ligament in acute dislocations of the patella. Arthroscopy. 2009;25(6):620–5.

124. Goyal D, Goyal A, Keyhani S, Lee EH, Hui JH. Evidence-based status of second- and third-generation autologous chondrocyte implantation over first generation: a systematic review of level I and II studies. Arthroscopy. 2013;29(11):1872–8.

Rehabilitation and Decision for Return to Play Following Cartilage Restoration Surgery

Francesco Della Villa, Filippo Tosarelli, Davide Fusetti, Lorenzo Boldrini, and Stefano Della Villa

27.1 Introduction

The post-surgical management of a sport patient undergoing cartilage restoration surgery is one of the most challenging scenarios in nowadays sport medicine practice. If compared to other sport's injury domain (e.g., Anterior Cruciate Ligament (ACL) injury), rehabilitation following cartilage procedures has received limited attention from a research perspective [1]. On the one hand, the continuous evolution of surgical techniques is constantly binging new opportunities and challenges in rehabilitation and on the other hand an optimized appreciation of neuromuscular function allows to better shape individualized protocols for each patient's needs following knee surgery [2, 3]. In this context, the sports rehabilitation team should consider the available evidence into the best clinical application, based also on experience. A complete functional recovery (physiological and psychological), respecting the biological of healing of the tissue is the sweet-spot that every patient deserve.

Return to play (RTP) following knee cartilage procedures is a long process, with an average length of 11 months (but up to 18 months) [4]. RTP at preinjury level percentages varies between studies (69–79%), but it is somewhat comparable with numbers following ACL reconstruction (ACLR). Systematic reviews report 72–79% RTP rate, with better results in regenerative techniques over microfractures [4–6]. However, details are often lacking in reference to progression in rehabilitation, and there is still no complete agreement about return-to-play criteria.

In this book chapter, the authors will discuss the principles (from logistic to clinical) of rehabilitation following knee cartilage procedures alongside the discussion of current concepts for cartilage rehabilitation [7], consisting of a customized criteria-based protocol to be applied in the day-by-day clinical practice. Key recent clinical additions will also be treated to allow the reader to live the present and the future of sports rehabilitation.

F. Della Villa (✉) · F. Tosarelli · S. Della Villa
Education and Research Department, Isokinetic Medical Group, FIFA Medical Centre of Excellence, Bologna, Italy
e-mail: f.dellavilla@isokinetic.com; s.dellavilla@isokinetic.com

D. Fusetti · L. Boldrini
Isokinetic Medical Group, FIFA Medical Centre of Excellence, Milan, Italy
e-mail: d.fusetti@isokinetic.com; l.boldrini@isokinetic.com

27.2 Principles of Rehabilitation Following Cartilage Restoration

The key principles of rehabilitation following knee surgery (e.g., cartilage restoration) may be divided into clinical and organizational ones. The

© ISAKOS 2021
A. J. Krych et al. (eds.), *Cartilage Injury of the Knee*,
https://doi.org/10.1007/978-3-030-78051-7_27

return-to-play process following cartilage restoration surgery is long (over 1 year in some cases) and demanding for the patient. To offer the best available treatment, logistic pitfalls should also be respected.

The clinical pitfalls of cartilage rehabilitation lays in the construct of the rehabilitation protocol. From basic science studies, we know that cartilage tissue respond to load and that mechanical loading (especially cyclical) is detrimentally important for cartilage and joint homeostasis, inducing positive adaptations, from stimulation of collagen and matrix production to increased diffusion of synovial fluid and optimization of cartilage nutrition [8–11]. Both *underloading* (e.g., prolonged immobilization) [12, 13] and *overloading* (excessive mechanical load, too much, too early) may be harmful after cartilage restoration. The clinical sweet-spot that should be pursued in an incremental mechanical loading through the months of rehabilitation. In this context, the clinician should always respect Scott Dye's theory of the envelope of function [14], with optimal and physiological loading varying in the different phases of rehabilitation.

Given this important and first rule, in the author's experience the rehabilitation protocol should be *personalized* (customized), *progressive*, and *supervised*.

To provide some examples and insights into the protocol *customization*, a patella-femoral cartilage lesion should be treated differently from a medial femoral condyle one and specific restriction of knee range of motion (ROM) exercises may vary in relation to the localization of the lesion [7]. The content of the protocol for each patient should be updated to the latest evidence, this point will be further discussed in the dedicated sub-paragraph.

As part of protocol supervision, in authors view, periodical clinical and functional evaluation are used to guide the functional progression towards RTP, briefly physical and psychological measures that should be measured are:

– **Muscle strength** (e.g., *Isometric or Isokinetic testing of knee extensors and flexors muscles*) [15]
– **Cardiovascular condition** (e.g., *aerobic and anaerobic threshold test*) [15]
– **Movement quality** (e.g., *jumping and cutting mechanics*) [16, 17]
– **Performance and Sport-specific measures** (e.g., *field testing and GPS metrics*) [18–21]
– **Psychological readiness** (e.g., *ACL-RSI scale*)

These functional data must be used to guide and adjust the rehabilitation protocol as will be discussed later in this chapter.

A quick scheme of the three features of the protocol is reported in Table 27.1.

Secondly, touching briefly on this point (that is often overlooked but critical), alongside an updated and evidence-based clinical method, *proper team* of specialists and *proper rehabilita-*

Table 27.1 *The three key features* of the rehabilitation protocol

Protocol feature	Details to be considered
Personalized (customized)	Clinical history Patient's gender Patient's activity level and functional expectations Primary sport Anthropometric data and general health (metabolic profile) Patient lower limb morphotype Type of lesion (chondral or osteochondral) Site of lesion (tibio-femoral (medial or lateral) or patellofemoral) Surgical technique (regenerative or reparative) Psychological aspects (personality traits)
Progressive	Rehabilitation in progressive phases depending on clinical and functional evaluation (criteria-based) with *incremental* loading; Progression according to joint responses (swelling and soreness) to rehabilitation stimuli (progress only with "clinically silent" knees)
Supervised	Rehabilitation should be supervised by a rehabilitation team; Periodical clinical (control consultations) and functional (testing) evaluation are warranted to objectively monitor the patient

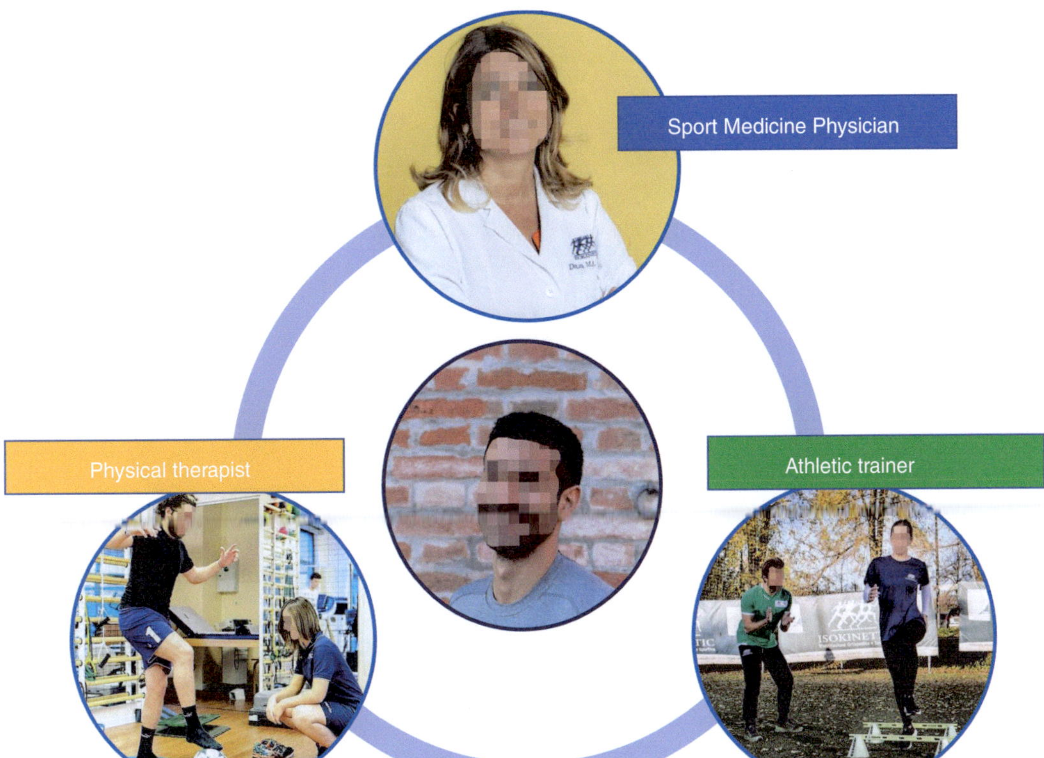

Fig. 27.1 *Proper team* for a patient-centered approach. To complete functional recovery following cartilage procedures, proper structures are needed, from medical offices to fields dedicated to rehabilitation

tion facilities are needed to schedule a complete and long-term recovery for an athlete following cartilage restoration surgery. A team (Fig. 27.1) including a sports medicine or rehabilitation physician (overseeing the process), a physiotherapist (engaged in the first phases of rehabilitation) and an athletic trainer (specialized in the last phase of On-Field Rehabilitation (OFR)) is necessary for an optimal patient's service. Having access to proper facilities is another aspect of rehabilitation (Fig. 27.2) as every phase of rehabilitation needs different and progressive stimuli, especially following cartilage restoration.

In this context, *rehabilitation pools* are important spaces mainly dedicated to the first rehabilitation phases. We recently underlined the benefit in pool rehabilitation (IPR) as applied to functional recovery after ACLR [22]. Early range of motion (ROM) and strength exercises may be commenced earlier, together with a gradual resumption of the correct gait cycle. The use of different water depths (progressing from deep to shallow) may allow a gradual and progressive increase in load. Also, this special environment allows implementation of early neuroplasticity exercises (e.g., heading on floating for the football (soccer) player) that mimic sport-specific gestures.

The *rehabilitation gym* remains the predominant environment in terms of total volume of rehabilitation sessions, while the other spaces support specific phases. The post-acute period as well most of the exercises for ROM recovery are undertaken in the gym. The crucial phase for the gym is the isolated strengthening period, an often-neglected period but crucial to develop the capability of the athlete to progress to more advanced rehabilitation phases. Both open kinetic chain (OKC) and closed kinetic chain (CKC) exercises, using both machines (e.g., Isokinetic

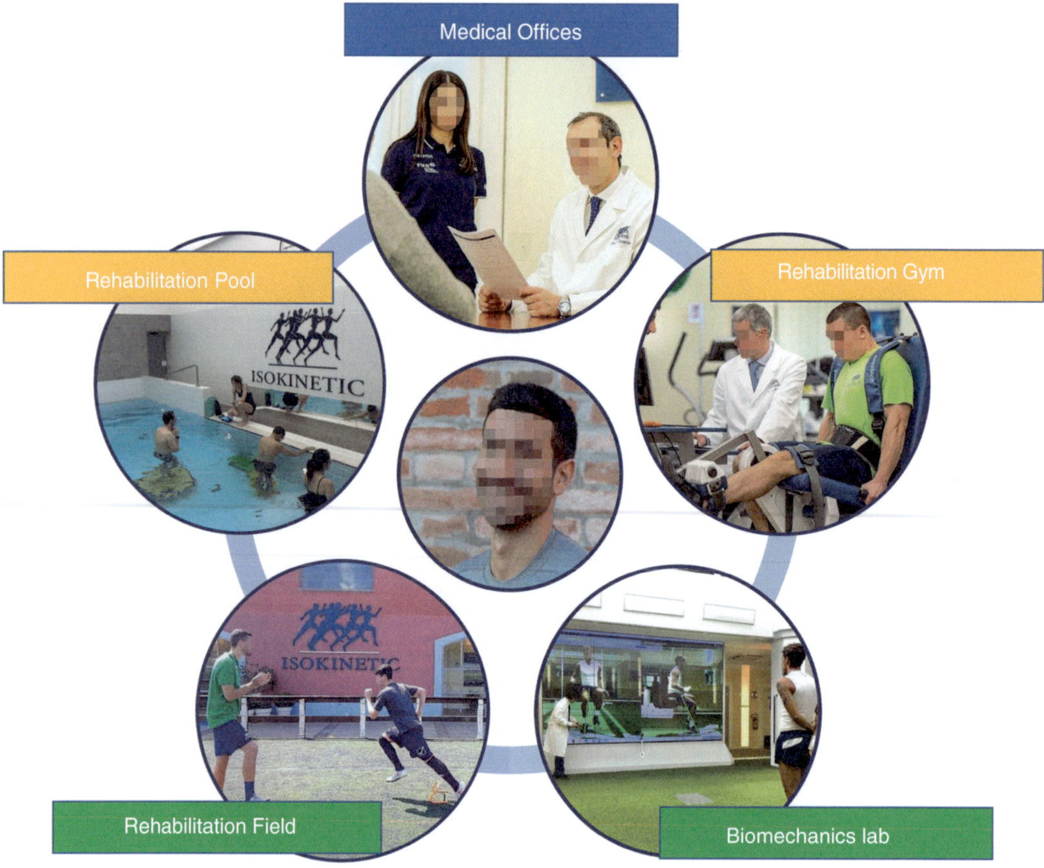

Fig. 27.2 *Proper facilities.* To complete functional recovery following cartilage procedures, proper structures are needed, from medical offices to fields dedicated to rehabilitation

dynamometers, leg press) and functional exercises are adopted to recover strength, tailored to the patient's specific responses.

The *biomechanics lab* (or other spaces dedicated to movements) is a recent addiction to the injury to the recovery process. It is suggested to consider the whole musculoskeletal (MSK) system and neuromuscular (NM) function following lower limb injuries. As such, re-integrating recently re-activated and strengthened muscles into proper and safe movement patterns is of paramount importance to allow long-term normal function and overall biomechanics.

Rehabilitation *sports fields* are dedicated to OFR. OFR stands as the very last phase of functional recovery, between standard rehabilitation and return to the team. It consists of a step-wise five sub-phases program of progressive return-to-sport activity [15, 18, 19]. With appropriate customization, this kind of service is applicable to all activity levels and sports. A multi-sports organization of this space in warranted to cover all the specific needs of the sports patients.

To deliver an updated service of sports rehabilitation, correct facilities need to be in place. The structural advances can facilitate, but not replace a correct application of the key clinical principles. Proper facilities "do not treat or cure" the patients, but facilitate the team guiding the application of innovative and evidence-based rehabilitation after cartilage restoration.

27.3 Return-to-Play Vision

To schedule a long-term recovery and increase the chances of successful RTP in athletes following cartilage restoration, the rehabilitation team should shift the focus *from the injured joint to the athlete*. This approach allows a serious consideration of many modifiable factors (muscle strength, physical conditioning, biomechanics, etc.) that can be optimized through specific intervention during rehabilitation.

Rehabilitation is generally and too often limited to the consideration of the first postoperative months and limited to resolution of pain, swelling, and ROM deficit (classical paradigm). This phase is crucial, but it is the foundation of what happen later in the process (mid and late phase rehabilitation).

When considering an expansion of the *ortho-bio-mechanic paradigm* (Fig. 27.3), we can move from the classical rehabilitation paradigm. Healing chondrocytes are part of tissue (cartilage) that is a part of the knee considered as an organ. The knee is controlled dynamically by knee spanning muscles and belongs to the lower limb (consider also distal and proximal joints). The lower limb kinetic chain is part of the MSK system. Finally, the system is a part of the patient as a person, with a certain physical conditioning and a unique personality trait and psychological response to injury status.

Shifting the focus on the athlete as a person allows to complete the functional recovery discussing about muscle strength recovery, cardiovascular conditioning, neuromuscular training, and restoring a sport-specific athletic profile using OFR.

The injury to recovery process starts immediately right after the injury and should continue until the return to the desired activity level (generally the preinjury level of sport participation). In our view, the same sport medicine team should oversee the process from the injury to the RTP (Fig. 27.4). As a medical community, we have a good control of the first phases, from diagnosis, through surgery (when required) until the recovery of activities of daily leaving. Then there is a slowly but progressive lack of control of the next rehabilitation phases (Fig. 27.4), when the process is less "medical" perceived in the classical definitions. This is a clinical mistake as a clinical "healed" knee (no symptoms) is not enough to restore an athlete's functional capacity to perform (that should rely on complete physiological and psychological functional recovery).

Even if the *strength recovery* is nowadays perceived as a key element of rehabilitation following knee surgery, there is still a sub-complete control of this phase that often is not completed, with strength deficit still present years after injuries [23]. This is the typical phase when the athlete has less symptoms, but underappreciated physical deficits are still present.

Finally, as explained in Fig. 27.4, there is a poor control towards the end of the process, when the patient is almost ready to RTP, in what it is generally called *late phase rehabilitation*. The sports rehabilitation team, alongside the sports surgery team should promote patient's compliance and adherence to this kind of approach to increase the likelihood to RTP [1, 24].

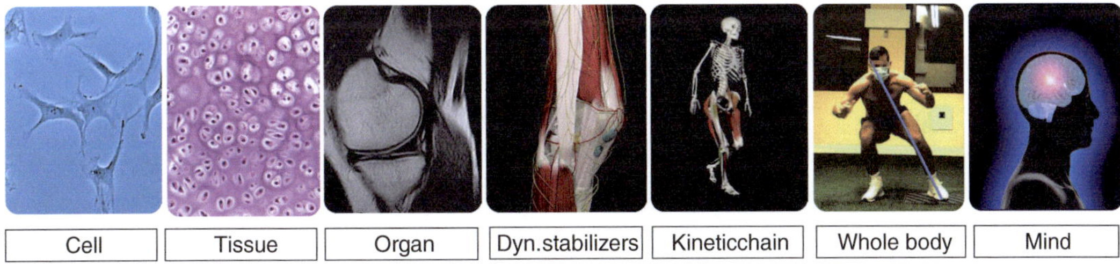

Fig. 27.3 *The ortho-bio-mechanic paradigm expanded.* The continuum from the cell (chondrocyte) to the patient as a person. Considering the whole picture is always important in rehabilitation. *Dyn* dynamic

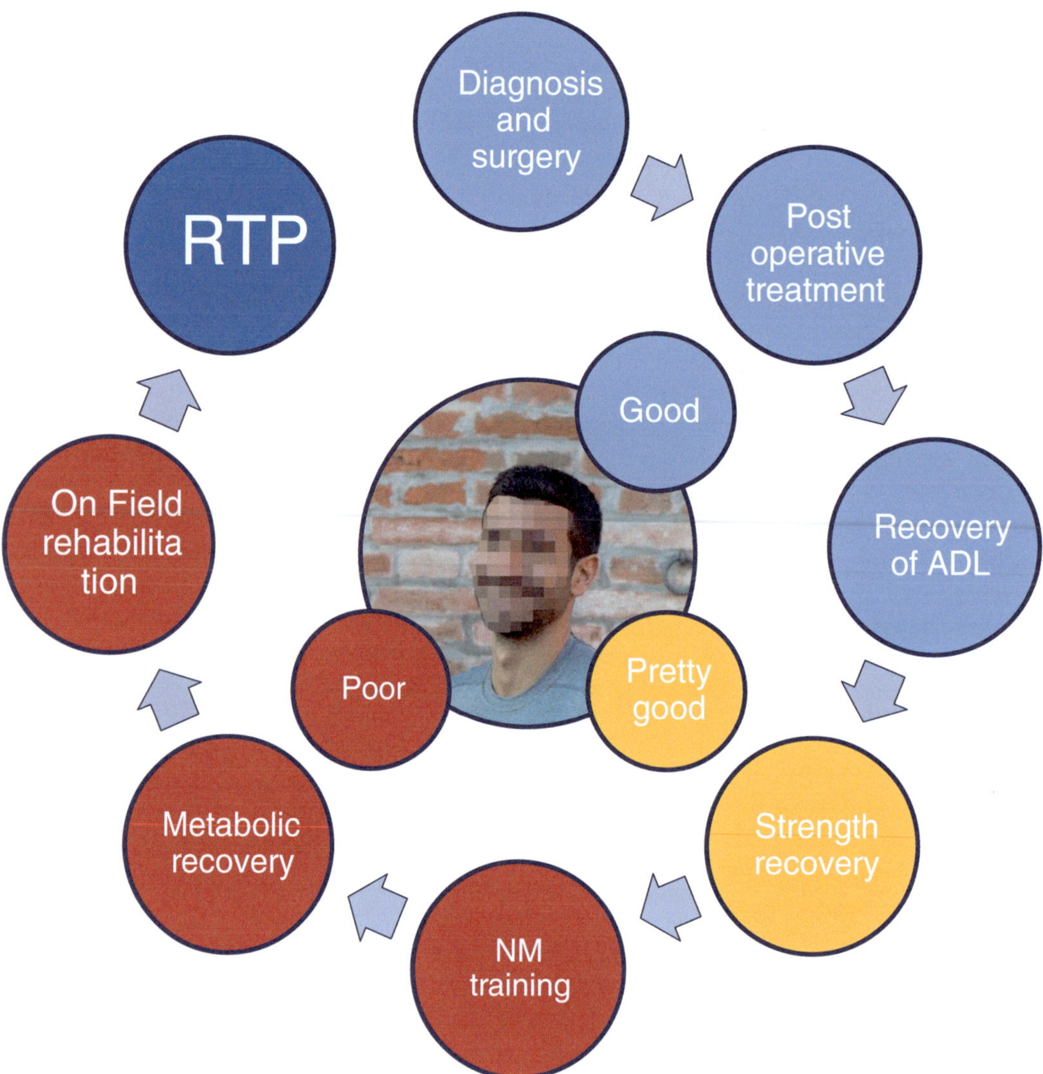

Fig. 27.4 *The injury to recovery process.* The injury to recovery process is a long and challenging journey. A lack of control of the last phase of rehabilitation is common and not acceptable. *ADL* activity of daily living, *NM* neuromuscular training, *RTP* return to play

27.4 Return-to-Play Protocol and Decision

As previously underlined in the chapter, the clinical approach to the patient is largely dependent on the contents of the rehabilitation protocol. In this sub-section, we will discuss the current concepts of rehabilitation following cartilage restoration surgery, with a special reference to rehabilitation after knee cartilage procedures. The basic concepts apply to any other joint.

Each patient is different, and protocol serves just as a general strategy. An example of a detailed current concept criterion-based protocol is presented in Table 27.2. The proposed protocol is divided into *five different stages* (with the recent addition of targeted neuromuscular training NMT in stage 4). Here after we discuss few key points

Table 27.2   Criteria-based RTP protocol following cartilage restoration procedure of the knee

Criteria-based protocol to RTP after cartilage restoration of the knee (times are indicative and should be measured ex post)						
	Predominant space	Goals	Weight bearing	ROM	Rehabilitation exercises	Criteria for progression
Stage 1 (From surgery to the third month)	Pool and gym	Pain and inflammation control Initial ROM recovery (Extension first) Recovery of normal gait cycle without crutches	No weight bearing for 2 weeks 2–6 weeks partial weight bearing 6–8 weeks progressive increase to full weight bearing without crutches	CPM (1 cycle/min 6–8/day for 2 to 4 weeks) Early self-assisted mobilization 0–90° Early patellar self-assisted mobilization Pendulum	Quadriceps isometric contractions Quadriceps electric stimulation Active ankle mobilization Posterior kinetic chain stretching Cryotherapy and physical therapies Proprioception without weight bearing From week 3 exercises in the water From week 6 stationary bike (seated)	No surgical contraindications No/minimal pain (NRS < 3/10) or swelling Full knee extension Recovery of the normal gait cycle
Stage 2 (fourth and fifth months)	Gym	Complete recovery of knee ROM (also flexion) Progressive recovery of strength	Full weight bearing (if the knee swells or is painful (NRS > 3/10) decrease the walking load and refer to the medical doctor)	Patellar mobilization	Eccentric strengthening of the triceps muscle Isomeric and isotonic exercises of hip muscles Bi-podalic proprioception exercises CKC strengthening exercises Aerobic reconditioning (stationary bike, treadmill, walking)	No/minimal pain or swelling Full knee ROM Adequate tone of trunk, thigh, and leg muscles
Stage 3 (sixth and seventh months)	Gym	Complete recovery of strength Return to running on a treadmill with normal running cycle	Full weight bearing	ROM should be already complete	Strengthening with isokinetic exercises (starts from high angular velocity 230–300°/s) Mono-podalic proprioception exercises OKC and CKC strengthening exercises (whole kinetic chain but focus on the knee) Core-stability exercises and initial NM control Continue aerobic reconditioning	Isokinetic test: strength >80% for knee extensors and flexors compared to the contralateral limb Good quality of SLS at 60° of knee flexion (with appropriate progression)

(continued)

Criteria-based protocol to RTP after cartilage restoration of the knee (times are indicative and should be measured ex post)						
	Predominant space	Goals	Weight bearing	ROM	Rehabilitation exercises	Criteria for progression
Stage 4 (eighth and ninth months)	Biomechanics lab (space dedicated to movement re-training)	Recovery of NM control and coordination Complete recovery of strength	Full weight bearing	ROM should be already complete	Continue strengthening exercises in the gym if needed (based on isokinetic testing results) Targeted NM training in biomechanics lab/space dedicated to movement training	Adequate NM training and proper movement quality (jumping and cutting mechanic) Be able to run on a treadmill at 8 km/h for at least 10′ (with good running quality)
Stage 5 (tenth to twelfth months)	Field	Return to training with the team Successful recovery of sport-specific athletic profile	Full weight bearing	ROM should be already complete	OFR periods [JOSPT 1 & 2] Continue targeted strengthening and/or NM training if needed	**Criteria to RTP** Surgeon consensus Complete knee ROM Complete recovery of muscle strength for knee extensors and flexors (isokinetic test 100%) Adequate CV reconditioning measured with aerobic (SA2) and anaerobic (SA4) threshold test [37, 38] Complete NM training with adequate movement quality (cutting and jumping mechanics) Complete OFR rehabilitation, with optimal GPS metrics progression

CPM continuous passive mobilization, *NRS* numeric rating scale, *ROM* range of motion, *CKC* closed kinetic chain, *OKC* open kinetic chain, *NM* neuromuscular, *OFR* on-field rehabilitation for each stage, whether the details are reported in Table 27.2.

27.4.1 First Stage (Early Rehabilitation)

The first stage can last 1–3 months. The main goals are: (1) recovery of joint homeostasis reducing pain and swelling, (2) progressive restoration of range of motion (knee extension first), and (3) recovery of the correct gait cycle. *Progression of weight bearing (WB)* (with the use of the rehabilitation pool) and *immediate mobilization* are key concept of this foundation stage. Restrictions in weight bearing are necessary in this postoperative stage. Progression to partial weight bearing is used to gradually increase the load walking without crutches. Timing to full WB varies in function of the type of surgery and the location of the lesion. On average, the range is from 40 days for microfractures (MF) to 2 months for Autologous Chondrocyte Implantation (ACI). There is no agreement at all on the exact timing for the full weight bearing. Studies that compared accelerated WB (6–8 weeks) to delayed WB (8–10 weeks) showing good clinical and functional outcome after 2 years in the group with the accelerated loading [25]. Accelerated WB does not seem detrimental but should be cautious. Continuous passive mobilization (CPM) should be introduced as soon as possible, also on the second day after surgery, to promote cartilage healing [26, 27]. Considering biomechanics is essential in targeting the ROM of CPM based on lesion localization. Other ROM exercises are added day after day to promote the full extension as soon as possible. This stage should not be aggressive, but progressive, respecting the joint responses (pain and swelling). The patient can progress in the protocol when certain criteria have been reached (Table 27.2).

At the end of first stage, the patient walks without crutches, without or with minimal symptoms and with an appropriate gait pattern.

27.4.2 Second Stage (Early Rehabilitation)

The second-stage duration is generally 1–2 months. The main goals are: (1) complete recovery of ROM (also knee flexion), (2) progressive recovery of muscles strength. *Loads progression* and *initial strengthening* are the basics of this stage. The patient keeps on working on the ROM recovery. Proprioceptive and NM activation exercises are introduced. The predominant location is the gym.

A proper tone of trunk (core-stability), thigh and leg muscles are crucial for shock absorption of loads during walking and running [28]. To facilitate load progression, exercises are both performed in open kinetic chain (OKC) and closed kinetic chain (CKC). The goal is avoiding overweight bearing on the graft and working in pain-free ROM. The approach to the patello-femoral-joint (PFJ) cartilage lesion is different from the femoral-tibial (FT) ones. For PFJ, the CKC exercises, such as free body weight or leg press, are preferred. Instead, for the TFJ, OKC exercises are preferred. Aerobic reconditioning is introduced as well using various exercises (stationary cycling, walking, etc.). The first strength test (isokinetic or isometric testing) is usually performed to quantify the side-to-side knee muscles strength deficit. Safety progression criteria are reported in Table 27.2.

At the end of this stage, the patient is ready to start running on the treadmill. Quality of loading during running is essential alongside quantity.

27.4.3 Third Stage (Mid Rehabilitation)

The third stage lasts about 2 months. The main goals are: (1) recovery of thigh muscles strength, (2) initial aerobic reconditioning, and (3) initial coordination and NM control. Proprioceptive and neuromuscular exercises, together with aerobic reconditioning and *strength exercises*, are the milestones of this stage. Recovery of muscle strength through various type of exercises (including isokinetic training) is the number one priority of this stage.

The progression of load in strength recovery is critical in this mid-stage. Advanced protocols including OKC and CKC exercises are warranted. Alongside strength recovery proprioception and NM control are implemented as well, looking for a good progression in task complexity and a very good frontal and sagittal plane control of basic movements (squat, single leg squat at 60°). Aerobic reconditioning is carried out with indoor running and a first aerobic and anaerobic threshold test can be performed to target the exercise prescription. As for all the stages progression criteria are reported in Table 27.2.

At the end of this stage, the patient should have a strength deficit lower than 20% compared to contralateral limb and should be able to perform basic movement with good quality (as a result of optimal progression).

27.4.4 Fourth Stage (Mid-to-Late Rehabilitation)

The fourth stage lasts about 1–2 months and the main goal of this stage is the inter-segmental control in basic to advanced sports movements. This stage consists of a *general or targeted (on a movement analysis test) NMT* to be carried out in a dedicated environment (space dedicated to movement training). Gym training can continue, with progressive strengthening and running progression.

At the beginning of this stage, it is useful to test patient's movement quality to target the intervention on the specific movement profile. Elements of corrective biomechanics focusing on lower limb, pelvis, and trunk control are implemented. Techniques of biofeedback can be used as well to teach safe movement patterns to the athlete prior coming back to the field. Optimization of frontal, transverse, and lateral plane biomechanics is the goal of this stage (Fig. 27.5). A customization of this stage is warranted as different lesion localization may need a slightly different approach. In the gym, the

patient continues to work on aerobic reconditioning and muscle strengthening.

At the end of this stage, strength and movement quality testing are repeated and the patient should display enough control of basic sports movements and improved strength.

27.4.5 Fifth Stage (Late Rehabilitation)

The goal of the final stage (that generally last 2 months) is return to training with the team. **Recovery of sport-specific gesture** is the milestone of this phase, which takes place mainly on the field (**OFR**). The transition between indoor and outdoor rehabilitation spaces until returning to sport is the key to this stage. NMT and strengthening can continue if specific deficits are still present.

The recovery of sport-specific movements can be introduced also in the previous stages through propaedeutic exercises in the other spaces to facilitate the neuroplasticity process, but it is only achieved on the field. Each rehabilitation session of OFR lasts about 90 min, from 3 to 5 times per week (depending on the patient's activity level) and for at least 8–10 weeks before returning to unrestricted sport participation.

The OFR program lays on four main pillars: *(1) Restoring movement quality, (2) Physical conditioning, (3) Restoring sport-specific skills, and (4) Progressively developing a chronic training load* [18]. The program is also divided into five specific sub-phases with increased physiological demands [19]. Progression though sub-phases is dictated by knee responses to load (no pain/no swelling and good progression). Monitoring the external player load may be useful during this last part of rehabilitation and should be done using GPS technology [19]. Building progressively a chronic workload while increasing the physical demands of each sport (context interactions and sport-specific movements) is warranted.

At the end of this process, based on previously reported objective data is useful to repeat all the

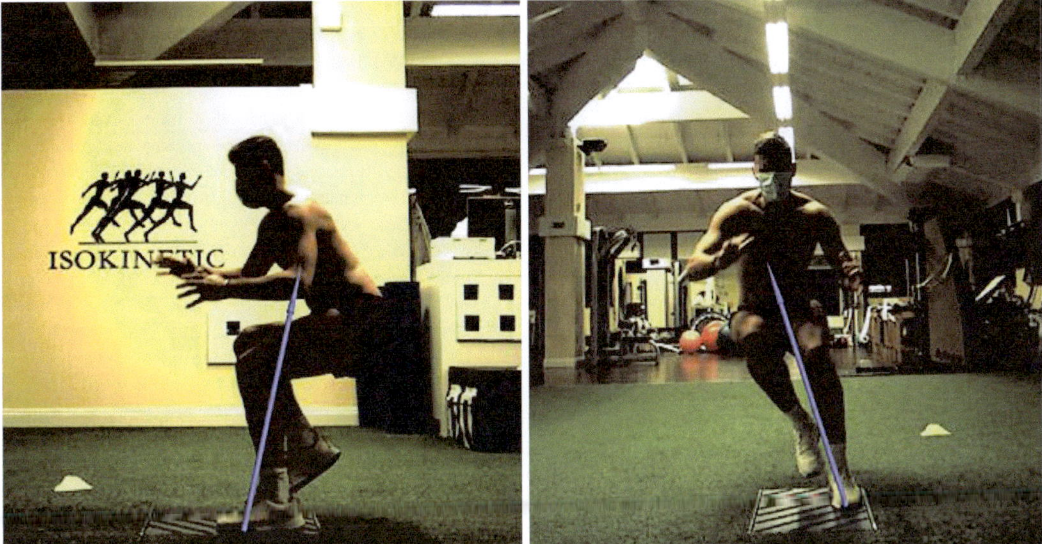

Fig. 27.5 *Movement analysis testing*. Example of frontal and lateral video-analysis of a patient displaying good quality of 90° sidestep cutting maneuver (proper knee alignment and proper knee-hip-trunk flexion on the lateral plane)

physical testing (strength, movement quality, and aerobic/anaerobic threshold test).

Good rehabilitation is about good progression. At the end of this protocol (that can last from 8 to 18 months following knee cartilage restoration procedure), the athlete should be ready to return to training with the team and gradually return to performance [29]. However, it is a current concept to apply criteria to RTP following knee procedures [7]. In Table 27.2, we report our proposed return to training (RTT) criteria.

That stated, each patient, lesion pattern, and surgical procedure is unique and in deciding when an athlete is ready to RTP, the sport medicine team should consider [29]:

- *Clinical criteria* (pain/swelling/stability)
- *Functional criteria* (muscle strength, aerobic/anaerobic conditioning)
- *Biomechanics and NM control* (movement quality)
- *Psychological criteria* (fear, readiness to RTS)
- *Sport-specific measures* (e.g., field testing or GPS metrics)

Additionally, the decision to RTP has not to be considered as an on/off button but should always be viewed as a continuum of increased physical and sports-specific demands, with RTT first followed by return to competition (RTC) afterwards [29]. Lastly, when dealing with professional athletes, performance-injury risk conflict should be considered as RTP is largely more important in elite level athletes, but a cautious approach should be maintained, and the patient should RTT with the team only if objectively ready.

27.5 Conclusions

In conclusion, successful RTS process following knee cartilage restoration is a complex issue that involves a patient and a whole sports medicine team for various months (8–18). Thinking beyond the knee is crucial, considering the athlete at 360° and especially taking into account each person unique response to injury. A criterion-based progression, using various rehabilitation spaces while controlling objective and clinically relevant parameters is suggested to increase the odds for a successful outcome.

Considering the state of the art in cartilage restoration rehabilitation (paucity of studies), embedding evidence with clinical experience is the clinical "sweet-spot" for the patient.

References

1. Della Villa S, Kon E, Filardo G, Ricci M, Vincentelli F, Delcogliano M, Marcacci M. Does intensive rehabilitation permit early return to sport without compromising the clinical outcome after arthroscopic autologous chondrocyte implantation in highly competitive athletes? Am J Sports Med. 2010;38(1):68–77.
2. Buckthorpe M, Della VF. Optimising the 'mid-stage' training and testing process after ACL reconstruction. Sports Med. 2020;50(4):657–78.
3. Buckthorpe M. Optimising the late-stage rehabilitation and return-to-sport training and testing process after ACL reconstruction. Sports Med. 2019;49(7):1043–58.
4. Campbell AB, Pineda M, Harris JD, Flanigan DC. Return to sport after articular cartilage repair in athletes' knees: a systematic review. Arthroscopy. 2016;32(4):651–68.
5. Nielsen ES, McCauley JC, Pulido PA, Bugbee WD. Return to sport and recreational activity after osteochondral allograft transplantation in the knee. Am J Sports Med. 2017;45(7):1608–14.
6. Mithoefer K, Hambly K, Della Villa S, Silvers H, Mandelbaum BR. Return to sports participation after articular cartilage repair in the knee: scientific evidence. Am J Sports Med. 2009;37(Suppl 1):167S–76S.
7. Mithoefer K, Hambly K, Logerstedt D, Ricci M, Silvers H, Della VS. Current concepts for rehabilitation and return to sport after knee articular cartilage repair in the athlete. J Orthop Sports Phys Ther. 2012;42(3):254–73.
8. Zhao Z, Li Y, Wang M, Zhao S, Zhao Z, Fang J. Mechanotransduction pathways in the regulation of cartilage chondrocyte homoeostasis. J Cell Mol Med. 2020;24(10):5408–19.
9. Shioji S, Imai S, Ando K, Kumagai K, Matsusue Y. Extracellular and intracellular mechanisms of Mechanotransduction in three-dimensionally embedded rat chondrocytes. PLoS One. 2014;9(12): e114327.
10. Leong DJ, Hardin JA, Cobelli NJ, Sun HB. Mechanotransduction and cartilage integrity. Ann N Y Acad Sci. 2011;1240:32–7.
11. Sanchez-Adams J, Leddy HA, McNulty AL, O'Conor CJ, Guilak F. The Mechanobiology of articular cartilage: bearing the burden of osteoarthritis. Curr Rheumatol Rep. 2014;16(10):451.
12. Säämänen AM, Tammi M, Jurvelin J, Kiviranta I, Helminen HJ. Proteoglycan alterations following immobilization and remobilization in the articular cartilage of young canine knee (stifle) joint. J Orthop Res. 1990;8(6):863–73.
13. Behrens F, Kraft EL, Oegema TR. Biochemical changes in articular cartilage after joint immobilization by casting or external fixation. J Orthop Res. 1989;7(3):335–43.
14. Dye SF. The knee as a biologic transmission with an envelope of function: a theory. Clin Orthop Relat Res. 1996;325:10–8.
15. Della Villa S, Boldrini L, Ricci M, Danelon F, Snyder-Mackler L, Nanni G, Roi GS. Clinical outcomes and return-to-sports participation of 50 soccer players after anterior cruciate ligament reconstruction through a sport-specific rehabilitation protocol. Sports Health. 2012;4(1):17–24.
16. Myer GD, Ford KR, Hewett TE. Tuck jump assessment for reducing anterior cruciate ligament injury risk. Athl Ther Today. 2008;13(5):39–44.
17. Dos'Santos T, McBurnie A, Donelon T, Thomas C, Comfort P, Jones PA. A qualitative screening tool to identify athletes with 'high-risk' movement mechanics during cutting: the cutting movement assessment score (CMAS). Phys Ther Sport. 2019;38:152–61.
18. Buckthorpe M, Della Villa F, Della Villa S, Roi GS. On-field rehabilitation part 1: 4 pillars of high-quality on-field rehabilitation are restoring movement quality, physical conditioning, restoring sport-specific skills, and progressively developing chronic training load. J Orthop Sports Phys Ther. 2019;49(8):565–9.
19. Buckthorpe M, Della Villa F, Della Villa S, Roi GS. On-field rehabilitation part 2: a 5-stage program for the soccer player focused on linear movements, multidirectional movements, soccer-specific skills, soccer-specific movements, and modified practice. J Orthop Sports Phys Ther. 2019;49(8):570–5.
20. Young W, Russell A, Burge P, Clarke A, Cormack S, Stewart G. The use of sprint tests for assessment of speed qualities of elite Australian rules footballers. Int J Sports Physiol Perform. 2008;3(2):199–206.
21. Sayers MGL. Influence of test distance on change of direction speed test results. J Strength Cond Res. 2015;29(9):2412–6.
22. Buckthorpe M, Pirotti E, Della VF. Benefits and use of acquatic therapy during rehabilitation after ACL reconstruction—a clinical commentary. Int J Sports Phys Ther. 2019;14(6):978–93.
23. Tayfur B, Charuphongsa C, Morrissey D, et al. Neuromuscular function of the knee joint following knee injuries: does it ever get back to normal? a systematic review with meta-analyses. Sports Med. 2021;51:321–38. https://doi.org/10.1007/s40279-020-01386-6.
24. Della Villa F, Andriolo L, Ricci M, Filardo G, Gamberini J, Caminati D, Della Villa S, Zaffagnini S. Compliance in post-operative rehabilitation is a key factor for return to sport after revision anterior cruciate ligament reconstruction. Knee Surg Sports Traumatol Arthrosc. 2020;28(2):463–9.
25. Wondrasch B, Zak L, Welsch GH, Marlovits S. Effect of accelerated weightbearing after matrix-associated autologous chondrocyte implantation on the femoral condyle on radiographic and clinical outcome after 2 years: a prospective, randomized controlled pilot study. Am J Sports Med. 2009;37(Suppl 1):88S–96S.

26. Rodrigo JJ, Steadman JR, Silliman JF, Fulstone HA. Improvement of full-thickness chondral defect healing in the human knee after debridement and micro fracture using continuous passive motion. Am J Knee Surg. 1994;7:109–16.

27. Salter RB. The biological concept of continuous passive motion of synovial joints: the first 18 years of basic research and its clinical application. In: Ewing JW, editor. Articular cartilage and knee joint function. New York: Raven Press; 1990.

28. LaStayo PC, Woolf JM, Lewek MD, Snyder-Mackler L, Reich T, Lindstedt SL. Eccentric muscle contractions: their contribution to injury, prevention, rehabilitation, and sport. J Orthop Sports Phys Ther. 2003;33(10):557–71.

29. Buckthorpe M, Frizziero A, Roi GS. Update on functional recovery process for the injured athlete: return to sport continuum redefined. Br J Sports Med. 2019;53(5):265–7.

Return to Sport Following Cartilage Treatment: Where Is the Evidence?

Naser Alnusif, Sarav S. Shah, and Kai Mithoefer

28.1 Introduction

Increasing sports participation—whether recreational or competitive—has been correlated with an increase in sport-related articular cartilage injuries of the knee. The reported prevalence of knee articular cartilage pathology in consecutive knee arthroscopies was found to be as high as 66%, with 11% of them may be suitable for a cartilage repair procedure [1]. Ciccotti et al. [2] reviewed 1010 knee arthroscopies performed for meniscectomy or meniscal repair in different age groups and reported knee articular cartilage injury in 5–22% patients younger than 20 years, 24–39% in patients between age 20–29, 48–54% in age 30–39 and higher the older the age group.

Due to the low propensity for intrinsic cartilage healing, the risk of progression to osteoarthritis specifically in athletes with repetitive joint loading sports is high. A recent systematic review suggested that patients with untreated focal chondral injuries are more likely to experience progression of the cartilage damage [3].Therefore, most patients with symptomatic chondral defects end up requiring surgery, especially young, active or high-level athletes.

Different surgical options have been utilized to manage knee articular cartilage injuries in athletes, and they are generally categorized into reparative and restorative procedures. Reparative procedures include marrow stimulation techniques (first- and second-generation microfracture) that aim to produce cartilage repair tissue using mesenchymal stem cells and the cell-based cartilage repair techniques (the different generations of autologous chondrocyte implantation (ACI) and matrix-induced autologous chondrocyte implantation (MACI)). Restorative procedures include osteochondral autograft transfer (OAT) and osteochondral allograft (OCA) implantation both procedures aim to restore the osteochondral defect without neocartilage repair tissue.

28.2 Return-to-Sport

One of the main outcome measures used to assess the success of an articular cartilage repair procedure is the patient's ability to return to their previous level of sports involvement. Therefore, more research has been focusing on the efficacy of the different surgical options in returning athletes to sports. The overall return-to-sport (RTS) rate in different cartilage restoration techniques was reported as 76% by a recent meta-analysis that

N. Alnusif · S. S. Shah
New England Baptist Hospital, Boston, MA, USA
e-mail: Naser.alnusif@mail.mcgill.ca

K. Mithoefer (✉)
Joint Preservation, Boston Sports and Shoulder Center, New England Baptist Hospital, Boston, MA, USA

© ISAKOS 2021
A. J. Krych et al. (eds.), *Cartilage Injury of the Knee*,
https://doi.org/10.1007/978-3-030-78051-7_28

included 2549 patients [4]. Another recent systematic review put the RTS at 78% with return to sport at pre-injury level at 72% at an average time to RTS of 11.2 months [5]. Across all surgical techniques (microfracture, ACI, OAT, or OCA), a high percentage of athletes have good outcomes scores after and may successfully return to athletic competition. Athletes who have a better prognosis are younger (<30 years), had smaller cartilage defects, underwent no previous surgical interventions, and participated in a more rigorous rehabilitation protocol. Furthermore, Mithoefer et al. [6] present data that suggests that untreated cartilage injuries (>12 months duration of symptoms) may create an unfavorable chemical environment for later cartilage repair. Early surgical intervention for articular cartilage injury is particularly important in the athlete's knee for the successful return to sports participation [7]. Below we will review the literature on RTS rate following each of the common cartilage restoration and reparation procedures as well as the estimated time needed for patients to return to sports postoperatively.

28.2.1 Marrow Stimulation Techniques (Microfracture, Microdrilling)

Microfracture is one of the oldest surgical options utilized in managing chondral defects in the knee and yet remains a valuable option when performed in the right patient population. However, one important point to note when reviewing the literature around microfracture procedures is that the surgical technique initially described was the first-generation microfracture with an awl diameter of 2.5 mm. This technique was found subsequently to have worse tissue fill and histological characteristics compared to the subchondral needling or microdrilling techniques using a 1 mm diameter K-wire [8]. The rationale behind the difference is that the larger diameter awls can seal off the channels by fractured and compacted bone compared to the smaller 1 mm channels. Multiple other factors have been reported in the literature to influence the outcomes of marrow

stimulation cartilage repair including: depth of subchondral perforation, number of subchondral perforations, and creation of vertical walls.

There are multiple studies that proved the strong efficacy and significant improvement in clinical outcomes after microfracture in patients with different levels of sports involvement. Good to excellent results were reported in 67% of athletes in a systematic review of 13 studies describing 821 athletes with 66% RTS at an average of 8 months after the microfracture surgery and 67% returning to competition at pre-injury level [7]. However, the same study showed deterioration in clinical outcomes and a drop in sports participation at the pre-injury level to 49% between 2 and 5 years after surgery. Another study noted 83% of National Basketball Association (NBA) players undergoing microfracture returned to professional basketball, including 73% in the NBA at 9.2 months. However, after microfracture, athletes played fewer games per season and with fewer points and steals per game versus pre-microfracture [9].

A recent study assessed return to sport in professional athletes after a microfracture procedure in four major leagues: NBA, Major Baseball League (MBL), National Hockey League (NHL), National Football League (NFL). Out of 131 athletes, 78% returned to play with significantly higher rates in MBL athletes 100% and lower rates in NFL athletes 71%. Average return time was 10.4 months. When comparing pre-surgery to post-surgery performance level, NBA athletes showed significantly lower performance in the first 2–3 seasons after surgery while MLB only showed lower performance in the first post-surgery season and NFL athletes showed no significant decrease in performance [10].

Several prognostic factors play a key role in identifying which patient would benefit the most from a microfracture procedure resulting in increased RTS [7]:

(a) Age < 40
(b) Duration of symptoms < 12 months
(c) Competitive athletes
(d) Lesion size < 2 cm^2
(e) Lesion involving the lateral femoral condyle

(f) Chondral defects not involving the subchondral bone

(g) Primary microfracture

(h) Better cartilage morphology

In terms of long-term follow-up, Gobbi et al. reported pain and swelling during strenuous activities only in nine patients by the end of 2 years, but in 35 out of 61 patients at final average follow-up of 15.1 years [11]. Overall, microfracture is still considered one of the main surgical options in managing articular cartilage defects with great early results and high RTS, keeping in mind the simplicity of the surgical technique, single-stage procedure, and low morbidity associated with it. However, the deterioration of patient reported outcomes as well as the gradual decline in sports performance over time (between 2- and 5-years post-treatment) is a disadvantage of this procedure. Limited cartilage repair tissue quality and quantity after microfracture have been described as reasons for the limited functional outcome after microfracture.

With the reported evidence on the time-dependent deterioration of outcomes and poor long-term durability of microfracture, this procedure would be an appropriate choice of repair in an older athlete that is at the end of his professional career and allows him to go back to sports relatively fast, while using it in a young athlete that is just starting his career would not be recommended. Therefore, using strict indications for the microfracture technique based on published outcome criteria, as well as second-generation augmented microfracture technologies, may be able to improve on the shortcoming observed with the first-generation technique and could result in more sustained return to sport following microfracture. However, clinical studies reporting on the outcomes and effect on RTS after those advanced microfracture techniques are still pending.

28.2.2 Cell-Based Cartilage Repair Techniques (ACI/MACI)

Since it was first reported by Brittberg in 1994 [12], ACI has undergone significant development, and it has been considered as an estab-lished treatment modality for symptomatic knee articular cartilage defects. The original technique was described as an injection of a suspension of cultured chondrocytes into a debrided chondral defect underneath a periosteal cover harvested from the proximal tibia (first generation) which evolved into the development of the bio-absorbable cover as an alternative to periosteum (second generation). In order to overcome some of the problems and complications related to the previous techniques (periosteal graft hypertrophy, calcification, and delamination as well as uneven distribution of chondrocytes within the defect and potential for cell leakage), a biodegradable scaffold seeded with chondrocytes in the form of membrane has been developed (third generation) referred to as matrix-induced autologous chondrocyte implantation (MACI) (Fig. 28.1). Therefore, when reviewing the literature, it is important to observe what technique was used, as different studies reported different outcomes and complication rates between the previous three surgical techniques.

Mithoefer et al. [13] reviewed the evolution of ACI procedures for articular cartilage defects of the knee in soccer athletes and showed the average time to return to soccer after first-generation ACI was 18 months while the combined effect of the newer second- and third-generation implantation techniques, along with the accelerated and sports-specific rehabilitation protocols, have reduced the time to return to sports to an average of 11 months [14]. The attributed reasoning behind that is the decreased invasiveness of the newer generation ACI which allows for faster neuromuscular recovery, joint mobilization, and restoration of joint biomechanics. Their review also found that return to soccer was 83% in competitive players and 16% in recreational players [15]. Eighty percent returned to same competitive level and 87–100% maintained their ability to play sports at 5 years postoperatively. Those numbers are considered the highest when compared to other cartilage restoration procedures. The same discussed paper reviewed the factors affecting return to sport (Table 28.1)

In a recent study of 150 patients [16], 85% of the entire cohort were satisfied with their ability

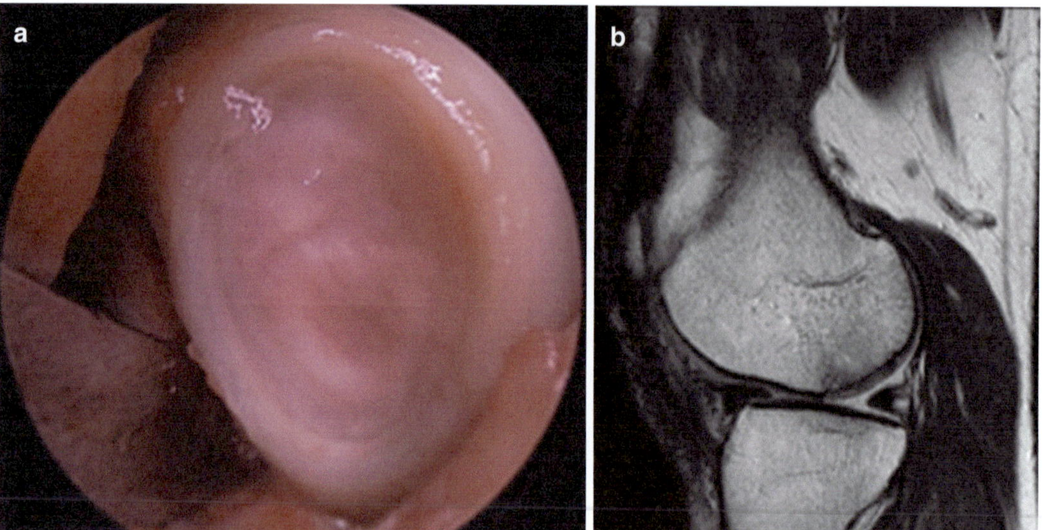

Fig. 28.1 Intraoperative appearance of a 3 cm² articular cartilage defect of the femoral condyle of an elite athlete treated with matrix-induced autologous chondrocyte implantation (MACI) (**a**). The player returned to full sports participation at 10 months after surgery. Routine postoperative MRI at 24 months (**b**) demonstrates intact cartilage repair under high athletic demand

Table 28.1 Factors affecting return to sport after autologous chondrocyte implantation [13]

Factor	Faster/Better return to play
Preoperative duration of symptoms	Duration < 12 months
Age	Age < 25 years
Addressing associated pathology	Simultaneous surgery
Athletic skill level	Competitive athletes
Rehabilitation	Individualized sport-related rehabilitation
Surgical invasiveness	Minimally invasive surgery

to return to recreational activities, while 66% were satisfied with their ability to participate in sports after MACI procedure. They also showed that outcome score (Tegner activity scale) improvement was correlated with younger age (<40 years) and duration of symptoms prior to surgery with no significant correlation with defect size and body mass index (BMI).

When looking at the midterm (5 year) outcomes in the average population of active patients after MACI procedure, a study by Zak et al. [17] reviewed their results on 70 patients with average recreational sports or competitive sports participation at baseline and their rate of RTS was 74.3%. They did not find a significant difference in clinical outcomes when comparing different age groups (<40 years versus >40 years). There was also no correlation between lesion size, duration of symptoms, and RTS rate.

Recent long-term studies have also shown maintenance of the significant improvements in clinical outcome measures after MACI procedure up to 10 and 15 years postoperatively [18, 19]. Zaffagnini et al. [20] reviewed the clinical outcomes and RTS rates of 31 competitive athletes (Tegner score 8, 9, 10) at 10 year after MACI procedure and showed remarkable improvements in multiple outcome measures at the 2-year follow-up with no significant change from then up to the 10 year mark. However, despite the overall 64.5% rate of RTS at a competitive level and 58.1% rate of the same pre-injury level, they found progressive decrease in those rates over time. Nevertheless, when different etiologies affecting this rate were investigated, they found that younger athletes (<20 years) presented 92.3% and 84.6% of RTS rates at competitive and pre-injury levels, respectively. Other factors found to have better results included traumatic lesions as well as having MACI as the primary surgery as opposed to revising a failure of other procedures. Similar promising results were found after ACI procedure in the adolescent athletes' population with 96% of athletes reporting good or excellent results and returned to high-impact sports and 60% returned to an athletic level equal or higher than that before knee injury with a mean follow-up of 47 months [21].

Despite the limited number of studies on return to sports after MACI procedure, the overall reported outcomes suggest promising results at both early, midterm, and long-term follow-ups, with varying prognostic factors between different studies. However, most studies correlate higher preoperative sports participation and younger age with a better chance of returning to same level of sports postoperatively, making this surgical option more suitable for younger competitive athletes in the beginning of their career due to better longevity and durability of the repair tissue.

28.2.3 Osteochondral Autograft Transfer (OAT)/Mosaicplasty

In cases of athletes with small osteochondral lesions (size < 2 cm^2) [22, 23], the OAT or mosaicplasty have shown to provide favorable outcomes in terms of high rate of RTS and relatively fast RTS participation.

A recent systematic review [24] determined the return-to-sport rate following different knee cartilage restoration procedures. Thirty-one studies were reviewed with 894 patients showing OAT as the highest rate of RTS 88.2% compared to the lowest being OCA 77.2%. As for the RTS at the same/higher level, 28 studies were reviewed with 895 patients and showed the highest rates with OAT 79.3% and ACI to have the lowest rates 57.3%. When they looked at the timing of RTS, the average reported time in OAT and ACI were 4.9 and 11.6 months, respectively.

Lynch et al. [23] performed a systematic review of level I and II studies reviewing outcomes after OAT/mosaicplasty. A total of nine studies were found with both minimal 12-month follow-up and 25 patients in each study. The overall RTS was as early as 6 months after the procedure. Additionally, they suggested that OAT/mosaicplasty might be more appropriate for lesions smaller than 2cm^2.

An interesting case series [25] of 20 competitive athletes (professional, collegiate, varsity high school, and regional or national competitive athletes) that underwent OAT/mosaicplasty procedure followed by an accelerated return-to-sport protocol described as up to 50% weight bearing immediately postoperatively with progression to full weight bearing at 2 weeks for patients with 1 or 2 plugs (14/20) otherwise 4 week. They reported 100% RTS rate with a mean time to return of 2.8 months. However, the reported mean pain score during ensuing athletic season was 4.4 ± 1.5 (out of 10). Half of the athletes reported moderate swelling or stiffness with a quarter of all patients requiring aspiration and/or injections. All 20 patients were able to perform the physical demands of their sports without significant instability. The criteria utilized to define an athlete returned to sports were the date that patients resumed full and unrestricted athletic activities.

The potential advantage of OAT over other cartilage repair techniques rendering its results in faster RTS is due to the direct incorporation of autologous bone with an already intact and healthy hyaline cartilage articular surface. In contrast, marrow stimulation or cell-based reparative techniques require growth of a repair tissue, as well as more prolonged protected weight bearing postoperatively with resultant slower recovery and RTS. One disadvantage of OAT that needs to be considered is the risk of donor-site morbidity that was reported to be as high as 6% after mosaicplasty [26]

Gudas et al. [22] performed one of the largest and longest term follow-up prospective randomized trials in the articular cartilage repair literature with a 10-year follow-up comparing mosaicplasty with microfracture in the high-level athletes population. There was significant clinical improvement found in both groups at 3 and 10 years comparted to preoperative scores; however, mosaicplasty had significantly better results at both time intervals compared to microfracture. More athletes in the mosaicplasty 75% than in the microfracture 37% group maintained the same physical activities at the long-term follow-up. This finding again demonstrates how microfracture outcomes tend to deteriorate over time. The average duration of return to previous sports was significantly longer in the mosaicplasty group. Positive prognostic factors favoring return to same level of sports were found to be younger age (<25 years) and lesion size (<2 cm^2), which correlates with the results of several other studies [23, 27].

Soccer is well known to be one of the high demand sports with increased risk in developing cartilage damage. Therefore, reviewing the results of OAT/mosaicplasty and their effect on RTS participation in this group of athletes provides important data about the long-term durability to withstand increased mechanical loads. Panics et al. [27] reviewed 61 high-level soccer athletes who underwent OAT/mosaicplasty and showed that 89% of the elite players returning to the same level of sports while only 62% of the competitive athletes did so. The average time to return to competition was 4.5 months. Their results also showed that younger age and smaller lesion size as positive prognostic factors with lesions involving the patellofemoral joint as worse outcomes when relating to return to sports.

Given the earlier reported time to RTS compared to other procedures, as well as the remarkably good long-term clinical outcomes, OAT is considered a suitable option for younger competitive athletes with small chondral or osteochondral lesions who wish to return to their sport the earliest possible.

28.2.4 Osteochondral Allograft Implantation (OCA)

When managing symptomatic osteochondral lesions in the knee that are larger than 2 cm^2, OCA implantation is considered the preferred surgical option as microfracture and OAT are correlated with poor outcomes when performed for lesions >2 cm^2 and ACI/MACI are suboptimal options for lesions involving both cartilage and subchondral bone.

A systematic review by Crawford et al. [28] that included 13 studies and 772 patients managed with OCA, found that most studies reported improvement in activity and most sport-related outcomes. However, only 3 in 13 studies provided RTS data with a rate of RTS ranging from 75 to 82%. A significant finding in the previous systematic review was the high reoperation rate, ranging from 34 to 53%. In most of the involved studies, the outcome was limited to less than 3 years, which makes it difficult to know if athletes maintain their level of sports involvement at longer follow-up.

In one study, the time to RTS for athletes after OCA transplantation was reported at 9.6 months, with 88% returning to sports and 79% return to previous level of sports [29]. No correlation of outcomes based on different types of sports participation was performed.

Balazs et al. [30] reviewed the RTS rate in professional and collegiate basketball players after OCA implantation, with a total of 11 athletes (4 NBA players and 7 collegiate players). Their overall return-to-play rate was 80%. Three of the 4 NBA players returned at the same level with a median RTS time of 20 months, while the fourth was cleared to play but remained an unsigned agent. Out of the 7 collegiate athletes, 1 was ineligible to return, but 5 out of the remaining 6 returned at a median 8 months after surgery. Despite the small cohort size, this study showed an overall good outcome in high-level athletes in a sport that is known to have a significantly high rate of knee chondral injuries. This is likely due to the repetitive jump landing with the high shear forces and peak loads on articular cartilage, as reported by an magnetic resonance imaging (MRI) study to be 81% and 50% in asymptomatic collegiate and professional basketball players, respectively [31, 32].

OCA implantation is considered one of the salvage operations that is commonly performed for larger osteochondral lesions that have failed other cartilage repair procedures. One of the debatable points when discussing OCA implantation is whether outcomes after primary implantation are superior to revisions from a failed prior cartilage repair surgery. Gracitelli et al. [33] showed no difference in functional outcomes between primary OCA implantation when compared to secondary implantation after a failed marrow stimulation procedure. Despite the higher reoperation rate in the secondary OCA 44% than the primary group 22%, there was no difference in graft survivorship at the 10-year follow-up (87.4% and 86%, respectively).

A reason of failure to return to same level of sport is unspecified in most of the reviewed literature. Key factors described in a paper assessing RTS after OCA implantation in high-level high school and intercollegiate athletes found that graduation from school or college 50%, fear of re-injury 38%, or continued pain 12% were present in the athletes unable to return to the same level of sports participation [34].

28.3 Effect of Different Rehabilitation Programs on Return to Sport

The role of the rehabilitation program—before and after any cartilage restoration procedure—has a big impact on the outcomes, as well as the RTS rates. The shared purpose of all different rehabilitation programs is to provide a mechanical environment for the local adaptation and remodeling of the repair tissue that will enable patients to safely return to their optimal level of function, without compromising the integrity or healing process of the repaired tissue [35]. Despite the various rehabilitation protocols observed in the literature, there is no clear consensus guidelines or criteria on a safe return-to-play protocol with significant differences in their speed of progression between the different phases of the rehabilitation program.

In a systematic review by Hurley et al. [24] assessing the different rehabilitation protocols after cartilage restoration procedures, they found that the vast majority of studies allowed early onset of range of motion (ROM) exercises within the first week postoperatively in all of the different procedures. This approach is supported by the basic science literature, as it improves cartilage healing with animal studies. These findings prove the efficacy of early ROM using continuous passive motion (CPM) device in improving chondro-

genesis, proteoglycan, and glycosaminoglycan synthesis in cartilage as well as decreasing collagen breakdown [36–38]. Other benefits of early initiation of ROM include preventing knee stiffness and muscle disuse atrophy.

Data from Hurley's review on the progression of weight bearing demonstrated variable protocols for initiation of partial weight bearing, ranging from 1 to 4 weeks after microfracture and ACI, while partial weight bearing was reported after OAT and OCA for up to 6 weeks postoperatively. Furthermore, the progression to full weight bearing was at the 6-week mark in the majority of the OAT and OCA studies, compared to between 6–10 weeks and 6–8 weeks in the ACI and microfracture studies, respectively. This can be explained by the bone to bone healing expected at 6 weeks in the OAT and OCA group, as compared to the primitive, unorganized, and soft initial repaired cartilage tissue observed in ACI, which makes it more vulnerable to mechanical overload and requires prolonged protection. However, a recent randomized controlled trial showed no difference in clinical outcomes when comparing full weight bearing at 6 versus 8 weeks after MACI procedure on 2-year follow-up [39]. Patient satisfaction with their ability to participate in sports was not significantly different between the two groups in this RCT; however, there are no studies comparing the effect of different protocols of progressing weight bearing status to the RTS rate in the athletes' population. The rationale behind targeting an earlier progression of weight bearing status is to enhance the cell loading stimulus to return patients to normal knee joint loading. In effect, they can resume their general daily activities and have sooner progression of further rehabilitation protocol phases.

The location of the cartilage defect is very important in the decision-making process of weight bearing and ROM progression after articular cartilage surgeries. In lesions located in the patella or trochlea, immediate full weight bearing with the brace locked in extension is recommended given the high joint reaction forces in the patellofemoral joint during ROM. In contrast, lesions involving the tibiofemoral joint typically have initial limitation of weight bearing, and accelerated resumption of ROM.

The RTS protocols are variable after different articular cartilage surgeries, with no clear individualized criteria on when to determine an athlete is safe to fully RTS. Most of the reviewed literature utilized time-based criteria for allowing RTS with 6 months being the quoted time in two-thirds of the studies reviewed by Hurley et al. [24]. While timing to RTS was relatively consistent for microfracture, OAT and OCA studies at around 6 months, timing after ACI was much more variable ranging between 6 and 18 months postoperatively. Despite the benefit of having predictable time-based criteria in progressing athletes between the different rehabilitation phases, individualized criteria should be developed to formulate guidelines on progressing patients based on their symptoms and clinical progress. While there has been a published protocol for MACI [14], there is no singular answer for cartilage repair, rather general principles that need to be applied to every individual case. Presence of pain and recurrent swelling for instance are considered indicators that rehabilitation is progressing too rapidly and overloading the healing tissue [35]. Other objective measures include restoration of full range of motion, return to functional strength, ability to perform sport-specific movements, and some even utilize MRI as an adjunct to assess tissue healing prior to releasing an athlete to RTS [20].

Overall, rehabilitation protocols should not be standardized for all patients alike, and rather need to be individualized to multiple different variables:

1. Athlete's age and type/level of sports involvement
2. Defect size and type of procedure performed
3. Location of the defect
4. Concomitant injuries and procedures performed along with the cartilage surgery

28.4 Key Points in Reviewing Return-to-Sport Evidence

Despite the limited number of studies focusing on RTS rates after articular cartilage surgeries, the overall findings have shown promising results with the majority of patients returning to play following cartilage repair procedures, regardless of the type of procedure used. However, when reviewing RTS studies, multiple important factors need to be taken into consideration that can change the way we interpret the data presented:

- There are multiple patient-reported outcome scores that have been used in studies investigating the return-to-sport rate. However, only International Knee Documentation Committee (IKDC) subjective score, Knee injury and Osteoarthritis Outcome Score (KOOS), and Lysholm Knee Score have been validated for use in patients with cartilage defects [40, 41]. Tegner Activity Scale and the Marx Activity Rating Scale are two commonly utilized outcomes measures that focus on sport-specific activity level. When looking at examples of the Tegner Scaling system, 9 represents the competitive soccer level while 7 represents the competitive basketball level. This makes it difficult to compare outcomes of different types of sports involvement as lower scores could correlate with the best outcome for certain level or type of sports and not necessarily a decrease in performance. Marx Scaling system, on the other hand, focuses on most challenging activities of the knee, regardless of the type of sport. The score includes four questions concerning four activities: running, cutting, deceleration, and pivoting. So having this score for specific athletes may not be beneficial, such as assessing the improvement of a professional cyclist or a cross-country skier. The KOOS is one of the most commonly used outcome scoring systems after articular cartilage repair procedures, but most of the questions involved are related to osteoarthritis with less emphasis on the higher level performance assessment of the young and active athletes.
- Concomitant pathology and procedures performed along with cartilage restoration techniques could affect the outcome, as well as the validity of the comparative studies. A recent meta-analysis showed 46% of patients undergoing cartilage repair surgery had concomitant surgeries with ligamentous reconstruction

making up the highest proportion of those procedures [4]. The results on the effect of concomitant procedures vary between studies; however, some studies do not incorporate those data with their results which could potentially skew the conclusion given the different rehabilitation protocols involved with different concomitant procedures.

- Comparing primary versus revision cartilage repair surgery has been shown to have contradicting results. Therefore, it is important to keep that in mind when interpreting the results of some of the comparative studies between two different cartilage repair procedures. In a meta-analysis that included 44 studies, only 27 out of them reported on previous surgeries prior to the index cartilage surgery [4]. An athlete with a history of multiple prior failed cartilage repair procedures is unlikely to gain the same improvements as an athlete undergoing a primary procedure.
- One of the main findings reported in multiple studies is the difference in RTS rate in the different levels of athletic involvement (recreational, competitive, collegiate, and professional). In a systematic review by Mithoefer et al., the RTS was 71–83% in competitive athletes and 16–29% in recreational athletes after microfracture and ACI procedures [42]. Despite this conclusion, the majority of studies focusing on RTS rates include a study population that has a mix of different levels of sports participation, which might affect the accuracy of the reported results.
- Choosing the indicated procedure for the proper patient is extremely important to obtain optimal outcomes. Procedure selection bias can be an issue in studies comparing the outcomes of two different cartilage repair procedures, as surgeons will aim to select a procedure that will best manage the athlete's lesion based on lesion characteristics. It is difficult to compare OAT, which is generally limited to smaller lesions to prevent donor-site morbidity, with ACI and OCA which are uncommonly used for smaller lesions. Also, microfracture is not typically recommended for deep osteochondral lesions or lesions ($>$2–4 cm^2), which makes it hard to compare with OAT and OCA. Another potential bias is seen in progressing athletes throughout the rehabilitation phases after the different cartilage repair procedures which is reliant on the type of procedure. For instance, autologous bone with an already intact and healthy hyaline cartilage articular surface allows for faster RTS protocols unlike marrow stimulation or cell-based reparative techniques that require more prolonged protected weight bearing postoperatively with resultant slower recovery and delayed RTS.

- The definition of RTS is variable in the literature with significant heterogeneity in the reported outcomes. Some report it as "clearance" to RTS while others define it as the athlete's ability to RTS participation or even same level of sports as prior to injury level. Hence, surgeons need to be cognizant when quoting those results to their patients. Also, RTS results do not necessarily mean better patient-reported outcomes, as some studies fail to show significant advantage of one cartilage restoration procedure over the other, regardless of the RTS outcome. Patient-reported outcomes focus on patients' symptoms and functional daily activities, which could be overlooked when purely addressing RTS as the outcome measure of the procedure.
- There are many socioeconomic factors that can affect athletes' ability to RTS regardless of how well the procedure was selected and performed and those factors are rarely addressed in the literature. Some of those factors were reported in a study by Nielsen et al. [43]:

1. Playing eligibility and contract status
2. Health issues unrelated to the knee
3. Loss of interest in sports participation
4. Starting a family
5. Change in jobs or career

Other psychological factors can also have an impact on the athlete's ability to perform at the same level of sport including fear of re-injury [34]

28.5 Summary

Cartilage repair techniques have demonstrated good to excellent outcomes with regard to RTS with an average rate of 76–78% amongst the combined different techniques. Each surgical option has its own pros and cons (Table 28.2) that surgeons need to be aware of when approaching patients with knee articular cartilage injury to achieve optimal outcomes based on both lesion characteristics and the patient's level of athletic involvement. While the scientific literature on RTS after cartilage repair is still evolving, a thorough understanding of the biology of each repair technique and differentiated knowledge of the indications and outcome of each technique specifically in the demanding athletic population is critical to optimize the rate of RTS. In addition, development of individualized, athlete-specific rehabilitation protocols based on the individual procedure type, defect location, type of sport, and level of competition is critical not only for a successful RTS but also to promote long-term sports participation after return. Based on all the presented date, we have formulated an algorithm that focuses on the specific demands in the athletic population, which would be different than the general population (Fig. 28.2).

Table 28.2 Summary of the Pros and Cons and RTS in the different cartilage repair techniques

Cartilage repair technique	RTS (Rate)	Time to RTS (months)	Pros	Cons	Positive prognostic factors
Marrow Stimulation Techniques (Microfracture, Microdrilling)	58%	9.1 ± 2.2	• Procedural technical simplicity • Readily available for incidental lesions • Single-stage procedure • Low morbidity • Cost-effective	• Clinical deterioration and decline in sports participation overtime (2–5 years) • Relies on fibrocartilage repair tissue (low stiffness, resilience, and wear resistance when compared to hyaline cartilage) • Potential for subchondral bony overgrowth	• Age < 40 years • Lesion size < 2 cm^2 • Competitive athletes compared to lower level athletes • Lesions involving the lateral femoral condyle • Primary compared to revision microfracture
Chondrocyte-based repair techniques (ACI/MACI)	82%	11.8 ± 3.8	• Potential for autologous hyaline cartilage repair tissue • Suitable for large chondral lesions	• Two-stage procedure (MACI) • Longer RTS rehabilitation process • High cost	• Age < 40 years • Duration of symptoms < 12 months • Competitive athletes compared to lower level athletes
Osteochondral Autograft Transfer (OAT/Mosaicplasty)	93%	5.2 ± 1.8	• Restoration for autologous hyaline cartilage articular surface • Single-stage procedure • Fastest and highest rate of RTS	• Donor-site morbidity • Limited to smaller lesions	• Lesion size < 2 cm^2 • Age < 25–30 years • Lesions involving the femoral condyles compared to patellofemoral joint lesions
Osteochondral Allograft	88%	9.6 ± 3.0	• Adequate option for larger lesions • Good salvage for failed cartilage repair surgeries • Restoration of hyaline cartilage articular surface along with the deficient subchondral bone	• Highest reoperation rate • High cost of allograft • Not readily available in all institutes • Immune response to the Allograft	• Lower BMI • Non-workers compensation claims • Age < 25 years • Competitive athletes compared to lower level athletes

RTS rate and time to RTS data [4]

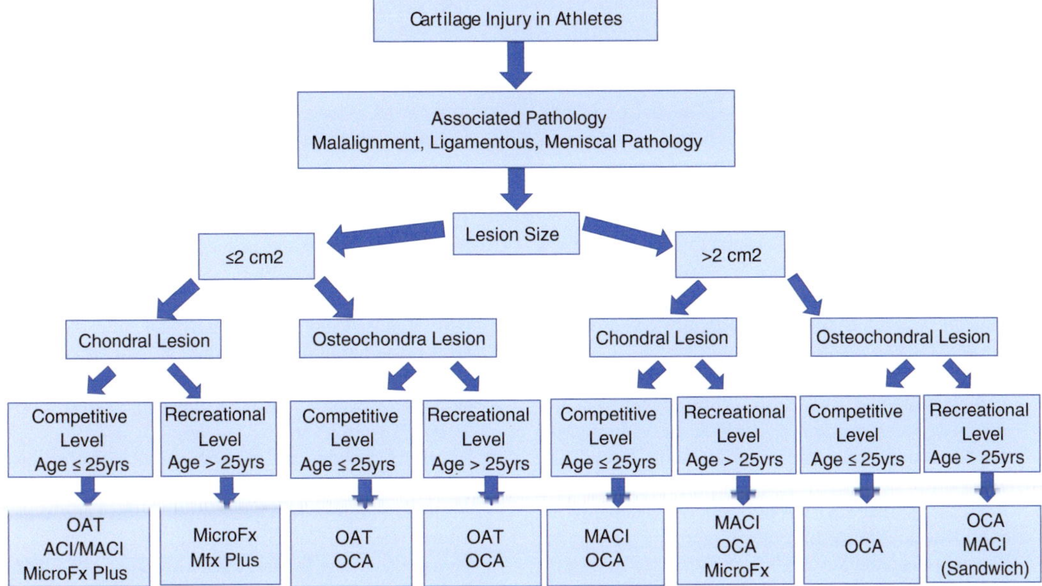

Fig. 28.2 Algorithm for the treatment options of articular cartilage repair in the athletic population. *OAT* osteochondral autograft transplantation, *ACI* autologous chondrocyte implantation, *MACI* matrix-induced chondrocyte implantation, *OCA* osteochondral allograft, *MicroFx Plus* augmented microfracture/second-generation microfracture

References

1. Årøen A, Løken S, Heir S, Alvik E, Ekeland A, Granlund OG, Engebretsen L. Articular cartilage lesions in 993 consecutive knee arthroscopies. Am J Sports Med. 2004;32(1):211–5.
2. Ciccotti MC, Kraeutler MJ, Austin LS, Rangavajjula A, Zmistowski B, Cohen SB, Ciccotti MG. The prevalence of articular cartilage changes in the knee joint in patients undergoing arthroscopy for meniscal pathology. Arthroscopy. 2012;28(10):1437–44.
3. Houck DA, Kraeutler MJ, Belk JW, Frank RM, McCarty EC, Bravman JT. Do focal chondral defects of the knee increase the risk for progression to osteoarthritis? A review of the literature. Orthop J Sports Med. 2018;6(10):2325967118801931.
4. Krych AJ, Pareek A, King AH, Johnson NR, Stuart MJ, Williams RJ. Return to sport after the surgical management of articular cartilage lesions in the knee: a meta-analysis. Knee Surg Sports Traumatol Arthrosc. 2017;25(10):3186–96.
5. Campbell AB, Pineda M, Harris JD, Flanigan DC. Return to sport after articular cartilage repair in athletes' knees: a systematic review. Arthroscopy. 2016;32(4):651–668.e651.
6. Mithoefer K, Williams RJ, Warren RF, Wickiewicz TL, Marx RG. High-impact athletics after knee articular cartilage repair: a prospective evaluation of the microfracture technique. Am J Sports Med. 2006;34(9):1413–8.
7. Mithoefer K, Gill TJ, Cole BJ, Williams RJ, Mandelbaum BR. Clinical outcome and return to competition after microfracture in the athlete's knee: an evidence-based systematic review. Cartilage. 2010;1(2):113–20.
8. Benthien JP, Behrens P. Reviewing subchondral cartilage surgery: considerations for standardised and outcome predictable cartilage remodelling. Int Orthop. 2013;37(11):2139–45.
9. Harris JD, Walton DM, Erickson BJ, Verma NN, Abrams GD, Bush-Joseph CA, Bach BR Jr, Cole BJ. Return to sport and performance after microfracture in the knees of National Basketball Association players. Orthop J Sports Med. 2013;1(6):2325967113512759.
10. Schallmo MS, Singh SK, Barth KA, Freshman RD, Mai HT, Hsu WK. A cross-sport comparison of performance-based outcomes of professional athletes following primary microfracture of the knee. Knee. 2018;25(4):692–8.
11. Gobbi A, Karnatzikos G, Kumar A. Long-term results after microfracture treatment for full-thickness knee chondral lesions in athletes. Knee Surg Sports Traumatol Arthrosc. 2014;22(9):1986–96.
12. Brittberg M, Lindahl A, Nilsson A, Ohlsson C, Isaksson O, Peterson L. Treatment of deep cartilage defects in the knee with autologous chondrocyte transplantation. N Engl J Med. 1994;331(14):889–95.
13. Mithoefer K, Peterson L, Saris DB, Mandelbaum BR. Evolution and current role of autologous chon-

drocyte implantation for treatment of articular cartilage defects in the football (soccer) player. Cartilage. 2012;3(1_suppl):31S–6S.

14. Villa SD, Kon E, Filardo G, Ricci M, Vincentelli F, Delcogliano M, Marcacci M. Does intensive rehabilitation permit early return to sport without compromising the clinical outcome after arthroscopic autologous chondrocyte implantation in highly competitive athletes? Am J Sports Med. 2010;38(1):68–77.

15. Mithöfer K, Peterson L, Mandelbaum BR, Minas T. Articular cartilage repair in soccer players with autologous chondrocyte transplantation: functional outcome and return to competition. Am J Sports Med. 2005;33(11):1639–46.

16. Ebert JR, Janes GC, Wood DJ. Post-operative sport participation and satisfaction with return to activity after matrix-induced autologous chondrocyte implantation in the knee. Int J Sports Phys Ther. 2020;15(1):1.

17. Zak L, Aldrian S, Wondrasch B, Albrecht C, Marlovits S. Ability to return to sports 5 years after matrix-associated autologous chondrocyte transplantation in an average population of active patients. Am J Sports Med. 2012;40(12):2815–21.

18. Kreuz PC, Kalkreuth RH, Niemeyer P, Uhl M, Erggelet C. Long-term clinical and MRI results of matrix-assisted autologous chondrocyte implantation for articular cartilage defects of the knee. Cartilage. 2019;10(3):305–13.

19. Zaffagnini S, Vannini F, Di Martino A, Andriolo L, Sessa A, Perdisa F, Balboni F, Filardo G, Committee EU. Low rate of return to pre-injury sport level in athletes after cartilage surgery: a 10-year follow-up study. Knee Surg Sports Traumatol Arthrosc. 2019;27(8):2502–10.

20. Williams RJ. Editorial commentary: are we really ready to talk about sports after osteochondral allograft transplantation? Arthroscopy. 2019;35(6):1890–2.

21. Mithöfer K, Minas T, Peterson L, Yeon H, Micheli LJ. Functional outcome of knee articular cartilage repair in adolescent athletes. Am J Sports Med. 2005;33(8):1147–53.

22. Gudas R, Gudaitė A, Pocius A, Gudienė A, Čekanauskas E, Monastyreckienė E, Basevičius A. Ten-year follow-up of a prospective, randomized clinical study of mosaic osteochondral autologous transplantation versus microfracture for the treatment of osteochondral defects in the knee joint of athletes. Am J Sports Med. 2012;40(11):2499–508.

23. Lynch TS, Patel RM, Benedick A, Amin NH, Jones MH, Miniaci A. Systematic review of autogenous osteochondral transplant outcomes. Arthroscopy. 2015;31(4):746–54.

24. Hurley ET, Davey MS, Jamal MS, Manjunath AK, Alaia MJ, Strauss EJ. Return-to-play and rehabilitation protocols following cartilage restoration procedures of the knee: a systematic review. Cartilage. 2019:1947603519894733.

25. Werner BC, Cosgrove CT, Gilmore CJ, Lyons ML, Miller MD, Brockmeier SF, Diduch DR. Accelerated return to sport after osteochondral autograft plug transfer. Orthop J Sports Med. 2017;5(4):2325967117702418.

26. Andrade R, Vasta S, Pereira R, Pereira H, Papalia R, Karahan M, Oliveira JM, Reis RL, Espregueira-Mendes J. Knee donor-site morbidity after mosaicplasty—a systematic review. J Exp Orthop. 2016;3(1):31.

27. Pánics G, Hangody LR, Baló E, Vásárhelyi G, Gál T, Hangody L. Osteochondral autograft and mosaicplasty in the football (soccer) athlete. Cartilage. 2012;3(1_suppl):25S–30S.

28. Crawford ZT, Schumaier AP, Glogovac G, Grawe BM. Return to sport and sports-specific outcomes after osteochondral allograft transplantation in the knee: a systematic review of studies with at least 2 years' mean follow-up. Arthroscopy. 2019;35(6):1880–9.

29. Krych AJ, Robertson CM, Williams RJ III, Cartilage Study Group. Return to athletic activity after osteochondral allograft transplantation in the knee. Am J Sports Med. 2012;40(5):1053–9.

30. Balazs GC, Wang D, Burge AJ, Sinatro AL, Wong AC, Williams RJ III. Return to play among elite basketball players after osteochondral allograft transplantation of full-thickness cartilage lesions. Orthop J Sports Med. 2018;6(7):2325967118786941.

31. Walczak BE, McCulloch PC, Kang RW, Zelazny A, Tedeschi F, Cole BJ. Abnormal findings on knee magnetic resonance imaging in asymptomatic NBA players. J Knee Surg. 2008;21(01):27–33.

32. Pappas GP, Vogelsong MA, Staroswiecki E, Gold GE, Safran MR. Magnetic resonance imaging of asymptomatic knees in collegiate basketball players: the effect of one season of play. Clin J Sports Med. 2016;26(6):483.

33. Gracitelli GC, Meric G, Briggs DT, Pulido PA, McCauley JC, Belloti JC, Bugbee WD. Fresh osteochondral allografts in the knee: comparison of primary transplantation versus transplantation after failure of previous subchondral marrow stimulation. Am J Sports Med. 2015;43(4):885–91.

34. McCarthy MA, Meyer MA, Weber AE, Levy DM, Tilton AK, Yanke AB, Cole BJ. Can competitive athletes return to high-level play after osteochondral allograft transplantation of the knee? Arthroscopy. 2017;33(9):1712–7.

35. Mithoefer K, Hambly K, Logerstedt D, Ricci M, Silvers H, Villa SD. Current concepts for rehabilitation and return to sport after knee articular cartilage repair in the athlete. J Orthop Sports Phys Ther. 2012;42(3):254–73.

36. Salter R, Simmonds D, Malcolm B, Rumble E, MacMichael D, Clements N. The biological effect of continuous passive motion on the healing of full-thickness defects in articular cartilage. An experimental investigation in the rabbit. J Bone Joint Surg Am. 1980;62(8):1232.

37. Sakamoto J, Origuchi T, Okita M, Nakano J, Kato K, Yoshimura T, Izumi S-i, Komori T, Nakamura H, Ida H. Immobilization-induced cartilage degen-

eration mediated through expression of hypoxia-inducible factor-1α, vascular endothelial growth factor, and chondromodulin-I. Connect Tissue Res. 2009;50(1):37–45.

38. Wang H-C, Lin T-H, Chang N-J, Hsu H-C, Yeh M-L. Continuous passive motion promotes and maintains chondrogenesis in autologous endothelial progenitor cell-loaded porous PLGA scaffolds during osteochondral defect repair in a rabbit model. Int J Mol Sci. 2019;20(2):259.

39. Ebert JR, Edwards PK, Fallon M, Ackland TR, Janes GC, Wood DJ. Two-year outcomes of a randomized trial investigating a 6-week return to full weightbearing after matrix-induced autologous chondrocyte implantation. Am J Sports Med. 2017;45(4):838–48.

40. Howard JS, Lattermann C, Hoch JM, Mattacola CG, Medina McKeon JM. Comparing responsiveness of six common patient-reported outcomes to changes following autologous chondrocyte implantation: a systematic review and meta-analysis of prospective studies. Cartilage. 2013;4(2):97–110.

41. Grant JA. Outcomes associated with return to sports following osteochondral allograft transplant in the knee: a scoping review. Curr Rev Musculoskelet Med. 2019;12(2):181–9.

42. Mithoefer K, Hambly K, Della Villa S, Silvers H, Mandelbaum BR. Return to sports participation after articular cartilage repair in the knee: scientific evidence. Am J Sports Med. 2009;37(1_suppl): 167–76.

43. Nielsen ES, McCauley JC, Pulido PA, Bugbee WD. Return to sport and recreational activity after osteochondral allograft transplantation in the knee. Am J Sports Med. 2017;45(7):1608–14.

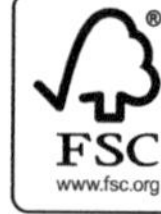

MIX
Papier aus verantwortungsvollen Quellen
Paper from responsible sources
FSC® C105338

If you have any concerns about our products,
you can contact us on
ProductSafety@springernature.com

In case Publisher is established outside the EU,
the EU authorized representative is:
Springer Nature Customer Service Center GmbH
Europaplatz 3, 69115 Heidelberg, Germany

Printed by Libri Plureos GmbH
in Hamburg, Germany